# Tumors of the Esophagus and Stomach

## Atlas
## of
## Tumor Pathology

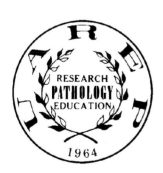

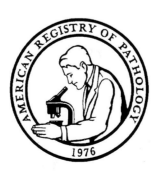

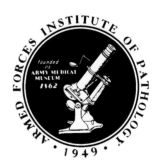

# ATLAS OF TUMOR PATHOLOGY

Third Series
Fascicle 18

# TUMORS OF THE ESOPHAGUS AND STOMACH

by

**KLAUS J. LEWIN, M.D. FRCPath**
Department of Pathology
UCLA School of Medicine
Los Angeles, California 90024

**HENRY D. APPELMAN, M.D.**
Department of Pathology
The University of Michigan Hospitals
Ann Arbor, Michigan 48109

With the Editorial Collaboration of
Patricia Lewin, M.D.

Published by the
ARMED FORCES INSTITUTE OF PATHOLOGY
Washington, D.C.

Under the Auspices of
UNIVERSITIES ASSOCIATED FOR RESEARCH AND EDUCATION IN PATHOLOGY, INC.
Bethesda, Maryland
1996

Accepted for Publication
1995

Available from the American Registry of Pathology
Armed Forces Institute of Pathology
Washington, D.C. 20306-6000
ISSN 0160-6344
ISBN 1-881041-27-1

# ATLAS OF TUMOR PATHOLOGY

## EDITOR
### JUAN ROSAI, M.D.
Department of Pathology
Memorial Sloan-Kettering Cancer Center
New York, New York 10021-6007

## ASSOCIATE EDITOR
### LESLIE H. SOBIN, M.D.
Armed Forces Institute of Pathology
Washington, D.C. 20306-6000

# EDITORS' NOTE

The Atlas of Tumor Pathology has a long and distinguished history. It was first conceived at a Cancer Research Meeting held in St. Louis in September 1947 as an attempt to standardize the nomenclature of neoplastic diseases. The first series was sponsored by the National Academy of Sciences-National Research Council. The organization of this Sisyphean effort was entrusted to the Subcommittee on Oncology of the Committee on Pathology, and Dr. Arthur Purdy Stout was the first editor-in-chief. Many of the illustrations were provided by the Medical Illustration Service of the Armed Forces Institute of Pathology, the type was set by the Government Printing Office, and the final printing was done at the Armed Forces Institute of Pathology (hence the colloquial appellation "AFIP Fascicles"). The American Registry of Pathology purchased the Fascicles from the Government Printing Office and sold them virtually at cost. Over a period of 20 years, approximately 15,000 copies each of nearly 40 Fascicles were produced. The worldwide impact that these publications have had over the years has largely surpassed the original goal. They quickly became among the most influential publications on tumor pathology ever written, primarily because of their overall high quality but also because their low cost made them easily accessible to pathologists and other students of oncology the world over.

Upon completion of the first series, the National Academy of Sciences-National Research Council handed further pursuit of the project over to the newly created Universities Associated for Research and Education in Pathology (UAREP). A second series was started, generously supported by grants from the AFIP, the National Cancer Institute, and the American Cancer Society. Dr. Harlan I. Firminger became the editor-in-chief and was succeeded by Dr. William H. Hartmann. The second series Fascicles were produced as bound volumes instead of loose leaflets. They featured a more comprehensive coverage of the subjects, to the extent that the Fascicles could no longer be regarded as "atlases" but rather as monographs describing and illustrating in detail the tumors and tumor-like conditions of the various organs and systems.

Once the second series was completed, with a success that matched that of the first, UAREP and AFIP decided to embark on a third series. A new editor-in-chief and an associate editor were selected, and a distinguished editorial board was appointed. The mandate for the third series remains the same as for the previous ones, i.e., to oversee the production of an eminently practical publication with surgical pathologists as its primary audience, but also aimed at other workers in oncology. The main purposes of this series are to promote a consistent, unified, and biologically sound nomenclature; to guide the surgical pathologist in the diagnosis of the various tumors and tumor-like lesions; and to provide relevant histogenetic, pathogenetic, and clinicopathologic information on these entities. Just as the second series included data obtained from ultrastructural (and, in the more recent Fascicles, immunohistochemical) examination, the third series will, in addition, incorporate pertinent information obtained with the newer molecular biology techniques. As in the past, a continuous attempt will be made to correlate, whenever possible, the nomenclature used in the Fascicles with that proposed by the World Health Organization's International Histological Classification of Tumors. The format of the third series has been changed in order to incorporate additional items and to ensure a consistency of style throughout. Close cooperation between the various authors and their respective liaisons from the editorial board will be emphasized to minimize unnecessary repetition and discrepancies in the text and illustrations.

To its everlasting credit, the participation and commitment of the AFIP to this venture is even more substantial and encompassing than in previous series. It now extends to virtually all scientific, technical, and financial aspects of the production.

The task confronting the organizations and individuals involved in the third series is even more daunting than in the preceding efforts because of the ever-increasing complexity of the matter at hand. It is hoped that this combined effort—of which, needless to say, that represented by the authors is first and foremost—will result in a series worthy of its two illustrious predecessors and will be a suitable introduction to the tumor pathology of the twenty-first century.

**Juan Rosai, M.D.**
**Leslie H. Sobin, M.D.**

# ACKNOWLEDGMENTS

We wish to express our sincere thanks to our many colleagues in pathology and clinical medicine, residents and students, without whose help, stimulation, and challenge over the years we would not have achieved our intellectual goals. Unfortunately, they are too numerous to list here. However, we would like to thank the anonymous reviewers of the Armed Forces Institute of Pathology (AFIP) Fascicle and Drs. Sanford Dawsey, Falko Fend, Elaine Jaffe, Felix Offner, and Leslie Sobin who have reviewed selected chapters of the Fascicle, for their most helpful constructive criticisms. In addition we wish to thank the numerous pathologists and other physicians who supplied gross and histologic material as well as endoscopic photographs. They are acknowledged in the legends. Ms. Carol Appleton and Mr. Luther Duckett are thanked for the excellent photographs they contributed.

One of us (KJL) had the great fortune of spending part of his sabbatical year at the National Cancer Center in Tokyo and at the Gastrointestinal Division of the AFIP in Washington, DC, to study cancers of the stomach and esophagus. I would like to thank the Foundation for Cancer Research and the National Cancer Center in Tokyo for their generous support and also to thank Drs. T. Hirota, M. Itabashi, A. Ochiai and K. Maruyama of the National Cancer Center for their hospitality and their generosity in sharing their material and experience with me. The AFIP and especially Dr. Leslie Sobin, Chief of the Gastrointestinal Division of the AFIP, were also most generous in placing the resources of the institute at my disposal. Finally, I would like to acknowledge the guidance of my clinical collaborator, Dr. Wilfred Weinstein, for the tremendous insight he has given me over the years regarding the clinical implications of biopsy material.

**Klaus Lewin, M.D.**
**Henry Appelman, M.D.**

Dedication:
To our families
Patricia, David, Nicky, and Bruno Lewin
and Peter Lewin
and
Harlene Appelman
Avery and Brett Appelman
Gabriel, Avi, and Naomi Adiv

# Contents

# TUMORS OF THE ESOPHAGUS AND STOMACH

## INTRODUCTION

Tumors of the esophagus and stomach are among the most common worldwide, but there are great differences in prevalence from one geographic area and one population to another. Thus, there are high prevalence areas in China and Iran for esophageal squamous cell carcinoma and high prevalence areas for tubule-forming gastric carcinoma in parts of the Far East, while in the United States both of these neoplasms have a relatively low prevalence. Presumably, this reflects significant differences in environmental factors and genetic predispositions, although quite often the specific issues are not yet known. Furthermore, even within local geographic areas, the prevalence of individual tumors has changed, sometimes dramatically, with time. The incidence of gastric carcinoma, one of the most common cancers and the most common cause of cancer deaths in adults in the United States in the third and fourth decades of this century, has declined greatly. Now it is not even among the top five cancers, either in terms of prevalence or cause of cancer deaths. However, in contrast to the rapid decline of the usual types of gastric cancer in some parts of the Western world, adenocarcinoma arising in Barrett's mucosa in the esophagus, virtually unheard of 30 years ago, and cardiac cancers arising in the most proximal stomach, now are increasingly common types of gastrointestinal tract cancer.

Over the last decade, a number of impressive new developments have occurred in the field of tumor biology in general as well as specifically related to gastrointestinal neoplasms, resulting in many advances and changes since the last Fascicle covering tumors of the esophagus and stomach was published. An exciting new discovery has been the recent evidence linking *Helicobacter pylori* infection to both a type of gastric lymphoma and the common type of gastric adenocarcinoma. Who would have thought, only a few years ago, that these tumors could be complications of an infection, and that some gastric lymphomas might even respond to antibiotics?

There has been an explosion of new studies that attempt to define the genetic alterations occurring within the precancer-cancer sequences for virtually all the common esophageal and gastric tumors, and an additional collection of studies linking genetic alterations to metastasis, extramural spread, and survival. We anticipate that these studies will be of increasing value, not only in determining prognosis and treatment, but also in the diagnosis and management of early neoplastic lesions.

A critically important issue is the demonstration that all gastrointestinal carcinomas develop from precursor lesions, some of which we recognize as dysplasias. Surveillance programs have been established for several types of carcinoma, with the main intent of detecting dysplasias before the carcinomas develop and secondarily to detect carcinomas in their incipient stages when they are unlikely to kill the patients.

Although this Fascicle is primarily aimed at illustrating and describing in detail the morphologic features of tumors and their precursors, we will also describe newer biologic and genetic advances and their applications to tumor diagnosis and management.

# 1
# HANDLING OF ESOPHAGEAL AND
# GASTRIC BIOPSY AND RESECTION SPECIMENS

The following paragraphs cover the recommended techniques for handling biopsy and resection specimens in general terms. Specific details relating to the handling of specimens of distinctive tumor types appear in the chapters discussing those tumors. There are no uniformly accepted standards for specimen handling: different gastrointestinal pathologists deal differently with their specimens, yet all are able to identify the important diagnostic and prognostic information from specimens handled in their favorite ways. There is already extensive literature on the proper handling of gastrointestinal biopsy and resection specimens, and the reader is referred to some of these for more details (1–5).

## BIOPSIES

**Types of Biopsy Samples and Orientation.** Biopsies of endoscopically visible tumors tend to contain variably sized pieces of neoplasm that are difficult to orient. Fortunately, they are usually easy to diagnose, and, are therefore less likely to require fastidious orientation than biopsies of inflammatory diseases or biopsies taken during surveillance endoscopy for early or superficial cancers and precancerous dysplasias. Obviously, accurate diagnosis depends upon having a representative fragment of the tumor. We recommend that the endoscopist take at least five samples from the bulk of the tumor, concentrating upon those areas that do not appear necrotic. For ulcerated tumors, biopsies should be obtained not only from the edges, where the tumor is most likely to be viable, but from the ulcer bed, since diagnostic tissue may be found at the base even when edge biopsies only contain hyperplastic or prolapsed mucosa. Intramural tumors, most of which are stromal and lymphoid, are the most difficult to sample adequately, unless giant biopsy forceps are used or unless the tumor is ulcerated and the biopsy forceps is sent deep into the ulcer to sample its depth. The biopsy fragments may be embedded within a single block, as long as they are placed in such a position to ensure that they will be cut together. It may be advisable to limit the number of such fragments to three or four in a single block to ensure proper embedding.

Biopsies are also taken for surveillance purposes in patients with Barrett's mucosa in the esophagus or gastric cancer precursors, such as extensive chronic atrophic gastritis, particularly in the parts of the world where gastric carcinoma is common. Unless jumbo biopsy instruments are used, these biopsies usually are irregular fragments that are difficult to orient, especially those from the esophagus. In such cases, we recommend embedding these fragments on edge and cutting them perpendicularly to the mucosal surface, but this is often difficult. When surveillance biopsies are taken with jumbo biopsy forceps, the resultant large specimens generally contain not only mucosa but superficial submucosa as well, and they are much easier to orient for perpendicular sectioning. We suggest that endoscopists or their support staff place the biopsies, submucosal side down, on a piece of support material, such as a Millipore filter, a small piece of file card, or Gelfoam, as soon as they are obtained. The specimens should then be placed upside-down in fixative (4). Handling of biopsies in this way makes it much easier to orient the specimen for perpendicular sectioning. In surveillance biopsies, it is ideal to separate and embed the specimens by site, although economic considerations may dictate that specimens from more than one level or site be blocked together.

**Cytologic Preparations.** Obtaining brush cytology specimens is a complementary technique that is likely to increase the diagnostic yield, especially for carcinomas. Balloon cytology is discussed in chapter 4. Endoscopic fine-needle aspiration of deep intramural tumors, such as stromal tumors, is becoming more widely used: a small bore needle is pushed into the tumor, and a sample is aspirated for cytologic analysis, including a cell block that often contains a microbiopsy.

**Fixation.** A most important step in handling all specimens, both biopsies and resections, is immediate fixation; this avoids any autolytic changes that may irreparably damage the cytologic features of the tumor. This is especially critical for lymphoid lesions because of the difficulties in differentiating lymphomas from benign lymphoid proliferations and in differentiating various lymphomas. Delayed fixation tends to make lymphocyte nuclei swell, so that small lymphocytes may appear to be large forms. We do not recommend a specific fixative. Exquisite nuclear detail may be obtained with picric acid fixatives such as Holande's, or mercury-based fixatives such as B5. However, these fixatives may lead to less desirable cytoplasmic differentiation, may be less satisfactory for immunocytochemistry, and unsatisfactory for genetic markers. Buffered formalin gives less nuclear but better cytoplasmic detail, and may be the best fixative for immunohistochemistry.

Snap frozen tissue may be obtained for immunocytochemistry, especially when lymphoma is suspected, since many antibodies work better with frozen than with fixed tissue. In our experience, unless careful attention is given to tissues obtained for a lymphoma workup and snap frozen immediately, the results are unreliable. Similar tissue may be used for gene rearrangements, although more and more such genetic determinants are being performed using the polymerase chain reaction on paraffin-embedded tissues.

**Cutting the Paraffin Blocks.** The number of microscopic sections necessary for biopsy diagnosis has not been established. Some pathologists prefer 5 to 10 serial sections from three or four different levels in the paraffin block, while others feel that they obtain optimal diagnostic information from 10 to 20 serial cuts without resorting to sampling different levels. Both camps are likely to be passionate in the support of their favorite sampling choices.

**Stains.** Hematoxylin and eosin (H&E) is the standard stain, and some laboratories add saffron for staining collagen and a mucin counter stain, such as Alcian blue (AB). The most commonly used special stains are mucin stains. AB at a pH of 2.5 is a good, general screening stain for acid mucins. Periodic acid–Schiff (PAS) stain with diastase pretreatment detects both acid mucins and neutral mucins. The combination of AB at a pH of 2.5 and PAS, with and without diastase pretreatment, picks up both neutral and acid mucins as well as glycogen: the AB stains the acid mucins, while the PAS counterstains the neutral mucins that AB does not detect. Mucicarmine detects only acid mucins. Endocrine cells are best detected using an immunocytochemical technique, such as the chromogranin A antibody. Histochemical, mainly argyrophilic, silver stains that identify endocrine granules, such as the Churukian-Schenck modification of the Grimelius stain, are used in some laboratories.

## SURGICAL (RESECTION) SPECIMENS

Most esophageal and gastric tumors are resected with variable quantities of adjacent esophagus or stomach; that is, they are incorporated within an esophagogastrectomy or gastrectomy specimen. Less commonly, they are "shelled out" so that the specimen only consists of the tumor. For those specimens that contain parts of the esophagus or stomach, we recommend that the viscus be opened in the fresh state. For most gastrectomy specimens, opening along the greater curvature gives the best view of most tumors; cutting through the tumor should be avoided in order to best see the lesion in its natural surroundings. This may mean that the stomach will not necessarily be opened along the greater curvature, the classic procedure for gross stomach specimens. The opened esophagus or stomach should be carefully evaluated in the fresh state. This is the time to obtain measurements such as size and distance from margins of resection and to check colors, since fixation results in shrinkage and muting of colors. This is usually the best time for photographing the tumor. In general, electron microscopy is rarely used for tumor diagnosis. However, if there is a hint that a tumor is unusual, either as a result of previous biopsies or of frozen sections at the time of resection, then samples fixed in glutaraldehyde may be taken for electron microscopy, since they may clarify the nature of the tumor.

This is also the time to take samples for flow cytometry and genetic studies, especially with lymphoid tumors. Best fixation is likely to be obtained if the specimen is stretched and pinned to a board of some type, such as cork board or Styrofoam. Big, bulky, solid tumors may be sliced in the fresh state to ensure that the fixative penetrates deeply into the mass. However, if it appears that the tumor extends to a margin of resection, either at the deepest point of invasion or peripherally, then that margin should be marked.

Once the specimen is fixed, better views can be obtained of the relationship of the tumor to the margins of resection and to the different layers of the esophagus or stomach. Lymph nodes may be more easily found at this time, although some pathologists prefer hunting for nodes in the unfixed specimen. Involvement of adjacent structures, such as the liver, pancreas, or omentum, should be assessed.

Microscopic samples should be taken to guarantee that three things are accomplished: diagnosis, if it has not been established by previous biopsy; resection margins clear of tumor; and staging for purposes of prognosis and determination of the need for ancillary radiation or chemotherapy. Four or five sections of large tumors are usually enough to ensure that the diagnosis is made. These can be chosen to obtain staging information as well, including the maximal depth of invasion and evidence of an intramucosal component, in the surrounding mucosa of a carcinoma. For large stromal tumors, additional sections may be needed to determine if there are sarcomatous areas. The margins of resection should be sampled for carcinomas and lymphomas, since such lesions in the stomach and especially the esophagus, have a tendency to spread intramurally, even at a considerable distance from the main mass. For stromal tumors, the only margin that should be sampled is that adjacent to the main mass, since stromal tumors usually grow by expansion rather than infiltration.

Regional lymph nodes should be counted, measured, and sampled, and their sites noted, as should any adjacent involved structures, since all of these are critical for accurate staging (13,18). (Refer to the information on staging later in this chapter.)

Microscopic analysis should include diagnosis and tumor grade when important, although, in general, histologic grading of carcinomas has not always given additional important prognostic information for all tumors. Other microscopic data include depth of invasion, involvement of adjacent structures, the presence or absence of lymph node metastases, and the number of nodes involved.

## THE TNM CLASSIFICATION AND CARCINOMA STAGING

There are many ways to describe the characteristics of tumors, such as anatomic site, clinical and pathologic extent of disease, tumor size, growth pattern, histologic type, histologic grade, duration of symptoms, and even age and sex of the patient. All of these variables may have an effect on the outcome of the disease, although some variables are of greater prognostic significance than others. In general, the most important prognostic factors for tumors of the esophagus and stomach relate to tumor stage, specifically to depth of invasion, regional lymph node involvement, and distant metastases.

The TNM (tumor, node, metastases) classification of the International Union Against Cancer (UICC), identical to the classification system of the American Joint Committee on Cancer (AJCC), is the most widely used system for staging of carcinomas, and its applicability in the treatment and prognostication of esophageal and gastric carcinomas has been validated (6–20). The current TNM classification is used in this Fascicle. The purpose of this system is: to provide a shorthand summary of tumor stage; give an indication of prognosis; assist the clinician in planning treatment; assist in evaluating the results of treatment; facilitate exchange of information among treatment centers; and contribute to the continuing investigation of tumors.

Furthermore, a comparison between clinical and pathologic staging permits an evaluation of the accuracy of the clinical classification (14).

The TNM classification compartmentalizes carcinomas according to the extent of the primary tumor, the absence or presence of regional lymph node metastases, and the absence or presence of distant metastases. These groups are subdivided numerically to describe tumor extent in terms of size or growth through anatomic structures, and extent of nodal and distant metastases. Classification of carcinomas by the TNM system with its four degrees of T, three degrees of N, and two degrees of M, results in 24 categories for analysis. This number of categories is too large for the meaningful evaluation of most tumors except in a few very large studies. Fortunately, cases with similar prognoses can be grouped into four stages (I, II, III, and IV). In addition, for each anatomic site there are two classifications, cTNM and pTNM. cTNM is based on the evidence acquired before treatment, namely physical exam, imaging (including ultrasound, computed tomography, and magnetic resonance imaging), endoscopy and ultrasonic endoscopy, biopsy, surgical exploration and other relevant examinations; pTNM is based on the clinical staging and the information obtained at surgery and pathologic examination of the resected specimen.

Two additional descriptors are useful in conjunction with the TNM classification. The first is the R classification which refers to the presence of residual carcinoma after treatment; the second system, G classification, is the inclusion of histologic grading (see Table 1-1).

At this time it remains to be proven whether histologic grading is an independent variable or parameter for prognosis in all esophageal and gastric carcinomas. If there is any doubt concerning the correct TNM category of a particular case, the lower category should be chosen. For multiple simultaneous tumors in one organ, the tumor with the highest T category should be classified and the classification of the other tumors should be indicated in parenthesis.

The following figures (figs. 1-1–1-20) are derived from the UICC TNM Atlas and illustrate in detail the TNM classification of esophageal and gastric carcinomas. The associated stages are defined in Tables 1-2 and 1-3. The individual TNM definitions are not always identical for esophageal and gastric tumors, and that is not surprising, since the TNM system analyzes each

Table 1-1

## R AND G TNM CLASSIFICATION SCHEMES

### R CLASSIFICATION SCHEME

RX  Presence of residual tumor cannot be assessed
R0  No residual tumor
R1  Microscopic residual tumor
R2  Macroscopic residual tumor

### G CLASSIFICATION SCHEME

GX  Grade of differentiation cannot be assessed
G1  Well differentiated
G2  Moderately differentiated
G3  Poorly differentiated
G4  Undifferentiated

Table 1-2

## TNM STAGING OF ESOPHAGEAL CARCINOMA

| Stage | T = Extent of the Primary Tumor | N = Metastases in Regional Lymph Nodes | M = Distant Metastases |
|---|---|---|---|
| | TX: primary tumor cannot be assessed | NX: nodes cannot be assessed | MX: distant metastases cannot be assessed |
| | T0: no primary tumor | N0: no nodal metastases | M0: no distant metastases |
| 0 | T1S: carcinoma in situ | N0 | M0 |
| I | T1: tumor invades lamina propria or submucosa | N0 | M0 |
| IIA | T2: tumor invades into, but not beyond, the muscularis propria | N0 | M0 |
| IIA | T3: tumor invades the adventitia | N0 | M0 |
| IIB | T1 | N1: regional lymph node metastases | M0 |
| IIB | T2 | N1 | M0 |
| III | T3 | N1 | M0 |
| III | T4: tumor invades adjacent structures | any N | M0 |
| IV | any T | any N | M1: distant metastases |

Table 1-3

## TNM STAGING OF GASTRIC CARCINOMA

| Stage | T = Extent of the Primary Tumor | | N = Metastases in Regional Lymph Nodes | | M = Distant Metastases | |
|---|---|---|---|---|---|---|
| | TX: | primary tumor cannot be assessed | NX: | nodes cannot be assessed | MX: | distant metastases cannot be assessed |
| | T0: | no primary tumor | N0: | no nodal metastases | M0: | no distant metastases |
| 0 | T1S: | carcinoma in situ | N0 | | M0 | |
| IA | TI: | tumor invades lamina propria or submucosa | N0 | | M0 | |
| IB | T1 | | N1: | metastases in perigastric nodes within 3 cm of the edge of the tumor | M0 | |
| 1B | T2: | tumor invades muscularis propria or subserosa | N0 | | M0 | |
| II | T1 | | N-2: | metastases in perigastric nodes over 3 cm from the edge of the tumor or along left gastric, common hepatic, splenic, or celiac arteries | M0 | |
| II | T2 | | N1 | | M0 | |
| II | T3: | tumor penetrates the serosa; no invasion of adjacent structures | N0 | | M0 | |
| IIIA | T2 | | N2 | | M0 | |
| IIIA | T3 | | N1 | | M0 | |
| IIIA | T4: | tumor invades adjacent structures | N0 | | M0 | |
| IIIB | T3 | | N2 | | M0 | |
| IIIB | T4 | | N1 | | M0 | |
| IV | T4 | | N2 | | M0 | |
| IV | Any T | | Any N | | M1: | distant metastases |

site independently. It is important to remember that the TNM system is applicable for esophagogastric carcinomas only. For lymphomas, the most widely used staging system is some modification of the Ann Arbor System for staging extranodal lymphomas (see chapter 13). However, a TNM system for gastric lymphomas has been published (17). Although the TNM system is used for the staging of sarcomas of the soft tissues, a specific staging system for visceral sarcomas, such as those arising in the esophagus and stomach, does not exist. Visceral sarcomas are simply staged by the presence or absence of metastases and invasion of adjacent organs.

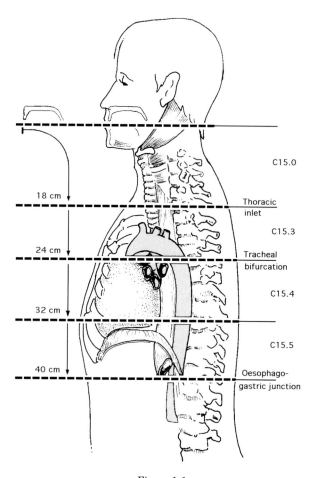

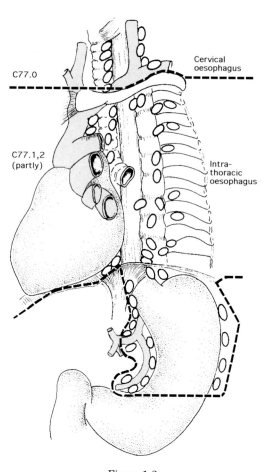

Figure 1-1
ESOPHAGUS: ANATOMIC SUBSITES

(Fig. 92 from Spiessl B, Beahrs OH, Hermanek P, et al. TNM atlas. Illustrated guide to the TNM/pTNM classification of malignant tumors. 3rd ed. International Union Against Cancer. Berlin: Springer-Verlag, 1992:63.)

Figure 1-2
ESOPHAGUS: REGIONAL LYMPH NODES

(Fig. 93 from Spiessl B, Beahrs OH, Hermanek P, et al. TNM atlas. Illustrated guide to the TNM/pTNM classification of malignant tumors. 3rd ed. International Union Against Cancer. Berlin: Springer-Verlag, 1992:64.)

Figure 1-3
ESOPHAGUS: T1 AND T2

(Figs. 94 and 95 from Spiessl B, Beahrs OH, Hermanek P, et al. TNM atlas. Illustrated guide to the TNM/pTNM classification of malignant tumors. 3rd ed. International Union Against Cancer. Berlin: Springer-Verlag, 1992:65.)

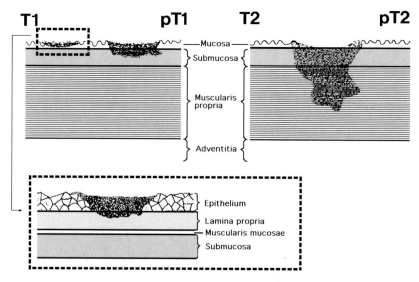

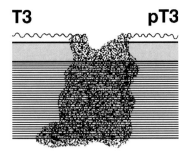

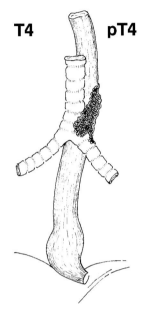

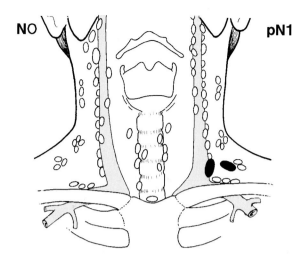

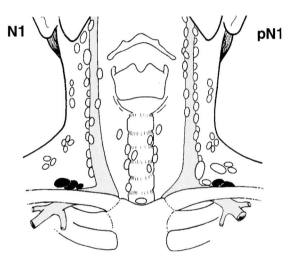

Figure 1-4
ESOPHAGUS: T3 AND T4

(Figs. 96 and 97 from Spiessl B, Beahrs OH, Hermanek P, et al. TNM atlas. Illustrated guide to the TNM/pTNM classification of malignant tumors. 3rd ed. International Union Against Cancer. Berlin: Springer-Verlag, 1992:66.)

FIGURE 1-5
CERVICAL ESOPHAGUS: N1

(Figs. 98 and 99 from Spiessl B, Beahrs OH, Hermanek P, et al. TNM atlas. Illustrated guide to the TNM/pTNM classification of malignant tumors. 3rd ed. International Union Against Cancer. Berlin: Springer-Verlag, 1992:67.)

**REFERENCES**

**Specimen Handling**

1. Goldman H, Antonioli DA. Mucosal biopsy of the esophagus, stomach, and proximal duodenum. Hum Pathol 1982;13:423–48.
2. Guinee DG Jr, Lee RG. Laboratory methods for processing and interpretation of endoscopic gastrointestinal biopsies. Lab Med 1990;21:13–6.
3. Haggitt RC. Handling of gastrointestinal biopsies in the surgical pathology laboratory. Lab Med 1982;13:272–8.
4. Lewin KJ, Riddell RH, Weinstein WM. Techniques. In: Lewin KJ, Riddell RH, Weinstein WM, eds. Gastrointestinal pathology and its clinical implications. New York: Igaku-Shoin, 1992:1–30.
5. Scott N, Quirke P, Dixon MF. ACP Broadsheet 133: November 1992. Gross examination of the stomach. J Clin Pathol 1992;45:952–5.

**TNM Staging**

6. American Joint Committee on Cancer. Manual for staging of cancer. 4th ed. Philadelphia: JB Lippincott, 1992.
7. Hermanek P, Gospodarowicz M, Henson DE, Hutter RV, Sobin LH, eds. Prognostic factors in cancer. Berlin: Springer-Verlag, 1995.
8. Hermanek P, Henson DE, Hutter RV, Sobin, LH, eds. TNM supplement. A commentary on uniform use. UICC International Union Against Cancer. Berlin: Springer-Verlag, 1993.
9. Hermanek P, Sobin LH. TNM classification of malignant tumours. 4th ed. UICC International Union Against Cancer. Berlin: Springer-Verlag, 1992.

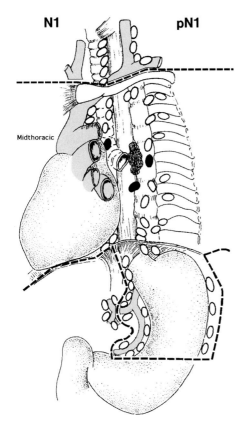

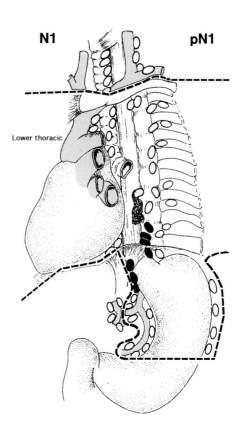

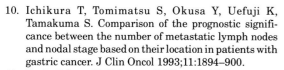

| Figure 1-6 | Figure 1-7 |
| --- | --- |
| MIDTHORACIC ESOPHAGUS: N1 | LOWER THORACIC ESOPHAGUS: N1 |

Figure 1-6
MIDTHORACIC ESOPHAGUS: N1
(Fig. 100 from Spiessl B, Beahrs OH, Hermanek P, et al. TNM atlas. Illustrated guide to the TNM/pTNM classification of malignant tumors. 3rd ed. International Union Against Cancer. Berlin: Springer-Verlag, 1992:68.)

Figure 1-7
LOWER THORACIC ESOPHAGUS: N1
(Fig. 101 from Spiessl B, Beahrs OH, Hermanek P, et al. TNM atlas. Illustrated guide to the TNM/pTNM classification of malignant tumors. 3rd ed. International Union Against Cancer. Berlin: Springer-Verlag, 1992:69.)

10. Ichikura T, Tomimatsu S, Okusa Y, Uefuji K, Tamakuma S. Comparison of the prognostic significance between the number of metastatic lymph nodes and nodal stage based on their location in patients with gastric cancer. J Clin Oncol 1993;11:1894–900.
11. Iizuka T, Isono K, Kakegawa T, Watanabe H. Parameters linked to ten-year survival in Japan of resected esophageal carcinoma. Japanese Committee for Registration of Esophageal Carcinoma Cases. Chest 1989;96:1005–11.
12. Iizuka T, The Japanese Committee for Registration of Esophageal Carcinoma Cases. A proposal for a new TNM classification of esophageal carcinoma. Jpn J Clin Oncol 1985;14:625–36.
13. Keller E, Stutzer H, Heitmann K, Bauer P, Gebbensleben B, Rohde H. Lymph node staging in 872 patients with carcinoma of the stomach and the presumed benefit of lymphadenectomy. German Stomach Cancer TNM Study Group. J Am Coll Surg 1994;178:38–46.
14. Kim JP, Yang HK, Oh ST. Is the new UICC staging system of gastric cancer reasonable? (Comparison of 5-year survival rate of gastric cancer by old and new UICC stage classification). Surg Oncol 1992;1:209–13.

15. Maruyama K. The most important prognostic factors for gastric cancer patients: a study using univariate and multivariate analyses. Scand J Gastroenterol 1987;22 (Suppl 133):63–8.
16. Miwa K, The Japanese Research Society for Gastric Cancer. Evaluation of the TNM classification of stomach cancer and proposal for its rational stage grouping. Jpn J Clin Oncol 1984;14:385–410.
17. Shimodaira M, Tsukamoto Y, Niwa Y, et al. A proposed staging system for primary gastric lymphoma. Cancer 1994;73:2709–15.
18. Siewert JR, Bottcher K, Roder JD, Busch R, Hermanek P, Meyer HJ. Prognostic relevance of systematic lymph node dissection in gastric carcinoma. German Gastric Carcinoma Study Group. Br J Surg 1993;80:1015–8.
19. Sobin LH, Ros PR. Radiology and the new TNM classification of tumors: the future. Radiology 1990;176:1–4.
20. Spiessl B, Beahrs OH, Hermanek P, et al. TNM atlas. Illustrated guide to the TNM/pTNM classification of malignant tumours. 3rd ed. UICC International Union Against Cancer. Berlin: Springer-Verlag, 1994.

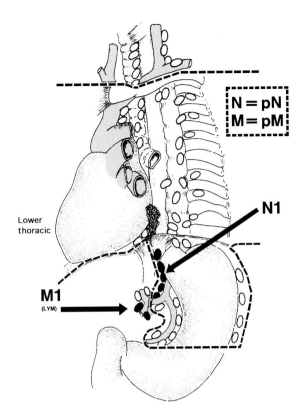

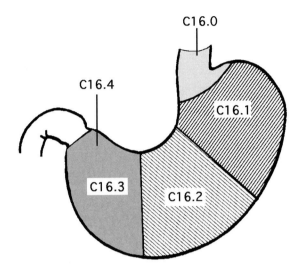

1. Cardia (C16.0)
2. Fundus (C16.1)
3. Corpus (C16.2)
4. Antrum (C16.3) and Pylorus (C16.4)

Figure 1-8
LOWER THORACIC ESOPHAGUS: N1 AND M1
(Fig. 102 from Spiessl B, Beahrs OH, Hermanek P, et al. TNM atlas. Illustrated guide to the TNM/pTNM classification of malignant tumors. 3rd ed. International Union Against Cancer. Berlin: Springer-Verlag, 1992:69.)

Figure 1-9
STOMACH: ANATOMIC SUBSITES
(Fig. 103 from Spiessl B, Beahrs OH, Hermanek P, et al. TNM atlas. Illustrated guide to the TNM/pTNM classification of malignant tumors. 3rd ed. International Union Against Cancer. Berlin: Springer-Verlag, 1992:71.)

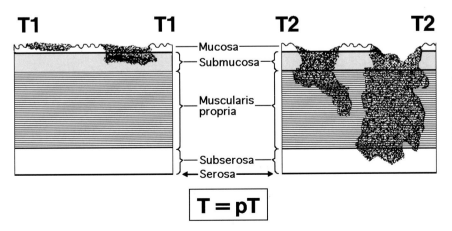

Figure 1-10
STOMACH: T1 AND T2
(Figs. 105 and 106 from Spiessl B, Beahrs OH, Hermanek P, et al. TNM atlas. Illustrated guide to the TNM/pTNM classification of malignant tumors. 3rd ed. International Union Against Cancer. Berlin: Springer-Verlag, 1992:74.)

11

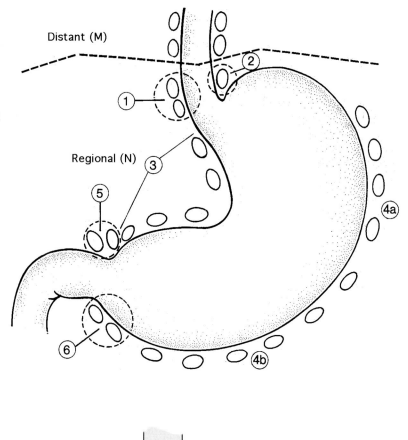

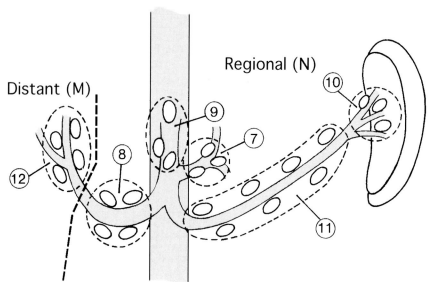

Figure 1-11

STOMACH: REGIONAL LYMPH NODES

Top: Nodes along the greater curvature (2, 4a, 4b, and 6) and along the lesser curvature (1, 3, and 5).

Bottom: Nodes along left gastric artery (7), common hepatic artery (8), celiac artery (9), splenic artery (10,11) and hepatoduodenal artery (12). (Fig. 104 from Spiessl B, Beahrs OH, Hermanek P, et al. TNM atlas. Illustrated guide to the TNM/pTNM classification of malignant tumors. 3rd ed. International Union Against Cancer. Berlin: Springer-Verlag, 1992:72–3.)

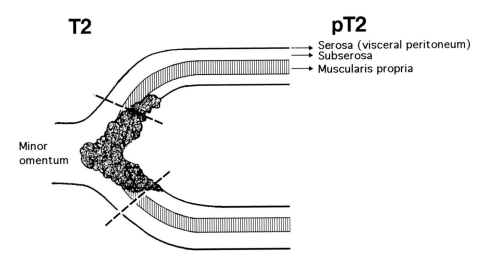

**T2**                    **pT2**

→ Serosa (visceral peritoneum)
→ Subserosa
→ Muscularis propria

Minor
omentum

Figure 1-12
STOMACH: T2 IN AREA
OF MINOR OMENTUM
(Fig. 107 from Spiessl B,
Beahrs OH, Hermanek P, et al.
TNM atlas. Illustrated guide to
the TNM/pTNM classification of
malignant tumors. 3rd ed. International Union Against Cancer. Berlin: Springer-Verlag,
1992:75.)

Figure 1-13
STOMACH: T3 AND T4
(Figs. 108 and 109 from
Spiessl B, Beahrs OH,
Hermanek P, et al. TNM atlas.
Illustrated guide to the
TNM/pTNM classification of
malignant tumors. 3rd ed. In-
ternational Union Against
Cancer. Berlin: Springer-Ver-
lag, 1992:76.)

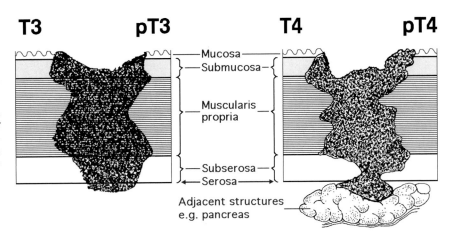

**T3**     **pT3**              **T4**     **pT4**

Mucosa
Submucosa

Muscularis
propria

Subserosa
Serosa

Adjacent structures
e.g. pancreas

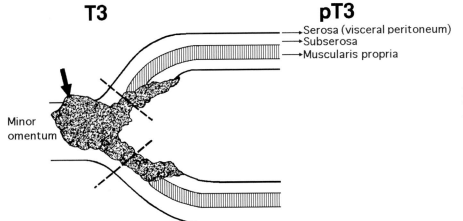

**T3**                    **pT3**

→ Serosa (visceral peritoneum)
→ Subserosa
→ Muscularis propria

Minor
omentum

Figure 1-14
STOMACH: T3 IN AREA
OF MINOR OMENTUM
(Fig. 110 from Spiessl B,
Beahrs OH, Hermanek P, et al.
TNM atlas. Illustrated guide to
the TNM/pTNM classification
of malignant tumors. 3rd ed.
International Union Against
Cancer. Berlin: Springer-Ver-
lag, 1992:76.)

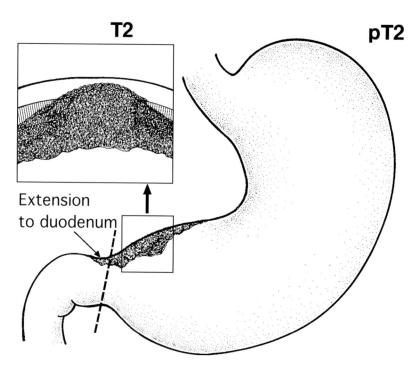

Figure 1-15
STOMACH: T2 WITH EXTENSION TO DUODENUM
(Fig. 111 from Spiessl B, Beahrs OH, Hermanek P, et al. TNM atlas. Illustrated guide to the TNM/pTNM classification of malignant tumors. 3rd ed. International Union Against Cancer. Berlin: Springer-Verlag, 1992:77.)

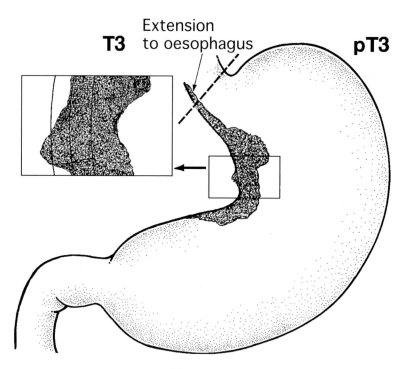

Figure 1-16
STOMACH: T3 WITH EXTENSION TO ESOPHAGUS
(Fig. 112 from Spiessl B, Beahrs OH, Hermanek P, et al. TNM atlas. Illustrated guide to the TNM/pTNM classification of malignant tumors. 3rd ed. International Union Against Cancer. Berlin: Springer-Verlag, 1992:78.)

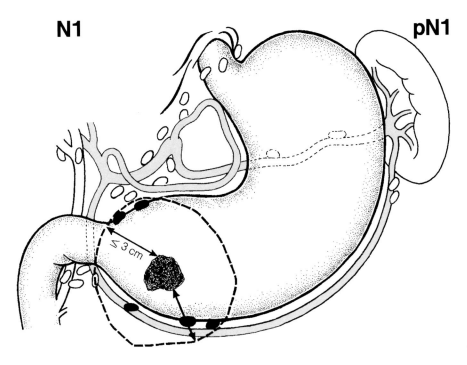

Figure 1-17
STOMACH: N1
(Fig. 113 from Spiessl B, Beahrs OH, Hermanek P, et al. TNM atlas. Illustrated guide to the TNM/pTNM classification of malignant tumors. 3rd ed. International Union Against Cancer. Berlin: Springer-Verlag, 1992:79.)

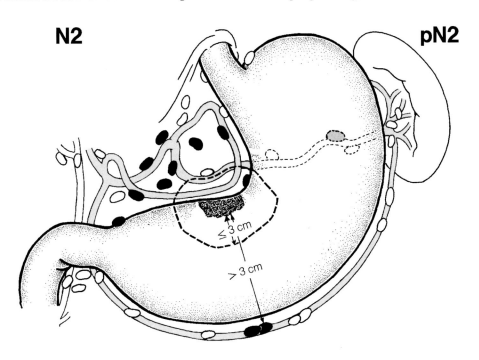

Figure 1-18
STOMACH: N2
(Fig. 114 from Spiessl B, Beahrs OH, Hermanek P, et al. TNM atlas. Illustrated guide to the TNM/pTNM classification of malignant tumors. 3rd ed. International Union Against Cancer. Berlin: Springer-Verlag, 1992:79.)

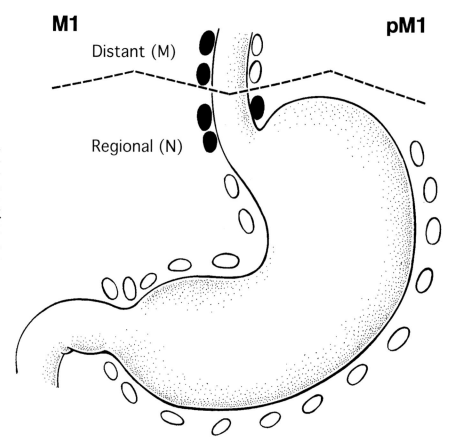

**M1**                                    **pM1**

Distant (M)

Regional (N)

Figure 1-19
STOMACH: M1
M1 with involvement of distant lymph nodes above the diaphragm along the lower esophagus. (Fig. 115 from Spiessl B, Beahrs OH, Hermanek P, et al. TNM atlas. Illustrated guide to the TNM/pTNM classification of malignant tumors. 3rd ed. International Union Against Cancer. Berlin: Springer-Verlag, 1992:80.)

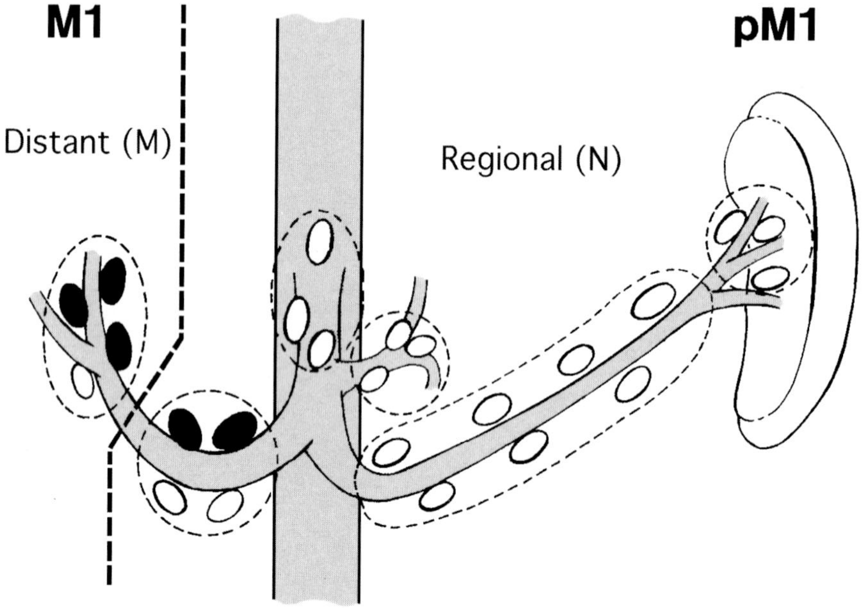

**M1**                                    **pM1**

Distant (M)          Regional (N)

Figure 1-20
STOMACH: M1
M1 with involvement of lymph nodes along celiac and hepatoduodenal arteries. (Fig. 116 from Spiessl B, Beahrs OH, Hermanek P, et al. TNM atlas. Illustrated guide to the TNM/pTNM classification of malignant tumors. 3rd ed. International Union Against Cancer. Berlin: Springer-Verlag, 1992:81.)

# 2
# NORMAL ANATOMY, EMBRYOLOGY, AND HISTOLOGY OF THE ESOPHAGUS

The esophagus is a hollow tube connecting the mouth and pharynx with the stomach; it is comprised of cervical, thoracic, and abdominal segments. It possesses no significant secretory or absorptive functions, and its only purpose is the transport of material from the mouth to the stomach. Unlike the rest of the gastrointestinal tract, the esophagus is not surrounded by a serosa; this is important clinically since once a tumor extends beyond the muscularis propria, it lies within the mediastinum.

## EMBRYOLOGY

The esophagus develops at about the twentieth day of gestation when septa arising from the lateral walls of the foregut fuse, thereby separating the trachea from the esophagus. The primitive esophagus is lined by columnar epithelium, which subsequently proliferates and occludes the lumen (16). By 7 weeks' gestation, the esophageal lumen reforms as a result of epithelial vacuolization and replacement by ciliated epithelium. At the fifth month, stratified squamous epithelium appears in the middle third of the esophagus and grows caudally and cephalad, replacing the ciliated epithelium (2,8). The esophageal mucosal glands form at 4 months' gestation by the downgrowth of the surface epithelium into the lamina propria. The submucosal glands do not develop until after development of the squamous epithelium (2,8,16,23). The muscularis propria first appears at about 6 weeks' gestation as a bundle of nonstriated circular muscle. The outer longitudinal coat develops at 9 weeks. However, the striated muscle, which is normally present in the upper third of the esophagus, is not fully formed until the fifth month (8).

## ANATOMY

The esophagus connects the pharynx to the stomach; it courses through the posterior mediastinum and extends several centimeters beyond the diaphragm. Its length varies with the height of the individual and ranges from 25 to 30 cm. The distance of the esophagogastric junction from the teeth averages 40 cm, but ranges from as little as 30 to 43 cm (18). In children, the esophageal length also is related to height (26). In the resting state the esophagus is collapsed and measures about 3 cm in lateral diameter and 2 cm in anterior-posterior diameter.

The esophagus begins at the level of the cricoid cartilage, at the apex of a funnel formed by the pharyngeal constrictors situated at the level of the sixth cervical vertebra (fig. 2-1). When viewed from above it appears as a transverse slit, with the pyriform sinus on either side. In its descent to the abdomen the esophagus follows the anteroposterior curvature of the vertebral column. It also has a reversed "S" configuration when viewed anteriorly. It exits the posterior mediastinum via the diaphragmatic hiatus through a tunnel approximately 5 centimeters in length. This diaphragmatic opening is relatively large and is located in the right crus of the diaphragm at the level of the seventh thoracic vertebra. It is filled with loose areolar tissue and contains the phrenoesophageal ligament which arises from the undersurface of the diaphragm and inserts into the esophagus about 3 cm above the hiatus. The ligament is thought to maintain a tight muscular seal between the diaphragm and the esophagus (6).

The esophagogastric junction is defined as the point at which the tubular esophagus joins the saccular stomach. The squamocolumnar junction, also known as the z-line or ora serrata, consists of an irregular serrated margin, and does not necessarily coincide with the esophagogastric junction. In fact, the squamocolumnar junction may lie anywhere within the distal 2 cm of the tubular esophagus (14); endoscopically, this junctional zone sometimes extends several centimeters on either side of the lower sphincter (fig. 2-2).

The International Union Against Cancer (UICC) has subdivided the esophagus into four regions: a cervical region and three intrathoracic and abdominal regions (Table 2-1).

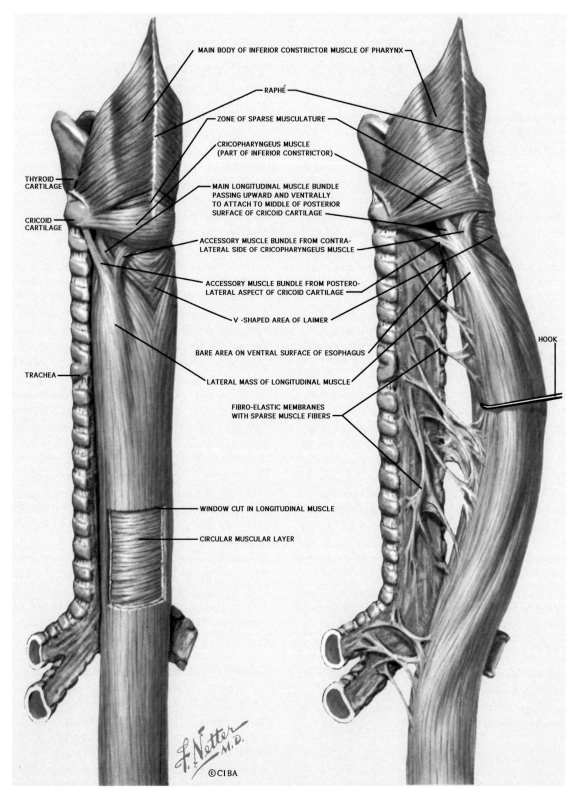

Figure 2-1
DIAGRAMMATIC ILLUSTRATION OF ESOPHAGEAL MUSCULATURE
(Plate 3 from Netter F. Ciba collection of medical illustrations, digestive system part 1. West Caldwell, NJ: Ciba Geigy, 1959:36.)

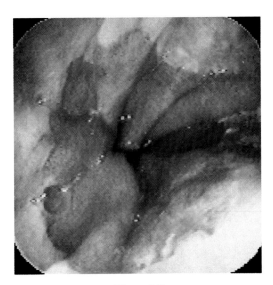

Figure 2-2
ENDOSCOPIC APPEARANCE
Endoscopic appearance of the z-line (the esophagogastric junction).

## Topographic Relationships and Normal Constrictions of the Esophagus

A knowledge of the relationship of the esophagus to neighboring structures is important, since tumors in these structures can affect the esophagus, and vice versa (21).

**Cervical Esophagus.** At its origin the esophagus lies on the vertebral bodies and is immediately posterior to the trachea. In the lateral grooves between the esophagus and trachea are the recurrent laryngeal nerves and adjacent to them are the right and left carotid sheaths and their contents. The lobes of the thyroid gland overlap the esophagus at the sides. At the root of the neck, on the left side of the esophagus, is the thoracic duct, which arches laterally behind the carotid sheath.

**Thoracic Esophagus.** Up until the bifurcation of the trachea (roughly around the fifth thoracic vertebra), the esophagus lies posterior to the trachea. At this point the trachea veers to the right and the esophagus is covered by the left main bronchus (fig. 2-1) and below this by the pericardium and left atrium. In the lowermost portion of the thorax the esophagus passes behind the diaphragm and into the esophageal hiatus. On the left side of the esophagus, in the upper thoracic region, lies the ascending segment of the left subclavian artery and the parietal pleura. Below this, at the level of the fourth thoracic vertebra, is the arch of the aorta which then runs alongside the esophagus until the eighth thoracic vertebra. The descending aorta then passes behind the esophagus (fig. 2-3). At this point the pleura is again in contact with the esophagus. On the right side the pleura lies adjacent to the esophagus along most of its length. Posteriorly the thoracic portion of the esophagus lies on the thoracic vertebrae up to the point where the descending aorta passes behind the esophagus. The azygos vein lies behind and to the right of the esophagus running up to the fourth thoracic vertebra; then it turns forward (fig. 2-4). The thoracic duct ascends on the right side of the lower esophagus. At the level of the fifth thoracic vertebra it passes behind the esophagus and then continues upwards on the left side, to the cervical esophagus.

**Abdominal Esophagus.** This is a very short segment which lies on the diaphragm, with the liver anterior to it.

**Normal Constrictions.** Normally, a number of indentations and constrictions can be found in the esophagus due to impingement from adjacent structures. These are potential sites at which food and pills may become lodged. These indentations occur at the following sites: at the level of the cricoid cartilage, caused by the cricopharyngeus muscle; at the aortic arch; at the level of the left atrium, where the left main bronchus crosses the esophagus; and at the diaphragmatic opening.

Below the tracheal bifurcation the esophageal plexus of nerves and anterior and posterior vagal nerves are close to the esophagus.

Table 2-1

## UICC ESOPHAGEAL REGIONS

1    **Cervical region:** extends from the cricoid cartilage to the level of the thoracic inlet

2–4   **Intrathoracic and abdominal regions:**

     2   Upper thoracic segment: extends from thoracic inlet to the tracheal bifurcation

     3   Mid-thoracic segment: consists of the proximal half of the esophagus between the tracheal bifurcation and the esophagogastric junction

     4   Lower abdominothoracic segment: is approximately 8 cm in length and is the distal half of the esophagus between the tracheal bifurcation and the esophagogastric junction; it includes the abdominal esophagus

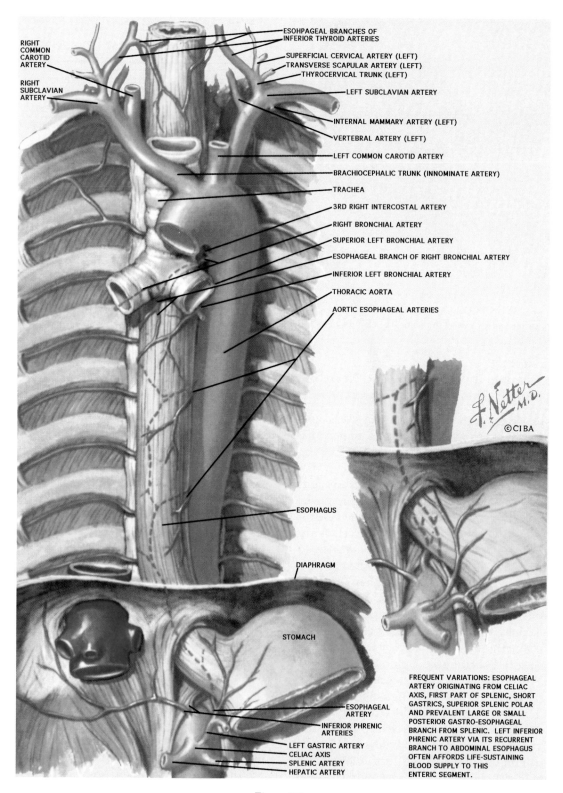

Figure 2-3

DIAGRAMMATIC ILLUSTRATION OF THE ESOPHAGEAL BLOOD SUPPLY

Diagrammatic representation of esophageal vasculature. (Plate 8 from Netter F. Ciba collection of medical illustrations, digestive system part 1. West Caldwell, NJ: Ciba Geigy, 1959:41.)

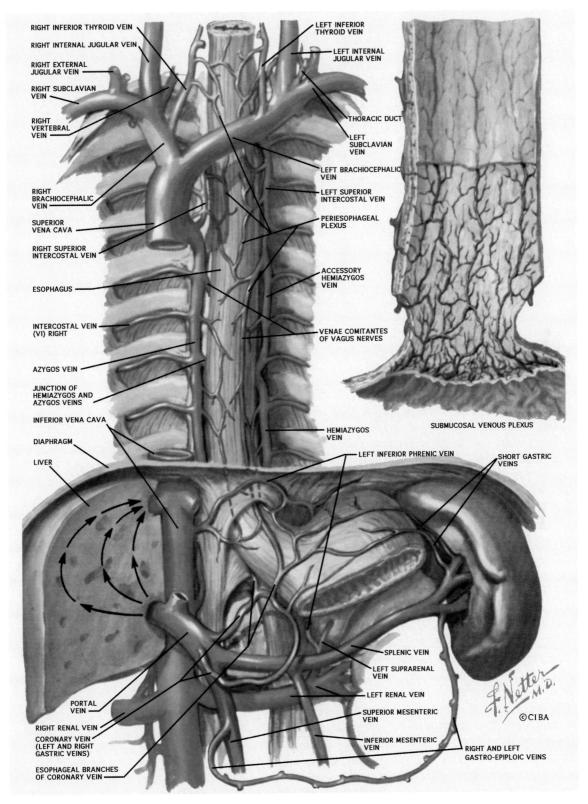

Figure 2-4

DIAGRAMMATIC ILLUSTRATION OF THE VENOUS DRAINAGE OF THE ESOPHAGUS

(Plate 9 from Netter F. Ciba collection of medical illustrations, digestive system part 1. West Caldwell, NJ: Ciba Geigy, 1959:42.)

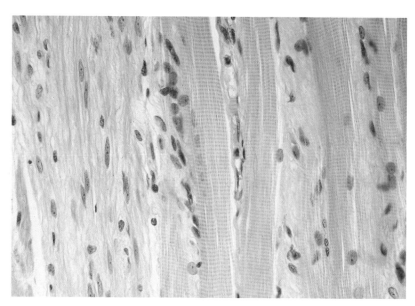

Figure 2-5
HISTOLOGIC APPEARANCE
OF THE ESOPHAGEAL
MUSCULATURE A THIRD OF
THE WAY DOWN
THE ESOPHAGUS
The left half of the field shows smooth muscle whereas the right half shows striated muscle. Faint cross striations are visible in the striated muscle.

### Esophageal Musculature and Sphincters

As in the rest of the gastrointestinal tract, the esophagus has an inner circular and an outer longitudinal muscle coat. The upper fourth of the esophagus consists entirely of striated muscle, the next quarter contains a mixture of striated and smooth muscle, and the lower half consists entirely of nonstriated muscle (fig. 2-5).

The longitudinal muscle coat arises from the cricopharyngeus muscle at the lateral aspect of the cricoid cartilage, and from two distinct bundles, one from each side of the posterior cricoid cartilage. These bundles spread laterally around the esophagus, where they interdigitate with one another in the dorsal midline. At the uppermost posterior level of the longitudinal muscle is a V-shaped gap between it and the cricopharyngeus muscle; this gap is covered anteriorly by the circular muscle (fig. 2-1). As the muscle fibers descend the esophagus, they form thick lateral masses and a thin anterior portion.

The inner circular muscle coat is usually thinner than the outer longitudinal muscle coat, a histologic feature that is the opposite of the rest of the gastrointestinal tract. The direction of the circular muscle fibers of the upper and lower third of the esophagus are more elliptical than circular; in the lowermost portion the fibers have a spiral configuration, with some bundles running vertically up and down.

Although both ends of the esophagus are closed under resting conditions, only the upper end has a clearly defined sphincter. This is formed by the cricopharyngeus muscle which is transversely oriented and inserted on the cricoid cartilage at the level of the sixth cervical vertebra. The tissue between the cricopharyngeus muscle and the inferior constrictors superiorly and the esophageal muscles inferiorly is relatively thin and is a potential site for esophageal diverticula.

Anatomically, the lower esophageal sphincter is difficult to see. In the lower esophagus, 1 to 2 cm above the hiatus, the circular and longitudinal muscle layers gradually become thickened and extend down to the cardia. Some investigators have suggested that there is an asymmetric thickening of the circular muscle that is arranged in a spiral fashion and blends with the inner oblique muscle of the stomach in the region of the physiologic sphincter (10,19). Contraction of these muscle fibers closes the lower esophagus.

### BLOOD SUPPLY

#### Arterial

The arterial blood supply is extremely variable (fig. 2-3) (8,21,25). On entering the esophagus, the arteries run within the muscular coat and give off branches which course within the submucosa and anastomose. The cervical portion of the esophagus is supplied primarily by the uppermost branches of the inferior thyroid artery, with minor contributions from the subclavian, common carotid, vertebral, and costocervical trunks. The thoracic esophagus is supplied mainly by branches of the bronchial and intercostal arteries, and by two unpaired branches of the aorta (a superior and inferior branch). The latter two vessels anastomose with branches of the inferior thyroid, bronchial, and left gastric arteries. The abdominal esophagus receives its blood supply mainly from the left gastric, the short gastrics, and the recurrent branch of the left inferior phrenic arteries.

### Venous

The venous drainage of the esophagus is mainly distributed within the mucosal folds (28). Radially arranged intraepithelial channels drain into a venous plexus, situated within the superficial submucosa, which then flows into three to five main venous channels situated in the deep submucosa. The latter communicate with a venous plexus on the adventitial esophageal surface via perforating vessels. The venous outflow from the adventitial venous plexus is illustrated in fig. 2-4, although this can vary among individuals and with site. In the cervical esophagus the plexus drains into the inferior thyroid, which empties into the brachiocephalic veins and the superior vena cava. The veins of the thoracic portion of the esophagus flow into the azygos vein, left inferior phrenic vein, and superior vena cava. The veins of the abdominal esophagus flow into the portal vein via the gastric vein. There are also connections with the short gastrics, gastroepiploic, and splenic veins. As is true for the arterial vasculature, there are numerous anastomotic connections between the veins, so that if any vein is blocked, as in portal hypertension, the blood flow is diverted to another venous branch.

### Lymphatic Drainage

This consists primarily of a rich network of lymphatics within the mucosa and submucosa that connect with lymphatics within the muscle and adventitial coats. The lymphatics within the muscle coats are predominantly oriented in a longitudinal direction (8). They freely connect with one another and these interconnections explain the frequency of intramucosal and submucosal spread of a primary tumor. In the cervical esophagus the adventitial lymphatics tend to drain into the paratracheal and internal jugular lymph nodes; the latter flow into the left thoracic duct. Lymphatics of the thoracic esophagus drain into the superior, middle, and lower mediastinal nodes; they then, in most instances, flow upwards into the thoracic duct on the left side and into the right lymph duct on the right side and into the right subclavian vein. The lymphatics of the abdominal esophagus drain into the superior gastric, celiac, common hepatic, and splenic artery lymph nodes. Because of the extensive interconnections of all the lymphatic channels, metastatic disease from the esophagus is frequently unpredictable: tumors of the lower esophagus which tend to metastasize to the upper abdominal lymph node chains mentioned above, also metastasize to the cervical lymph nodes in some cases (1).

## INNERVATION OF THE ESOPHAGUS

The nerve supply of the esophagus consists of parasympathetic (vagus) and sympathetic nerves, which innervate the epithelium and glands, the vasculature, and the muscle coats. The parasympathetic nerves originate in the neck from the cervical and thoracic paravertebral sympathetic trunks; these fibers then join the vagus nerve. The vagus itself consists of both afferent and efferent fibers that end in the dorsal vagal nucleus. The nerve fibers supplying the striated muscles of the upper esophagus and pharynx originate in the dorsal motor nucleus.

At the root of the neck on the right side and opposite the aortic arch on the left side, the vagus gives rise to the right and left recurrent laryngeal nerves. These run upward in a groove between the trachea and esophagus, giving off nerve twigs to the cervical esophagus. In the thorax, the right and left vagi descend posterior to the lung roots. At this point they break into a number of branches and form a meshwork of nerves on the anterior and posterior surfaces of the esophagus. Just above the esophageal hiatus the meshwork of vagal nerves reunite into one or several vagal trunks located on the anterior and posterior surfaces of the esophagus.

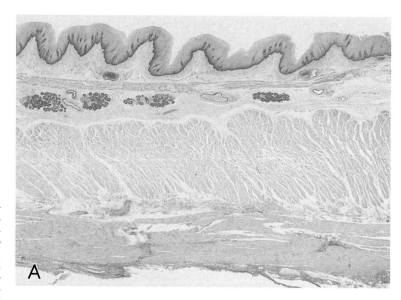

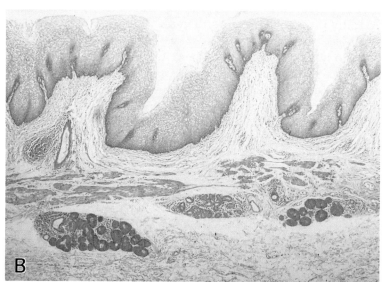

Figure 2-6
HISTOLOGIC FEATURES
OF THE ESOPHAGUS

A: Scanning-power view of the full thickness of the esophagus. The mucosa is composed of squamous epithelium, lamina propria, and muscularis mucosae. The latter separates the mucosa from the submucosa. The muscularis propria consists of two layers, namely the inner circular and the outer longitudinal coats. Note that the circular muscle coat is thicker than the longitudinal coat. Also visible are lymphoid follicles just above the muscularis mucosae.

B: Higher power magnification shows the three layers of the mucosa and the submucosal glands stained by hematoxylin and eosin and Alcian blue stains.

The intrinsic innervation of the esophagus consists of mucosal (Meissner's) and intermyenteric (Auerbach's) plexuses, made up of ganglia interconnected by a meshwork of nerve fibers. The latter consist of postganglionic sympathetic, and preganglionic and postganglionic parasympathetic fibers (22).

## HISTOLOGY

### Mucosa

The esophageal mucosa has three components: an outer stratified squamous epithelium; a thin muscle coat, the muscularis mucosae; and the lamina propria which is sandwiched in between the two (fig. 2-6). In addition, glands similar to those of the gastric cardia and known as esophageal cardiac glands, consisting of mucous cells that secrete neutral mucin (9), are commonly found in the lamina propria of the distal esophagus (fig. 2-7).

The squamous epithelium is nonkeratinized, although occasionally rare keratohyaline granules are present. It is composed of three zones: the basal, prickle, and functional layers; the latter refers to the flattened surface epithelium devoid of nuclei (fig. 2-8).

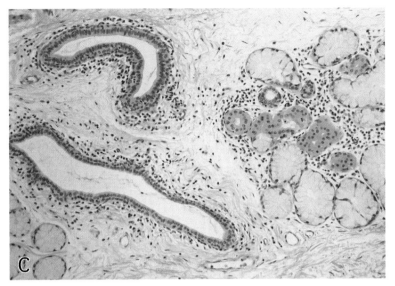

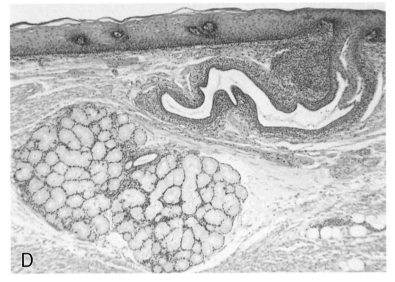

Figure 2-6 (continued)

C: Higher power magnification of the submucosal glands and their ducts stained with hematoxylin and eosin.

D: Section of esophageal mucosa shows a duct originating from the submucosal glands penetrating the squamous epithelium.

The basal cell layer is about three cells thick and comprises up to 15 percent of the thickness of the squamous epithelium, except for the most distal 3 cm of the esophagus (15,29). It is composed primarily of basal cells with scattered mitoses, interspersed with rare argyrophilic cells and melanocytes (5,27). The latter two cells are the sources of the rare primary small cell (oat cell) carcinoma (5) and malignant melanoma of the esophagus in which melanosis often is found around the melanoma (5,7). Pseudomelanosis of the esophagus has also been reported but the cells of origin are unknown (11). The basal cells have hyperchromatic nuclei and scant cyto-

plasm, and they blend with the prickle cell layer. A rule of thumb used to define the lower edge of the prickle cell layer is to determine where nuclei are separated by a distance of at least one nuclear diameter (17).

The cells of the prickle cell layer contain flattened nuclei and a glycogen-rich cytoplasm; the latter stains with periodic acid–Schiff (PAS) and Lugol's iodine solution. As these cells move up towards the luminal surface, they become progressively flatter and their cytoplasm becomes clearer.

In the cervical esophagus, just below the upper esophageal sphincter, may be a patch of heterotopic gastric mucosa known as the "inlet

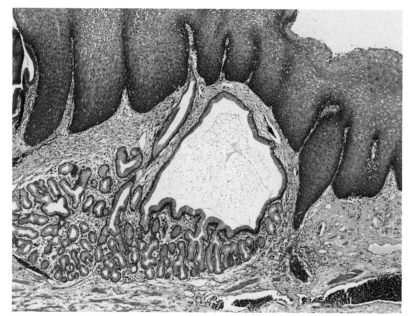

Figure 2-7
ESOPHAGEAL CARDIAC GLANDS
Low-power view of the esophageal mucosa just above the esophagogastric junction shows the mucosal glands.

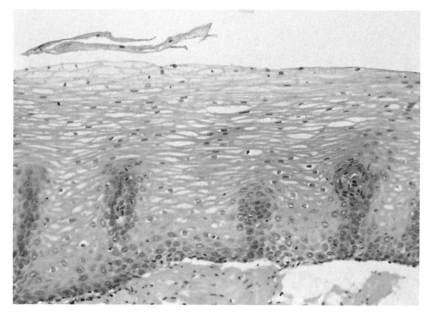

Figure 2-8
NORMAL ESOPHAGEAL SQUAMOUS EPITHELIUM
The epithelium is non-keratinized and has a thin basal zone; a prickle cell zone composed of glycogen-rich flattened cells that occupy most of the epithelium; and a few flattened cells on the surface that are devoid of nuclei.

patch." This consists of heterotopic gastric fundic or antral mucosa (fig. 2-9). In most instances this heterotopic mucosa is benign, but on rare occasions may result in peptic ulceration or carcinoma.

Phenotypic T-cell lymphocytes are frequently scattered throughout the squamous cell layer (3, 11, 12,24) and Langerhans cells are occasionally present (11,24). Sometimes the lymphocytic nuclei are compressed or lobulated and may be mistaken for neutrophils (the so-called squiggle cells) (fig. 2-10) (4).

The lamina propria invaginates the basal cell zone to produce dermal papillae that extend one third to half the thickness of the epithelium. These papillae contain capillaries which are sometimes engorged with blood. The lamina propria consists of loose connective tissue containing mononuclear cells, lymphocytes, occasional plasma cells, and rare lymphoid follicles. In the distal esophagus, sparsely distributed mucous glands are present in the lamina propria between the muscularis mucosae and the overlying squamous epithelium.

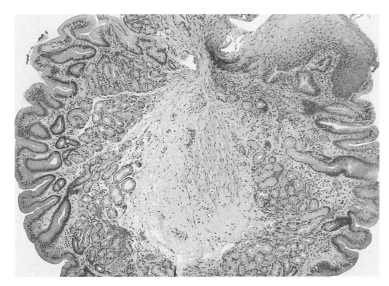

Figure 2-9
ESOPHAGEAL INLET PATCH
Mucosal biopsy showing antral type mucosa
and a small fragment of squamous epithelium.

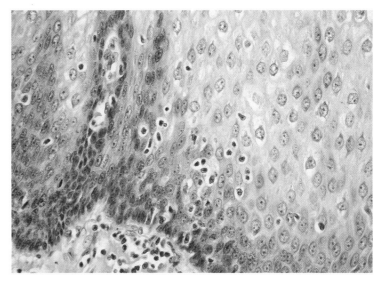

Figure 2-10
SQUAMOUS EPITHELIUM WITH
INTRAEPITHELIAL LYMPHOCYTES

These can occur normally within the epithelium and do not necessarily indicate esophagitis.

Top: Low-power view of squamous epithelium containing scattered lymphocytes just above the basal layers.

Bottom: High-power magnification showing lymphocytes with round nuclei surrounded by a clear halo. A "squiggle cell" is in the center of the field.

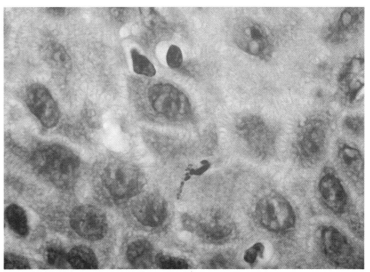

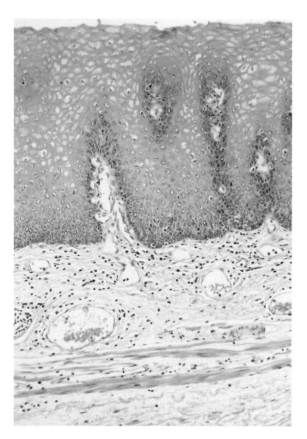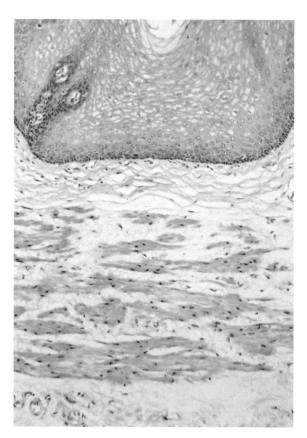

Figure 2-11
ESOPHAGEAL MUCOSA
Sections of esophageal mucosa show the variability in the thickness of the muscularis mucosae.
Left: A rather thin layer of muscularis mucosae.
Right: A thicker layer than on the left.

These glands may communicate with the luminal surface and have sometimes been misdiagnosed as Barrett's esophagus. It should be stressed that these glands almost never give rise to esophageal adenocarcinoma (fig. 2-7).

The muscularis mucosae consists of a thin band of longitudinally oriented smooth muscle separating the lamina propria from the submucosa (13). It becomes progressively thicker in the distal part of the esophagus and may be mistaken for the muscularis propria in biopsy specimens (fig. 2-11).

## Submucosa

The submucosa consists of loose connective tissue, blood vessels, nerve fibers, scattered lymphocytes, and small lymphoid follicles. In addition it contains distinct mucous gland complexes, which are most prominent at the upper and lower ends of the esophagus, and which communicate with the surface through ducts lined by cuboidal epithelium. Occasionally, the glands and ducts show focal cystic dilatation (20).

## REFERENCES

1. Akiyama H, Tsurumaru M, Kawamura T, Ono Y. Principles of surgical treatment for carcinoma of the esophagus: analysis of lymph node involvement. Ann Surg 1981;194:438–46.

2. Berardi RS, Devaiah KA. Barrett's esophagus. Surg Gynecol Obstet 1983;156:521–38.

3. Cooper HS, Dayal Y, Gourley WK, et al. Proceedings of the 1988 Subspecialty Conference on Gastrointestinal Biopsy Pathology at the United States and Canadian Academy of Pathology. Diagnostic nonproblems in gastrointestinal biopsy pathology. Mod Pathol 1989;2:244–59.

4. Dawsey SM, Lewin KJ, Liu FS, Wang GQ, Shen Q. Esophageal morphology from Linxian, China. Squamous histologic findings in 754 subjects. Cancer 1994;73:2027–37.

5. De La Pava S, Nigogosyan G, Pickren JW, Cabrera A. Melanosis of the esophagus. Cancer 1963;16:48–50.

6. Delattre JF, Palot JP, Ducasse A, Flament JB, Hureau J. The crura of the diaphragm and diaphragmatic passage. Applications to gastroesophageal reflux, its investigation and treatment. Anat Clin 1985;7:271–85.

7. DiCostanzo DP, Urmacher C. Primary malignant melanoma of the esophagus. Am J Surg Pathol 1987;11:46–52.

8. Enterline H, Thompson J. Pathology of the esophagus. New York: Springer-Verlag, 1984.

9. Fenoglia-Preiser CM, Lantz PE, Listrom MB, Davis M, Rilke FO. Gastrointestinal pathology. An atlas and text. New York: Raven Press, 1989.

10. Friedland GW. Progress in radiology: historical review of the changing concepts of lower esophageal anatomy: 430 BC-1977. AJR Am J Roentgenol 1978;131:373–88.

11. Geboes K, De Wolf-Peeters C, Rugeerts P, Janssens J, Vantrappen G, Desmet V. Lymphocytes and Langerhans cells in the human esophageal epithelium. Virchows Arch [A] 1983;401:45–55.

12. Goldman H, Antonioli DA. Mucosal biopsy of the esophagus, stomach and proximal duodenum. Hum Pathol 1982;13:423–48.

13. Goyal RK. Columnar cell-lined (Barrett's) esophagus: a historical perspective. In: Spechler SJ, Goyal RK, eds. Barrett's esophagus. Pathophysiology, diagnosis and management. New York: Elsevier, 1985:1–18.

14. Hayward J. The lower end of the oesophagus. Thorax 1961;16:36–41.

15. Ismail-Beigi F, Horton PF, Pope CE II. Histological consequences of gastroesophageal reflux in man. Gastroenterology 1970;58:163–74.

16. Johns BA. Developmental changes in the oesophageal epithelium. J Anat 1852;86:431–42.

17. Johnson LF, DeMeester TR, Haggitt RC. Esophageal epithelial response to gastroesophageal reflux. A quantitative study. Am J Dig Dis 1978;23:498–509.

18. Kalloor GJ, Deshpande AH, Collis JL. Observations on oesophageal length. Thorax 1976;31:284–8.

19. Liebermann-Meffert D, Allgower M, Schmid P, Blum AL. Muscular equivalent of the lower esophageal sphincter. Gastroenterology 1979;76:31–8.

20. Medeiros LJ, Doos WG, Balogh K. Esophageal intramural pseudodiverticulosis: a report of two cases with analysis of similar, less extensive changes in "normal" autopsy esophagi. Hum Pathol 1988;19:928–31.

21. Netter FH. Upper digestive tract. In: Anonymous digestive system, Part 1 of CIBA collection of medical illustration, vol 3. Summit, New Jersey: CIBA-Geigy, 1959.

22. Pope CE II. Normal anatomy and developmental anomalies. In: Sleisenger MH, Fordtran JS, eds. Gastrointestinal disease, pathophysiology, diagnosis and management. Philadelphia: WB Saunders, 1994.

23. Rector LE, Connerley ML. Aberrant mucosa in the esophagus in infants and children. Arch Pathol 1941;31:285–94.

24. Seefeld U, Krejs GJ, Siebenmann RE, Blum AL. Esophageal histology in gastroesophageal reflux. Morphometric findings in suction biopsies. Am J Dig Dis 1977;22:956–64.

25. Shackelford RT. Surgery of the alimentary tract. Philadelphia: WB Saunders, 1978.

26. Strobel CT, Byrne WJ, Ament ME, Euler AR. Correlation of esophageal lengths in children with height: application to the Tuttle test without prior esophageal manometry. J Pediatr 1979;94:81–4.

27. Tateishi R, Taniguchi H, Wada A, Horai T, Taniguchi K. Argyrophil cells and melanocytes in esophageal mucosa. Arch Pathol 1974;98:67–89.

28. Vianna A, Hayes PC, Moscoso G, et al. Normal venous circulation of the gastroesophageal junction. A route to understanding varices. Gastroenterology 1987;83:876–89.

29. Weinstein WM, Bogoch ER, Bowes KL. The normal human esophageal mucosa: a histological reappraisal. Gastroenterology 1975;68:40–4.

# 3

# BENIGN EPITHELIAL NEOPLASMS, SALIVARY GLAND-LIKE TUMORS, NON-NEOPLASTIC EPITHELIAL PROLIFERATIONS, AND OTHER NON-NEOPLASTIC EPITHELIAL TUMOR-LIKE CONDITIONS

The three most common neoplasms of the esophagus are ordinary squamous cell carcinoma, adenocarcinoma complicating Barrett's mucosa, and tiny well-differentiated leiomyomas. Nevertheless, esophageal neoplasms are seemingly limitless: almost every type of neoplasm, both benign and malignant, has been reported as a primary in the esophagus. However, neoplasms other than the three mentioned above are rare, and reports are generally limited to small series and single cases. Non-neoplastic epithelial lesions that present as lumps, masses, or tumors are referred to as tumor-like conditions, and are also rare. This chapter deals with unusual benign epithelial masses of the esophagus, both neoplastic and not. The descriptions are frequently limited or incomplete because published reports are few.

## SQUAMOUS PAPILLOMA AND CONDYLOMA-LIKE PROLIFERATIONS

**Definition.** Squamous papillomas are benign polyps characterized microscopically by a core of lamina propria covered by mature stratified squamous epithelium.

**Clinical and Endoscopic Features.** These uncommon lesions have no characteristic clinical features and no distinctive demographic relationships (5). In two different reports from Italy, there was a considerable difference in prevalence (3,11): in one study, only 15 papillomas were found in 20,000 upper endoscopic exams, a prevalence of 0.075 percent, while in the second study, 35 papillomas were found in about 8,100 exams, a six times higher prevalence of 0.45 percent. In a study from Spain, only 6 papillomas were found in about 15,000 upper endoscopic exams, a prevalence of 0.04 percent, about half of the lower prevalence of the Italian study. Thus, there may be some geographic differences in frequency, but the reasons for these differences are unknown.

Squamous papillomas are invariably incidental findings at upper endoscopy. Patients are more likely to be men, with a median age of between 45 and 50 years (5,8,11); women tend to be older than men. These age and sex data presumably reflect the population that has esophagogastroscopic exams: the endoscopic exams, during which the papillomas are found, are performed for common indications, including heartburn, dysphagia, and upper gastrointestinal bleeding, none of which are caused by the papillomas (6). Removal of the papillomas does not alleviate the symptoms (8).

Endoscopically, the lesions are polyps, sometimes with irregular surfaces, the results of the frond-like microscopic morphology. Most are small, sessile or partly pedunculated, white to pink and soft, and usually 5 mm or less in maximum measurement. Rare cases of giant papillomas have been reported, with sizes as large as 5 cm (14). The distribution within the esophagus varies somewhat depending upon the study, but generally it is the same as that for squamous carcinoma, with most occurring in the middle and lower thirds. Upper esophageal papillomas account for less than a fifth of the total. Most papillomas are solitary, but in about 10 to 15 percent of cases they are multiple, but generally no more than three or four. A few case reports of *papillomatosis,* that is, many papillomas, mostly in children, have been published (1,7,10,15). There is no indication that these are associated with laryngotracheal papillomatosis, a much more common condition.

**Histologic Findings.** There are different types of papilloma, based upon differences in the configuration of the stroma. The most common form has a branching core of lamina propria, producing fronds that are covered by squamous epithelium (fig. 3-1). This form sometimes appears to have a narrow stalk by which the polyp is attached to the mucosa. The squamous epithelium may be of any thickness, but is usually

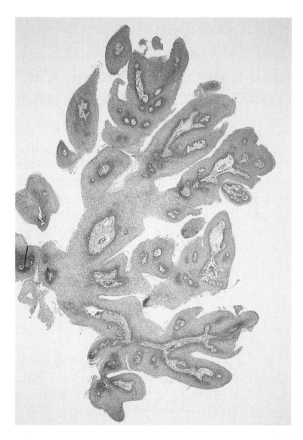 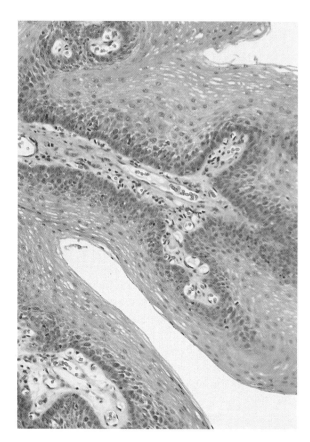

Figure 3-1
SQUAMOUS CELL PAPILLOMA

Left: This is an exaggerated version of the common form. It has an elaborate branching core of lamina propria that is covered by mature squamous epithelium.

Right: This is a high-power view of the mature squamous epithelium and the cores of lamina propria that contain thin-walled vessels and little else. The squamous epithelium is no thicker than that in the normal mucosa, and, in spots, it is even thinner.

normal or slightly thinned. The number of branches varies: some polyps have only two or three, while others have a complex system of many branches. A second type of papilloma has a bulbous lamina propria core that is covered by squamous epithelium; thick rete-like squamous cell extensions from the epithelium project down into the stromal core (fig. 3-2). This gives the polyp an inverted look, somewhat akin to inverted papillomas of the nose and paranasal sinuses. This has been referred to as the *endophytic type* (8). Some of these vaguely resemble cutaneous acrochordons or anal tags, and they may be given comparable names, such as *fibroepithelial polyps.* A third variant, the least common, is sessile and has a lamina propria that forms stromal spikes that are covered by hyperplastic, usually keratinized squamous epithelium (fig. 3-3) (7).

Occasionally, the squamous epithelium of all types has koilocytotic changes, with crinkled nuclei surrounded by clear cytoplasmic halos resembling the squamous cells of condylomas. In some papillomas there are proliferative changes resembling low-grade squamous dysplasia with increase in the basal cell thickness, cellular crowding, increased numbers of mitoses, and a few hyperchromatic or pleomorphic nuclei. Only one invasive carcinoma has been reported to develop in a proven squamous papilloma, and that papilloma was a giant form that was associated with human papilloma virus (13).

**Etiology, including Relation of Papillomas to Human Papilloma Virus Infection.** Squamous papillomas arise in the same parts of the esophagus as do squamous carcinomas, and they tend to be found in patients about 10 years

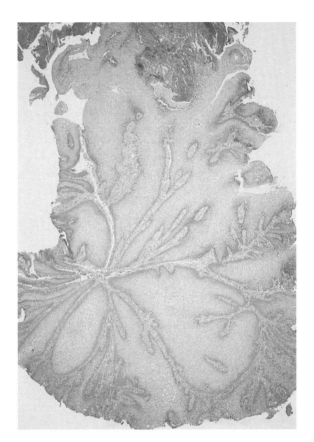
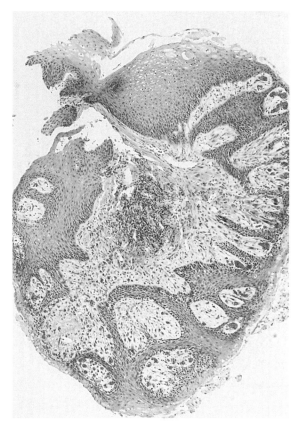

Figure 3-2
SQUAMOUS CELL PAPILLOMA

A second type of squamous papilloma, in which thick, irregular prongs of mature stratified squamous epithelium extend into the core of lamina propria. Left and right are different polyps. The lesion on the right vaguely resembles an acrochordon or fibroepithelial polyp of the skin.

younger than those with carcinomas. However, the risk factors for carcinomas do not apply for papillomas. There are no data to indicate that the patients are smokers or drinkers, and papillomas do not seem to occur with unusual frequency in the parts of the world where squamous cell cancer is endemic. There have been suggestions that some papillomas are related to gastroesophageal reflux, but this has not been substantiated (3,5,9,11). Several studies have focused upon the possibility that papillomas may be induced by longstanding human papilloma virus (HPV) infection (4,8,10, 12,16). The results of these studies have varied, possibly because of differences in sensitivity of HPV detection systems and possibly because of differences in HPV infection rates in different populations. In a study from the United States, two papillomas showed histologic changes suggesting HPV infection, but neither contained HPV proteins using immunohistochemical analysis (16). Of

33 papillomas in a Swiss study, none had typical light microscopic HPV changes, and only 6 had HPV DNA types 31-33-35 using in situ hybridization as the detection system (4). Two studies from the United States in which the polymerase chain reaction was used to detect HPV DNA reported amazingly different results: in one study, from Boston, half of the papillomas, mainly the common type with the branched appearance, had HPV DNA, mostly type 16 (8); in the second study of 17 patients from Washington, D.C., only one with papilloma had HPV DNA, and that was type 6-11 (2). It is also possible that some, or even most papillomas develop as the result of multiple factors acting in concert, including reflux or other irritants as well as HPV infection. The relationship among squamous papillomas, squamous cell carcinomas, and HPV has yet to be worked out, but it seems clear that papillomas are not frequent precursors of invasive carcinoma.

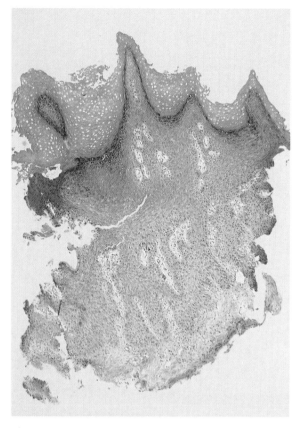

Figure 3-3
SQUAMOUS CELL PAPILLOMA: SPIKE FORM
This small plaque is characterized by spires of lamina propria that elevate the variably thick squamous epithelium. (Courtesy of Drs. Robert Odze and Donald Antonioli, Boston, MA.)

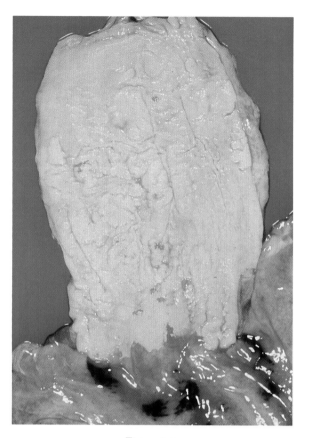

Figure 3-4
GLYCOGEN ACANTHOSES
In this lower esophagus, there are slightly elevated longitudinal plaques.

## GLYCOGEN ACANTHOSIS (GLYCOGENIC ACANTHOSIS)

Glycogen acanthosis usually is a white plaque mostly found in the distal esophagus, commonly oriented longitudinally paralleling the longitudinal axis of the esophageal wall (figs. 3-4, 3-5). From an endoscopic standpoint, this lesion is part of the differential diagnosis of endoscopic white plaques in the esophagus: other possibilities include candidiasis, ulcers covered by exudate, and no histologic abnormality, that is, "disappearing white patches." Glycogen acanthosis may be single or multiple, and there is no predictable clinical association with any other condition; they are therefore discovered serendipitously. The only exception was a case of Cowden's syndrome in which mucosal polyps of the stomach were associated with esophageal lesions that appeared to be glycogen acanthoses (20,22).

Glycogen acanthoses are common. In one study, they were found in 15 percent of 160 consecutive esophagoscopies (24). In another study, they were found in 27 consecutive adult autopsies (23). They can be detected by careful radiographic studies, using double contrast views of a well-distended esophagus, as uniform fine nodules, usually less than 3 mm, sometimes producing a cobblestone appearance when multiple, and they are frequently multiple (18,19). In one radiographic study, they were found in over a fourth of 300 consecutive double-contrast esophagrams (19). In fact, since they are so common, they may even be considered a normal variant (21).

The microscopic features are simple and characteristic. The superficial squamous epithelial

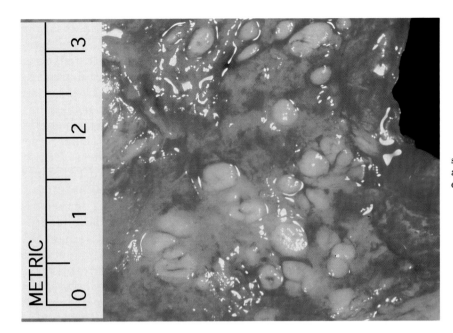

Figure 3-5
GLYCOGEN ACANTHOSES
Numerous glycogen acantho-ses stand out as white islands against the background of hyper-emic mucosa.

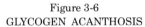

Figure 3-6
GLYCOGEN ACANTHOSIS
The superficial squamous epi-thelium is thicker than normal and contains enlarged squamous cells that have abundant pale to clear cytoplasm.

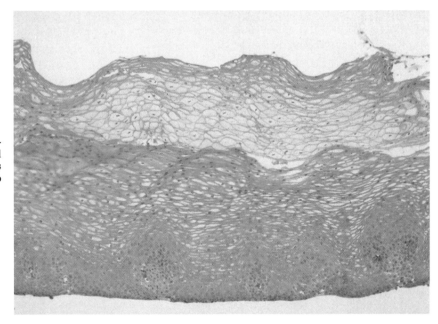

layers are thicker than normal and contain un-usually large cells with pale or clear cytoplasm filled with glycogen (fig. 3-6) (17). The glycogen is best demonstrated by staining the epithelium with the periodic acid–Schiff (PAS) reagent. This stain colors the glycogen granules in the clear cells dark red; pretreating a duplicate slide with diastase (amylase) prior to staining with PAS results in loss of staining, indicating that the material in the cytoplasm of the clear cells is glycogen. Sometimes, it is difficult to tell glyco-gen acanthosis from normal mucosa when the lesion is less than fully developed, when the top of the epithelium has been stripped during the biopsy process, or when normal mucosa is cut at a bias, so that the superficial layers appear to be unusually thick (see Normal Mucosa in chapter 2 for comparison). In all situations, the diagnosis is questionable and is best avoided if the biopsy is not from an endoscopic plaque.

## PSEUDOEPITHELIOMATOUS HYPERPLASIA AT THE EDGES AND BASES OF ULCERS

Chronic ulcers, almost always induced by severe chronic gastroesophageal reflux, are common. As an ulcer heals, squamous epithelium creeps along the surface of the granulation tissue at the base of the ulcer. As this epithelium migrates along the surface, it sends prongs of undifferentiated cells into the granulation tissue. These prongs elongate, resulting in parallel columns of primitive squamous cells mixed with granulation tissue, an appearance that can be easily confused with invading squamous cell carcinoma nests, especially when the prongs are cut across. The granulation tissue of the ulcer base may resemble an inflamed fibrosing stroma, much like the inflammatory desmoplasia of invasive squamous cell carcinoma. This proliferation is discussed in more detail and is illustrated in the section on differential diagnosis of esophageal squamous cell carcinoma in chapter 4.

## CYSTS

### Developmental Cysts and Duplications

The esophagus occasionally contains one or more cysts that seem to be developmental because they contain epithelial and stromal elements that are either part of the normal esophagus or part of the normal foregut other than the esophagus. Some of these cysts are intramural, while others lie mainly in the mediastinum, attached to the adventitial or outer muscularis of the esophagus. How they develop is not known, although there are several theories, among the most popular of which is the theory of misplaced epithelial cells during embryogenesis. The cysts may present in childhood or adulthood. Some are large and cause obstructive symptoms, such as dysphagia, but many, even large cysts, are asymptomatic and are found by accident during chest X-ray or barium swallow exams (32). The lack of symptoms may result from their pliability. Some of these cysts are lined by ciliated columnar or respiratory epithelium and have smooth muscle, mucous glands, and cartilage in their walls (fig. 3-7). For these the designation *bronchogenic cysts* is appropriate (29). Others are lined by stratified squamous epithelium and

have a muscularis mucosae and submucosal mucous glands, and are aptly named *esophageal cysts* (25). However, when esophageal cysts occur within the esophageal wall and share muscularis propria with the esophagus proper, they may really be intramural duplication anomalies.

Duplications (duplication anomalies) are defined as either cysts or elongated tubular structures lined by esophageal squamous; gastric, especially fundic; primitive; or ciliated columnar or small intestinal epithelium. They also contain other layers of the gut, including muscularis mucosae, submucosa, and muscularis propria. When they form intramural cysts, rather than extramural elongated duplications, they are also referred to as *gastroenteric* or *enteric cysts* (28). Identical cysts in the stomach are discussed in chapter 9. Such duplications are more common in the esophagus than in the stomach, but they still only account for 10 to 15 percent of all gastrointestinal duplications (27). They usually involve the lower third of the esophagus, especially on the right side, although longer segments, even the full length of the esophagus, may be involved (27). Some esophageal duplications communicate with gastric duplications below the diaphragm, but about 90 percent do not communicate with the esophageal lumen. Most present in childhood, especially in the first year of life (31). Associated vertebral anomalies are common when the duplications are extrinsic to the esophageal wall (28,30), but rare when the duplication is intramural (26). In contrast to most gastric duplications that share muscle coats with the normal stomach, most esophageal duplications are generally surrounded by their own muscularis, so they can be dissected away from the esophagus proper (32). The split notochord theory is the favored theory of duplication development: this suggests that abnormal splitting of the notochord during the first several weeks of gestation may induce gut duplications (28,31).

### Pseudodiverticulosis (Intramural Diverticulosis)

Dilatation of the ducts of the submucosal esophageal glands, possibly as a result of inflammation, is common. Such dilatations are generally microscopic findings and are clinically insignificant by themselves, although the inflammations that may have induced them may be important.

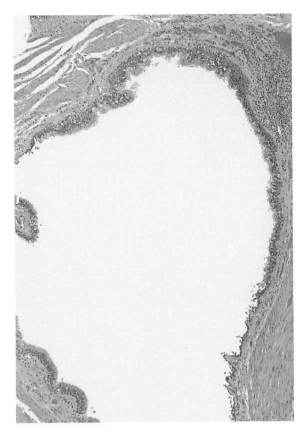 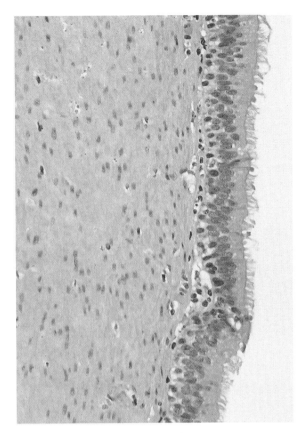

Figure 3-7
DEVELOPMENT CYST
Left: Low-power view of a cyst lined by pseudostratified, ciliated, columnar epithelium, beneath which is a thin layer of collagen fibers and small vessels. The entire cyst is surrounded by smooth muscle that blends with the muscularis propria.
Right: High magnification view.

However, there is no evidence that the most common inflammation in the esophagus, that due to chronic gastroesophageal reflux, predisposes to dilatation. When one of the authors studied over 40 patients with esophageal achalasia, ductal dilatations were found in about half, but they were never grossly apparent as cysts. These dilated ducts are lined by the typical ductal epithelium, that is, several layers of cuboidal epithelium. Obstruction of the gland ducts cannot be implicated, since these ductal cysts have open communication with the esophageal lumen.

On rare occasions, dilatations of these ducts become huge, producing grossly visible intramural cysts, a condition called *intramural pseudo-diverticulosis* (36). An identical process is named *esophagitis cystica* (39). This process resembles the Rokitansky-Aschoff sinuses that occur in the gall bladder, possibly as a response to increased intraluminal pressure. In fact, in some cases, there has been an abnormality in esophageal motility (33). Except for a few reported cases in children, this is a disease of adults, but there are no known predilections. There are less than 100 published cases and most of the reports are in the radiologic literature so that there is little detailed morphologic information.

The cysts vary in number and size, and in some cases they almost fill the submucosa, producing lumps that distort the esophageal mucosa (fig. 3-8). Such cases may give rise to obstructive symptoms, particularly dysphagia, but the dysphagia is almost always mild and long-standing, and there is usually a good symptomatic response to mechanical dilatation (34). The area of involvement may be segments of any

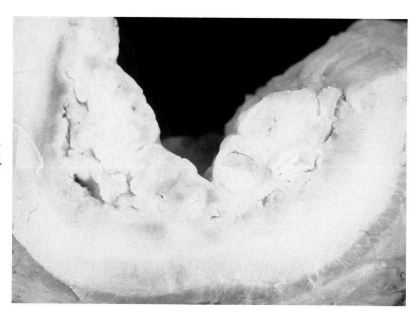

**Figure 3-8**
**INTRAMURAL**
**PSEUDODIVERTICULOSIS**
The esophageal wall is thick, due to the expanded submucosa that contains numerous collapsed cysts, some of which appear as irregular slits.

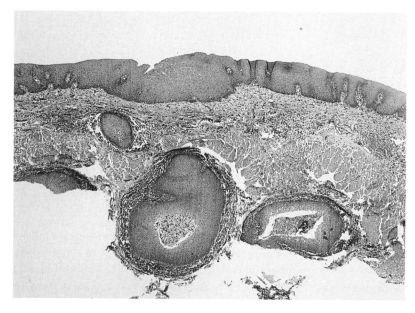

**Figure 3-9**
**PSEUDODIVERTICULOSIS**
In the superficial submucosa there are two dilated ducts lined by thick metaplastic squamous epithelium. Perhaps it is ducts such as these that are the precursors of the full-blown cystic disease.

length, and any part of the esophagus is at risk, although most occur in the upper part (34). The cysts communicate with the lumen through narrow stomas. In some cases, careful barium radiographic studies demonstrate that the intramural cysts are flask-shaped outpouchings with very narrow necks, a result of their communication with the lumen (34,38). Contraction of the esophageal muscularis may obliterate the narrow neck.

Superinfection with *Candida albicans* is common, but there is no indication that this organism has any role in producing the abnormality.

Endoscopic exams may detect the tiny openings of the dilated ducts, and biopsies of the mucosa will usually produce normal mucosa or possibly some of the superinfecting *Candida* (35). One reported case involved a segment covered by Barrett's mucosa (37).

The cysts are commonly lined by stratified squamous epithelium (figs. 3-9, 3-10). They may develop complex extensions or outpouchings, so that in florid cases, the whole submucosa and even part of the muscularis propria seems filled with squamous cysts. The cysts may become

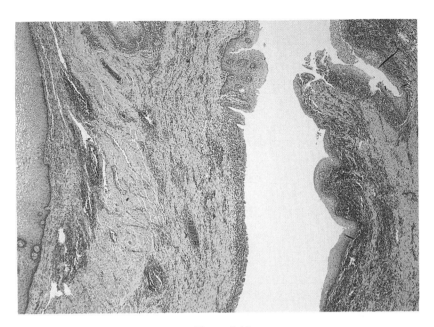

Figure 3-10
PSEUDODIVERTICULOSIS
The mucosa is at the far left. Within the submucosa is a large squamous-lined cyst surrounded by scar containing lymphoid aggregates.

infected or inflamed for other reasons, leading to variously intense secondary inflammation, ulceration, and scar around the cysts. There are a few cases in which cysts perforated, thereby forming fistulae that extended into the mediastinum (33).

## INTRAMURAL EPITHELIAL TUMORS, INCLUDING SALIVARY GLAND–TYPE TUMORS, AND OTHER EPITHELIAL TUMORS AND TUMOR-LIKE LESIONS

Some rare intramural epithelial tumors seem to be salivary gland–type tumors; these probably arise in the submucosal glands since these glands resemble salivary glands. Some of these are *mucoepidermoid tumors,* with a mixture of squamous and mucous cells (41,43,49,50). It is not clear how many of the reported cases of mucoepidermoid tumor of the esophagus are of the salivary gland type and how many actually are squamous cell carcinomas with glandular or mucous cell differentiation, since many have a surface abnormality, such as an ulcer. Presumably, tumors that have intact overlying mucosa, suggesting that they arose within the esopha-

geal wall and not from the surface epithelium, are more likely to be bona fide mucoepidermoid carcinomas. If this criterion is rigorously applied, then only a few of the reported cases of mucoepidermoid tumors actually fulfill the diagnostic requirements.

*Pleomorphic adenomas* have also been reported, but they total less than 20 cases, and the histologic documentation of that diagnosis, based upon published photomicrographs, is often tenuous (40). *Adenoid cystic carcinomas* also have been reported, but almost all reported cases are not the typical low-grade salivary gland variety but are high-grade tumors. These are discussed in detail in chapter 4.

Other one-of-a-kind tumors include a multicystic submucosal tumor in which the cysts were lined by cuboidal epithelium that contained neither glycogen nor mucin. This was reported as a *serous cystadenoma,* and was apparently such a problem in classification that it required eight authors to report this single tumor (48).

There have been individual case reports of ectopic tumors of thyroid and parathyroid tissue in the cervical esophagus. In one of these reports,

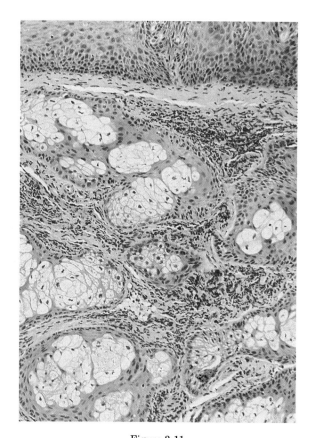

Figure 3-11
ECTOPIC SEBACEOUS GLANDS
Ectopic sebaceous glands in the lamina propria, in this case surrounded by a lymphocyte-rich infiltrate.

a patient with hypercalcemia and high parathormone levels had a *parathyroid adenoma* in the submucosa of the upper esophagus (45). The authors questioned whether this was just a curiosity. Another case was that of a *follicular tumor of thyroid type* with large numbers of oxyphil or Hürthle cells that occurred in the cervical esophagus (42). The tumor cells contained immunoreactive thyroglobulin.

*Ectopic* or *heterotopic sebaceous glands* have been found in the esophagus, perhaps in as much as 2 percent of adult autopsies (fig. 3-11) (51). They occur at all levels, and they may be multiple. They are located in the lamina propria. Although they are designated as ectopias, there is some suggestion that they may be metaplasias of submucosal gland ducts.

There was an individual report of a *hamartomatous polyp* of the upper esophagus containing cartilage, adipose tissue, and columnar epithelium, resembling the chondromatous hamartoma of the lung (44). Another lesion was described as an adenoma that contained gastric glands with parietal cells that probably deserved to be called an ectopia. Finally, a localized submucosal papillary glandular and tubular lesion that resembled both the papillary syringoadenoma of the skin and the intraductal papilloma of the breast was reported (43,46,47).

**REFERENCES**

**Squamous Papilloma**

1. Brinson RR, Schuman BM, Mills LR, Thigpen S, Freedman S. Multiple squamous papillomas of the esophagus associated with Goltz syndrome. Am J Gastroenterol 1987;82:1177–9.
2. Carr NJ, Bratthauer GL, Lichy JH, Taubenberger JK, Monihan JM, Sobin LH. Squamous cell papillomas of the esophagus: a study of 23 lesions for human papillomavirus by in situ hybridization and the polymerase chain reaction. Hum Pathol 1994;25:536–40.
3. Fernández-Rodríguez CM, Badia-Figuerola N, Ruiz del Arbol L, Fernández-Seara J, Dominguez F, Avilés-Ruiz JF. Squamous papilloma of the esophagus: report of six cases with long-term follow-up in four patients. Am J Gastroenterol 1986;81:1059–62.
4. Fontolliet C, Hurlimann J, Monnier P, Ollyo JB, Levi F, Savary M. Le papillome de l'oesophage est-il une lesion preneoplasique? Etude de 33 cas. Schweiz Med Wochenschr 1991;121:754–7.
5. Franzin G, Musola R, Zamboni G, Nicolis A, Manfrini C, Fratton A. Squamous papillomas of the esophagus. Gastrointest Endosc 1983;29:104–6.
6. Javdan P, Pitman ER. Squamous papilloma of esophagus. Dig Dis Sci 1984;29:317–20.
7. Nuwayhid NS, Ballard ET, Cotton R. Esophageal papillomatosis: case report. Ann Otol Rhinol Laryngol 1977;86:623–6.
8. Odze R, Antonioli D, Shocket D, Noble-Topham S, Goldman H, Upton M. Esophageal squamous papillomas. A clinicopathologic study of 38 lesions and analysis for human papillomavirus by the polymerase chain reaction. Am J Surg Pathol 1993;17:803–12.
9. Parnell SA, Peppercorn MA, Antonioli DA, Cohen MA, Joffe N. Squamous cell papilloma of the esophagus. Report of a case after peptic esophagitis and repeated bougienage with review of the literature. Gastroenterology 1978;74:910–3.

10. Politoske EJ. Squamous papilloma of the esophagus associated with the human papillomavirus. Gastroenterology 1992;102:668–73.
11. Sablich R, Benedetti G, Bignucolo S, Serraino D. Squamous cell papilloma of the esophagus. Report on 35 endoscopic cases. Endoscopy 1988;20:5–7.
12. Syrjänen K, Pyrhönen S, Aukee S, Koskela E. Squamous cell papilloma of the oesophagus: a tumour probably caused by human papilloma virus (HPV). Diagnostic Histopathol 1982;5:291–6.
13. Van Cutsem E, Geboes K, Vantrappen G. Malignant degeneration of esophageal squamous papilloma associated with the human papillomavirus [Letter]. Gastroenterology 1992;103:1119–20.
14. Walker JH. Giant papilloma of the thoracic esophagus. Am J Roentgenol 1978;131:519–20.
15. Waterfall WE, Somers S, Desa DJ. Benign oesophageal papillomatosis. A case report with a review of the literature. J Clin Pathol 1978;31:111–5.
16. Winkler B, Capo V, Reumann W, et al. Human papillomavirus infection of the esophagus. A clinicopathologic study with demonstration of papillomavirus antigen by the immunoperoxidase technique. Cancer 1985;55:149–55.

### Glycogen Acanthosis

17. Bender MD, Allison J, Cuaratas F, Montgomery C. Glycogenic acanthosis of the esophagus: a form of benign epithelial hyperplasia. Gastroenterology 1973;65:373–80.
18. Ghahremani GG, Rushovich AM. Glycogenic acanthosis of the esophagus: radiographic and pathologic features. Gastrointest Radiol 1984;9:93–8
19. Glick SN, Teplick SK, Goldstein J, Stead JA, Zitomer N. Glycogenic acanthosis of the esophagus. AJR Am J Roentgenol 1982;139:683–8.
20. Haggitt RC, Reid BJ. Hereditary gastrointestinal polyposis syndromes. Am J Surg Pathol 1986;10:871–87.
21. Hamilton SR. Esophagitis. In: Ming SC, Goldman H, eds. Pathology of the gastrointestinal tract. Philadelphia: WB Saunders, 1992:385–6.
22. Lashner BA, Riddell RH, Winans CS. Ganglioneuromatosis of the colon and extensive glycogenic acanthosis in Cowden's disease. Dig Dis Sci 1986;31:213–6.
23. Rywlin AM, Ortega R. Glycogenic acanthosis of the esophagus. Arch Pathol 1970;93:439–43.
24. Stern Z, Sharon P, Ligumsky M, Levij IS, Rachmilewitz D. Glycogen acanthosis of the esophagus. A benign but confusing endoscopic lesion. Am J Gastroenterol 1980;74:261–3.

### Developmental Cysts and Duplications

25. Abell MR. Mediastinal cysts. Arch Pathol 1956;61:360–79.
26. Dehner LP. Pediatric surgical pathology. Baltimore: Williams & Wilkins, 1987:334.
27. Dresler CM, Patterson GA, Taylor BR, Moote DJ. Complete foregut duplication. Ann Thorac Surg 1990;50:306–8.
28. Enterline H, Thompson J. Pathology of the esophagus. New York: Springer-Verlag, 1984:31–4.
29. Harmand D, Grosdidier J, Hoeffel JC. Multiple bronchogenic cysts of the esophagus. Am J Gastroenterol 1981;75:321–3.
30. Herman TE, Oser AB, McAlister WH. Tubular communicating duplications of esophagus and stomach. Pediatr Radiol 1991;21:494–6.
31. Milsom J, Unger S, Alford BA, Rodgers BM. Triplication of the esophagus with gastric duplication. Surgery 1985;98:121–5.
32. Postlethwait RW. Benign tumors and cysts of the esophagus. Surg Clin North Am 1983;63:925–31.

### Pseudodiverticulosis

33. Braun P, Nussle D, Roy CC, Cuendet A. Intramural diverticulosis of the esophagus in an eight-year-old boy. Pediatr Radiol 1978;28:235–7.
34. Castillo S, Aburashed A, Kimmelman J, Alexander LC. Diffuse intramural esophageal pseudodiverticulosis. New cases and review. Gastroenterology 1977;72:541–5.
35. Graham DY, Goyal RK, Sparkman J, Cagan ME, Pogonowska MJ. Diffuse intramural diverticulosis. Gastroenterology 1975;68:781–5.
36. Medeiros LJ, Doos WG, Balogh K. Esophageal intramural pseudodiverticulosis: a report of two cases with analysis of similar, less extensive changes in "normal" autopsy esophagi. Hum Pathol 1988;19:928–31.
37. Mendl K, Montgomery RD, Stephenson SF. Segmental intramural diverticulosis associated with and confined to a spastic area of muscular hypertrophy in a columnar lined oesophagus. Clin Radiol 1973;24:440–4.
38. Montgomery RD, Mendl K, Stepthenson SF. Intramural diverticulosis of the oesophagus. Thorax 1975;30:278–84.
39. Voirol MW, Welsh RA, Genet EF. Esophagitis cystica. Am J Gastroenterol. 1973;59:446–53.

### Miscellaneous Epithelial Tumors

40. Banducci D, Rees R, Bluett MK, Sawyers JL. Pleomorphic adenoma of the cervical esophagus: a rare tumor. Ann Thorac Surg 1987;44:653–5.
41. Bell-Thomson J, Haggitt RC, Ellis FH Jr. Mucoepidermoid and adenoid cystic carcinomas of the esophagus. J Thorac Cardiovasc Surg 1980;79:438–46.
42. Mansour KA, Zaatari GS, Krick JG. Oxyphilic granular cell adenoma (oncocytoma) of the esophagus. Ann Thorac Surg 1986;42:705–7.
43. Sasajima K, Watanabe M, Takubo K, Takai A, Yamashita K, Onda M. Mucoepidermoid carcinoma of the esophagus: report of two cases and review of the literature. Endoscopy 1990;22:140–3.

44. Shah B, Unger L, Heimlich HJ. Hamartomatous polyp of the esophagus. Arch Surg 1975;110:326–8.
45. Sloane JA, Moody HC. Parathyroid adenoma in submucosa of esophagus. Arch Pathol Lab Med 1978;102:242–3.
46. Spin FP. Adenomas of the esophagus: a case report and review of the literature. Gastrointest Endosc 1973;20:26–7.
47. Takubo K, Esaki Y, Watanabe A, Umehara M, Sasajima K. Adenoma accompanied by superficial squamous cell carcinoma of the esophagus. Cancer 1993;71:2435–8.
48. Tsutsumi M, Mizumoto K, Tsujiuchi T, et al. Serous cystadenoma of the esophagus. Acta Pathol Jpn 1990;40:153–5.
49. Weitzner S. Mucoepidermoid carcinoma of the esophagus. Report of a case. Arch Path 1970;90:271–3.
50. Woodard BH, Shelburne JD, Vollmer RT, Postlethwait RW. Mucoepidermoid carcinoma of the esophagus: a case report. Hum Pathol 1978;9:352–4.
51. Zak FG. Sebaceous glands in the esophagus. Arch Dermatol 1976;112:1153–4.

# 4

# SQUAMOUS CELL CARCINOMA

## USUAL (TYPICAL) SQUAMOUS CELL CARCINOMA

Squamous cell carcinoma is the most common esophageal neoplasm as well as one of the most common cancers worldwide. It is a cancer of developing rather than developed countries. It has peculiar epidemiologic characteristics suggesting that there are strong environmental factors critical for carcinogenesis, yet these factors are elusive. It is a carcinoma which, unfortunately, usually is detected only when advanced, and as a result, is infrequently cured. Populations at high risk have been identified, and surveillance programs to either deter the development of the cancer or at least to detect it in its nonfatal early or low stages have been established in those populations. In low-risk populations, the carcinoma is of such low frequency that surveillance programs are not cost effective.

**Prevalence and Incidence.** In 1980, it was estimated that, worldwide, esophageal cancer was the sixth most common cancer in men, the ninth most common in women, and the seventh most common overall for both sexes, with an estimated 310,400 new cases per year (34). In almost all populations, squamous cell carcinoma accounts for most cases of esophageal cancer, although adenocarcinoma complicating Barrett's mucosa is on the rise in some areas, such as in the United States (54). In all parts of the world it is predominantly a disease of men, with men outnumbering women by about 3 to 1. In the United States, squamous cell carcinoma is not among the 10 most common malignancies, nor is it among the 10 most common fatal cancers, when all segments of the population are considered together; however, in 1989 it was the fifth most common fatal cancer in men from 55 to 74 years of age (7). It has been estimated that in the United States in 1993 all cases of carcinoma of the esophagus, including both squamous cell and adenocarcinomas, accounted for about 11,300 new cases and about 10,200 cancer deaths (7). This makes esophageal carcinoma the least prevalent of all gastrointestinal cancers except for those of the small intestine and anus, both of

which are rare. Unfortunately, statistics such as these fail to distinguish between squamous cell carcinomas and adenocarcinomas arising in Barrett's esophagus. The latter cancer may be increasing in incidence. In a study in Canada from 1970 to 1980, the incidence of new cases of esophageal cancer among men varied from 2.4 cases per 100,000 people in Saskatchewan to 5.8 cases in the Northwest Territories and Yukon (2). This study did not separate the two major types of carcinoma, nor did it separate different populations, such as whites, blacks, and native Americans.

There is great variation in the geographic distribution of esophageal squamous cell cancer. There is high frequency in the People's Republic of China; Singapore; Iran around the Caspian sea; Kazakhstan; Puerto Rico; temperate South America including Chile, Uruguay, northern Argentina, and Brazil; parts of western Europe such as Switzerland and France; and the Transkei region of South Africa (12,17,34). It was estimated that in 1980, 54 percent of all new cases of esophageal carcinoma worldwide would occur in China, a country in which this cancer is second only to gastric cancer as a cause of cancer deaths (12,34). In a Chinese study published in 1982, 24.5 percent of all cancer deaths in men and 18.1 percent in women were caused by squamous cancer of the esophagus (52). The incidence was highest along the Taihang mountain range in North China, especially in the Henan and Shanxi provinces, where the age-adjusted incidence from 1971 to 1974 was 161.3 cases per 100,000 men and 102.9 per 100,000 women (39). Even the local chickens have a remarkably high incidence of esophageal and pharyngeal cancers (12). The incidence in developing countries is four times that of developed countries. In northeast Iran around the Caspian sea, the incidence of squamous cell esophageal carcinoma is second only to that in China. In South Africa, the incidence in the black population has been increasing rapidly since World War II to the point where it is the most common cancer among men and the second most common among women (27).

Population differences also exist even within one country. In the United States in 1991, carcinoma of the esophagus, virtually all of which was squamous cell, was the sixth most common cancer and the fourth leading cause of cancer deaths among blacks (6). The annual incidence of squamous cell carcinoma among the general population in the United States, based upon an analysis of nine cancer registries, for the years 1973 through 1982 was clearly racially biased (54). The annual incidence was 15.1 cases per 100,000 black men compared to only 2.9 cases per 100,000 white men. Furthermore, the incidence among black women was four times that for white women.

**Pathogenesis.** *Risk Factors.* Since squamous cell carcinoma has such a striking variation in incidence in different parts of the world and even among different population groups within the same country, it is to be expected that there are different risk factors in different areas. Diet seems to be most important in China, Iran, and South Africa, the highest risk areas in the world, while alcohol and tobacco seem to be more significant in the West. As a result, it is possible that squamous cell carcinoma of the esophagus is not a single disease but a family of diseases that are related by site and cell type, but not by pathogenesis. The various risk factors may be interdependent, and they may be modified by social habits, so that it may be impossible to separate specific dietary components or deficiencies from alcohol use and tobacco smoking, established behavioral norms in certain high-risk populations. In addition, there are limited data suggesting that the risk factors may be different, quantitatively if not qualitatively, for carcinomas arising in different parts of the esophagus. The risk factors that have been analyzed most include alcohol consumption, tobacco use, staple foods, vitamin and mineral deficiencies some of which may be soil related, thermal injury from eating hot food, viruses, and exposure to potentially carcinogenic nitrosamines and other nitrogenous compounds. Many of these factors appear to be so interrelated that it is often impossible to analyze them independently. The reader is referred to several recently published long and detailed summaries analyzing the risk factors for esophageal squamous cell carcinoma (12,39). The following discussion summarizes the current data derived from such comprehensive analyses.

Alcohol. One of the strongest associations in Western developed countries is that between squamous cell cancer of the esophagus and alcohol consumption. The risk of developing this tumor is 25 times greater for chronic liquor drinkers than for nondrinkers; for chronic beer drinkers, the risk is 10 times that of nondrinkers (43). However, this interaction may be somewhat different for cancers arising in different parts of the esophagus. As an example, in a Swedish study, 59 percent of the patients with cervical esophageal carcinoma were alcohol abusers, while this dropped to 43 percent for carcinomas in the upper thorax, 37 percent in the mid-thorax, and 25 percent in the lower thorax (26). Presumably alcohol is not important in the high-risk population of Iran which is Islamic and therefore has little chronic alcoholism (39).

Tobacco. In the West, tobacco has been implicated as a risk factor, although not with the intensity of alcohol. However, it may also play a role in carcinogenesis in some underdeveloped countries. As an example, in the Transkei of South Africa, the population at risk has a long tradition beginning in adolescence of smoking locally grown tobacco (39). In this population, risk factors for esophageal cancer are smoking and use of traditional medicines, but not consumption of beer. Also, the nitrosamine-rich tobacco juice that accumulates in the pipe stem is swallowed. In the high-risk areas of Iran, opium use is common among the population at risk, and not only is the opium smoked, but the tars in the pipes are often eaten (12). In Kerala, India, tobacco smoking or chewing is one of the most significant risk factors, along with alcohol, but only in men, not women (41). Even in low-risk populations, tobacco sometimes surfaces as the most important risk factor, as it did in a study of esophageal cancer in women in northern Italy (44). Finally, some studies suggest that tobacco and alcohol act synergistically to increase the risk (46).

Dietary Factors. In the high-risk areas, there are dietary characteristics that combine deficiencies of vitamins and minerals with the dominant foodstuffs to produce situations that are potentially conducive for cancer development. Many of these combinations lead to an exaggerated nitrosamine content in the daily diet of the inhabitants of the various localities. This chemical may be the most important carcinogen for squamous cell carcinoma.

Specific Foods. Certain foods, many of which are dietary staples, have been implicated in the etiology of esophageal cancer. A common thread is a diet rich in cereals or grains but poor in fresh fruits and fresh vegetables (39). A study comparing the diet of patients with and without esophageal cancer in northern China found that the cancer patients were more likely to have a diet containing millet gruel, millet soup with noodles, boiled vegetables, moldy foods, and pickled vegetable juice, while soybean consumption was associated with a decreased risk (49). In northern Iran, the diet includes homemade bread, and in Transkei in South Africa, maize is the dietary staple (39). In this region, fermented maize, which is rich in nitrosamines, is the basic ingredient of the local beer. In all of these high-risk areas, the grains are likely to be contaminated by a variety of fungi which produce nitrosamines (12). There are obviously other factors that contribute to the cancers in the high-risk areas since not everyone has cancer. In a case-controlled study from Transkei, those with esophageal cancer ate significantly more of a particular wild vegetable, *Solanum nigrum,* or nightshade than did a cancer-free age- and sex-matched control group (40).

Vitamins and Minerals. Studies from high-risk areas have shown that vitamin deficiencies are more common among high-risk populations: riboflavin deficiency is common in China and Iran, while intake of vitamins A and C is low in northern Iran (31). The results of a double-blind controlled study of a high-risk population in China indicated that there were no differences in the development of squamous dysplasia and carcinoma between one group given a combination of riboflavin, retinol, and zinc and a second group that received placebos. (31) However, the study period was only 13.5 months, which may be far too short to determine the value of such dietary supplements in the inhibition of dysplasia and cancer. However, two recent multi-year prospective randomized interventional studies in high-risk Chinese adults showed some protective effect for several combinations of vitamins and minerals against esophageal squamous cell cancer incidence and mortality, but only the combined effect of beta carotene, vitamin E, and selenium significantly decreased cancer incidence (6a). In Transkei, the soil has low concentrations of zinc and molybdenum, and this may be important in the very high rate of esophageal cancer in that region (39). A study of esophageal cancer patients who were heavy smokers and drinkers in Washington, D.C. indicated that as a group they had significantly lower levels of plasma zinc than did a group of nonalcoholic controls and a nonalcoholic group with non-squamous cell carcinoma (30). They also had lower levels of vitamin A than did two control groups without cancer, one alcoholic and one not. These results suggested that zinc and vitamin A deficiencies may be carcinogenic co-factors for human esophageal squamous cell cancer in this American population.

Water Contaminants. In high-risk parts of northern China, the well water is often contaminated with animal and human wastes, and it contains levels of nitrites that are much higher than in low-risk areas (39).

*Genetic Factors.* In general, esophageal squamous cell carcinoma does not appear to be a familial cancer, although heredity may have some effect. In a Chinese study, there was an increased cancer risk if there was a family history in one high-risk geographic area, but family history was not important in a second high-risk area (49). Perhaps a third of family members with the rare, hereditary, dominantly transmitted condition, tylosis palmaris et plantaris, have esophageal carcinoma, in addition to the abnormal cutaneous keratinization involving the palms, soles, and ventral surfaces of the fingers and toes (28,43). In a study of an American family with the syndrome, the esophageal cancer risk among affected members was at least 90 percent (28).

*Infectious Agents.* Human Papilloma Virus (HPV). Viruses including herpes simplex virus, cytomegalovirus, Ebstein-Barr virus, and HPV have been implicated in human tumorigenesis. Of these, HPV is important in the evolution of several squamous cell or squamous-like carcinomas, especially those arising in the uterine cervix, vulva, vagina, and the anal transitional zone. The most commonly implicated viral types are 16 and 18. It is logical to look for viral material in other squamous cell cancers, and the esophageal tumors are obvious targets.

Table 4-1

**HUMAN PAPILLOMA VIRUS IN ESOPHAGEAL SQUAMOUS CARCINOMAS
AND IN ASSOCIATED LESIONS AND ADJACENT MUCOSAE**

| Country | Ref | Technique | Tumor | Dysplasia | Nontumor | Types |
|---------|-----|-----------|-------|-----------|----------|-------|
| China | 11 | ISH* | 2/51 | 8/36 | 13/36 | 16, 18, 30 |
| China | 12 | ISH | 85/363** | | 23/363[+] | 16, 18 |
| France | 4 | ISH, D-B | 4/12 | | 5/12 | 16, 18 |
| France | 45 | PCR | 1/8 | | | 16 |
| Japan | 45a | PCR | 3/45 | | | 16, 18 |
| Japan | 45 | PCR | 1/4 | | | 16 |
| S Africa[§] | 50 | PCR | 6/13 | | 6/9 | NS[‡] |
| S Africa | 45 | PCR | 3/18 | | | 16 |
| USA | 51 | PCR, ISH | 0/15 | | 0/15 | |
| USA | 45 | PCR | 2/15 | | | 16 |
| Iran | 45 | PCR | 1/8 | | | 18 |
| Italy | 45 | PCR | 2/20 | | | 16 |

*ISH: in situ hybridization; PCR: polymerase chain reaction; D-B = dot-blot.
**No relation between HPV and degree of differentiation. HPV was detected in 7 of 57 nodal metastses.
[+]Includes both hyperplasia and dysplasia.
[‡]NS = not stated.
[§]6 of 41 biopsies from esophagi without carcinoma were also positive for HPV DNA, including 3 of 9 with glycogen acanthosis.

Several techniques have been used to detect different components of the virus. Immunohistochemical staining of tissue using antibodies to viral proteins is the least sensitive. More sensitive is in situ hybridization (ISH) to detect viral DNA. The most sensitive technique uses the polymerase chain reaction (PCR) to detect minute amounts of viral DNA. The frequency of HPV DNA in squamous cancers differs greatly in different studies; but not all studies used the same detection system. Therefore, these differences may reflect either true differences in the prevalence of HPV infection in esophageal cancer patients, differences in sensitivity of the detection systems, or both. Results of most published studies are summarized in Table 4-1. In all studies in which HPV was found, the common types were 16 and 18. In a study using ISH in Linxian, a high-risk part of China, the investigators found HPV DNA in 22 nonmalignant foci adjacent to carcinomas, most of which also had histologic changes of HPV infection, such as koilocytosis, multinucleation, and dyskeratosis so that they commonly resembled flat condylomas (11). When hyperplasias and dysplasias were analyzed separately, HPV DNA was detected in 36 percent of the hyperplasias but only in 22 percent of the dysplasias. In a study 3 years later by the same authors from the same region in China using the same techniques, HPV DNA was found in biopsies from 23.4 percent of 363 cancers but in only 6.3 percent of the adjacent dysplastic or hyperplastic epithelium (13). Why the discrepancies between these two studies occurred was not explained. The same group of investigators studied balloon cytology preparations from patients with previously diagnosed esophageal dysplasia, also from a high-risk Chinese area, also using ISH (10). They found HPV DNA in 53 of 80 cases, with the greatest prevalence in squamous cells that were moderately to severely dysplastic or carcinomatous. Perhaps the cytologic detection system was more sensitive than the system using paraffin sections in the previously described study, and HPV infection may be even more of a factor in squamous carcinogenesis in this population. Using ISH and dot blot techniques, HPV DNA was found in the nontumor mucosa of 5 of 12 squamous cell cancer patients from France (4). Tumor tissue also contained HPV DNA in 4 cases. No viral DNA was found in the esophageal mucosa in 17 control patients matched for age, sex, and alcohol and tobacco consumption. Japanese investigators analyzed 45 biopsies of esophageal squamous cell cancer by PCR and found that 3 contained HPV DNA (45a). This study did not specifically analyze the marginal mucosa, but viral DNA in any mucosa included in the biopsy would have been detected by PCR. In a South African study, HPV DNA was found by PCR in 6 of 13 carcinomas and in adjacent mucosa in 6 of 9 cases (50). Viral DNA was also found in 6 of 41 esophageal biopsies in noncarcinoma patients, 3 of whom had glycogen acanthosis. When 72 squamous cell carcinomas from different parts of the world were analyzed in a single laboratory by PCR, HPV DNA was detected in only 10 (14 percent). There was no difference in prevalence of HPV DNA in the cancers among the various countries that included Italy, France, Japan, Iran, South Africa, and the United States, but the number of cases tested from each country was small (45). Finally, in a study from the United States, no HPV DNA was detected in 15 squamous cell carcinomas or in the adjacent mucosa by both ISH and PCR (51). Thus, HPV is probably an important factor in the evolution of some, but not all, squamous cell cancers in some, but not all, parts of the world. In South Africa, HPV may be a significant factor, with less importance in northern China and some parts of France and minimal importance elsewhere, especially in parts of the world with low risk for squamous cancer. However, the mode of transmission is unknown. Standardized HPV DNA detection system use in future studies may produce more meaningful data about population differences.

*Candida* Infection. The most common fungus infecting the esophagus is *Candida* species, usually *Candida albicans*. In a cytologic study from the high incidence areas of China, the presence of *Candida* correlated with progressive degrees of squamous cell dysplasia, beginning with a 31 percent infection rate among those with normal cells or mild dysplasia to a 72 percent rate among those with severe dysplasia to a 90 percent rate among those with carcinoma (12). However, this association has not been confirmed in other populations.

*Predisposing Conditions.* Esophagitis. In many of the epidemiologic studies of esophageal carcinoma, there is repeated reference to an inflammation of the esophagus that is prevalent in the high-risk populations. This inflammation is referred to simply as "esophagitis" or "chronic esophagitis" with no qualification. It is asymptomatic and not related to gastroesophageal reflux. However, in one study from Sweden, there was a strong association between squamous cell carcinoma of the lower thoracic esophagus, hiatal hernia, and clinical, but not histologic, reflux esophagitis, while there was no such associadion between upper esophageal cancer and reflux (26). The nonreflux type of esophagitis in high-risk populations has been described as the most frequent finding in esophageal biopsies in these regions. This esophagitis has a combination of histologic features, including papillomatosis with papillae of lamina propria extending close to the surface, basal cell hyperplasia, and a mixed inflammatory infiltrate with lymphocytes, plasma cells, and neutrophils (21,48). It may be multifocal, and it is usually in the middle and lower esophagus, where the cancers predominate (15). It also tends to occur in relatively young people in the high-risk areas. In a survey in both low-risk and high-risk areas of China, endoscopic and histologic esophagitis occurred with almost equal frequency in both, but the squamous hyperplasias and dysplasias were far more common in the high-risk area, especially the dysplasias which were almost eight times as common in the high-risk region (21). In another study from a high-risk area in China, histologic esophagitis of this generic type occurred in about 40 percent of people 26 years of age and younger, but the prevalence only increased with age in females over 20 years old; the process did not increase in severity with age (48). In this study, the esophagitis was significantly associated with the consumption of very hot beverages, a family history of esophageal cancer, and a diet low in fresh fruit and dietary staples other than maize. A follow-up of these same patients 30 to 78 months later showed that 34 percent who had histologic dysplasia initially developed invasive cancer, but only 4 percent who did not have dysplasia, but who only had histologic esophagitis, developed invasive cancer (35). Other studies of Chinese patients followed endoscopically for 42 months also showed that 34 percent of patients with dysplasia developed invasive cancer, but only 3 percent of those with esophagitis developed carcinoma (19). In still another study from a high-risk Chinese area, endoscopic biopsies were taken in 754 patients who had a prior cytologic diagnosis of dysplasia based upon screening balloon cytology (18). The follow-up biopsies were taken from endoscopic lesions or blindly from the middle third of the esophagus. No atrophy was found and esophagitis occurred in only 4.6 percent, suggesting that esophagitis was not an important premalignant condition in this high-risk population. Although this asymptomatic, possibly irritant-induced esophagitis may occur in high-risk populations, it is not the direct precursor of squamous cell cancer. Some additional steps or factors must be operative to produce the true precursor, squamous dysplasia, and it is in this area that very little is known.

Achalasia. Achalasia is an idiopathic esophageal motility disease characterized by a nonrelaxing lower esophageal sphincter and a nonperistaltic body. Morphologically, the esophagus has no neurons in the myenteric plexus, but the mechanism for this neuronal destruction is unknown. Because of the functional obstruction at the lower sphincter and the lack of peristalsis, the esophagus does not empty well and dilates, all muscular layers undergo hypertrophy, and it becomes the equivalent of a stagnant loop with ingested material accumulating. The squamous mucosa is commonly acanthotic and inflamed. In this setting, possibly as a result of the stasis, squamous cell dysplasias and carcinomas have been reported. Because both achalasia and the complicating carcinoma are so uncommon, reports of the combination have mainly included single cases, with a very few series. The occurrence of carcinoma among achalasia patients is impossible to determine from the reported series: it was none in one American study (53), 0.9 percent in a second American study, 1.5 percent in a Dutch study (29), 3.5 percent in a third American series (20), 7.2 percent in a Japanese series (20), and 8.6 percent in a French series (20). Some of these were really incidence studies based upon follow-up of achalasia patients for different periods, others were prevalence studies, while still others were combined, based upon cases of cancer found at the beginning of the study mixed with those found during follow-up. Thus, these numbers are based upon different data bases, and are not comparable. In one long-term study of 195

patients with achalasia, 3 developed squamous cell cancer, an incidence of 3.4 cases per 1,000 patients per year (29). The authors of the study calculated the risk to be 33 times the risk for squamous cell carcinoma in the general population. In contrast, in an American study of 1,318 patients with alchalsia followed for an average of 13 years, only 7 developed carcinoma, an incidence of 0.41 per 1,000 patients per year (53). However, that low incidence figure was still about 7 times the rate for the general population. The carcinomas are discovered about 20 years after the onset of symptoms of the achalasia (20).

Since the patients already have an esophageal disease characterized by the same symptom common to most esophageal cancers, namely, dysphagia, beginning carcinomas are impossible to differentiate clinically from achalasia. The symptoms of carcinoma are increasing dysphagia and bleeding; they are usually diagnosed when they are advanced and unlikely to be cured by resection. Morphologically, the associated carcinoma is high stage and typical squamous cell, both grossly and microscopically. There are no clinical markers of high risk, so any surveillance program to detect both the preinvasive dysplasias and the incipient cancers must include esophageal biopsy, probably with cytology, on a regular schedule, although schedules have not been established.

Barrett's Mucosa. Barrett's mucosa is a known precursor of adenocarcinoma, and is a common phenomenon. If for no other reason than the high frequency of Barrett's mucosa, there are likely to be cases of squamous cell carcinoma occurring in the same esophagus as Barrett's mucosa. In fact, several cases of this association have been reported, mainly from three series: one from the United States (36), one from France (33), and one from Sweden (38). In the Swedish and American studies, the squamous cell cancers all arose in the squamous mucosa proximal to the Barrett segments, sometimes with adjacent squamous dysplasia, suggesting that the two diseases had little relationship (36,38). In the French study, two squamous cell cancers arose within the proximal squamous mucosa, while two others arose at the squamocolumnar junction. A fifth carcinoma, which arose within the Barrett's segment, may have been an adenosquamous carcinoma, since it had areas of differentiated adenocarcinoma. In all three studies, there were certain linkages. The squamous cancers in all the American cases arose in white men, much like Barrett's adenocarcinomas. In contrast there is a predominance of usual esophageal squamous cell cancers in black men in the United States. Heavy tobacco use and alcoholic intake are suspected factors linking squamous cell cancer and the Barrett's lesion. In the French study, three tumors arose in men and two in women, and all of the men had a history of alcohol and tobacco use. However, the two women had no such history. In the Swedish study, which used very meticulous sampling of the entire esophagus, Barrett's mucosa was found in the distal esophagus in 13 of 32 consecutive resections for squamous cell carcinoma, an unusually high prevalence for Barrett's mucosa. The reason for this association was not analyzed by the authors. Although squamous metaplasia of the Barrett mucosa, the process known as "pseudoregression," occurs, as of yet, squamous carcinoma has not been reported to occur in this metaplasia. Squamous cell carcinomas may occur in the same esophagi that have Barrett's mucosa, and there may be some shared etiologic factors, such as alcoholic use and smoking.

Plummer-Vincent (Patterson-Kelly) Syndrome. This syndrome, also known as *sideropenic dysphagia,* was described by the four individuals after whom it was named between 1914 and 1922. It is characterized by cervical dysphagia, mostly in postmenopausal women, who may have cervical esophageal webs, iron deficiency anemia, and poor nutrition, probably secondary to impaired oral intake; formerly, this led to cheilosis, glossitis, and nail changes (32). The syndrome occurs mostly in Scandinavia and Great Britain. Close to 10 percent of the patients develop carcinomas of the hypopharynx, mouth, and esophagus, but this may be decreasing, especially in Sweden (43).

Other Diseases. Esophageal squamous cell carcinoma has been reported as a complication of acid and lye burns with resultant strictures (1,43). In one report from Finland, there were 63 such carcinomas complicating lye corrosion injuries among 2,414 patients with esophageal carcinomas admitted to one hospital in a 43-year period. The carcinomas occur after a long latent period, usually 30 years or more, but the latent period may decrease as the age at lye ingestion increases. However, since almost all cases of lye ingestion are during childhood, the age of the patient when the carcinoma develops is still lower than for the usual or common carcinomas. Since lye strictures are most common in the upper thoracic portion of the esophagus behind the tracheal bifurcation, the complicating carcinomas occur there, in contrast to the usual site of squamous cell carcinoma, which is the middle or distal esophagus (1).

*Genetic Alterations.* Very little information has been published about the genetic alterations that occur in the esophageal squamous mucosa prior to the development of dysplasia, during any transitions from low- to high-grade dysplasia, and preceding the first invasive events. The limited literature mostly covers the p53 tumor suppressor gene and *ras* oncogenes, both of which have been implicated in the evolution of a variety of cancers, most notably colonic adenocarcinoma. The data suggest that esophageal squamous cell carcinoma has different genetic changes than do other gastrointestinal cancers. In two Japanese studies, mutations of the p53 gene were found in 4 of 5 cases of invasive squamous cell carcinoma using PCR analysis; p53 gene overexpression suggesting mutations was detected in 17 of 20 carcinomas by immunohistochemistry (24,42). However, not all studies have found equally high frequencies, so there may be geographic differences. For instance, in a study of 34 cases from two high incidence areas, Uruguay and Normandy in France, only 15 cases had p53 point mutations using PCR analysis (22). This is about half the rate of the two Japanese studies. In a study from a high incidence area in China, the p53 mutation rate was about 50 percent, also much lower than the rate in the Japanese studies (5).

The family of *ras* oncogenes, commonly mutated in many cancers including adenocarcinomas of pancreas, colon, lung, and thyroid, have also been analyzed in esophageal squamous cell carcinomas by PCR techniques (8). In contrast to the frequent p53 mutations, no ras oncogene mutations of any type were found in all 16 carcinomas from Uruguay (22), 25 carcinomas from a high-risk area of China (25), and 41 carcinomas from France (23). In the study from France, amplification of the epidermal growth factor receptor gene was detected in 2 of 25 carcinomas using hybridization techniques and in 3 of 12 carcinomas there were higher levels of epidermal growth factor RNA than in the surrounding squamous mucosa (23).

**Experimental Models.** The most spectacular animal model for squamous cell carcinoma of the esophagus is not experimentally induced but naturally occurring. In some of the high-risk areas of China, the chickens and the humans share the same high frequency of esophageal carcinoma (12,39). This suggests that there are some contaminants in either the water or food, or deficiencies in the soil in which food is grown that affect man and chicken.

Experimentally, esophageal squamous cell carcinoma has been induced in several different rodents by nitrosamines. Study results suggest that in these models, benign squamous cell tumors or nontumorous squamous dysplasias precede the carcinomas, and the transformation from benign to malignant may involve activation of an oncogene.

Methyl-n-amylnitrosamine injected intraperitoneally into Wistar rats induces squamous papillomas in almost all animals and squamous carcinomas in over half, depending upon the dose. This suggests that both benign and malignant squamous tumors can have the same stimulus, and it further suggests that benign tumors may be precursors of malignant ones, although detailed histologic descriptions of the papillomas and the carcinomas were not given (9). Mice fed a diethylated nitrosamine in drinking water had the whole gamut of dysplasias through in situ to invasive carcinoma, but the author could not determine if the invasive carcinomas arose in papillomas or in flat dysplasias (37). Activation of H-*ras* oncogene occurred in two thirds of squamous papillomas induced in rats by another nitrosamine (3).

In another study, the tumorigenic effects in rats of a related nitrosamine, N-nitroso-methyl-benzylamine, were reduced by half by the simultaneous oral administration of a protease inhibitor derived from soybeans (47). This inhibitor may work by reducing the number of chromosomal abnormalities that occur during carcinogenesis. The protease appears to decrease the incidence not only of carcinomas, but of squamous hyperplasias, papillomas, and dysplasias; this suggests that it exerts its effects very early in the precursor-carcinoma sequence.

In an important study in primates, 1-methyl-1-nitrosourea was fed to monkeys daily, beginning one week after birth (16). The whole spectrum of dysplasias, carcinomas in situ, invasive carcinomas, and squamous papillomas occurred, but they were not dose dependent. Peculiarly, in this model, males were much more susceptible than females, and, in addition, cancers of the entire upper aerodigestive tract occurred. Both of these features indicate that the primate experimental model is remarkably similar to spontaneously occurring human disease.

**Clinical Features.** Patients with esophageal squamous cell carcinoma are usually men, whether the population is at high or low risk. However, the male to female ratio varies somewhat and tends to be lower in high-risk areas. Overall, this ratio is about 3 or 4 to 1. Although most patients are in their sixth and seventh decades of life when the tumors become symptomatic, many are diagnosed in their eighth decade. The most common presenting symptom is dysphagia, beginning with solid foods and then progressing to liquids. The duration of symptoms prior to diagnosis is often a few months. Concurrently with the dysphagia, there is weight loss, far in excess of that which might be attributable to the difficulty in swallowing. A small group of patients with significant hypercalcemia have been reported both from Japan and the United States (122,127). This is probably due to a parathyroid hormone–related protein produced by the tumors (127). As many as 10 percent of patients with esophageal squamous cell carcinoma have synchronous or metachronous squamous cell carcinomas in upper aerodigestive sites, such as lip, tongue, mouth, tonsil, and larynx. (67). These may occur before, at the same time as, or after the esophageal tumor is discovered. In a few cases, especially in those few patients who survive for several years, second primary carcinomas of the esophagus may occur.

## SQUAMOUS EPITHELIAL DYSPLASIA INCLUDING SQUAMOUS CELL CARCINOMA IN SITU

Invasive esophageal squamous cell carcinoma evolves through a series of preinvasive lesions, known as dysplasias or intraepithelial neoplasias, although the esophagus has its own unique types which may differ from those occurring in other squamous sites, such as cervix and skin. In studies from China, these precursor lesions

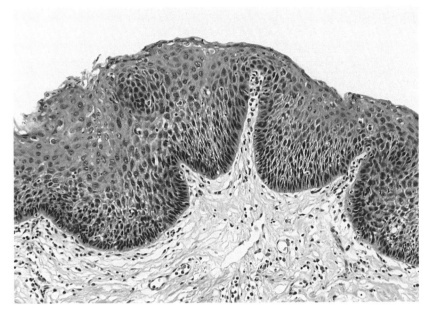

Figures 4-1
SQUAMOUS INTRAEPITHELIAL
NEOPLASIA/DYSPLASIA
Figures 4-1 to 4-4 show increasing epithelial disorganization with progressive loss of maturation and involvement of the surface, accompanied by progressive loss of orientation, pleomorphism and cell crowding. This figure has obvious squamous differentiation in the upper half.

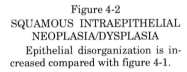

Figure 4-2
SQUAMOUS INTRAEPITHELIAL
NEOPLASIA/DYSPLASIA
Epithelial disorganization is increased compared with figure 4-1.

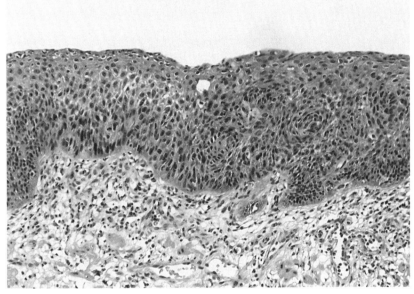

were about eight times more common in high cancer-risk areas than in the low-risk areas (111); also there is an increased proliferation of cells in the upper layers of the esophageal squamous epithelium in people who live in these areas (99). The preinvasive lesions, or dysplasias, contain abnormal epithelia which vary from that closely caricaturing the normal squamous mucosa to epithelium so disorganized that its malignant cytologic and architectural features are obvious.

In the 1990 monograph on esophageal and gastric tumors from the World Health Organization (WHO), the term dysplasia includes most precancerous lesions; it includes both architectural and cytologic abnormalities, and also involves aberrant differentiation. The nuclei are larger and more hyperchromatic than normal, and there is increased mitotic activity (135). The lower grades of dysplasia have a larger component of mature-appearing squamous cells, some of which may be keratinized, and the abnormal

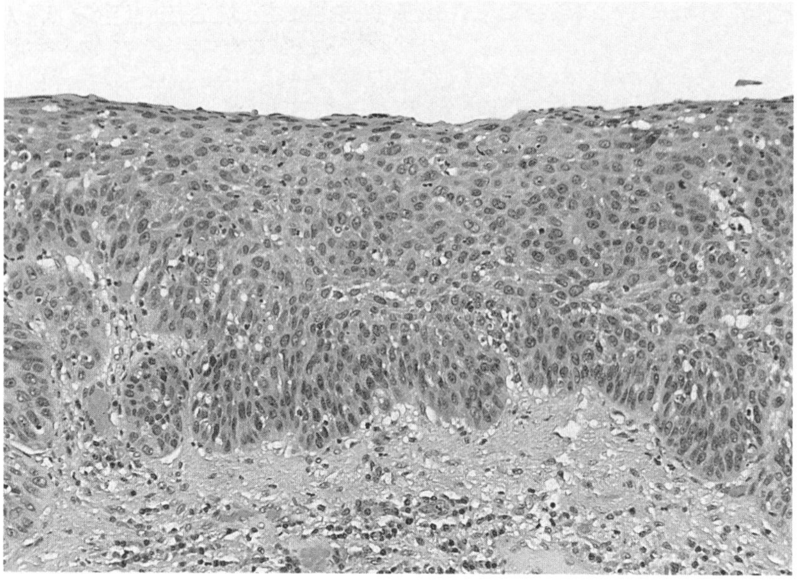

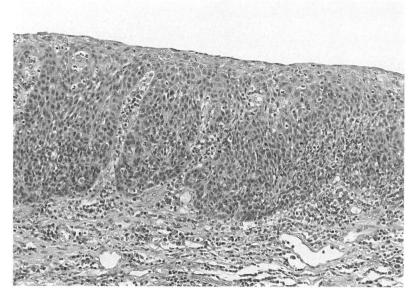

Figure 4-3
SQUAMOUS INTRAEPITHELIAL
NEOPLASIA/DYSPLASIA
Further increased epithelial disorganization.

Figure 4-4
SQUAMOUS INTRAEPITHELIAL
NEOPLASIA/DYSPLASIA
There is little squamous maturation
in this epithelium.

cells are often limited to the lower half of the epithelium (figs. 4-1–4-4). The highest grade of dysplasia is squamous cell carcinoma in situ or intraepithelial carcinoma. In this proliferation, the epithelial cells have the cytologic features of invasive carcinoma cells, and the epithelium is disorganized in ways which resemble invasive carcinoma nests (fig. 4-4). Most dysplasias and in situ carcinomas occur in either normally thick or hyperplastic epithelium; however, there are unusual cases in which the epithelium is thinner than normal or atrophic. In situ carcinoma is usually described as a full-thickness abnormality and the neoplastic cells are present throughout the epithelium (91). However, there is at least one type of dysplasia and in situ carcinoma in which the abnormal cells are confined to the basal half or two thirds of the epithelium (figs. 4-5–4-8) (68). In rare cases, the normal basal layer may be partially preserved with the neoplastic squamous cells situated above it, thus imparting a pagetoid appearance to the lesion (fig. 4-9). Although lower grades of dysplasia are usually described as partial-thickness abnormalities, involving less than

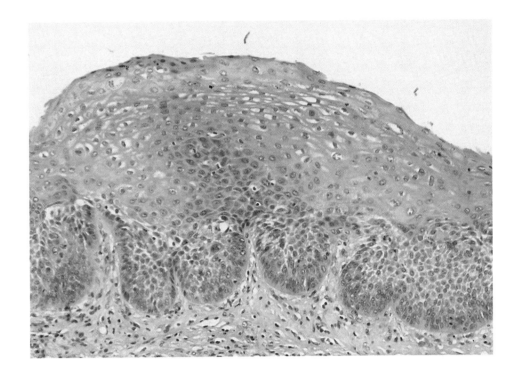

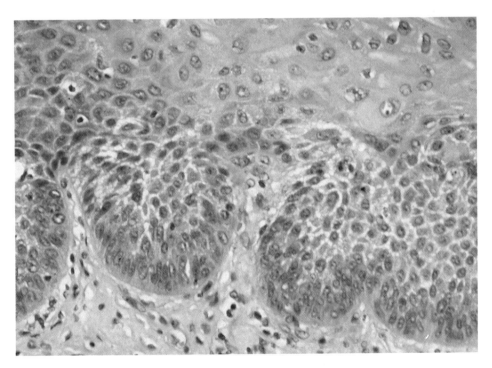

Figure 4-5
BASAL SQUAMOUS DYSPLASIA
Low (top) and high (bottom) magnification views of basal epithelium. The basal half of this epithelium is composed of tightly packed, small dysplastic basaloid cells, while the upper half has clear-cut squamous differentiation.

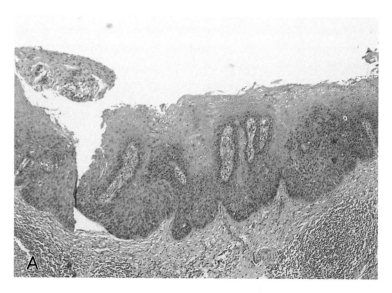

Figure 4-6
BASAL SQUAMOUS DYSPLASIA
Low (A), medium (B), and high (C) magnification views of the basal epithelium. The basal two thirds of this epithelium is composed of primitive cells, while the upper third has differentiated stratified squamous cells.

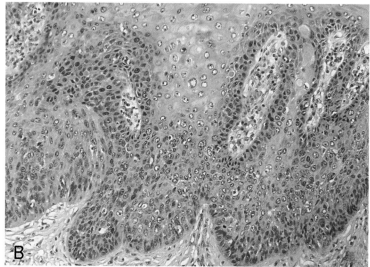

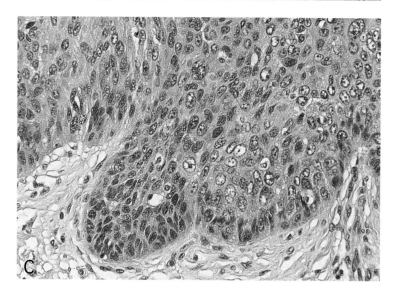

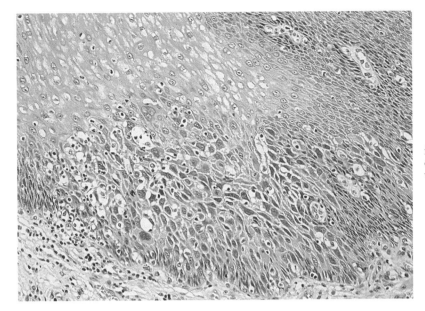

Figure 4-7
INTERMEDIATE
GRADE DYSPLASIA
Intermediate grade dysplasia involving the basal half of the epithelium. The cells at the base are pleomorphic with variably enlarged, hyperchromatic nuclei.

Figure 4-8
INTERMEDIATE
GRADE DYSPLASIA
Intermediate grade dysplasia with cellular crowding and nuclear pleomorphism involving the basal two thirds of the epithelium. In rare cases, the normal basal layer may be partially preserved, with the neoplastic squamous cells situated above it, thus imparting a pagetoid appearance to the lesion (see figure 4-9).

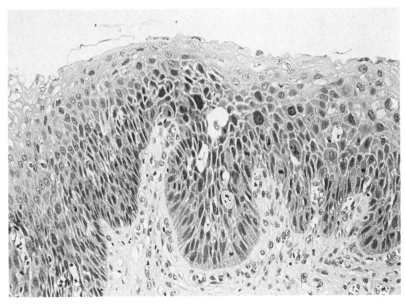

half of the epithelial thickness and higher grades as involving more than half, separating grades of dysplasia on the basis of level of involvement is not always reliable (91). Also, separating one grade of dysplasia from another is frequently difficult, since there are no clear lines of demarcation. As a result, even with a two-grade system that includes low and high grades, there are occasional dysplasias that seem to be borderline or intermediate between the two grades. In the future, all intraepithelial proliferations might be grouped into a spectrum that could be designated esophageal intraepithelial neoplasia (EIN), comparable to the terms in use for the uterine cervix, the vagina, and the vulva, or into a two-grade dysplasia system comparable to that used in ulcerative colitis. In such systems, high-grade dysplasia and in situ carcinoma are incorporated within the same group.

The dysplastic and in situ foci are variable in size and are not always found at the margins of invasive carcinomas. However, in one French study of nonirradiated carcinomas, in situ carcinoma and lower grades of squamous dysplasia

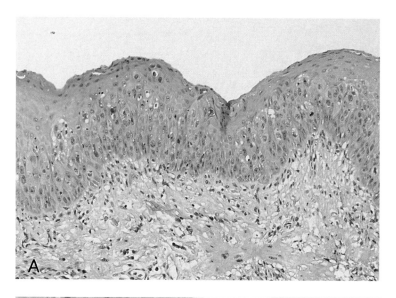

Figure 4-9
PAGETOID HIGH-GRADE
SQUAMOUS CELL DYSPLASIA

A: The dysplastic cells fill the middle of the epithelium, with a relatively intact basal layer below and normal epithelium above.

B: Higher magnification view.

C: Another example of squamous cell dysplasia with a pagetoid appearance.

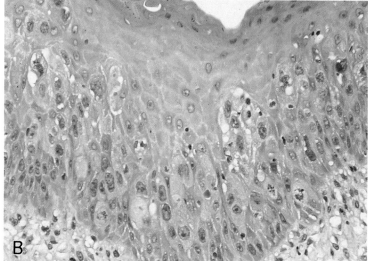

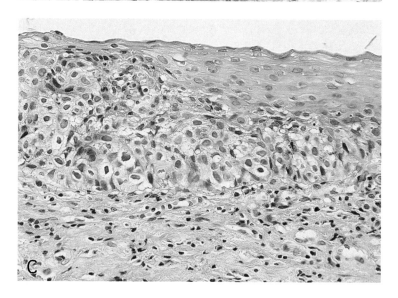

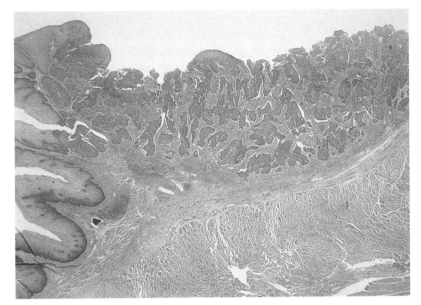

Figure 4-10
SUPERFICIAL SQUAMOUS
CELL CARCINOMA
The deepest invasion is in the middle of the submucosa. There is a thin layer of submucosa between the carcinoma and the muscularis propria.

were found adjacent to the invasive tumors in about two thirds of the cases (91). Intraepithelial carcinoma may involve the ducts of the submucosal glands as they penetrate into the mucosa, and it can even extend into the glands proper (131). There are no published data concerning whether lower grade dysplasias can also involve the ducts and glands or whether this phenomenon is limited to carcinomatous epithelium.

Unfortunately, not all studies of esophageal squamous cell dysplasia have used the same morphologic criteria. Low-grade dysplasia in one study may be interpreted as hyperplasia in another. Some investigators do not consider in situ carcinoma to be part of the dysplasia spectrum (100). Furthermore, in some studies cytologic and architectural changes are not evaluated; other studies are biopsy or resection based and include both cytologic and architectural changes. These issues are discussed in more detail in the section on diagnosis.

In esophagi with invasive carcinomas, the amount of dysplastic epithelium of all grades, including in situ carcinoma, and its proximity to the invasive carcinoma are unpredictable. However, dysplastic epithelium is more likely to be found when the cancer is low stage and small (83). One uncommon variant of in situ carcinoma has been described as "superficial spreading," and is defined as in situ change extending a minimum of 2 cm from the invasive lesion (119).

Peculiarly, when this extensive in situ lesion occurs, the invasive carcinoma, even when no deeper than the submucosa, has an unusually high rate of nodal metastasis.

A study from Linxian, China, an area with one of the highest rates of squamous cell carcinoma, attempted to determine if there were endoscopic lesions that correlated with dysplasias and early carcinomas (62). The results indicated that moderate or higher grade dysplasias and early cancers had endoscopic changes of friability, focal red areas, erosions, plaques, and nodules in over 80 percent of the cases. Low-grade dysplasias showed similar endoscopic features about half the time. Biopsying only such areas would have uncovered moderate and high grades of dysplasia and early cancers in almost all cases, suggesting that random sampling of normal mucosa is unnecessary in surveillance programs in this high-risk area.

**Multicentricity.** There are conflicting data about the frequency of multicentricity in esophageal squamous cancer, probably related to geographic variability and to the fastidiousness with which the studies were done, that is, whether detailed sampling of the entire esophageal mucosa was undertaken or whether random samples were used. In one analysis of 11 patients with superficial and in situ cancers from Japan, 4 patients had more than one cancer: 2 had 2 cancers, 1 had 3, and 1 had 4 (95). In another Japanese study, second carcinomas occurred in about one fourth of cases, and this was more likely if there was intraepithelial carcinoma at the margin of the main tumor (86). In a third Japanese study, multifocal dysplasias occurred in about a third of esophagi resected for carcinoma (102). In a French study, separate foci of in situ carcinoma were found in 14 percent of esophagectomy specimens that contained invasive carcinomas, and patches of lower grade dysplasias were found in over 20 percent (91).

## SUPERFICIAL SQUAMOUS CELL CARCINOMA

**Definition.** Any carcinoma of the esophagus that extends no deeper than the submucosa is referred to as a *superficial esophageal carcinoma* in most publications from Western countries (fig. 4-10). This designation is used whether or not there are lymph node metastases. Superficial esophageal carcinoma is stage I or IIB in the TNM system. In some studies, in situ or intraepithelial carcinomas are included within the superficial category, while in other studies, only invasive lesions are included. In terms of depth of invasion, superficial carcinoma is the esophageal equivalent of *early gastric cancer*, a designation that also is used regardless of nodal status. In China and Japan, the term *early esophageal carcinoma* is often used for a carcinoma that invades no deeper than the submucosa but that has not metastasized, in other words, a superficial cancer without nodal metastases (87,95). In this discussion, superficial esophageal carcinoma is defined as invasive carcinoma extending no deeper than the submucosa, regardless of node status. Since prognosis is to a great extent determined by depth of invasion of a squamous cell cancer of the esophagus, as is the risk of nodal metastasis, superficial carcinomas have a better prognosis and fewer positive nodes than more deeply invasive tumors.

Table 4-2 lists the results of several studies of superficial carcinomas from different parts of the world. Except for one large series from France, an area of relatively high risk for esophageal squamous cell carcinoma, most of the published data on superficial carcinoma come from Japan. There is only one small series from the United States (118). As is true for early gastric carcinoma, the frequency of detecting superficial esophageal cancer depends upon having a surveillance program for cancer prevention or early detection. In several studies from Japan, superficial carcinomas accounted for 10 to 20 percent of all resected carcinomas (79,133,138). In a French study, there were 72 superficial cancers in a total of 341 resected cancers, or 21 percent (58). There are also changes in incidence over time. In a huge study from Japan, between 1965 and 1969, superficial carcinomas accounted only for 3 percent of 305 resected carcinomas. This gradually increased so that between 1985 and 1989, the rate rose to 23 percent of 530 resected tumors (125). In a report from a large metropolitan center, Memphis, Tennessee, in the United States, there were no superficial carcinomas among 43 carcinomas resected between 1975 and 1980, but there were 7 (13 percent) among 54 resected carcinomas between 1981 and 1984 (118). These differences in temporal and geographic distribution may reflect more rigorous endoscopic screening, the use of iodine staining for minimally suspicious endoscopic lesions, and more fastidious biopsy sampling in high frequency areas. Preoperative chemotherapy and radiation therapy for biopsy-proven squamous cell carcinoma often destroys most of the invasive component. Tumors, including superficial cancers, so treated can not be staged accurately, and the prevalence of superficial carcinomas may be underestimated in the future.

**Clinical Features.** Since superficial and advanced carcinomas are simply different stages of the same disease, the clinical features are similar. The age and sex distributions for superficial carcinoma are comparable to those for advanced cancer, with a male predominance of 10 to 1 in some studies, and a mean age in the seventh decade (58,79,138). There are no differences in risk factors. Dysphagia is the main symptom of superficial carcinoma as it is for more advanced carcinomas, although there are more asymptomatic patients, up to 40 or 50 percent in some series, since many of the tumors are so small (79, 138). Tumor location within the esophagus is also identical to that of advanced disease.

**Gross Findings.** Although all superficial carcinomas are small, measuring a few centimeters at most, several gross patterns have been defined. In a Chinese study, there were four gross patterns: the occult type, the least common, is an

Table 4-2

## SUPERFICIAL SQUAMOUS CELL CARCINOMA

| Reference | Country | Years Included | Superf/* Total | Mean Age (years) | Depth/Nodal Metastases LP-MM | Submucosa |
|---|---|---|---|---|---|---|
| 58** | France | 1979-87 | 72/341 (22%) | 56 | 19/1 (5%) | 53/16 (30%) |
| 138 | Japan | 1975-89 | 56/395 (15%) | 62 | 15/0 (0%) | 38/18 (47%) |
| 70 | Japan | 1981-91‡ | 42/NS | NS | 12/1 (8%) | 30/15 (50%) |
| 79+ | Japan | 1968-88 | 92/1006 (9%) | NS | 24/1 (4%) | 68/24 (35%) |
| 133 | Japan | 1979-89‡ | 39/199 (20%) | 66 | 11/0 (0%) | 28/8 (29%) |
| 125 | Japan | 1965-89§ | 233/2130 (11%) | 60 | 36/3 (8%) | 197/64 (32%) |
| | | 1965-69 | 8/305 (3%) | | | |
| | | 1970-74 | 17/373 (5%) | | | |
| | | 1975-79 | 31/403 (8%) | | | |
| | | 1980-84 | 65/519 (13%) | | | |
| | | 1985-89 | 122/530 (23%) | | | |
| 65 | Japan | NS | 109/NS | | 14/2 (14%) | 95/42 (44%) |
| 118 | USA | 1981-84 | 7/54 (13%) | 60 | 1/0 ( 0%) | 6/2 (33%) |

*Superf/total = number of superficial carcinomas and the total number of carcinomas of all depths of invasion that were resected; LP-MM = number of carcinomas that invade only the lamina propria and muscularis mucosae; NS = not stated.
**This study included 5 adenoid cystic and 6 pseudosarcomatous carcinomas.
+This study included all histologic types of superficial cancer, 76% of which were squamous.
‡The authors of these studies evaluated all cases resected in the "previous 10 years," but they did not specify the dates. The dates given above are estimates based upon the dates the manuscripts were accepted for publication.
§This study is broken down into 5-year increments.

intraepithelial lesion and may appear as nothing more than a slightly congested focus in a fresh specimen; the erosive type is a sharply marginated, irregularly shaped, depressed, finely granular area (figs 4-11–4-13); the papillary type is a small polyp; and the plaque type, the most common, is an elevated, granular, often superficially eroded macule (87). Most carcinomas that invade the submucosa are plaques. In a French study of 76 cases, five gross appearances were defined: the normal flat type, comparable to the occult type in the Chinese classification, is so subtle that it only is detected by negative staining with Lugol's iodine; the coarse type, comparable to the Chinese erosive and plaque types, has red, slightly raised or depressed mucosa; the verrucous type is either a plateau-like lesion with an irregular surface or a convoluted lesion with nodules and depressions; the polypoid type is an elevated mass, comparable to the papillary type in the Chinese system; and the ulcerating infiltrating type, with no Chinese counterpart, is a mixture of fungating, infiltrating and ulcerating patterns common to advanced cancer (58). A third macroscopic classification from Japan has three primary types: protruded, flat, and excavated; the flat type is further divided into five subtypes: slightly elevated, flat, slightly depressed, mixed, and extended (138).

There is some correlation between the gross and microscopic changes. Both exophytic and ulcerating gross patterns, regardless of the names, usually indicate that the submucosa has been invaded (58,138). The flat pattern usually is a tumor confined to the mucosa.

Perhaps the most useful system is that proposed by Japanese investigators in which superficial esophageal carcinoma is classified endoscopically, like early gastric cancer, into polypoid, plateau-like, flat (with three subtypes), erosive, ulcerative, and mixed types (65). The utility of this system is that these endoscopic classes are comparable to those in the gross classification.

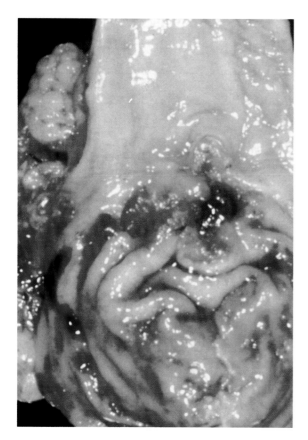

Figure 4-11
SUPERFICIAL CARCINOMA
OF THE DISTAL ESOPHAGUS
This appears as a small ulcer or depression covered by a
blood clot. Depending upon the gross classification scheme,
this is either the erosive type, the coarse type, or the excavated type. (See text for classification details.)

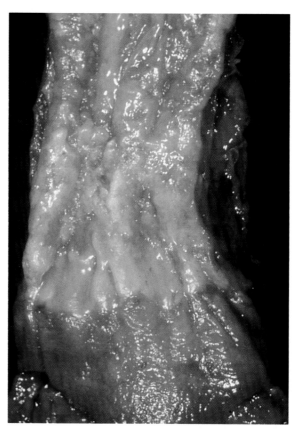

Figure 4-12
SUPERFICIAL CARCINOMA
In this plaque-like gross appearance the carcinoma forms
an irregular, slightly elevated lesion, covering most of the
field. This is classified as plaque type, coarse type, or the
slightly elevated flat type, depending upon the classification
scheme used.

However, perhaps 20 percent of what seem to be
superficial cancers by endoscopic exam actually
have invaded into the muscularis propria when
viewed histologically (55).

**Microscopic Findings.** These small tumors
may be multicentric, and they are likely to be next
to foci of dysplasia of any grade (55). Carcinoma
invading the lamina propria, that is, intramucosal
carcinoma, is characterized by small nests of carcinoma cells, or even single carcinoma cells which
have broken through the basement membrane of
the intraepithelial component (fig. 4-14). One helpful histologic hint is that the invasive focus may
have larger, more squamous-appearing cells, even
with keratinization, while the surface component
may be more basaloid and nonkeratinizing. This
histologic diagnosis is often difficult to make with

confidence. First, intraepithelial carcinoma that
extends along the ducts of submucosal glands
may mimic invasion, much like the comparable
situation in the uterine cervix where intraepithelial carcinoma often extends into the
endocervical crypts. Second, tiny foci of invasion
into the lamina propria may be difficult to detect.
Third, if the intraepithelial lesion is papillary or
undulating, less than perfectly perpendicular
microscopic sections may catch numerous islands of carcinoma which are really at the base
of the squamous surface between the projections.

Some carcinomas have been described as
"basaloid" and are characterized by small cells
with little keratinization and an expansile pattern of growth resembling the nodular patterns
of cutaneous basal cell carcinoma (133). In one

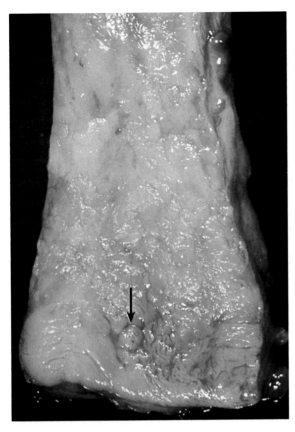

Figure 4-13
SUPERFICIAL CARCINOMA
The bulk of this lesion is a plaque, but at the base, there is a small polyp (arrow). That polyp fits the description of the papillary type, the polypoid type, and the protruded type, depending on the classification.

study from Japan, this pattern was seen only in superficial carcinomas, and when it was pure, that is, not mixed with another pattern, it was associated with 100 percent survival in 14 patients, some of whom were followed for as long as 84 months (133). However, basaloid carcinomas, also known as basaloid squamous cell carcinomas, do not seem to be so superficial and so innocuous in most studies. These are discussed in detail toward the end of this chapter.

**Metastasis and Prognosis.** Superficial carcinoma is a potentially curable disease, which is rarely the case in advanced carcinoma. In one report from China of nonmetastatic superficial and in situ carcinomas together, survival following resection alone was 86 percent at 5 years and 56 percent at 10 years; most of the deaths were not due to the tumor (71).

As can be seen from Table 4-2, about 5 percent of superficial carcinomas that have invaded no deeper than the lamina propria metastasize. This metastatic rate is much higher than that for gastric cancers confined to the mucosa (70). When the esophageal carcinoma invades into the submucosa, the risk of nodal metastasis jumps dramatically to about 35 percent, a risk three times that of gastric cancer of similar depth. Therefore, superficial esophageal cancer extending into the submucosa is, in fact, an advanced lesion (125). In a Japanese study, there was a 5-year survival rate for patients with carcinomas confined to the mucosa of 88 percent, including in situ carcinomas, regardless of node status, but it was only 55 percent for those with carcinomas reaching the submucosa (125). Furthermore, as is expected, the risk of metastasis increases as the carcinoma extends deeper into the submucosa, leading to decreased survival. In a Japanese study, the 5-year survival for those with superficial cancer without nodal metastses was 62 percent; this dropped to 17 percent when nodes were involved (65).

Survival and metastasis also may be related to the amount or bulk of invasive carcinoma in the submucosa, which is a manifestation of size, although it is not clear whether size is independent of depth (101). In one study, none of 5 superficial cancers 1 cm or less in diameter metastasized, 8 of 27 cancers between 1.1 and 2 cm metastasized, and 36 of 81 cancers larger than 2 cm metastasized (65).

Outcome for patients with submucosal carcinoma may also be related to DNA content, at least as defined by histograms using image analysis. In one Japanese study of 30 carcinomas that had invaded into the submucosa, there was an increasing risk of nodal metastasis, postoperative tumor recurrence, and death from tumors with increasing DNA abnormalities (124). Of the 9 patients with multiple DNA peaks on their histograms, the most abnormal histogram pattern, 6 had nodal metastases, 5 developed recurrences, and 5 died from the tumor.

Cure rates are higher if adjuvant cancer therapy is used in addition to resection. However, since these modalities often destroy most or even all of the primary lesion, it is difficult to stage these lesions accurately. Superficial carcinomas extending deeply into the submucosa may be impossible to distinguish from advanced cancers that have

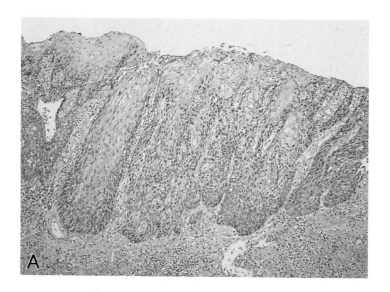

Figure 4-14
SQUAMOUS CELL CARCINOMA
WITH POSSIBLE
INCIPIENT INVASION AT THE BASE

A: The long prongs of dysplastic epithelium extend deeply into the lamina propria, but only at the base of the epithelium. In the center there is invasion with irregularity of the basal epithelium and separation of small clusters of cells from the main prongs. Serial sections might be necessary to ensure that these nests are truly separated from the basal epithelium.

B: High magnification view.

C: Another case with clusters of dysplastic squamous cells in the superficial lamina propria that seem detached from the surface dysplasia, yet with no change in the stroma to assist in determining if this is true invasion.

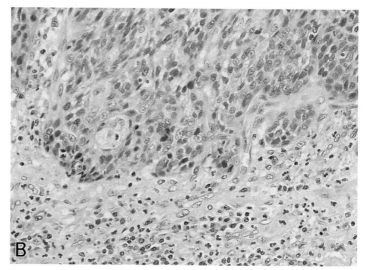

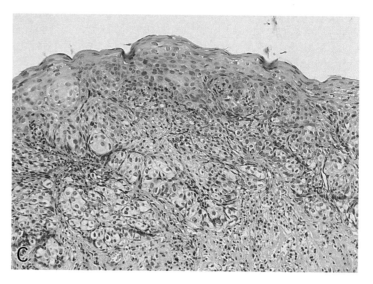

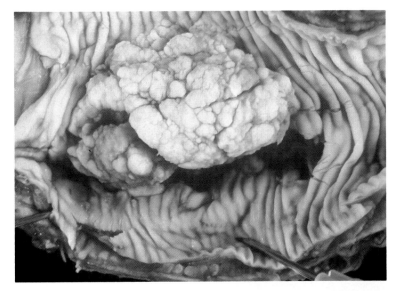

Figure 4-15
EXOPHYTIC OR
FUNGATING CARCINOMA
The lesion is in the middle third of the esophagus. (Courtesy of Dr. William Blamey, Oakland County, MI.)

Figure 4-16
FUNGATING CARCINOMA
Fungating carcinoma in the upper esophagus, immediately below and behind the larynx.

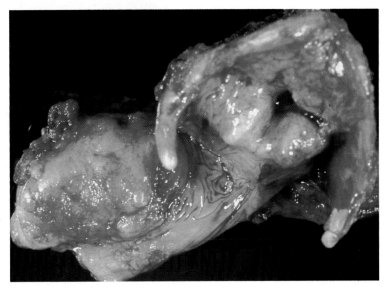

invaded the inner muscularis propria. In such cases, it is difficult to know whether the therapy was directed against a superficial or an advanced carcinoma. At the moment, there are no data from large series evaluating the effect of adjuvant therapy on survival of patients with superficial carcinomas.

## DEEPLY INVASIVE
## SQUAMOUS CELL CARCINOMA

**Gross Findings.** In almost all areas of the world, the carcinomas are located predominantly in the middle and lower portions of the thoracic esophagus, with the middle usually the more common site (94). In almost all series, the upper esophagus is the site of origin of less than 20 percent, and often less than 10 percent of tumors, although in a few parts of the world almost 40 percent occur there.

There are several classifications for the gross appearance of advanced, large esophageal squamous cell cancers. One system has three major patterns: fungating, ulcerative, and infiltrating (figs. 4-15–4-22) (94). The fungating pattern, said to be the most common, has a dominant exophytic or intraluminal growth. In the ulcerative pattern, the growth of the tumor is mainly intramural,

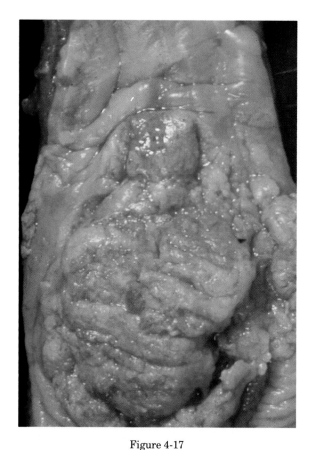

Figure 4-17
EXOPHYTIC CARCINOMA
This exophytic carcinoma forms a broad sessile plaque in the lower third of the esophagus.

with an ulcer in the center, surrounded by tumor-filled, slightly protuberant edges. The infiltrative form, the least common, has a large amount of intramural tumor with, at most, only a minor mucosal defect; it is likely to produce a stricture. There may be mixtures of these primary patterns as well. Large, advanced cancers usually involve long segments of the esophagus.

In a Chinese classification system, the large tumors are split into five types: medullary, fungating, ulcerative, scirrhous (stenosing), and intraluminal (polypoid) (87). The fungating, ulcerative, and scirrhous types correspond to the three types mentioned above. The medullary type, the most common by far in several Chinese studies, is a transmural, circumferential, centrally ulcerated tumor which intensely thickens the wall. It seems to be a combination of the ulcerative and infiltrating patterns, but is more advanced. The intraluminal or polypoid type is described as a round to oval mass which protrudes into the lumen, sort of a mix of fungating and infiltrative types. Small, low-stage tumors may appear as plaques, some with superficial erosions.

Many invasive esophageal carcinomas are treated with preoperative irradiation or chemotherapy, which severely distorts the gross appearance, and often destroys the tumor completely or almost completely. As such modalities are used more routinely, the standard gross description and classification are likely to become meaningless.

Figure 4-18
SMALL ULCERATING
CARCINOMA
This carcinoma is in the middle third of the esophagus.

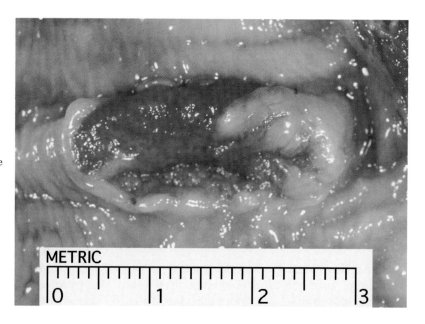

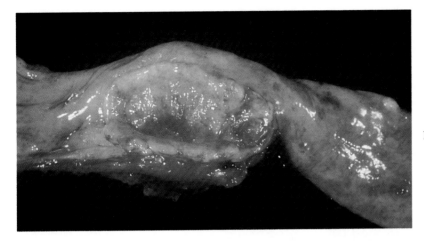

Figure 4-19
ULCERATING CARCINOMA
Prominent edges are seen in this large ulcerating carcinoma.

Figure 4-20
ULCERATING CARCINOMA
Huge ulcerating carcinoma with necrotic, hemorrhagic, nodular base and piled-up edges.

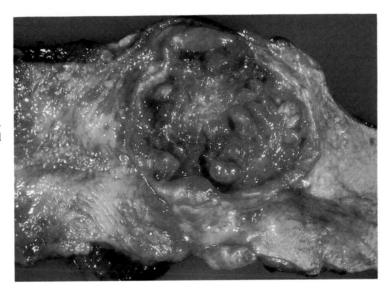

**Microscopic Findings.** *Intramural Spread.* Beginning from the in situ focus, squamous cell carcinoma invades the lamina propria, and as long as it is confined to that layer, it is an intramucosal carcinoma. The invasion commonly takes the form of elongation of rete-like projections which push into the lamina propria, sometimes budding and eventually breaking free of the surface (fig. 4-14). In general, there is very little, if any, accompanying desmoplasia. The neoplasm then penetrates the muscularis mucosae and enters the submucosa, where it pushes deeply and expands circumferentially, thereby undermining mucosa at its periphery (figs. 4-23, 4-24). This is quite a different growth pattern when compared to colorectal carcinoma which

invades deeply but rarely grows peripherally. This submucosal component may have a desmoplastic stroma, but that is unpredictable. As long as the esophageal carcinoma is confined to the mucosa and submucosa, it is designated as "superficial carcinoma." More will be said about superficial carcinoma in the discussion of staging. It also appears that in situ carcinoma can invade along submucosal gland ducts, so that it is possible for there to be a focus of submucosal invasion with no invasion of the mucosa (figs. 4-25, 4-26) (131).

The carcinoma commonly invades submucosal and lamina propria lymphatics, and this can lead to intralymphatic carcinomatous emboli, some of which may be found several centimeters beyond the gross tumor (fig. 4-27) (103). In two recent

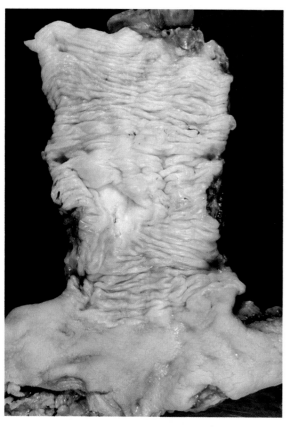

Figure 4-21
INFILTRATIVE PATTERN
The infiltrative pattern is characterized by an elevated plaque that obliterates the folds and thickens the wall.

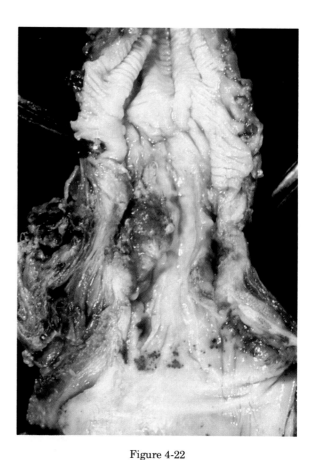

Figure 4-22
INFILTRATIVE PATTERN
A large tumor with a predominantly infiltrative pattern has produced a carcinomatous stricture. The surface has ulcerated foci and nodular areas, so that this tumor actually has features of all three primary gross types, although the infiltrative pattern dominates.

Figure 4-23
SUBEPITHELIAL INVASION
Subepithelial invasion by carcinoma that has filled the lamina propria. The site of origin was to the right of this field, about three high-power fields away.

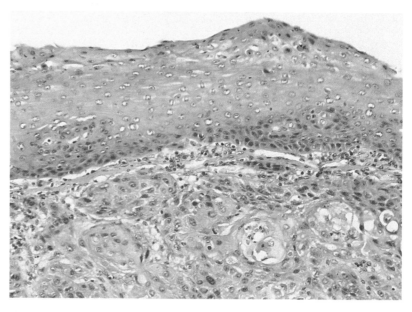

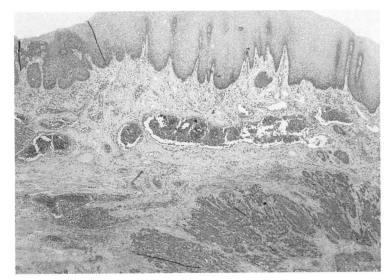

Figure 4-24
SQUAMOUS CELL CARCINOMA
Squamous cell carcinoma invades the submucosa on the right, undermining normal mucosa and muscularis mucosae. At the left, there is a small focus of in situ carcinoma. The dilated veins in the superficial submucosa are stuffed with carcinomatous thromboemboli.

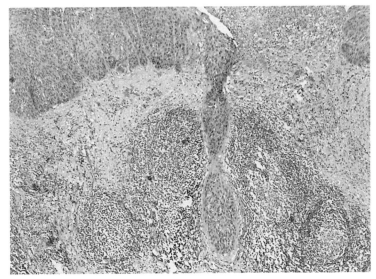

Figure 4-25
IN SITU CARCINOMA
In situ carcinoma involving a submucosal gland duct from its opening onto the in situ lesion on the surface to its origin in the submucosa. Invasion occasionally begins here.

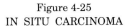

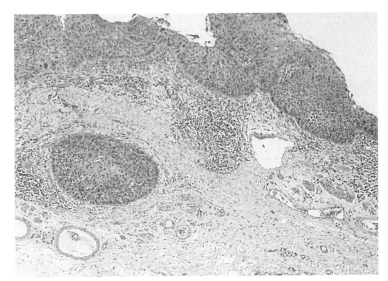

Figure 4-26
IN SITU CARCINOMA
In the submucosa below a carcinoma that only invades into the lamina propria, there is in situ carcinoma that distends a submucosal gland duct, seen here in cross section.

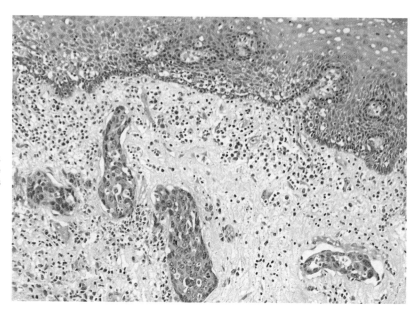

Figure 4-27
INTRAMUCOSAL
CARCINOMATOUS EMBOLI
In the lamina propria beneath a surface epithelium with low-grade basal dysplasia, there are numerous lymphatics filled with carcinoma.

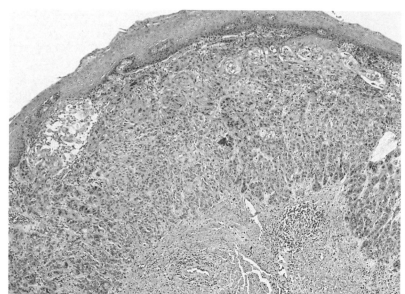

Figure 4-28
INTRAMURAL METASTASES
Secondary foci (intramural metastases) of carcinoma are seen beneath intact squamous mucosa. These probably developed from intramural lymphatic spread, such as occurred in figure 4-27.

studies from Japan, the authors described the phenomenon of intramural metastases, in which submucosal masses of carcinoma separated from the main mass; these were found in about 15 percent of the cases of invasive carcinoma, especially those carcinomas that invaded the adventitia (fig. 4-28) (78,130). Presumably these metastases result from intramural lymphatic spread with the establishment of secondary intramural tumor deposits. In these Japanese studies, over three quarters of the metastases were found either preoperatively or by examination of the gross resected esophagus. Patients with intramural metastases had more mediastinal lymph node and liver metastases, a shorter survival, and significantly larger primary tumors. Although this seems to be a common aberration among this Japanese population, it is virtually never mentioned in other detailed analyses of esophageal squamous cell cancer. In our experience, small microscopic intramural metastases occur, and sometimes they invade the base of the mucosa. However, they are rarely large enough to be detected grossly. Intramural

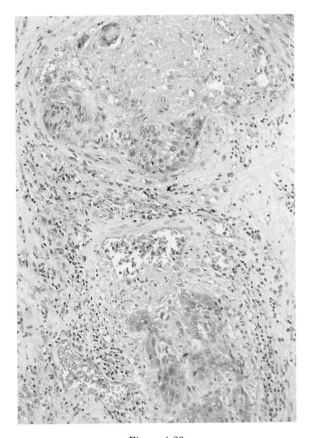

Figure 4-29
INTRAMURAL VENOUS INVASION
These submucosal veins are filled with a mixture of tumor cells and fibrin clot.

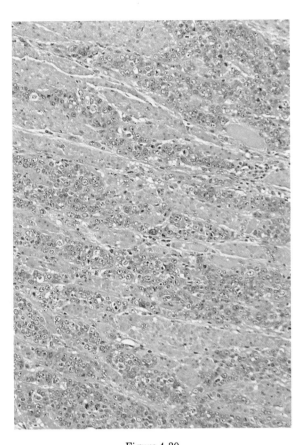

Figure 4-30
CARCINOMA WITHOUT DESMOPLASTIC STROMA
This carcinoma without desmoplastic stroma invades the muscularis propria. The tumor strands interdigitate with muscle fibers.

venous invasion may also contribute to intramural metastases (fig. 4-29).

As the carcinoma grows more deeply, it pierces the muscularis propria and begins to follow the direction of the muscle fibers, so that in the inner circular layer the cancer grows perpendicularly, while in the area of the myenteric plexus and the outer longitudinal muscle layer it expands peripherally, much as it did in the submucosa. Even at this depth, the carcinoma may not have a desmoplastic stroma, so the nests of invasive carcinoma interdigitate with the muscle fiber (fig. 4-30).

The last layer for the carcinoma to enter is the loose fibrous adventitia. Here the carcinoma tends to stimulate a dense, heavily collagenized desmoplasia (fig. 4-31). Once the tumor invades beyond the adventitia, all adjacent structures are at risk, especially the trachea and bronchi for upper and middle thoracic tumors. Carcinomatous fistulae between the esophagus and the airways are not unusual. Extension into the gastric cardia from lower thoracic primaries also occurs, as does perineural invasion. In one Japanese study, perineural invasion was seen in 23 percent of 129 cases, and the frequency was directly related to the depth of invasion (132).

*Differentiation.* Squamous cell carcinoma of the esophagus covers the entire range of differentiation from the best to the worst (figs. 4-32–4-35). Furthermore, it is common for a given carcinoma to have different degrees of differentiation in different areas. The classification of differentiation is based upon the mix of undifferentiated or primitive, relatively small, basal-type or generative cells; large flat cells that are identifiable as squamous cells; and keratinized foci. The greater the basal cell component the higher

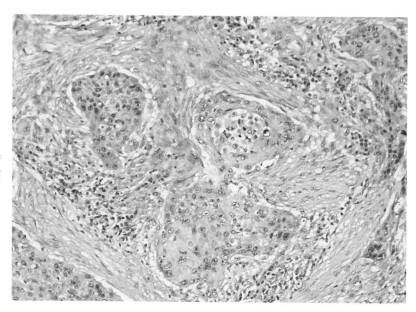

Figure 4-31
CARCINOMA WITH
DESMOPLASTIC STROMA
Carcinoma with a desmoplastic
stroma in the adventitia. Desmoplasia
can also be found in the submucosa and
muscularis propria, but with less regularity than in the adventitia.

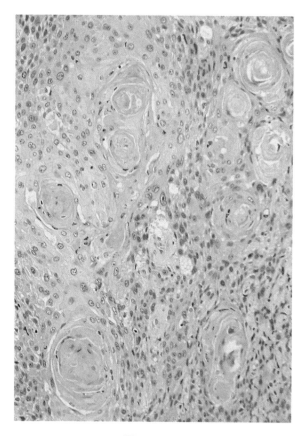

Figure 4-32
WELL-DIFFERENTIATED
SQUAMOUS CARCINOMA
Well-differentiated carcinoma with large squamous
pearls and a small component of basaloid cells.

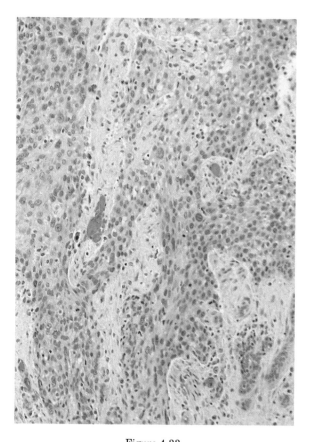

Figure 4-33
MODERATELY DIFFERENTIATED CARCINOMA
Moderately differentiated carcinoma with a trabecular
growth pattern. The trabeculae contain mostly small primitive cells, but there are large differentiated squamous cells
scattered throughout.

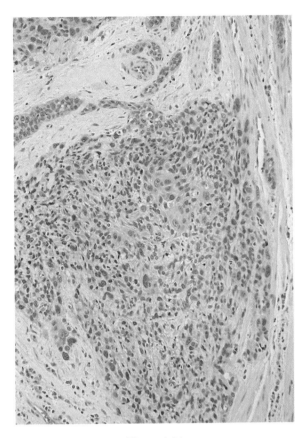

Figure 4-34
MODERATELY TO POORLY
DIFFERENTIATED CARCINOMA
Most of the tumor is composed of basaloid cells, but there is a small focus of larger squamous cells.

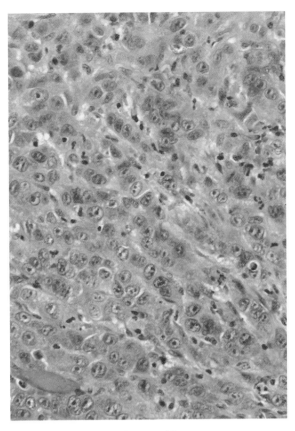

Figure 4-35
POORLY DIFFERENTIATED
SQUAMOUS CARCINOMA
Poorly differentiated carcinoma composed of rounded cells without clear-cut squamous differentiation.

the mitotic rate, since these cells are the predominant proliferative component. The best differentiated tumors have few basal cells, which means a lower mitotic rate, many squamous cells, and abundant keratin. The most poorly differentiated tumors have many basal cells resulting in a higher mitotic rate, few squamous cells, and no keratinization. In between these extremes lies a whole range of moderately or intermediately differentiated carcinomas, and, as is true for all carcinomas throughout the gastrointestinal tract, the moderately differentiated carcinomas are the most common, accounting for about two thirds of the total. For practical purposes, defining the level of differentiation for any tumor is not critical, since this adds little prognostic information, unless the tumor is anaplastic. The point of separation between well and moderately differentiated carcinomas and moderately and

poorly differentiated carcinomas is not sharp, so unless a pathologist is experienced in grading many such carcinomas on a regular basis, the intraobserver variability is likely to be great and the reproducibility low.

*Glandular (Adenocarcinomatous) and Small Cell Differentiation.* Carcinomas that are almost completely squamous may have small foci of other types of differentiation. Glandular differentiation, consisting of either scattered mucin-containing tumor cells or tubules with lumens, occur in as much as 20 percent of all cases (figs. 4-36, 4-37) (64,84,86,129). At one time it was postulated that this indicated that the tumor partly arose in the submucosal glands or ducts. However, these foci are often found beneath or extending from in situ purely squamous cell carcinoma, and an in situ adenocarcinoma in the glands or ducts has never been found. This glandular alteration only

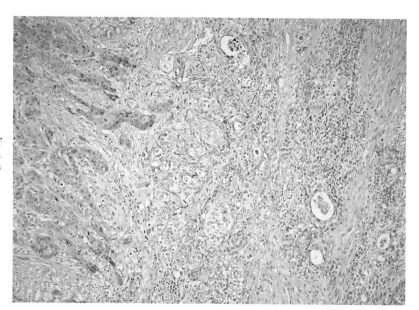

Figure 4-36
SQUAMOUS CELL CARCINOMA
WITH GLANDULAR COMPONENT
At the left, there are trabeculae of
invasive squamous carcinoma, while on
the right, the adenocarcinomatous
component forms lumens.

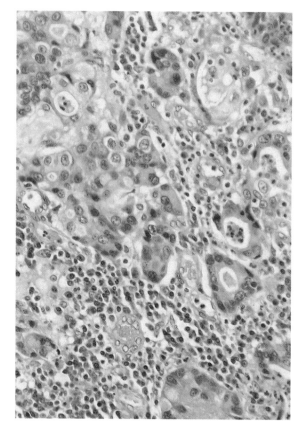

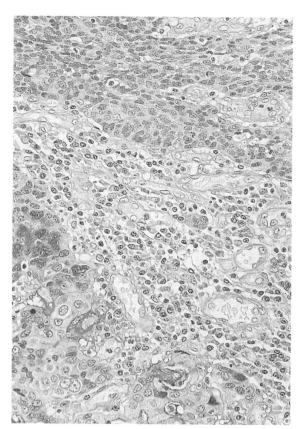

Figure 4-37
SQUAMOUS CELL CARCINOMA WITH AN ADENOCARCINOMATOUS FOCUS
Left: In this field, the squamous component is in the left center. It gives way subtly to lumen-forming adenocarcinoma.
Right: Alcian blue-PAS stain with diastase predigestion of the same tumor. The unstained squamous component is at the
top. The Alcian blue stains the goblet cells and outlines some lumens of the adenocarcinomatous component at the bottom.

occurs in the invasive component, and is usually limited to tumor in the lamina propria or superficial submucosa (85). However, when this component is roughly equal to the squamous component, then the carcinoma can be designated as "adenosquamous." (See also chapter 5, Adenocarcinoma of the Esophagus.)

Even less common is the presence of small foci that resemble small cell undifferentiated carcinoma (64,129). Little information has been published concerning the presence or absence of endocrine markers in such foci.

*Other Morphologic Modifications.* A poorly differentiated squamous cell carcinoma with abundant lymphocytic stroma, both surrounding and permeating the nests of cancer, has been reported (96). This tumor somewhat resembles similar lymphoepithelial carcinomas that occur in the nasopharynx, breast, and stomach. Another reported tumor is composed mostly of basaloid cells which form nests partly surrounded by massive amounts of basement membrane material (128).

Special variants with unusual gross or microscopic features have been designated as pseudosarcomatous, basaloid, and verrucous squamous cell carcinomas and are described separately at the end of this chapter. Some differ from typical squamous cell carcinoma not only histologically but prognostically.

**Diagnosis.** *Biopsy.* Except for the parts of the world where screening with balloon cytology is conducted, the diagnosis of esophageal squamous cell carcinoma is almost always made from a biopsy of an endoscopically suspicious lesion in a symptomatic patient. Occasionally, the endoscopic lesion does not appear to be malignant, and the diagnosis of carcinoma in such cases is a surprise to the endoscopist. In high-risk populations or when there is an endoscopic lesion that is subtle but suspicious, Lugol's iodine may be sprayed on the mucosa. The normal squamous mucosa is sufficiently glycogenated to react with the iodine and stain the surface brown. Dysplastic and carcinomatous foci are glycogen poor and do not stain, but they are outlined by the positive staining of the normal squamous epithelium around them (143,151). In a Japanese study, patients with head and neck cancers were screened for esophageal cancers using the iodine method (156). Among 178 patients screened, 9

patients had 13 esophageal cancers, only 9 of which were visible with the iodine alone. In addition, in another 22, dysplastic foci were detected using iodine staining. Endoscopic iodine staining has even been used to determine the resection margin prior to esophagectomy (149). Toluidine blue has also been used as an endoscopic stain, but the mechanism of staining has not been worked out (143). The dysplastic and carcinomatous foci stain blue, while the normal mucosa remains unstained. Both of these stains are not specific for neoplastic mucosa, since ulcers and esophagitis may also stain.

The optimal number of biopsies that should be taken from a lesion is obviously the number required to make the diagnosis. In one study from the United States which attempted to determine this number, seven biopsies were obtained from each of 27 esophageal carcinomas (144). The first biopsy was diagnostic in 25 cases, while three more biopsies added one more positive case. The last three additional biopsies did not alter this number, but cytologic examination picked up the last carcinoma. In another study from India, eight biopsies were taken from each of 48 carcinomas (150). The first two were positive in 46 cases. Two additional biopsies picked up another one, and two more biopsies detected the final cancer, so six biopsies was the magic number for 100 percent detection with no false negatives. These data indicate that five to six biopsies from the non-necrotic and nonulcerated edges and from the base of an endoscopically suspected carcinoma are diagnostic almost all of the time. Cytologic samples may pick up any cancer that is missed by the biopsies.

There are other considerations than simply the number of biopsies needed for diagnosis. Some of these factors may account for the variability in accuracy of biopsies. In one study from Spain, 170 or 90 percent of 189 squamous cell carcinomas of esophagus were diagnosed on biopsy, but the number of biopsies was not stated (140). An additional 36 carcinomas could not be biopsied, usually because the cancers were obstructing access of the biopsy forceps to the diagnostic areas. The volume of sample taken varies with the biopsy instrument. A large volume in a single sample may be as adequate as several small volume samples. Interpretation of the sample depends on the experience and diagnostic skill of the pathologist, so some

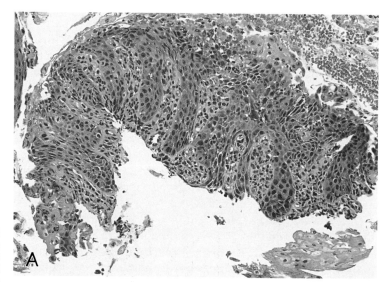

Figure 4-38
ULCER-ASSOCIATED
FLORID REGENERATIVE
SQUAMOUS PROLIFERATION

Two examples of the ulcer-associated florid regenerative squamous proliferation that may be confused with carcinoma. In both examples, long prongs of undifferentiated cells, generally arranged in parallel, penetrate the granulation tissue of the base and edges of an ulcer. The cells in these prongs have a high nuclear to cytoplasmic ratio, nuclear hyperchromasia, nuclear pleomorphism, and large nucleoli. A and C: low magnification; B and D: high magnificaton.

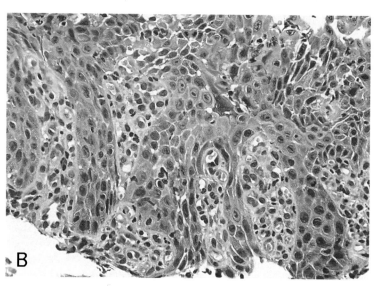

biopsies that appear negative to an inexperienced pathologist may be interpreted as positive by someone more experienced.

The biopsy appearance of a squamous cell carcinoma is comparable to that of the resection specimen, except in those cases in which preoperative chemotherapy or radiation therapy was given. Any extension into the lamina propria indicates that the carcinoma is invasive. However, detecting minor infiltration into the lamina propria may be difficult, especially in biopsies that contain inflamed tissue or are bias-cut. However, detecting invasion on the biopsy may not be critical, since endoscopic and imaging studies are likely to demonstrate invasion, and since the usual treatment for in situ and invasive carcinoma is the same (see Treatment, below).

*Differential Diagnosis in Biopsies.* The most important differential diagnostic consideration in a biopsy is the squamous epithelial proliferation that occurs at the edges and bases of chronic reflux-induced ulcers. These appear as uniformly thick, parallel prongs of primitive squamous cells that penetrate the granulation tissue of the ulcer bed. Early in the healing process, the cells in these prongs do not look like typical basal cells. Instead, they are cuboidal, with little cytoplasm and large, often misshapen, hyperchromatic nuclei and a very high nuclear/cytoplasmic ratio (fig. 4-38). Mitotic figures are often prominent. The

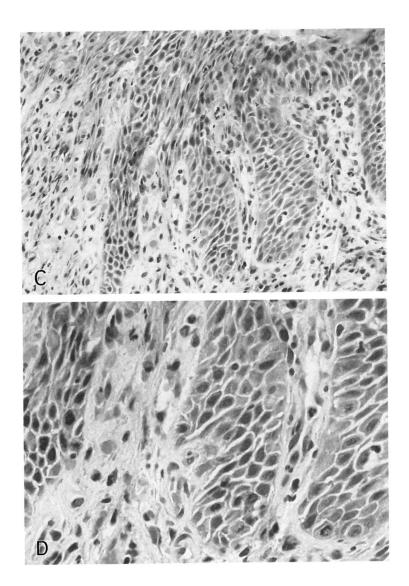

Figure 4-38 (Continued)

prongs arise from the base of thin, immature surface squamous epithelium. As long as these foci are sectioned perfectly, the diagnosis is not difficult because the parallel arrangement of the uniform prongs is obvious, and squamous cancers do not produce this uniformity. However, in bias-cut samples, the prongs are often sectioned across so that they appear trapped and separated within the inflamed stroma, thus resembling nests of invasive carcinoma. As the epithelium and granulation tissue mature, the prongs become separated by collagen rather than by granulation tissue, the cuboidal epithelial cells become smaller, the nuclei become more normochromatic, the mitoses disappear, and the epithelium on the surface becomes thicker and more mature.

The second differential diagnosis is radiation change or chemotherapy-induced change in squamous mucosa. Clearly, this diagnosis is easiest when the history of previous irradiation or chemotherapy is known. Sometimes, there is an associated ulcer. The altered squamous epithelium may retain the structure of its normal counterpart with smaller, basal-like cells and larger, superficial cells, but the cells tend to be of variable shapes and sizes in all layers, and the nuclei are strangely shaped and vary from hyperchromatic to normochromatic to smudged (fig. 4-39). Some nuclei have large eosinophilic nucleoli. Mitoses are usually not present. In general, when the nuclei are enlarged, the cytoplasmic volume is also expanded so that there is little

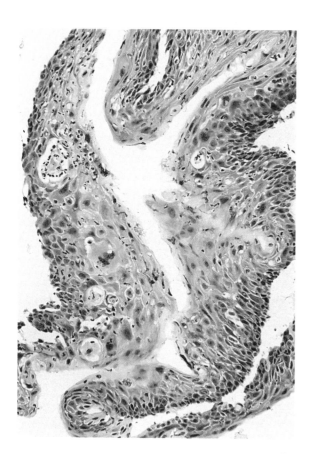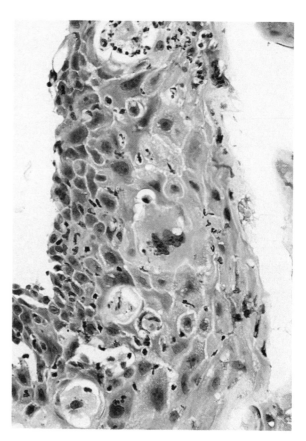

Figure 4-39
RADIATION CHANGE IN ESOPHAGEAL SQUAMOUS EPITHELIUM
Left: The overall orientation of the epithelium is normal, and the epithelium is thinner than normal, but there are bizarre cells at all levels.
Right: High magnification view.

change in the nuclear/cytoplasmic ratio. Virtually identical changes occur in the columnar mucosa of the stomach or in Barrett's mucosa (154).

The third differential diagnostic problem is granulation tissue in an ulcer bed or in a polyp that contains bizarre stromal cells that assume epithelioid shapes (139,147,153,155). The ulcerative and polypoid gross features may suggest malignancy to the endoscopist. These strange stromal cells are not limited to the esophagus but are found throughout the gut. They have large, hyperchromatic or coarsely chromatinated, often angulated nuclei that resemble malignant nuclei; mitoses are rare, however. These are the same cells that may mimic sarcoma cells. They are discussed and illustrated in detail in chapter 6. They usually have a rim of pink, slightly foamy or vacuolated cytoplasm. These bizarre cells occur singly and in small clusters or nests, and

they are mixed with the vessels, edematous stroma, and inflammatory cells of the granulation tissue. The endothelial cells of the capillary buds also may be unusually hypertrophied and have large dark nuclei. The whole complex forms a disorganized mass resembling a carcinoma with an inflamed desmoplastic stroma. The bizarre stromal cells can be differentiated from carcinoma cells by immunohistochemical means. They do not contain cytokeratins or carcinoembryonic antigen, but do contain vimentin and occasionally actin. These findings, coupled with ultrastructural evidence indicating that the cells have no epithelial features, suggest that they are fibroblasts or myofibroblasts (148).

**Cytology.** Several techniques have been developed to capture cells from gastrointestinal lesions for cytologic examination. In endoscopically directed brush cytology, the specimens are obtained during direct endoscopic visualization of the lesion. In indirect brush cytology, the specimens are taken blindly after the patient swallows a nasogastric tube containing the cytology brush. Using either brushing technique, the whole esophageal mucosa may be sampled. In one study, both brush procedures resulted in a positive diagnosis in 78 percent of 49 carcinomas of various stages and sizes that were a mixture of squamous cell, undifferentiated, and adenocarcinoma (142). Both techniques were 95 percent accurate in diagnosing malignancy in 86 cases and 100 percent accurate in correctly identifying 68 normal esophagi. In all cases the ultimate diagnoses were made by biopsy, examination of resected specimens, or at autopsy. In a Spanish study, the correct diagnosis was made in 216 (96 percent) of 225 squamous cell carcinomas by endoscopic brush cytology (140). The combination of biopsy and cytology yielded positive results in 223 or 99 percent of the 225 cases. Furthermore, brush cytology was able to obtain material for diagnosis in 36 squamous cell cancers that could not be adequately biopsied, mostly because the cancers were obstructive: the brushes could pass the obstruction, but the endoscope could not. Thus, the use of brush cytology may be critical for diagnosis in obstructing esophageal lesions.

A variation of indirect brush cytology uses a compressed cytology brush placed inside a gelatin capsule which the patient swallows (152). The gelatin capsule melts, the brush expands, and the entire esophagus is sampled as the brush is withdrawn. The positive diagnostic rate using this technique was 92 percent for cancers over 20 mm in diameter, but only 50 percent for those that were smaller.

The balloon cytology technique is used in some studies from China. A tube with an inflatable balloon is swallowed and an abrasive mesh covering the balloon functions like the cytology brush (157). In China, this balloon collecting technique has been reported to diagnose more than 80 percent of the cancers in mass screening programs and over 90 percent in symptomatic outpatients. A substantial number of small or early cancers, perhaps as many as 20 percent, were detected by the balloon cytology, including some that were missed by radiologic and endoscopic examinations (146,157). Balloon cytologic screening was also able to detect those at increased risk for developing carcinoma by identifying many patients with dysplasias (141). The procedure can be used to determine the site of the cancer by sampling multiple levels in the esophagus. Although it is used in high-risk areas for screening, there are some false negative results. Its use in outpatients in low cancer frequency populations is not established.

As with biopsies, the major differential cytologic diagnosis is reparative epithelium, which shares many features with malignant cells, such as multiple nucleoli, macronucleoli, and loss of nuclear polarity in cell clusters (145).

**Prognosis.** Survival of American patients with squamous cell carcinoma of the esophagus, if all stages and all treatments are included together, is abysmal, with 5-year survival for whites of 9 percent and 6 percent for blacks in the period from 1983 through 1988 (58a). However, these figures are a great improvement over the 4 percent and 1 percent survival rate 25 years earlier. The reasons for this change probably include better access to the medical care system, better and earlier detection, better surgical techniques, and adjuvant therapy. In some series from high-risk areas in China, the 5-year survival is much higher, approaching 45 percent for cases treated surgically (89).

*Morphologic Prognosticators.* Different morphologic characteristics of esophageal squamous cell carcinoma have been analyzed as potential prognosticators, including stage, grade, DNA content, growth pattern, venous invasion, lymphatic invasion, cellular host response, and growth factor receptor content. However, there is little information on the significance of any of these features independently when studied in large series using multivariate statistical analysis. Furthermore, the impact of specific types of surgical approaches and adjuvant chemoradiation therapy on all of these morphologic features has yet to be defined, so that any specific survival data based upon any factor or factors mentioned below may be significantly altered in the future.

*Stage.* The single most important prognosticator is stage (87). The most widely used staging system is the TNM classification as defined by the American Joint Committee on Cancer and the International Union Against Cancer (see chapter 1) (57,74). Because overall survival is so poor, and because most carcinomas are of such high stage when first diagnosed, it is difficult to find survival data for each T and N status. All studies indicate that the depth of invasion and the presence of nodal or distant metastases are prognostically related. This was discussed in part in the section on superficial carcinoma. Unfortunately, superficial carcinomas comprise only a small fraction of the total number of cases; the rest are advanced cancers. Tumors that extend beyond the adventitia are unlikely to be resectable for cure. Of patients with tumors resected for cure, the 5-year survival varies from 40 percent to 60 percent in different studies as long as the tumor is confined to the muscularis propria (66). This figure drops to 10 to 20 percent for resected tumors invading the adventitia and beyond. These percentages do not include the large number of patients with unresectable disease. Depending upon the series, between 30 and 65 percent of patients are not even surgically explored, and, of those who are, another 15 to 30 percent are found to have unresectable tumors (66). In addition to depth of invasion, intramural metastasis is associated with more frequent nodal and distant metastases and with diminished survival (130). In a Japanese study of carcinomas invading the adventitia and beyond, regardless of metastatic status, the 5-year survival was about 10 percent when there were intramural metastases, whereas it was about 15 percent when there were not (130).

Lymph node involvement, regardless of the extent of the primary tumor, also reflects poorer survival. The numbers vary from study to study, but the trends are obvious. Five-year survival rates of 32 percent without nodal metastases and 5 percent with nodal metastases have been reported (114); others have found 5-year survival rates in resected cases of 40 to 50 percent for patients without positive nodes and 10 to 15 percent for those with them (66).

*Histologic Grade.* As is true for most carcinomas of different types arising in different sites, squamous cell esophageal cancer may be separated into histologic grades based upon the relative proportions of keratinization, intercellular bridges, and primitive basal-like cells. A three-grade system is usual: well-differentiated or grade I, moderately differentiated or grade II, and poorly differentiated or grade III. However, it is likely that different investigators analyzing tumor grade do not interpret the histologic fea-

tures similarly. One report analyzed the association between grade and staining of tumor with a monoclonal antibody, AE1, against low molecular weight cytokeratins (136): well-differentiated carcinomas stained poorly for AE1, poorly differentiated tumors stained well and diffusely, and moderately differentiated tumors had a mixed staining pattern. Anaplastic tumors did not stain. There was no attempt to relate the staining patterns to survival. The authors of this study stated that unpublished data of theirs indicated that there was no relationship between grade and staining for high molecular weight keratins, using the antibody AE3.

There is no agreement upon the value of grade as a prognostic factor. In a study from the United States, patients with well- and moderately differentiated tumors combined had a 5-year survival rate of 54 percent, a significantly better rate than the 6 percent for poorly differentiated tumors (114). In contrast, an English study showed that moderately and poorly differentiated carcinomas were associated with longer survival periods than well-differentiated ones (64). Some Chinese studies suggest that grade is an important prognosticator, while others indicate it is not (87). In a Swedish study of patients treated both surgically and with radiation, there was no difference in survival whether the tumor was well, moderately, or poorly differentiated (73). Based upon all available data and our experience, it is our impression that for usual squamous cell carcinomas, tumor grade is not reproducible and of no clinical use. Most tumors deserve the grade of moderately differentiated, leaving few in the other categories. Most truly high-grade tumors are special variants, such as small cell undifferentiated and basaloid squamous cell carcinomas.

*DNA Ploidy.* Unfortunately, published studies that relate ploidy to survival are not comparable: some use flow cytometry on either fresh or fixed tissues and on biopsies or resection specimens, while others use image analysis on fixed tissues. Furthermore, tumors may be heterogeneous in their DNA content: in about 40 percent of the tumors it varies from one area to another (117). Nevertheless, all studies from different parts of the world, regardless of technique and substrate, show that most squamous cell cancers, 70 percent or more in some series, are aneuploid somewhere; often multiple aneuploid populations are seen

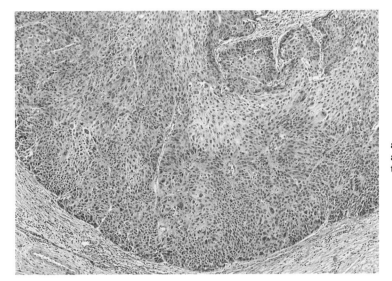

Figure 4-40
EXPANSILE GROWTH PATTERN
The invasive edge is smooth, and the tumor appears to expand into the surrounding tissues along a broad front. There is no lymphocyte infiltration of the tumor at its advancing edge.

Figure 4-41
INFILTRATIVE GROWTH PATTERN
The tumor sends individual tongues and nests into the adjacent tissue. There is an intense lymphocytic infiltrate within and around the invasive cords and nests.

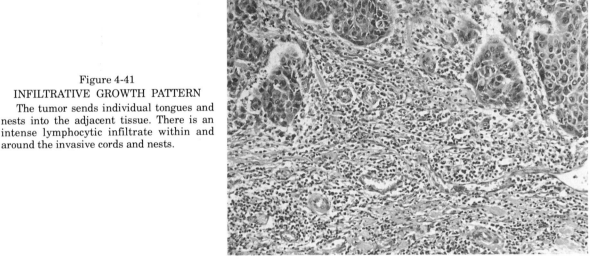

(59,75,76,93,107,110,113,114,116,121,124). Aneuploidy tends to correlate with nodal metastases, advanced stage, periesophageal invasion, poor differentiation, high mitotic rates, and postoperative recurrence. In general, patients with diploid tumors survive longer than do those with aneuploid tumors, but the difference is rarely statistically significant. When DNA histograms are generated by image analysis, tumors with increasing DNA content have a significantly poorer prognosis than do those with lower DNA (59,93,126). Finally, tumors that have been preoperatively irradiated are much less likely to be aneuploid than are those that were not irradiated (110). In summary, DNA analysis may correlate with other histologic and clinical parameters, but it may not offer independently important prognostic information, and it need not be performed as part of the routine evaluation.

*Other Morphologic and Molecular Prognosticators.* A number of additional factors have been analyzed to determine if they have prognostic significance. In terms of microscopic growth pattern, a tumor with an expansile edge may have a more favorable prognosis than one that is raggedly infiltrating (figs. 4-40, 4-41). Venous invasion may indicate a worse outcome, although lymphatic invasion may be less important (64). In one study, peritumoral lymphocytic reaction, an indication of host response, was a statistically significant index of prolonged survival (figs. 4-40, 4-41) (64). Prominent infiltration of tumor by Langerhans' cells has been associated with prolonged survival (92). A complex malignancy grading scheme, using eight parameters to relate tumor cells to tumor-host interactions, was developed: those whose tumors had the highest scores, that is, the more anaplastic tumors with the most aggressive growth characteristics and the least host response, had a statistically worse survival than those with lower scoring tumors (73). Amount of tumor receptor for epidermal growth factor, a powerful growth stimulator for a variety of cells, has been measured in esophageal squamous cell cancers by chemical analysis or immunostaining. In all studies, a high content of the receptor was associated with a statistically significant poorer survival (98,106,137). Finally, in one Japanese study, gene amplification at the int-2 locus in DNA tumor extracts correlated with a tendency for deeper invasion and decreased survival (97).

**Preoperative Staging and Determination of Resectability.** Endoscopy is done for almost every patient, and during this procedure biopsies and brush cytology specimens are obtained for diagnosis. The size of the tumor can be determined if the endoscope can be passed completely past it. The remainder of the esophagus and the proximal stomach are evaluated for additional disease. In tumors that produce strictures through which the endoscope cannot be passed, barium swallow may outline the tumor and assist with size estimation, but this often gives a falsely exaggerated impression (66). Computed tomography (CT) gives the best preoperative views of the esophageal wall, mediastinal structures, enlarged lymph nodes, lungs, liver, and adrenal glands (66). Chest X ray may help outline the tumor and detect local spread and metastases, but is not nearly as useful as CT. Endoscopic ultrasound can define the esophageal wall thickness and detect nodal metastases; in some centers, it produces views that may be superior to CT (115,134). Bronchoscopy is often used to detect airway involvement if the tumor is near the tracheobronchial tree. Magnetic resonance imaging (MRI) and bone scanning to detect bone metastases are less frequently used, and data on their value for staging are not available. Such scans have a high false positive rate.

Data from these modalities help determine the size, local spread, and metastases of the tumor. Unfortunately, they do not provide all the necessary information, so tumors initially thought to be resectable are further staged at the time of surgery, and the final decision whether to resect for cure is made at that time. Resectability rates vary greatly from one population to another, and this variability may be due, at least in part, to the general health of the patient population. In one large French series, only 10 percent of the patients with symptomatic cancer were considered to have tumors that could be resected for cure, while in a Chinese study, this figure was about 40 percent (89). Cases for which resection for cure is the preferred treatment include those with a depth of invasion no greater than into the adventitia without involvement of adjacent structures, and those with no nodal metastases (66). However, some cases with only regional node metastases are also surgically treated.

**Treatment.** There has been a gradual series of changes in the treatment of esophageal carcinoma. Simultaneously, the mortality and morbidity associated with resection has declined. Over 30 years, the postoperative death rate from esophageal squamous cell carcinoma in the United States fell from 30 percent in the 1950s to 10 percent in the 1970s (77). There are a variety of surgical options, ranging from transthoracic approaches with fastidious dissections of the tumor and removal of regional lymph nodes to transhiatal esophagectomy. The transthoracic approaches are done through incisions in the chest and include standard esophagectomy for palliation of symptoms of tumors that have spread transmurally or metastasized to radical en bloc esophagectomy for potentially curable disease (66). This latter approach is aimed at removing not only the entire tumor but all the immediately surrounding tissue, including the entire lymphatic drainage system. In the transhiatal approach, the chest is never entered during the operation, but instead, incisions are made in the upper abdomen and in the neck and the esophagus is bluntly dissected with the fingers. Then it is pulled out through the abdominal incision, and an esophagogastric anastomosis is constructed in the neck (104). This procedure has even lower surgical mortality, about 6 percent in one large series (104). However, this approach does not allow direct visualization of the esophagus in situ so that fastidious dissection of the tumor with its extensions and all the regional lymph nodes is not possible.

Studies analyzing the value of adjuvant therapy, either radiation or chemotherapy in conjunction with resection, are beginning to appear (63,69,80,105,108,109,123). Survival following such combined therapy seems to be superior to that following resection alone. Currently, there are many studies being conducted worldwide to evaluate new regimens, so at this time, survival data are undergoing constant change. In vitro sensitivity testing of certain chemotherapeutic regimens upon endoscopically obtained cancer cells in cell cultures may be useful in picking the proper agents to be used prior to resection (81).

Not all carcinomas are resectable. For those that are not, a variety of palliative procedures are available, including laser destruction of tumor in patients with obstruction as well as chemotherapy, radiation therapy, or both (80,88,108,112). These treatments improve the quality of life for the patients for the short term, but they do not seem to offer any significant improvement in survival.

Local therapy has been considered for superficial carcinomas. In a recent Japanese trial, an anticancer agent, peplomycin, was adsorbed on activated carbon particles and injected endoscopically into six superficial cancers (72). Five patients survived without recurrence. The sixth patient had a recurrence that was treated by a second course of the drug, with no further recurrence.

*Morphologic Effects of Chemotherapy and Irradiation.* Esophageal squamous carcinoma is frequently treated by irradiation or chemotherapy prior to resection. When adjuvant modalities are used, both the gross and microscopic appearances of the carcinomas are often dramatically altered (61). Commonly, particularly following radiation, the tumor is not even grossly apparent (57a). All that may be left is a large, shallow, chronic ulcer with sharp margins instead of the lumpy or nodular margins that are so common in ulcerative carcinomas (figs. 4-42, 4-43).

Microscopically, such ulcer beds contain superficial granulation tissue and deep scar. There may be residual carcinoma in the ulcer bed, and it is sometimes difficult for the pathologist to decide whether the carcinoma cells are viable or not. The residual cancer cells may have changes of severe damage, including cytoplasmic enlargement with abundant red cytoplasm and bizarre nuclei, ar-

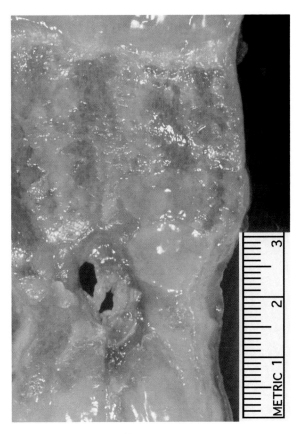

Figure 4-42
IRRADIATED CARCINOMA
The radiation destroyed the tumor and all of the in situ component as well, resulting in a sharply circumscribed erosion with a deep ulcer, presumably where the tumor had infiltrated the deepest.

ranged singly or in small clusters. Many such nuclei may be pyknotic (fig. 4-44). If these cells are the only ones that remain, then the tumor may not be viable post-treatment. Sometimes, mixed with these large bizarre squamous cells are isolated or small collections of basal-type cells; these may have mitoses, possibly a marker of viability, but even that is not certain. Occasionally, all that remains of the carcinoma are small nodules of keratin or dyskeratotic cells, sometimes inciting a foreign-body response (fig. 4-45). Recent data from a study of squamous cell cancers treated with a mixture of mitomycin, ifosfamide, and cisplatin suggest that patients whose cancers respond to chemotherapy, as measured by a decrease in the proportion of tumor to stroma, have better 1-year survival rates than do those without such a tumor response (61).

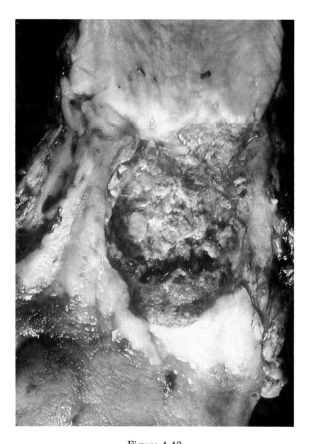

Figure 4-43
IRRADIATED CARCINOMA

In this irradiated carcinoma the deep ulcer with the necrotic base is due to the destruction of a large and deeply invasive tumor.

**Metastasis and Recurrence.** The regional lymph nodes are the most common sites of metastasis, and the risk of metastasis increases with increasing depth of invasion by the tumor (91). The node groups affected differ, depending upon the site of the tumor. Carcinomas of the cervical esophagus metastasize mostly to the cervical and superior mediastinal nodes; those in the upper and middle thoracic esophagus spread to the mediastinal nodes at all levels and to the superior gastric nodes; and those in the lower thoracic part most frequently involve the lower mediastinal, superior gastric, celiac artery, and splenic artery nodes (66). The most common extranodal metastatic sites in all reported series are the liver and lung (56,60,90,120). Either or both sites contain metastases in about 50 percent of cases. Less common metastatic sites (10 percent of cases) are the adrenal gland, kidney, pleura, and bone. The stomach is involved in 8 percent of resected cancers, either by direct extension, intramural metastases, or secondary spread from involved perigastric nodes (82).

Local recurrences are common following resection. In an autopsy study published in 1986, over 35 percent of patients surviving at least 3 months postresection developed recurrences (60). It is conceivable that the number of recurrences may drop dramatically when adjuvant therapy is used.

Figure 4-44
IRRADIATED
SQUAMOUS CARCINOMA

The cells have large bizarre nuclei, some of which have vacuoles or granules. There are no small dark basaloid cells. It is unclear if these nests are viable.

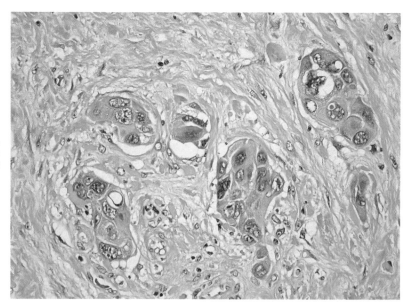

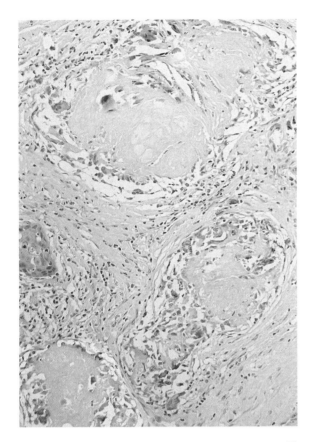 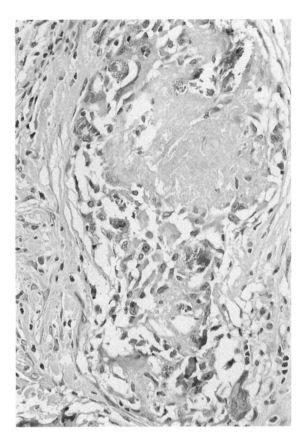

Figure 4-45
IRRADIATED SQUAMOUS CANCER

Left: Scattered throughout the deep submucosa are clumps of keratin without epithelium, but with surrounding foreign body reaction. The surrounding scar tissue has obliterated both the submucosa and the muscularis propria.
Right: High magnification.

## SPECIAL VARIANTS OF SQUAMOUS CELL CARCINOMA

### Pseudosarcomatous Squamous Cell Carcinoma (Spindle Cell Carcinoma, Polypoid Carcinoma, Carcinosarcoma, Polypoid Tumor)

The unusual malignancy that goes by all of the names listed in the title above is composed of variable quantities of differentiated squamous cell carcinoma and sarcoma-like stroma. No matter what the name, this tumor has a characteristic gross polypoid configuration, hence the designation polypoid carcinoma. In this Fascicle, all of these tumors are designated as pseudosarcomatous squamous cell carcinoma, abbreviated as PSCC.

These tumors are common enough that many pathologists have had experience with them. In one study from China, there were 4 such tumors among a total of 850 resected carcinomas of the esophagus and gastric cardia (172). In a study from Japan, 7 polypoid squamous cell carcinomas were found among 101 resected squamous cell carcinomas. However, since specific histologic descriptions were not given in the report, it is not clear how many, if any, PSCCs were included in the 7 polypoid tumors (169). They are uncommon enough that their literature consists of single case reports and small series, eight cases at most. There are no large series from single institutions; therefore, meaningful data are difficult to obtain. This discussion is, by necessity, a compilation of the limited experiences of others covering almost all the reported cases in the English language literature from 1951 through mid-1992, a total of about 80 cases (158,160,164,169, 172). Not all reported cases

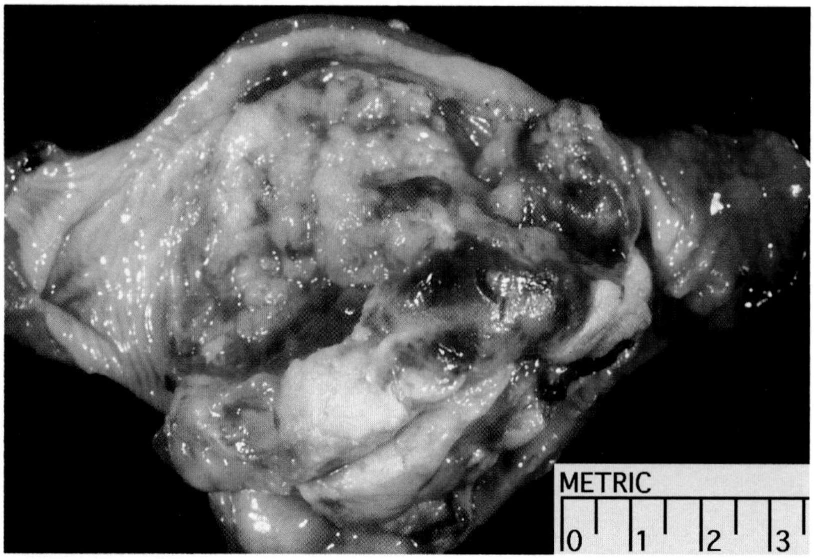

Figure 4-46
PSEUDOSARCOMATOUS
SQUAMOUS CELL CARCINOMA
The tumor forms a large, long, lob-
ulated polypoid mass.

included all the important demographic and descriptive information, and only about half had useful follow-up information.

**Clinical Features.** PSCC is a tumor that occurs in men about 5 1/2 times as often as it occurs in women. Peak patient age is in the late sixth decade. Both the sex and age distribution are identical to that of usual squamous cell carcinoma. Patients present with the same symptoms as usual carcinomas, namely progressive dysphagia and, less frequently, chest pain and weight loss. The duration of symptoms varies from days to months, but is usually 3 months or less. It is surprising that these bulky, solid neoplasms, almost all of which are polyps, can reach enormous sizes, 10 cm in diameter or more, and only produce symptoms for 3 months or less. They are discovered in the same way as all other esophageal neoplasms, with radiographic studies or during endoscopy. About 60 percent arise in the mid-esophagus, close to one third are in the distal part, and the rest, less than 10 percent, occur proximally. This roughly parallels the distribution of usual squamous cell carcinoma. A few reports of multiple tumors have been published.

**Gross Findings.** The typical PSCC is a polypoid mass, commonly attached to the wall by a short, thick pedicle and usually oriented with its long axis longitudinally (figs. 4-46–4-48). Sometimes, there is no pedicle. The surface is slightly knobby or scalloped, although it may be smooth. In most cases, this surface is almost completely eroded superficially. The surrounding mucosa usually is grossly normal. The lumen is dilated and the wall is stretched. This mural and luminal expansion may indicate that these peculiar tumors are slow growing, and this may explain why symptoms occur so late, when many of the tumors are so large. The combination of a bulky polypoid tumor expanding but not obstructing the lumen of the esophagus is characteristic radiographically (161,165). Only two ulcerative, nonpolypoid PSCCs have been described; the rest have been typical polypoid lesions (159,160).

**Microscopic Findings.** These are biphasic tumors: there is a sarcomatous and a carcinomatous component (figs. 4-49–4-53). Most PSCCs contain a pleomorphic spindle and stellate cell sarcoma-like proliferation, and this may dominate every histologic field. Many tumor cells are huge, with strangely shaped nuclei and bizarre mitoses, but there is also a population of smaller spindle cells (figs. 4-49–4-51). These cells are embedded in an undifferentiated matrix that commonly is edematous and contains scattered collagen fibers and abundant acid mucopolysaccharides. Stromal differentiation has been reported, usually with the formation of tumor bone, but cartilaginous and rhabdomyoblastic foci have also been described (fig. 4-52) (162,164). In some tumors, parts of the stroma resemble malignant fibrous histiocytoma (fig. 4-53). About 10 percent of PSCCs have been reported to have such differentiation, but the actual rate is probably higher.

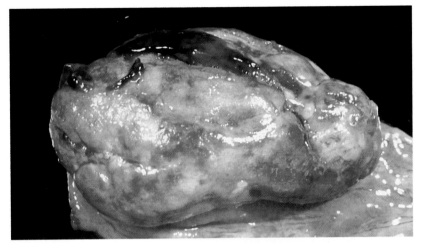

Figure 4-47
PSEUDOSARCOMATOUS
SQUAMOUS CELL CARCINOMA
Another large, elongated polypoid mass that appears to be tacked onto the mucosa. This tumor has a smooth surface.

Figure 4-48
PSEUDOSARCOMATOUS
SQUAMOUS CELL CARCINOMA
The esophageal wall is at the bottom. The lower border of the tumor is in the superficial submucosa and is extraordinarily well circumscribed. Thus, this is a large, yet very low stage neoplasm. The cyst in the mass is lined by squamous cell carcinoma.

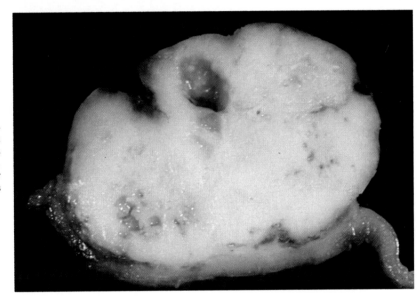

PSCCs are often very large, and foci of stromal differentiation may be tiny, so that compulsive sampling is needed to find them.

The second component is carcinomatous, almost always squamous cell, although a few tumors with adenocarcinomatous foci have been reported (159,167). In virtually every case, the carcinomatous component is much less prominent than the sarcomatous one. The squamous carcinoma may be mixed with the sarcomatous-appearing stroma, or it may be separate. In some cases, the only carcinoma is in situ in the flat mucosa at the edges of the polypoid lesion. Because the surfaces of PSCCs are diffusely eroded, it is almost impossible to find the focus where the in situ carcinoma gives rise to the invasive component.

Because of this combination of sarcoma and carcinoma, debate has centered upon whether the two components are truly independent, so that the designation "carcinosarcoma" is the best one, or if the sarcomatous part evolves by metaplasia from the carcinomatous component, necessitating some other name. Identical tumors occur throughout the upper aerodigestive tract, and there the same debate recurs with each new report. Attempts have been made to solve this dilemma, but the resulting data are mixed. In some immunohistochemical studies, some of the pleomorphic sarcoma-like stromal cells contain the same cytokeratins that are present in the carcinoma cells, suggesting that they are epithelial derivatives, but in other studies the stromal

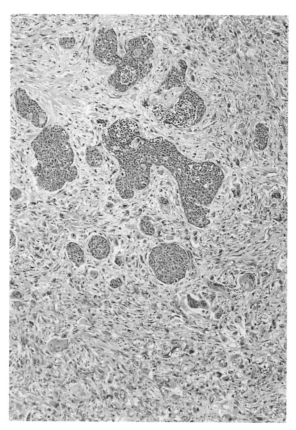

Figure 4-49
PSEUDOSARCOMATOUS
SQUAMOUS CELL CARCINOMA
There is a mixture of epithelial and stromal elements. At the top are small nests of differentiated squamous carcinoma, while the rest of the field contains the stromal component with its bizarre spindle and giant cells.

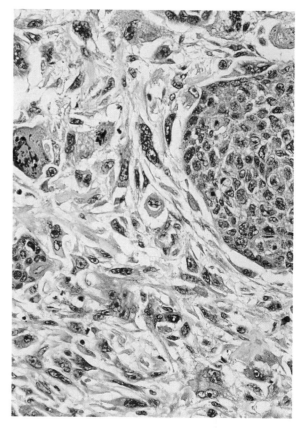

Figure 4-50
PSEUDOSARCOMATOUS
SQUAMOUS CELL CARCINOMA
In this high-power field, there is a nest of poorly differentiated squamous cancer at the right, while the entire left has the bizarre stroma.

cells contain only vimentin or even alpha-1-antitrypsin or alpha-1-antichymotrypsin and no cytokeratins, suggesting that they are not epithelial but purely stromal (160,163,164,170). In some electron microscopic studies, some of the stromal cells have tonofilaments and intercellular junctions much like squamous epithelial cells, but in other such studies, the stromal cells have no epithelial features (159,164,166–168,170,171). Most authors have concluded that the spindle and stellate cells are epithelial cells that gradually undergo metaplasia, losing the ultrastructural and microfilamentous characteristics of squamous cells, so that eventually they have no squamous cell features and become undifferentiated stromal cells. Presumably, such cells may subsequently undergo maturation to specialized stromal cells, such as bone, cartilage, and skeletal muscle cells.

**Prognosis and Survival.** As a group, PSCCs have a much better prognosis than common squamous cell carcinomas of comparable size, because PSCCs often remain at low stage until reaching enormous size. They have a peculiar tendency to grow into the lumen rather than the wall. Some are huge tumors that invade no deeper than the lamina propria or the submucosa. In general, however, the depth of invasion is related to the size, and size, in turn, is associated with site. The largest tumors occur in the mid-esophagus: PSCCs of 7 cm and larger are common here but rare in the upper and lower regions. Peculiarly, however, the lower esophageal tumors, in spite of their smaller

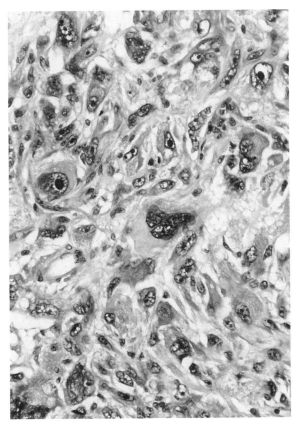

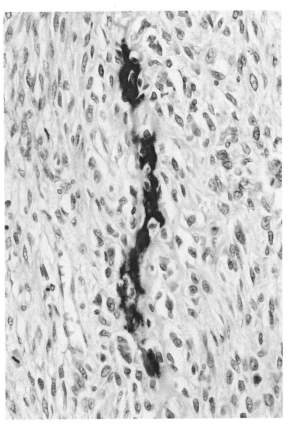

**Figure 4-51**
**PSEUDOSARCOMATOUS**
**SQUAMOUS CELL CARCINOMA**
Most of this tumor was composed of bizarre stromal and spindle cells such as these. The entire surface was ulcerated. The only carcinoma was a small patch of superficially invasive tumor at the junction between the mass and the esophageal mucosa.

**Figure 4-52**
**STROMAL DIFFERENTIATION**
**IN A PSEUDOSARCOMATOUS**
**SQUAMOUS CELL CARCINOMA**
The dark foci are where membranous bone formation has occurred within the undifferentiated stromal component.

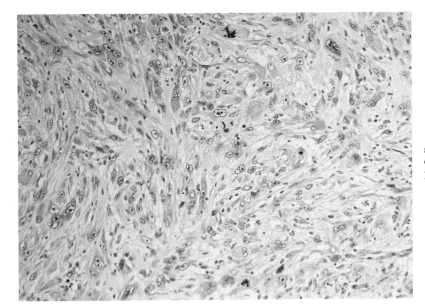

**Figure 4-53**
**PSEUDOSARCOMATOUS**
**SQUAMOUS CELL CARCINOMA**
Part of the stromal component resembled a malignant fibrous histiocytoma with its characteristic storiform pattern.

size, seem to have a higher frequency of metastasis, both to nodes and distant sites, than those arising elsewhere. The larger tumors also tend to invade more deeply than the smaller ones. Finally, depth of invasion is associated with metastasis: roughly 10 percent of PSCCs confined to the lamina propria metastasize, about 25 percent of those in the submucosa and muscularis propria do, and 75 percent of those that reach the adventitia metastasize. These metastatic rates are identical to those of the usual squamous cell carcinomas with comparable depths of invasion. The metastases may be purely carcinomatous, purely sarcomatous, or mixed, much like the primary. The preferred metastatic sites are the regional lymph nodes followed by the lungs and pleura.

## Basaloid Squamous Carcinoma (The Commonly Misnamed Adenoid Cystic Carcinoma)

The esophagus is the site of origin of two very different tumors, both of which have been given the name "adenoid cystic carcinoma." One of these is the typical slow-growing adenoid cystic carcinoma, identical to the tumor of salivary glands, while the second is a highly malignant neoplasm. These two tumors share some growth patterns, but otherwise, they are completely different, both morphologically and behaviorally.

The typical adenoid cystic carcinoma contains the characteristic uniform basaloid cells with small nuclei and rare mitoses. These cells grow in cords, cribriform arrangements, tubules, and solid nests, all of which are surrounded by abundant hyaline material that is excess basement membrane. This material also fills the holes between the epithelial bridges in the cribriform pattern. These strange tumors have very irregular or jagged invasive edges, and often extend along nerves. As a result, they are difficult to eradicate and tend to recur multiple times. They metastasize in about half of the cases, sometimes late in the course. Metastasis is mostly to lungs and not to lymph nodes.

A tiny group of primary esophageal, typical, salivary gland–type adenoid cystic carcinomas have been reported as single cases (175,182). These were intramural tumors that may have arisen within the submucosal glands. They had the characteristic small, uniform, basaloid cells arranged in small clusters and cribriform structures with the typical hyalinized or myxoid ma-

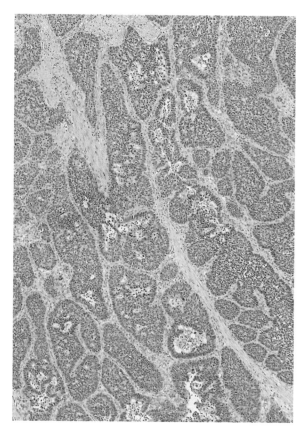

Figure 4-54
BASALOID SQUAMOUS CELL CARCINOMA
The small dark carcinoma cells form strands, trabeculae, and nests, some with central holes. The stromal spaces separating the cell groups are often uniform, as in typical adenoid cystic carcinomas.

terial around and within the nests; they exhibited the typical behavior of salivary gland tumors. There are so few of these tumors that it is impossible to analyze their clinical and epidemiologic characteristics.

In contrast to the slow-growing behavioral characteristics of typical salivary gland adenoid cystic carcinoma, most of the esophageal tumors reported as adenoid cystic carcinoma are aggressive, deeply invasive, and rapidly fatal following diagnosis. The basaloid cells are much larger than in the salivary gland tumors, the nuclei are high grade, and mitoses are common (173,176–182,184). The cells form cords and cribriform structures, but they also form solid nests in which central necrosis is common (figs. 4-54–4-57). Small foci of clear-cut squamous differentiation are often present (fig. 4-56) (178). In the only two

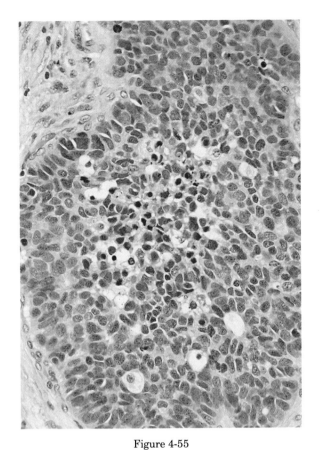

Figure 4-55
TYPICAL NEST FROM A
BASALOID SQUAMOUS CELL CARCINOMA
This is an imperfect palisade of peripheral basal-type cells. The nest has multiple small holes, giving it a cribriform look.

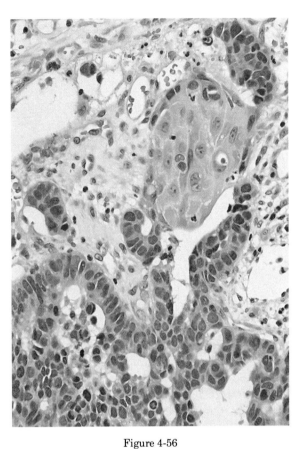

Figure 4-56
BASALOID SQUAMOUS CELL CARCINOMA
In this basaloid squamous carcinoma, a focus of squamous differentiation is present in the upper center, while the rest of the tumor forms strands of primitive cells.

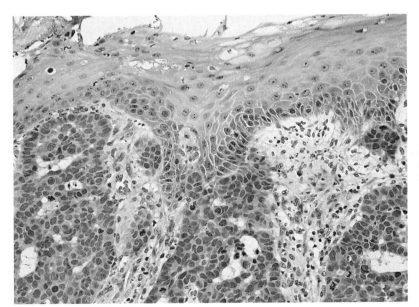

Figure 4-57
BASALOID SQUAMOUS
CELL CARCINOMA
These nests of basaloid squamous carcinoma touch the basal squamous esophageal mucosa, but this is not the site of origin.

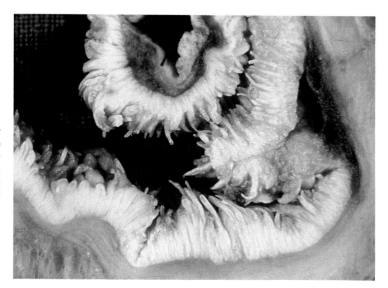

Figure 4-58
VERRUCOUS SQUAMOUS
CELL CARCINOMA

In this gross view, there is a very long plaque of carcinoma with its base in the lamina propria. Its luminal aspect has many spike-like projections: these are the epithelial spikes covered by thick keratin. (Courtesy of Dr. Karel Geboes, Leuven, Belgium.)

published ultrastructural studies, the basaloid cells had little cytoplasmic differentiation, although in one study, a few neurosecretory-like granules were found (181,184). Occasional distorted microvilli were found projecting into intercellular spaces. However, in neither study were the cells enveloped by massively duplicated basement membrane, a feature characteristic of adenoid cystic carcinoma of salivary glands.

It appears that these tumors arise from an in situ component on the surface, and dysplasia of different grades has been found in the overlying or marginal mucosa in several reported cases (178,181). Sometimes this is a full-thickness basaloid cell dysplasia, but in other cases, the invasive component appears to descend as single strands from the basal layer of an otherwise intact squamous surface (fig. 4-57).

This misnamed adenoid cystic carcinoma of the esophagus is probably nothing more than another unusual histologic variant of squamous cell carcinoma of the esophagus. The reported cases have the same male predominance; age distribution, with most patients in the sixth and seventh decades; location mainly in the middle esophagus, with fewer in the lower esophagus; symptoms of progressive dysphagia; and miserable prognosis of usual squamous cell carcinoma.

These unusual carcinomas appear to be identical to the recently described basaloid squamous cell carcinomas of the upper aerodigestive tract (174,182,183). They have the same histologic features, including cell type, in situ component, and aggressive behavior.

## Verrucous Squamous Cell Carcinoma

In the WHO classification of esophageal cancers, verrucous squamous cell carcinoma, an unusual neoplasm originally described in the oral cavity by Ackerman in 1948, is defined as "a malignant papillary tumor composed of well-differentiated squamous epithelium with minimal cytologic atypia and blunt, pushing margins rather than insinuating, tentacular growth" (figs. 4-58, 4-59) (190). To this definition should be added the fact that these tumors are covered by a thick layer of keratin (186,188). Verrucous carcinomas are slow growing. They may be locally aggressive but do not metastasize, unless they convert to a more aggressive carcinoma, a change that may follow radiation therapy. Most such tumors occur in the upper aerodigestive tract, the female genitalia, and the skin, especially of the feet.

There is one reported series of five esophageal verrucous carcinomas; otherwise, the literature only contains scattered case reports. There are less than 25 total cases reported in the English language literature in the past 30 years (189). Furthermore, some of the reported cases may not even be verrucous carcinomas, either because they appear to lack one or more of the required diagnostic features or because the diagnosis was

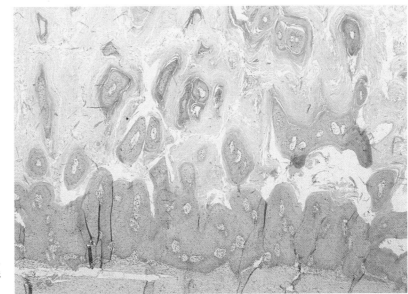

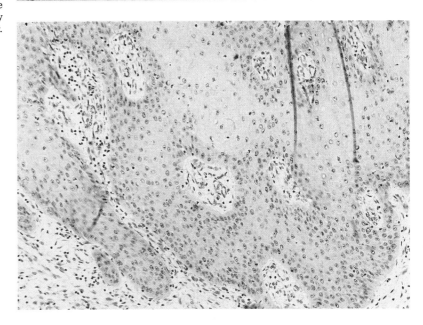

Figure 4-59
VERRUCOUS SQUAMOUS
CELL CARCINOMA

Top: A low-power view of the squamous spikes covered by keratin that also covers dips between them.

Bottom: High-power view of the blunted base. The tumor is unusually well differentiated. (Courtesy of Dr. Karel Geboes, Leuven, Belgium.)

made on small biopsies which may not capture enough of the tumor for a secure diagnosis. Nevertheless, if we assume that all reported cases are truly valid examples of the entity, then the following conclusions may be made. They share with usual squamous cell carcinoma of the esophagus the roughly 3 to 1 male predominance, an age range beginning with the fourth decade, and a median age in the seventh decade (185). They differ in that about a third arise in the upper esophagus. Peculiarly, the reported cases occurred in patients who had some of the more unusual risk factors for esophageal carcinoma. In two patients, the verrucous carcinomas were complications of achalasia, two others had esophageal diverticula, two more had histories of caustic esophageal strictures, and another had a postcricoid web, although the carcinoma was in the lower esophagus (185,187). Most were described as polypoid, cauliflower-like masses on endoscopy.

# REFERENCES

## Prevalence, Pathogenesis

1. Appelqvist P, Salmo M. Lye corrosion carcinoma of the esophagus. A review of 63 cases. Cancer 1980;45:2655–8.
2. Ayiomamitis A. Epidemiology of cancer of the esophagus in Canada: 1931-1984. Gastroenterology 1988;96:374–80.
3. Barch, DH, Jacoby RF, Brasitus TA, Radosevich JA, Carney WP, Iannaccone PM. Incidence of Harvey ras oncogene point mutations and their expression in methylbenzylnitrosamine-induced esophageal tumorigenesis. Carcinogenesis 1991;12:2373–7.
4. Benamouzig R, Pigot F, Quiroga G, et al. Human papillomavirus (HPV) infection in esophageal squamous-cell carcinoma in western countries. Int J Cancer 1992;50:549–52.
5. Bennett WP, Hollstein MC, He A, et al. Archival analysis of p53 genetic and protein alterations in Chinese esophageal cancer. Oncogene 1991;6:1779–84.
6. Blot WJ, Li JY, Taylor PR, et al. Nutrition intervention trials in Linxian, China: supplementation with specific vitamin/mineral combinations, cancer incidence, and disease-specific mortality in the general population. JNCI 1993;85:1483–92.
6a. Boring CC, Squires TS, Heath CW Jr. Cancer statistics for African Americans. CA Cancer J Clin 1992;42:7–17.
7. Boring CC, Squires TS, Tong T. Cancer statistics, 1993. CA Cancer J Clin 1993;43:7–26.
8. Bos JL. Ras oncogenes in human cancers: a review. Cancer Res 1989;49:4682–9.
9. Bulay O, Mirvish SS. Carcinogenesis in rat esophagus by intraperitoneal injection of different doses of methyl-n-amylnitrosamine. Cancer Res 1979;39:3644–6.
10. Chang F, Shen Q, Zhou J, Wang D, Syrjänen S, Syrjänen K. Detection of human papillomavirus DNA in cytologic specimens derived from esophageal precancer lesions and cancer. Scand J Gastroenterol 1990;25:383–8.
11. Chang F, Syrjänen S, Shen Q, Ji H, Syrjänen K. Human papillomavirus (HPV) DNA in esophageal precancer lesions and squamous cell carcinomas from China. Int J Cancer 1990;45:21–5.
12. Chang F, Syrjänen S, Shen Q, Wang L, Syrjänen K. Screening for human papillomavirus infections in esophageal squamous cell carcinomas by in situ hybridization. Cancer 1993;72:2525–30.
13 Chang F, Syrjänen S, Wang L, Syrjänen K. Infectious agents in the etiology of esophageal cancer. Gastroenterology 1992;103:1336–48.
14. Chuong JJ, DuBovik S, McCallum RW. Achalasia as a risk factor for esophageal carcinoma. A reappraisal. Dig Dis Sci 1984;39:1105–8.
15. Correa P. Precursors of gastric and esophageal cancer. Cancer 1982;50:2554–65.
16. Correa P, Seiber SM, Adamson RH, Dalgard DW, Rodriguez E, Santamaria C. Are there models in non-human primates of precursor lesions and squamous cell carcinoma of the esophagus? In: Giuli R, McCallum RW, eds. Benign lesions of the esophagus and cancer. Berlin: Springer-Verlag, 1989:798–808.
17. Crespi M, Munoz N, Grassi A, et al. Oesophageal lesions in northern Iran: a premalignant condition? Lancet 1979;2:217–20.
18. Dawsey SM, Lewin KJ, Liu FS, Wang GQ, Shen Q. Esophageal morphology from Linxian, China. Squamous histologic findings in 754 subjects. Cancer 1994;73:2027–37.
19. Dawsey SM, Lewin KJ, Wang GQ, et al. Esophageal squamous histology and subsequent risk of squamous cell carcinoma of the esophagus. A prospective follow-up study from Linxian, China. Cancer 1994;74:1686–92.
20. Ellis FH, Endo M, Giuli R. Degeneration of mega-esophagus. Is there a particular symptomatology? In: Giuli R, McCallum RW, eds. Benign lesions of the esophagus and cancer. Berlin: Springer-Verlag, 1989:705–9.
21. Guanrei Y, Songliang Q. Endoscopic surveys in high-risk and low-risk populations for esophageal cancer in China with special reference to precursors of esophageal cancer. Endoscopy 1987;19:91–5.
22. Hollstein MC, Peri L, Mandard AM, et al. Genetic analysis of human esophageal tumors from two high incidence geographic areas: frequent p53 base substitutions and absence of ras mutations. Cancer Res 1991;51:4102–6.
23. Hollstein MC, Smits AM, Galiana C, et al. Amplification of epidermal growth factor receptor gene but no evidence of ras mutation in primary human esophageal cancers. Cancer Res 1988;48:5119–23.
24. Imazeki F, Omata M, Nose H, Ohto M, Isono K. p53 gene mutations in gastric and esophageal cancers. Gastroenterology 1992;103:892–6.
25. Jiang W, Kahn SM, Guillem JG, Lu SH, Weinstein IB. Rapid detection of ras oncogenes in human tumors: applications for colon, esophageal, and gastric cancer. Oncogene 1989;4:923–8.
26. Kuylenstierna R, Munck-Wikland E. Esophagitis and cancer of the esophagus. Cancer 1985;56:837–9.
27. Mannell A, Murray W. Oesophageal cancer in South Africa. A review of 1926 cases. Cancer 1989;64:2604–8.
28. Marger RS, Marger D. Carcinoma of the esophagus and tylosis. A lethal genetic combination. Cancer 1993;72:17–9.
29. Meijssen MA, Tilanus HW, van Blankenstein M, Hop WC, Ong GL. Achalasia complicated by oesophageal squamous cell carcinoma: a prospective study in 195 patients. Gut 1992;33:155–8.
30. Mellow MH, Layne EA, Lipman TO, Kaushik M, Hostetler C, Smith JC Jr. Plasma zinc and vitamin A in human squamous carcinoma of the esophagus. Cancer 1983;51:1615–20.
31. Munoz N, Wahrendorf J, Bang LJ, et al. No effect of riboflavin, retinol, and zinc on prevalence of precancerous lesions of oesophagus. Randomized double-blind intervention study in high-risk population of China. Lancet 1985;2:111–4.
32. Orringer MB. Miscellaneous conditions of the esophagus. In: Orringer MB, ed. Shackelford's surgery of the alimentary tract, Vol. I. Philadelphia: WB Saunders, 1991:464–6.
33. Paraf F, Flejou JF, Potet F, Molas G, Fekete F. Esophageal squamous carcinoma in five patients with Barrett's esophagus. Am J Gastroenterol 1992;87:746–50.
34. Parkin DM, Laara E, Muir CS. Estimates of the worldwide frequency of sixteen major cancers in 1980. Int J Cancer 1988;41:184–97.
35. Qiu SL, Yang GR. Precursor lesions of esophageal cancer in high-risk populations in Henan province, China. Cancer 1988;62:551–7.

36. Rosengard AM, Hamilton SR. Squamous carcinoma of the esophagus in patients with Barrett esophagus. Mod Pathol 1989;2:2–7.

37. Rubio CA. Epithelial lesions antedating oesophageal carcinoma. I. Histologic study in mice. Path Res Pract 1983;176:269–75.

38. Rubio CA, Aberg B. Barrett's mucosa in conjunction with squamous carcinoma of the esophagus. Cancer 1991;68:583–6.

39. Sagar PM. Aetiology of cancer of the oesophagus: geographical studies in the footsteps of Marco Polo and beyond. Gut 1989;30:561–4.

40. Sammon AM. A case-control study of diet and social factors in cancer of the esophagus in Transkei. Cancer 1992;69:860–5.

41. Sankaranarayanan R, Duffy SW, Padmakumary G, Nair SM, Day NE, Padmanabhan TK. Risk factors for cancer of the oesophagus in Kerala, India. Int J Cancer 1991;49:185–9.

42. Sasano H, Guokon Y, Nishihira T, Nagura H. In situ hybridization and immunohistochemistry of p53 tumor suppresser gene in human esophageal carcinoma. Am J Pathol 1992;141:545–50.

43. Sons HU. Etiologic and epidemiologic factors of carcinoma of the esophagus. Surg Gynecol Obstet 1987;165:183–90.

44. Tavani A, Negri E, Franceschi S, La Vecchia C. Risk factors for esophageal cancer in women in northern Italy. Cancer 1993;72:2531–6.

45. Togawa K, Jaskiewicz K, Takahashi H, Meltzer SJ, Rustgi AK. Human papillomavirus DNA sequences in esophagus squamous cell carcinoma. Gastroenterology 1994;107:128–36.

45a. Toh Y, Kuwano H, Tanaka S, et al. Detection of human papillomavirus DNA in esophageal carcinoma in Japan by polymerase chain reaction. Cancer 1992;70:2234–8.

46. Tuyns AJ. Epidemiology of esophageal cancer in France. In: Pfeiffer CJ, ed. Cancer of the esophagus, Vol. 1. Boca Raton: CRC Press 1982:3–18.

47. von Hofe E, Newberne PM, Kennedy AR. Inhibition of N-nitrosomethylbenzylamine-induced esophageal neoplasms by the Bowman-Birk protease inhibitor. Carcinogenesis 1991;12:2147–50.

48. Wahrendorf J, Chang-Claude J, Liang QS, et al. Precursor lesions of oesophageal cancer in young people in a high-risk population in China. Lancet 1989;2:1239–41.

49. Wang YP, Han XY, Wang YL, et al. Esophageal cancer in Shanxi province, People's Republic of China: a case-control study in high and moderate risk areas. Cancer Causes Control 1992;3:107–13.

50. Williamson AL, Jaskiesicz K, Gunning A. The detection of human papillomavirus in oesophageal lesions. Anticancer Res 1991;11;263–6

51. Wilson R, Tickman R, Unger E, Varma V, Cohen C. Human papillomavirus infection and esophageal carcinoma: analysis by immunohistochemistry, in situ hybridization, and polymerase chain reaction. Mod Pathol 1990;3:107A.

52. Wu YK, Huang GJ, Shao LF, Zhang YD, Lin XS. Honored guest's address: progress in the study and surgical treatment of cancer of the esophagus in China, 1940-1980. J Thorac Cardiovasc Surg 1982;84:325–33.

53. Wychulis AR, Woolam GL, Andersen HA, Ellis FH Jr. Achalasia and carcinoma of the esophagus. JAMA 1971;215:1638–41.

54. Yang PC, Davis S. Incidence of cancer of the esophagus in the US by histologic type. Cancer 1988;61:612–7.

## Clinical and Morphologic Aspects, including
### Superficial Carcinoma, Dysplasias, Carcinoma In Situ, and Advanced Carcinoma

55. Anani PA, Gardiol D, Savary M, Monnier P. An extensive morphological and comparative study of clinically early and obvious squamous cell carcinoma of the esophagus. Pathol Res Pract 1991;187:214–9.

56. Anderson LL, Lad TE. Autopsy findings in squamous-cell carcinoma of the esophagus. Cancer 1982;50:1587–90.

57. Beahrs LH, Henson DE, Hutter RV, Myers MH. Manual for staging of cancer. 3rd ed. American Joint Committee on Cancer. Philadelphia: JB Lippincott, 1988.

57a. Berry B, Miller RR, Luoma A, et al. Pathologic findings in total esophagectomy specimens after intracavitary and external beam radiotherapy. Cancer 1989;64:1833–7.

58. Bogomoletz WV, Molas G, Gayet B, Potet F. Superficial squamous cell carcinoma of the esophagus. A report of 76 cases and review of the literature. Am J Surg Pathol 1989;13:535–46.

58a. Boring CC, Squires TS, Tong T. Cancer statistics, 1993. CA Cancer J Clin 1993;43:7–26.

59. Böttger T, Störkel S, Stöckle M, et al. DNA image cytometry: a prognostic tool in squamous cell carcinoma of the esophagus? Cancer 1991;67:2290–4.

60. Chan KW, Chan EY, Chan CW. Carcinoma of the esophagus. An autopsy study of 231 cases. Pathology 1986;18:400–5.

61. Darnton SJ, Allen SM, Edwards CW, Matthews HR. Histopathological findings in oesophageal carcinoma with and without preoperative chemotherapy. J Clin Pathol 1993;46:51–5.

62. Dawsey SM, Wang GQ, Weinstein WM, et al. Squamous dysplasia and early esophageal cancer in the Linxian region of China: distinctive endoscopic lesions. Gastroenterology 1993;105:1333–40.

63. Diehl LF. Radiation and chemotherapy in the treatment of esophageal cancer. Gastroenterol Clin North Am 1991;20:765–74.

64. Edwards JM, Hillier VF, Lawson RA, Mousalli H, Hasleton PS. Squamous carcinoma of the oesophagus: histological criteria and their prognostic significance. Br J Cancer 1989;59:429–33.

65. Endo M, Takeshita K, Yoshida M. How can we diagnose the early stage of esophageal cancer? Endoscopic diagnosis. Endoscopy 1986;18:11–8.

66. Ferguson MK, Skinner DB. Carcinoma of the esophagus and cardia. In: Orringer MB, ed. Shackelford's surgery of the alimentary tract, Vol. I. Philadelphia: WB Saunders, 1991:246–74.

67. Fogel TD, Harrison LB, Son YH. Subsequent upper aerodigestive malignancies following treatment of esophageal cancer. Cancer 1985;55:1882–5.

68. Gardiol D, Hurlimann J, Anani P. What is known about precursor and squamous cell carcinoma? Are there different nomenclatures in different parts of the world for these lesions? In: Giuli R, McCallum RW, eds. Benign lesions of the esophagus and cancer. Berlin: Springer-Verlag, 1989:790–8.

69. Gill PG, Denham JW, Jamieson GG, Devitt PG, Yeoh E, Olweny C. Patterns of treatment failure and prognostic factors associated with the treatment of esophageal carcinoma with chemotherapy and radiotherapy, either as sole treatments or followed by surgery. J Clin Oncol 1992;10:1037–43.

70. Goseki N, Koike M, Yoshida M. Histopathologic characteristics of early stage esophageal carcinoma. Cancer 1992;69:1088–93.

71. Guojun H, Lingfang S, Dawei Z, et al. Diagnosis and surgical treatment of early esophageal carcinoma. Chin Med J 1981;94:229–32.

72. Hagiwara A, Takahashi T, Kojima O, et al. Endoscopic local injection of a new drug-delivery form of peplomycin for superficial esophageal cancer: a pilot study. Gastroenterology 1993;104:1037–43.

73. Hambraeus GM, Mercke CE, Willen R, et al. Prognostic factors influencing survival in combined radiotherapy and surgery of squamous cell carcinoma of the esophagus with special reference to a histopathologic grading system. Cancer 1988;62:895–904.

74. Hermanek P, Sobin LH, eds. TNM classification of malignant tumours. 4th ed. Berlin: Springer-Verlag 1987:40–2.

75. Jin-Ming Y, Li-Hua Y, Guo-Qian, et al. Flow cytometric analysis DNA content in esophageal carcinoma. Correlation with histologic and clinical features. Cancer 1989;64:80–2.

76. Kaketani K, Saito T, Kobayashi M. Flow cytometric analysis of nuclear DNA content in esophageal cancer. Aneuploidy as an index for highly malignant potential. Cancer 1989;64:887–91.

77. Katlic MR, Wilkins EW Jr, Grillo HC. Three decades of treatment of esophageal squamous carcinoma at the Massachusetts General Hospital. J Thorac Cardiovasc Surg 1990;99:929–38.

78. Kato H, Tachimori Y, Watanabe H, et al. Intramural metastases of thoracic esophageal carcinoma. Int J Cancer 1992;50:49–52.

79. Kate H, Tachimori Y, Watanabe H, Yamaguchi H, Ishikawa T, Itabashi M. Superficial esophageal carcinoma. Surgical treatment and the results. Cancer 1990;66:2319–23.

80. Kelsen D. Chemotherapy for esophageal cancer. In: Orringer MB, ed. Shackelford's surgery of the alimentary tract, Vol. I. Philadelphia: WB Saunders, 1991:299–313.

81. Kondo K, Okuma T, Yoshioka M, Torigoe Y, Miyauchi Y, Katsuki T. Preoperative in vitro chemosensitivity test of esophageal cancer with endoscopic specimens. Cancer 1993;71:661–6.

82. Kuwano H, Baba K, Idebe M, et al. Gastric involvement of oesophageal squamous cell carcinoma. Br J Surg 1992;79:328–30.

83. Kuwano H, Matsuda H, Marsuoka H, Kai H, Okudaira Y, Sugimachi K. Intra-epithelial carcinoma concomitant with esophageal squamous cell carcinoma. Cancer 1987;59:783–7.

84. Kuwano H, Nagamatsu M, Ohno S, Matsuda H, Mori M, Sugimachi K. Coexistence of intraepithelial carcinoma and glandular differentiation in esophageal squamous cell carcinoma. Cancer 1988;62:1568–672.

85. Kuwano H, Ohno S, Matsuda H, Mori M, Sugimachi K. Serial histologic evaluation of multiple primary squamous cell carcinomas of the esophagus. Cancer 1988;61:1635–8.

86. Kuwano H, Ueo H, Sugimachi K, Inokuchi K, Toyoshima S, Enjoji M. Glandular or mucin-secreting components in squamous cell carcinoma of the esophagus. Cancer 1985;56:514–8.

87. Liu FS, Wang QL. Squamous cell carcinoma of the esophagus. In: Ming SC, Goldman H, eds. Pathology of the gastrointestinal tract. Philadelphia: WB Saunders, 1992:439–58.

88. Loizou LA, Rampton D, Atkinson M, Robertson C, Brown SG. A prospective assessment of quality of life after endoscopic intubation and laser therapy for malignant dysphagia. Cancer 1992;70:386–91.

89. Mandard AM. Tumors of the squamous epithelium. In: Whitehead R, ed. Gastrointestinal and oesophageal pathology. New York: Churchill Livingstone, 1989:663–8

90. Mandard AM, Chasle J, Marnay J, et al. Autopsy findings in 111 cases of esophageal cancer. Cancer 1981;48:329–35.

91. Mandard AM, Marnay J, Gignoux M, et al. Cancer of the esophagus and associated lesions: detailed study of 100 esophagectomy specimens. Hum Pathol 1984;5:660–9.

92. Matsuda H, Mori M, Tsujitani S, Ohno S, Kuwano H, Sugimachi K. Immunohistochemical evaluation of squamous cell carcinoma antigen and S-100 protein-positive cells in human malignant esophageal tissues. Cancer 1990;65:2261–5.

93. Matsuura H, Kuwano H, Morita M, et al. Predicting recurrence time of esophageal carcinoma through assessment of histologic factors and DNA ploidy. Cancer 1991;67:1406–11.

94. Ming SC. Tumors of the esophagus and stomach. Atlas of Tumor Pathology. 2nd Series, Fascicle 7. Washington: Armed Forces Institute of Pathology, 1973:30–43.

95. Misumi A, Harada K, Murikami A, et al. Early diagnosis of esophageal cancer. Analysis of 11 cases of esophageal mucosal cancer. Ann Surg 1989;210:732–9.

96. Mori M, Matsuda H, Kuwano H, Matsuura J, Sugimachi K. Oesophageal squamous cell carcinoma with lymphoid stroma. Virchows Arch [A] 1989;415:473–9.

97. Mori M, Tokino T, Yanagisawa A, Kanamori M, Kato Y, Nakamura Y. Association between chromosome 11q13 amplification and prognosis of patients with oesophageal carcinomas. Eur J Cancer 1992;28A:755–7.

98. Mukaida H, Toi M, Hirai T, Yamashita Y, Toge T. Clinical significance of the expression of epidermal growth factor and its receptor in esophageal cancer. Cancer 1991;68:142–8.

99. Munoz N, Lipkin M, Crespi M, Wahrendorf J, Grassi A, Lu SH. Proliferative abnormalities of the oesophageal epithelium of Chinese populations at high and low risk for oesophageal cancer. Int J Cancer 1985;36:187–9.

100. Nagamatsu M, Mori M, Kuwano H, Sugimachi K, Akiyoshi T. Serial histologic investigation of squamous epithelial dysplasia associated with carcinoma of the esophagus. Cancer 1992;69:1094–8.

101. Ohno S, Mori M, Tsutsui S, et al. Growth patterns and prognosis of submucosal carcinoma of the esophagus. A pathologic study. Cancer 1991;68:335–40.

102. Ohta H, Nakazawa S, Segawa K, Yoshino J. Distribution of epithelial dysplasia in the cancerous esophagus. Scand J Gastroenterol 1986;21:392–8.

103. Orringer MB. Complications of esophageal surgery. In: Orringer MB, ed. Shackelford's surgery of the alimentary tract, Vol. I. Philadelphia: WB Saunders 1991: 434–59.

104. Orringer MB. Transhiatal esophagectomy without thoracotomy. In: Orringer MB, ed. Shackelford's surgery of the alimentary tract, Vol. II. Philadelphia: WB Saunders, 1991:408–33.

105. Orringer MB, Forastiere AA, Perez-Tamayo C, Urba S, Takasugi BJ, Bromberg J. Chemotherapy and radiation therapy before transhiatal esophagectomy for esophageal carcinoma. Ann Thorac Surg 1990;49:348–55.

106. Ozawa S, Ueda M, Ando N, Shimizu N, Abe O. Prognostic significance of epidermal growth factor receptor in esophageal squamous cell carcinomas. Cancer 1989;63:2169–73.

107. Patil P, Redkar A, Patel SG, et al. Prognosis of operable squamous cell carcinoma of the esophagus. Relationship with clinicopathologic features and DNA ploidy. Cancer 1993;72:20–4.

108. Perez-Tamayo C. Radiation therapy in dhe treatment of carcinoma of the esophagus. In: Orringer MB, ed. Shackelford's surgery of the alimentary tract, Vol. II. Philadelphia: WB Saunders, 1991:275–98.

109. Petrovich Z, Lam K, Langholz B, Formenti S, Luxton G, Tildon T. Surgical therapy and radiotherapy for carcinoma of the esophagus. Treatment results in 195 patients. J Thorac Cardiovasc Surg 1989;98:614–7.

110. Porschen R, Bevers G, Remy U, Schauseil S, Borchard F. Influence of preoperative radiotherapy on DNA ploidy in squamous cell carcinomas of the oesophagus. Gut 1993;34:1086–90.

111. Qiu S, Yang G. Precursor lesions of esophageal cancer in high-risk populations in Henan province, China. Cancer 1988;62:551–7.

112. Resbeut M, Le Prise-Fleury E, Ben-Hassel M, et al. Squamous cell carcinoma of the esophagus. Treatment by combined vincristine-methotrexate plus folinic acid rescue and cisplatin before radiotherapy. Cancer 1985;56:1246–50.

113. Robaszkiewicz M, Reid BJ, Volant A, Cauvin JM, Rabinovitch PS, Gouerou H. Flow-cytometric DNA content analysis of esophageal squamous cell carcinomas. Gastroenterology 1991;101:1588–93.

114. Robey-Cafferty S. El-Naggar A, Sahin A, Bruner J, Ro J, Cleary K. Prognostic factors in esophageal squamous carcinoma: a study of clinicopathologic features, blood group expression, and DNA ploidy [Abstract]. Mod Pathol 1990;3:84.

115. Rosch T, Lorenz R, Zenker K, et al. Local staging and assessment of resectability in carcinoma of the esophagus, stomach and duodenum by endoscopic ultrasonography. Gastrointest Endosc 1992;38:460–7.

116. Ruol A, Segalin A, Panozzo M, et al. Flow cytometric DNA analysis of squamous cell carcinoma of the esophagus. Cancer 1990;65:1185–8.

117. Sasaki K, Murakami T, Murakami T, Nakamura M. Intratumoral heterogeneity in DNA ploidy of esophageal squamous cell carcinomas. Cancer 1991;68;2403–6.

118. Schmidt LW, Dean PJ, Wilson RT. Superficially invasive squamous cell carcinoma of the esophagus. A study of seven cases in Memphis, Tennessee. Gastroenterology 1986;91:1456–61.

119. Soga J, Tanaka O, Sasaki K, Kawaguchi M, Muto T. Superficial spreading carcinoma of the esophagus. Cancer 1982;50:1641–5.

120. Sons HU, Borchard F. Esophageal cancer. Autopsy findings in 171 cases. Arch Pathol Lab Med 1984;108:983–8.

121. Stephens JK, Bibbo M, Dytch H, Maiorana A, Ruol A, Little AG. Correlation between automated karyometric measurements of squamous cell carcinoma of the esophagus and histopathologic and clinical features. Cancer 1989;64:83–7.

122. Stephens RL, Hansen HH, Muggia FM. Hypercalcemia in epidermoid tumors of the head and neck and esophagus. Cancer 1973;31:1487–91.

123. Stewart FM, Harkins BJ, Hahn SS, Daniel TM. Cisplatin, 5-fluorouracil, mitomycin C, and concurrent radiation therapy with and without esophagectomy for esophageal carcinoma. Cancer 1989;64:622–8.

124. Sugimachi K, Ide H, Okamura T, Matsuura H, Endo M, Inokuchi K. Cytophotometric DNA analysis of mucosal and submucosal carcinoma of the esophagus. Cancer 1984;53:2683–7.

125. Sugimachi K, Kitamura K, Matsuda H, Mori M, Kuwano H, Ide H. Proposed new criteria for early carcinoma of the esophagus. Surg Gynecol Obstet 1991;173:303–8

126. Sugimachi K, Koga Y, Mori M, Huang J, Yang K, Zhang RG. Comparative data on cytophotometric DNA in malignant lesions of the esophagus in Chinese and Japanese. Cancer 1987;59:1947–50.

127. Tachimori Y, Watanabe H, Kato H, et al. Hypercalcemia in patients with esophageal carcinoma. The pathophysiologic role of parathyroid hormone-related protein. Cancer 1991;68:2625–9.

128. Takubo K, Mafune K, Tanaka Y, Miyama T, Fujita K. Basaloid-squamous carcinoma of the esophagus with marked deposition of basement membrane substance. Acta Pathol Jpn 1991;41:59–64.

129. Takubo K, Sasajima K, Yamashita K, Tanaka Y, Fujita K. Prognostic significance of intramural metastasis in patients with esophageal carcinoma. Cancer 1990;65:1816–9.

130. Takubo K, Sasajima K, Yamashita L, et al. Morphologic heterogeneity of esophageal carcinoma. Acta Pathol Jpn 1989;39:180–9.

131. Takubo K, Takai A, Takayama S, Sasajima K, Yamashita K, Fujita K. Intraductal spread of esophageal amous cell carcinoma. Cancer 1987;59:1751–7.

132. Takubo K, Takai A, Yamashita K, et al. Light and electron microscopic studies of perineural invasion by esophageal carcinoma. JNCI 1985;74:987–93.

133. Tauchi K. Kakudo K, Machimura T, Makuuchi H, Mitomi T. Superficial esophageal carcinoma. With special reference to basaloid features. Pathol Res Pract 1990;186:450–4.

134. Tio TL, Cohen P, Coene PP, et al. Endosonography and computed tomography of esophageal carcinoma. Preoperative classification compared to the new (1987) TNM system. Gastroenterology 1989;96:1478–86.

135. Watanabe H, Jass JR, Sobin LH. Histological typing of oesophageal and gastric tumours. Berlin: Springer-Verlag, 1990:3,17–18.

136. Yang K, Lipkin M. AE 1 cytokeratin reaction patterns in different differentiation states of squamous cell carcinoma of the esophagus. Am J Clin Pathol 1990;94:261–9.

137. Yano H, Shiozaki H, Kobayashi K, et al. Immunohistologic detection of the epidermal growth factor receptor in human esophageal squamous cell carcinoma. Cancer 1991;67:91–8.

138. Yoshinaka H, Shimazu H, Fukumoto T, Baba M. Superficial esophageal carcinoma: a clinicopathological review of 59 cases. Am J Gastroenterol 1991;86:1413–18.

**Diagnosis and Differential Diagnosis**

139. Berry GJ, Pitts WC, Weiss LM. Pseudomalignant ulcerative change of the gastrointestinal tract. Hum Pathol 1991;22:59–62.

140. Cusso X, Mones-Xiol J, Vilardell F. Endoscopic cytology of cancer of the esophagus and cardia: a long-term evaluation. Gastrointest Endosc 1989;35:321–3.

141. Dawsey SM, Yu Y, Taylor PR, et al. Esophageal cytology and subsequent risk of esophageal cancer. A prospective follow-up study from Linxian, China. Acta Cytol 1994;38:183–92.

142. Dowlatshahi K, Skinner DB, DeMeester TR, Zachary L, Bibbo M, Weid GL. Evaluation of brush cytology as an independent technique for detection of esophageal carcinoma. J Thorac Cardiovasc Surg 1985;89:848–51.

143. Endo M, Takeshita K, Yoshida M. How can we diagnose the early stage of esophageal cancer? Endoscopic diagnosis. Endoscopy 1986;18:11–8.

144. Graham DY, Schwartz JT, Cain GD, Gyorkey F. Prospective evaluation of biopsy number in the diagnosis of esophageal and gastric carcinoma. Gastroenterology 1982;82:228–31.

145. Hoover L, Berman JJ. Epithelial repair versus carcinoma in esophageal brush cytology. Diagn Cytopathol 1988;4:217–23.

146. Huang GJ, Shen Q. An evaluation of balloon cytology in the early detection of carcinoma of the esophagus. Jpn J Cancer Res 1986; 31:99–103.

147. Isaacson P. Biopsy appearances easily mistaken for malignancy in gastrointestinal endoscopy. Histopathology 1982;6:377–89.

148. Jessurun J, Paplanus SH, Nagle RB, Hamilton SR, Yardley JH, Tripp M. Pseudosarcomatous changes in inflammatory pseudopolyps of the colon. Arch Pathol Lab Med 1986;110:833–6.

149. Kuwano H, Kitamura K, Baba K, et al. Determination of the resection line in early esophageal cancer using intraoperative endoscopic examination with Lugol staining. J Surg Oncol. 1992;50:149–52.

150. Lal N, Bhasin DK, Malik AK, Gupta NM, Singh K, Mehta SK. Optimal number of biopsy specimens in the diagnosis of carcinoma of the oesophagus. Gut 1992;33:724–6.

151. Misumi A, Harada K, Murikami A, et al. Early diagnosis of esophageal cancer. Analysis of 11 cases of esophageal mucosal cancer. Ann Surg 1989;210:732–9.

152. Nabeya K, Hanaoka T, Onozawa K, Ri S, Kimura O. New measures for early detection of carcinoma of the esophagus. In: Siewert JR, Holscher AH, eds. Berlin: Springer-Verlag, 1987:105– 09.

153. Nash S. Benign lesions of the gastrointestinal tract that may be misdiagnosed as malignant tumors. Semin Diag Pathol 1990;7:102–14.

154. Petras RE, Hart WR, Bukowski RM. Gastric epithelial atypias associated with hepatic arterial infusion chemotherapy. Its distinction from early gastric carcinoma. Cancer 1985;56:745–50.

155. Shekitka KM, Helwig EB. Deceptive bizarre stromal cells in polyps and ulcers of the gastrointestinal tract. Cancer 1991;67:2111–7.

156. Shiozaki H, Tahara H, Kobayashi K, et al. Endoscopic screening of early esophageal cancer with the Lugol dye method in patients with head and neck cancers. Cancer 1990;66:2068–71.

157. Shu YJ. Cytopathology of the esophagus. An overview of esophageal cytopathology in China. Acta Cytolog 1983;27:7–16.

**Pseudosarcomatous Squamous Cell Carcinoma**

158. Appelman HD. Stromal tumors of the esophagus, stomach, and duodenum. In: Appelman HD, ed. Pathology of the esophagus, stomach, and duodenum. New York: Churchill Livingstone, 1984:198–201.

159. Du Boulay CE, Isaacson P. Carcinoma of the oesophagus with spindle cell features. Histopathology 1981;5:403–14.

160. Gal AA, Martin SE, Kernen JA, Patterson MJ. Esophageal carcinoma with prominent spindle cells. Cancer 1987;60:2244–50.

161. Halvorsen RA, Foster WL, Williford ME, Roberts L Jr, Postlethwait RW, Thompson WM. Pseudosarcoma of the esophagus: barium swallow and CT findings. J Can Assoc Radiol 1983;34:278–81.

162. Haratake J, Jimi A, Horie A, Inokuma T, Ohno M. Malignant mesenchymoma of the esophagus. Acta Pathol Jpn 1984;34:925–33.

163. Kuhajda FP, Sun TT, Mendelsohn G. Polypoid squamous cell carcinoma of the esophagus. A case report with immunostaining for keratin. Am J Surg Pathol 1983;7:495–9.

164. Linder J, Stein RB, Roggli VL, et al. Polypoid tumor of the esophagus. Hum Pathol 1987;18:692–700.

165. Olmsted WW, Lichtenstein JE, Hyams VJ. Polypoid epithelial malignancies of the esophagus. AJR Am J Roentgenol 1983;140:921–5.

166. Ooi A, Kawahara E, Okada Y, et al. Carcinosarcoma of the esophagus. An immunohistochemical and electron microscopic study. Acta Pathol Jpn 1986;36:151–9.

167. Orsatti G, Corvalan AH, Sakurai H, Choi H-SH. Polypoid adenosquamous carcinoma of the esophagus with prominent spindle cells. Report of a case with immunohistochemical and ultrastructural studies. Arch Pathol Lab Med 1993;117:544–7.

168. Osamura RY, Watanabe K, Shimamura K, et al. Polypoid carcinoma of the esophagus. A unifying term for "carcinosarcoma" and "pseudosarcoma." Am J Surg Pathol 1978;2:201–8.

169. Sasajima K, Takai A, Taniguchi Y, et al. Polypoid squamous cell carcinoma of the esophagus. Cancer 1989;64:94–7.

170. Takashi T, Ito H, Ogawa I, Miyauchi M, Ijuhin N, Nikai H. Spindle cell squamous carcinoma of the oral region. An immunohistochemical and ultrastructural study on the histogenesis and differential diagnosis with a clinicopathological analysis of six cases. Virchows Arch [A] 1991;419:177–82.

171. Takubo K, Tsuchiya S, Nakagawa H, Futatsuki K, Ishibashi I, Hirata F. Pseudosarcoma of the esophagus. Hum Pathol 1982;13:503–5.

172. Xu LT, Sun CF, Wu LH, Chang ZR, Liu TH. Clinical and pathological characteristics of carcinosarcoma of the esophagus: report of four cases. Ann Thorac Surg 1984;37:197–203.

## Basaloid Squamous (so-called Adenoid Cystic) Carcinoma

173. Akamatsu T, Honda T, Nakayama J, Nakamura Y, Katsuyama T. Primary adenoid cystic carcinoma of the esophagus. Report of a case and its histochemical characterization. Acta Pathol Jpn 1986;36:1707–17.

174. Banks ER, Frierson HF Jr, Mills SE, George E, Zarbo RJ, Swanson PE. Basaloid squamous cell carcinoma of the head and neck. A clinicopathologic and immunohistochemical study of 40 cases. Am J Surg Pathol 1992;16:939–46.

175. Bell-Thomson J, Haggitt RC, Ellis FH Jr. Mucoepidermoid and adenoid cystic carcinomas of the esophagus. J Thorac Cardiovasc Surg 1980;79:438–46.

176. Benisch B, Toker C. Esophageal carcinomas with adenoid cystic differentiation. Arch Otolaryng 1972;96:260–3.

177. Cerar A, Jutersek A, Vidmar S. Adenoid cystic carcinoma of the esophagus. A clinicopathologic study of three cases. Cancer 1991;67:2159–64.

178. Epstein JI, Sears DL, Tucker RS, Eagan JW Jr. Carcinoma of the esophagus with adenoid cystic differentiation. Cancer 1984;53:1131–6.

179. Kim JH, Lee MS, Cho SW, Shim CS. Primary adenoid cystic carcinoma of the esophagus: a case report. Endoscopy 1991;23:38–41.

180. Nelms DC, Luna MA. Primary adenocystic carcinoma (cylindromatous carcinoma) of the esophagus. Cancer 1972;29:440–3.

181. Sweeney EC, Cooney T. Adenoid cystic carcinoma of the esophagus: a light and electron microscopic study. Cancer 1980;45:1516–25.

182. Tsang WY, Chan JK, Lee KC, Leung AK, Fu YT. Basaloid-squamous carcinoma of the upper aerodigestive tract and so-called adenoid cystic carcinoma of the oesophagus: the same tumour type? Histopathology 1991;19:35–46.

183. Wain SL, Kier R, Vollmer RT, Rosen EH. Basaloid-squamous carcinoma of the tongue, hypopharynx, and larynx: report of 10 cases. Hum Pathol 1986;17:1158–66.

184. Zardawi IM, Talbot IC. Primary adenoid cystic carcinoma of the oesophagus. Diagnost Histopathol 1983;6:39–46.

## Verrucous Carcinoma

185. Agha FP, Weatherbee L, Sams JS. Verrucous carcinoma of the esophagus. Am J Gastroenterology 1984;79:844–9.

186. Ferlito A, Recher G. Ackerman's tumor [verrucous carcinoma] of the larynx: a clinicopathologic study of 77 cases. Cancer 1980;46:1617–30.

187. Jasim KA, Bateson MC. Verrucous carcinoma of the oesophagus—a diagnostic problem. Histopathology 1990;17:473–5.

188. Kraus FT, Perezmesa C. Verrucous carcinoma. Clinical and pathologic study of 105 cases involving oral cavity, larynx and genitalia. Cancer 1966;19:26–9.

189. Minielly JS, Harrison EG Jr, Fontana RS, Payne WS. Verrucous squamous cell carcinoma of the esophagus. Cancer 1967;20:2078–87.

190. Watanabe H, Jass JB, Sobin LH. Histological typing of oesophageal and gastric tumours. 2nd ed. Berlin: Springer-Verlag, 1990:12.

# 5
## BARRETT'S ESOPHAGUS, COLUMNAR DYSPLASIA, AND ADENOCARCINOMA OF THE ESOPHAGUS

Primary adenocarcinoma of the esophagus is a relatively uncommon tumor, accounting for between 1 and 50 percent of all malignant esophageal tumors, depending upon geographic location. In the United States, however, its incidence in the last 20 years has risen faster than that of any other cancer (8). Almost all cases of primary esophageal adenocarcinoma arise from Barrett's esophagus, although occasional cases arise from heterotopic mucosa of the upper esophagus, the esophageal mucosal glands, the ducts of submucosal glands, or the submucosal glands of the middle and lower third of the esophagus; proof of the latter three associations is tenuous, however. It is sometimes difficult to determine the exact site of origin of tumors at the cardioesophageal region, but it is thought that about 60 percent are probably of gastric origin (16) (see Carcinoma of the Gastric Cardia).

Because of the importance of Barrett's esophagus and dysplasia in the pathogenesis of esophageal adenocarcinoma, these entities are discussed before describing adenocarcinoma.

## BARRETT'S ESOPHAGUS

**Etiology and Pathogenesis.** In Barrett's esophagus the normal stratified squamous epithelium lining the esophagus is replaced by columnar epithelium for variable lengths from the lower esophageal sphincter region cephalad (figs. 5-1–5-3). The importance of this disorder is that it is associated with an increased risk of adenocarcinoma of the esophagus (3,95,120,139).

The most common predisposing factor for Barrett's esophagus is chronic gastroesophageal reflux. Evidence in support of this comes from the following observations: 1) patients with clinical gastroesophageal reflux have a much higher prevalence of Barrett's esophagus when compared with patients undergoing endoscopy for other reasons (13,54,76); 2) patients with reflux-associated conditions, such as scleroderma and achalasia after esophagomyotomy, have an increased prevalence of Barrett's esophagus

(1,46,73,88), and one patient with Zollinger-Ellison syndrome developed Barrett's esophagus and esophageal adenocarcinoma (125); 3) most children with Barrett's esophagus have a history of regurgitation in infancy and reflux symptoms, and many have gastroesophageal reflux as documented on radiography or by pH monitoring (21,47); and 4) the geographic variation in the prevalence of Barrett's esophagus parallels a similar variation in gastroesophageal reflux.

Other factors may also be associated with Barrett's esophagus, albeit much less commonly. These include esophageal bile reflux associated with the postgastrectomy state (73), esophageal injury following lye ingestion, and genetic predisposition. The common link appears to be esophageal acid reflux as it has been shown that alkaline reflux parallels acid reflux and can be largely abolished with potent acid antisecretory therapy (5,20,122,133b). It has also been suggested that there is a relationship between *Helicobacter pylori* infection in the stomach and Barrett's esophagus. However, reports regarding this relationship are contradictory and remain unproven (7,80,128). It is still possible that in some patients, Barrett's esophagus has a congenital basis. Congenital rests of gastric epithelium usually occur in the cervical epithelium but occasionally may be found in the distal esophagus (89). It is theoretically possible that some cases of Barrett's esophagus occur when these small rests expand in response to gastroesophageal reflux.

The sequence of events leading to Barrett's esophagus has not been clearly defined. It is probable that ulceration of the squamous epithelium occurs in response to gastroesophageal reflux of acid, bile, and duodenal contents and that reepithelialization occurs via multipotential stem cells which in turn differentiate into the variety of epithelial cells found in Barrett's esophagus. There may, however, be other mechanisms. It is possible, although unproven, that metaplasia occurs simply by the upward migration and overgrowth of columnar epithelium from the gastric cardia, in response to gastroesophageal reflux.

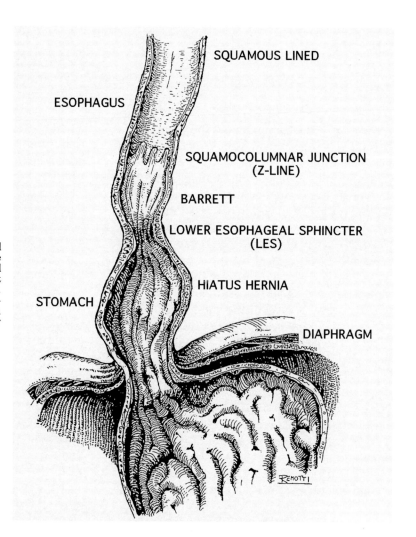

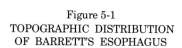

Figure 5-1
TOPOGRAPHIC DISTRIBUTION
OF BARRETT'S ESOPHAGUS

The lower esophageal sphincter is located in the chest above the diaphragm because Barrett's esophagus is invariably associated with a sliding hiatus hernia. The lowermost constriction marks the site of the diaphragm. Additional esophageal narrowing may sometimes be seen due to strictures associated with esophagitis with ulceration. (Illustration by Fabrizio Remotti, M.D.)

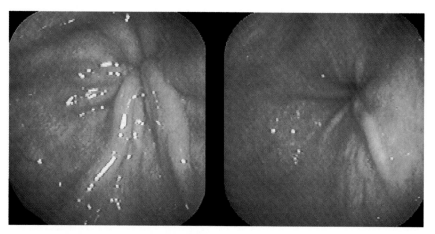

Figure 5-2
ENDOSCOPIC APPEARANCE OF A HIATUS HERNIA MIMICKING BARRETT'S ESOPHAGUS

If the lower esophagogastric sphincter is patulous, the landmarks of the lower esophagus may not be clearly visible. In these patients the location of the lower esophageal sphincter may be identified by insufflating air in order to demarcate the saccular hernia. The endoscopic view on the left is the regular view of a hiatus hernia and on the right the appearance after insufflation. Note the presence of the gastric folds, indicating that this is gastric mucosa. The folds radiate towards the esophagogastric junction.

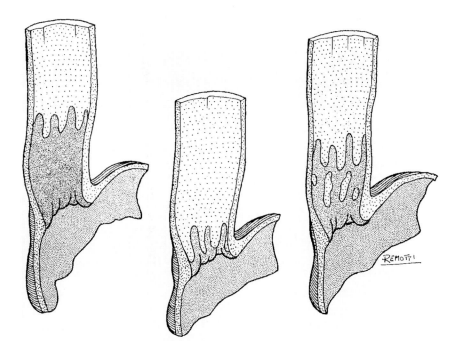

Figure 5-3
PATTERNS OF
BARRETT'S ESOPHAGUS
i) circumferential involvement; ii) short segment with tongues only; iii) circumferential involvement with residual whitish squamous islands. (Illustration by Fabrizio Remotti, M.D.)

Alternatively, as was postulated in the past, Barrett's esophagus may arise from congenital rests of gastric columnar epithelium, which usually occur in the cervical esophagus but have also been documented in the distal esophagus. Although these rests may account for rare cases of childhood Barrett's esophagus, there is no evidence of this mechanism in adults (25,63,84).

**Columnar Dysplasia in Barrett's Esophagus and Its Association with Esophageal Adenocarcinoma.** There is good evidence that the most important risk factor for esophageal columnar dysplasia is prolonged gastroesophageal reflux complicated by Barrett's esophagus. Most patients with dysplasia have a history of clinical gastroesophageal reflux (20,35,46,139), and dysplasia almost invariably develops in Barrett's epithelium (68). The international variation in the prevalence of esophageal columnar dysplasia parallels a similar variation in gastroesophageal reflux.

Dysplasia, especially high grade, is considered to be a precursor lesion for adenocarcinoma, based largely on retrospective histologic studies of adenocarcinoma in which dysplasia is commonly found in the adjacent mucosa. In addition, some patients with Barrett's esophagus followed by serial endoscopy appear to progress to low-grade dysplasia, then to high-grade dysplasia,

and on to cancer. It is presumed that low-grade dysplasia reflects a heightened cancer risk but this risk is less well defined than for high-grade dysplasia (15). Thus, the finding of dysplasia in a given patient may not only be a marker of heightened cancer risk but may itself already be associated with early invasive carcinoma elsewhere (68, 96). However, it should be stressed that the time sequence for the progression of dysplasia to carcinoma is variable, that it is not inevitable, and that even when dysplasia develops, it commonly does not progress further (44,68,96).

The pathogenic factors responsible for the transformation of epithelium in Barrett's esophagus to dysplasia and carcinoma remain unclear. It is most likely that they are multifactorial and include hereditary factors, infections with *H. pylori,* and continued reflux injury. It remains unclear whether it is the exposure to refluxing gastric acid or to the bile which predisposes this epithelium to dysplasia and carcinoma. There are some reports which have suggested that patients with Barrett's esophagus and complications, ulcers, strictures, or dysplasia, are more likely to have alkaline reflux than those with uncomplicated Barrett's disease (5). Some patients have developed dysplasia and carcinoma following antireflux therapy (16a,43,84,97,107,110,124).

However, this could be because acid suppression was incomplete. In fact, we and others have seen columnar-lined mucosa showing squamous metaplasia (suggesting possible regression of Barrett's esophagus) with maximal medical therapy or antireflux surgery (16a,43,55,107,113–115,125). Whether such therapies reduce the risk of adenocarcinoma in the esophagus is as yet unknown.

**Regression of Dysplasia in Barrett's Esophagus.** There have been sporadic reports of the regression of dysplasia in Barrett's esophagus (15,31,90,91,97,107,115). Since it has been shown that the development of dysplasia is accompanied by genomic instability and progressive genetic changes, it is hard to visualize regression of this process. To us it seems more likely that if dysplasia truly disappears, it may result from the body's immunologic response or the progression of the clonal process to a point of nonviability (i.e., necrosis). Other possible explanations for apparent regression of dysplasia are that the histologic changes diagnosed as dysplasia were in fact reactive atypia rather than true dysplasia; that dysplasia is still present but not detectable endoscopically; and that dysplasia was entirely removed by biopsy.

**DNA and Oncogene Markers.** Flow cytometry studies of epithelial DNA content in Barrett's esophagus with dysplasia (and also occasionally without) and carcinoma have clarified the sequence of events leading up to carcinoma at the cellular level. Barrett's esophagus is only rarely associated with abnormal nuclear DNA content (aneuploidy) or cell cycle abnormalities; however, such abnormalities are common in dysplasia and carcinoma (31,71,71a,94). Studies by Rabinovitch et al. (85) and others (31) have shown that the dysplasia of Barrett's esophagus commonly encompasses several different populations of aneuploid cells, but that early adenocarcinomas usually have only a single clone of aneuploid cells. These findings indicate that Barrett's esophagus is prone to genomic instability, which can result in multiple aneuploid populations; some patients develop a clone of cells that is capable of invasion (15,33,41,44,45).

Only a few oncogene studies have been performed on patients with Barrett's esophagus with and without dysplasia and carcinoma. Studies of p53 gene mutations have demonstrated different clones in mucosae from patients with Barrett's

dysplasia and patients with adenocarcinoma (9, 18,55a,59a,109). In addition, point mutations affecting the adenomatous polyposis coli (APC) suppressor gene, which were previously described for familial polyposis, have now also been demonstrated in both adenocarcinoma and squamous cell carcinoma of the esophagus (11). These findings support the concept that several genetic alterations are required for tumorigenesis to occur in Barrett's esophagus.

In another oncogene study, it was found that c-*myc* expression was consistently observed in all grades of dysplasia and carcinoma and the H-*ras* gene was consistently expressed in higher grades of dysplasia and carcinoma but absent in nondysplastic epithelium. H-*ras* expression may be a helpful marker for identifying dysplastic lesions that can progress to carcinoma (78). However, the potential clinical utility of specific oncogenes in predicting heightened cancer risk remains to be clarified (40).

**Prevalence and Incidence.** Barrett's esophagus is a complication that occurs in 10 to 20 percent of all patients with prolonged gastroesophageal reflux (15,80,110,118); these statistics come from studies of patients who had endoscopic evaluations for gastroesophageal reflux disease (120). However, a number of studies have indicated that Barrett's esophagus is probably more common than was previously thought. One study based on a review of all the records of patients with known Barrett's esophagus treated at the Mayo Clinic and other health providers in Olmsted county, Minnesota, found that the incidence of clinically apparent Barrett's esophagus was 18 cases per 100,000 population (17). Another study, based upon a prospective review of all autopsies performed at the Mayo Clinic, found that the frequency of Barrett's esophagus was 376 per 100,000 population (118). These two studies suggest that for each case of Barrett's esophagus being treated, there may be as many as 20 unrecognized cases in which dysplasia or carcinoma never develop (118). Many cases are not detected because only one third of patients with Barrett's esophagus in some series are symptomatic (19,116,124) and there is some evidence the Barrett mucosa is less sensitive to refluxed acid than is normal squamous mucosa (52,116).

The reported prevalence of dysplasia in Barrett's esophagus varies from 14 percent to as high as 40 percent (22). However, true prevalence figures for dysplasia are as difficult to obtain as they are for Barrett's esophagus, for the reasons given above. Furthermore, difficulty arises because most studies tend to lump together the findings of dysplasia and carcinoma. Thus, although it is true that most cases of adenocarcinoma of the esophagus are associated with dysplasia, there are a significant number of cases of dysplasia of the esophagus, especially low-grade dysplasia, without carcinoma.

The frequency of malignant change in Barrett's esophagus remains unclear. The prevalence rate of adenocarcinoma at the time of diagnosis of Barrett's esophagus is 7 to 15 percent (79). Based on retrospective studies, the incidence of adenocarcinoma of the esophagus developing in patients with Barrett's esophagus without evidence of dysplasia has been estimated at between 1 in 440 and 1 in 52 patient years, a risk that is 30 to 125 times greater than that in the population without Barrett's esophagus. Speckler (119,121) has extrapolated these data to calculate an incidence of 500 cancers per 100,000 patients with Barrett's esophagus per year. These figures imply that the risk of developing carcinoma in the lifetime of a patient who has Barrett's esophagus at age 50 is 5 to 10 percent (16a,50,84,120,121,124). The wide range of estimates reflects the retrospective nature of most of the studies or the bias related to the selection process of patients sent to referral centers (118,120). For example, in one referral population of 50 patients, 7 had dysplasia at the beginning of the study, 13 developed dysplasia, and 5 developed invasive carcinoma in a follow-up period averaging 5.2 years, an incidence of carcinoma 125 times over that of the general population. It is also possible that the patients who developed cancer already had it at the initial presentation but it was histologically undetected (42).

There are only a few prospective studies evaluating the true cancer incidence in Barrett's esophagus. In a study conducted by the American College of Gastroenterology, 6 of 220 patients with Barrett's esophagus developed adenocarcinoma (1 case per 150 person years). The mean length of follow-up was about 4 years (range, 0.1 to 19.1 years) (84). In two other studies, the incidence was 1 per 175 person years (120) and 1 per 441 person years (16a). Thus, although high-grade dysplasia is a good indicator for high risk

of adenocarcinoma, better prospective long-term follow-up is needed to determine the proportion of patients who do develop adenocarcinoma.

The risk of carcinoma developing in short-segment Barrett's esophagus, defined as a 1- to 2-cm affected segment in the distal esophagus, is unknown (37,41). The risk of developing cancer appears to be similar to that with usual cases of Barrett's esophagus and is unrelated to the length of the columnar lined segment (45,68).

Another problem lies in separating these cases from carcinomas of the gastric cardia (see Differential Diagnosis of Esophageal Adenocarcinoma). However, increasing evidence suggests that adenocarcinoma of the gastric cardia belongs to the same spectrum of disease as Barrett-associated adenocarcinoma (53,66,137).

There is marked geographic variation in the prevalence of Barrett's esophagus with dysplasia, which parallels the prevalence of gastroesophageal reflux. It is much less common in Japan and China, where reflux esophagitis is rare, than in Europe and North America.

**Clinical Features.** Barrett's esophagus, with or without dysplasia, is most commonly diagnosed between the ages of 40 and 60 years (23), but it can also occur in children (47). There is a clear-cut predominance in white males over females, in the order of 4 to 1 (84). The disorder is uncommon in blacks: less than 2 percent of blacks with gastroesophageal reflux have Barrett's esophagus (84). There is an association with heavy cigarette smoking and alcohol abuse. In one study, 85 percent of patients with Barrett's esophagus were heavy cigarette smokers and 16 percent were alcohol abusers (120).

Most patients with Barrett's esophagus and dysplasia are asymptomatic. Those with symptoms exhibit no unique clinical features beyond those of chronic gastroesophageal reflux disease. These clinical features include regurgitation, heartburn, dysphagia, and odynophagia (pain on swallowing) which is usually due to ulceration or stricture. A change in symptoms, such as progressive dysphagia, is likely to portend the development of advanced esophageal cancer (116,124).

Squamous cell carcinoma and adenosquamous tumors of the esophagus have been reported in patients with Barrett's esophagus (103,105). In one study, Barrett's esophagus was found in 13 of 42 cases (40 percent) of squamous cell carcinoma of the esophagus, however, the dysplasia and carcinoma were separated from the Barrett's esophagus by normal squamous epithelium, supporting the view that the two are not pathogenetically related (105). It is probable that the simultaneous occurrence of Barrett's esophagus and squamous cell cancer is related to common risk factors, such as alcohol and smoking.

Data on whether the incidence of colonic adenomas and adenocarcinomas is increased in patients with Barrett's esophagus is conflicting (86,99,117,132).

**Gross and Endoscopic Findings.** Barrett's esophagus almost always occurs in conjunction with a sliding esophageal hernia (fig. 5-1). The endoscopic features and the gross appearance of resected specimens are quite distinctive. The squamocolumnar junction is displaced, with a salmon-pink mucosa extending proximally from its usual location at the esophageal sphincter (fig. 5-4A,B). Whitish squamous islands are commonly seen in the proximal few centimeters (fig. 5-4C,D). Ulcerations may be seen anywhere in the zone of metaplasia. Segments of Barrett mucosa shorter than 5 cm may not exhibit circumferential involvement but may appear as tongues of red mucosa extending cephalad (fig. 5-4D,E).

In almost all cases, the endoscopic and gross appearances of Barrett's esophagus with dysplasia or early cancer cannot be distinguished from those of simple Barrett's metaplasia, so multiple biopsies are usually necessary. However, on rare occasions dysplasia has presented as small, sometimes multiple, pedunculated adenomas (44,57,70,130,137).

Originally it was thought that dysplasia was a multifocal process. However, mapping studies that we and others have done show that it is commonly a unifocal process, as is the invasive carcinoma when present. The dysplastic process may involve the entire Barrett's mucosa or a limited area (68,96).

**Microscopic Findings.** By definition, Barrett's esophagus is a metaplastic process in which columnar epithelium, usually accompanied by underlying mucous glands, replaces the normal esophageal squamous epithelium for variable lengths from the lower esophageal sphincter region cephalad (figs. 5-5, 5-6). The metaplastic epithelium is typically characterized by the presence of a variety of cells such as goblet cells, gastric and intestinal (small bowel and colonic) columnar cells, intermediate cells (with mixed features of gastric and intestinal cells), Paneth cells, and endocrine cells. Pancreatic acinar metaplasia may also be found in about 10 percent of individuals, primarily in the region of the lower esophageal sphincter (figs. 5-6–5-12) (55b, 61,143). The presence of goblet cells is the most useful feature for diagnosis of Barrett's esophagus since these cells are not normally present in gastric cardiac or fundic mucosa. This is especially important since the gastroesophageal junction, which is the point at which the tubular esophagus joins the saccular stomach, does not always coincide with the squamocolumnar junction. The latter may lie anywhere within the region of the lower esophageal sphincter which occupies approximately the distal 2 cm of the esophagus. As a result, the finding of gastric cardiac or fundic mucosa within the lower esophageal sphincter should not be considered indicative of Barrett's metaplasia whereas goblet cells should. Goblet cells also help distinguish between an eccentric esophagogastric junction and a short Barrett segment. However, from a practical point, the exact site of the goblet cells within the gastroesophageal region is not that critical since this metaplastic change denotes an increased risk of cancer both in the esophagus and the gastric cardia (36,37,122a). The metaplastic epithelium has been given a variety of names such as specialized epithelium (45), which we favor; distinctive epithelium (80); and Barrett's mucosa. Histologically, it is identical to intestinal metaplasia of the incomplete type (type II and III) in the stomach (69).

Another problem sometimes results from misinterpretation of the finding of fundic-type mucosa. Fundic mucosa does not occur in Barrett's esophagus but is the result of a hiatus hernia, which is almost invariably associated with Barrett's esophagus. In some patients the landmarks of the lower esophagus may not be clearly visible especially if the lower esophagogastric sphincter is patulous (36). In such patients the location of the lower esophageal sphincter may be identified by gently insufflating air to demarcate the saccular hernia from the tubular esophagus and to demonstrate the proximal margins of the gastric folds which end at the sphincter (36,37).

There are two major epithelial components of Barrett's esophagus: the surface epithelium and

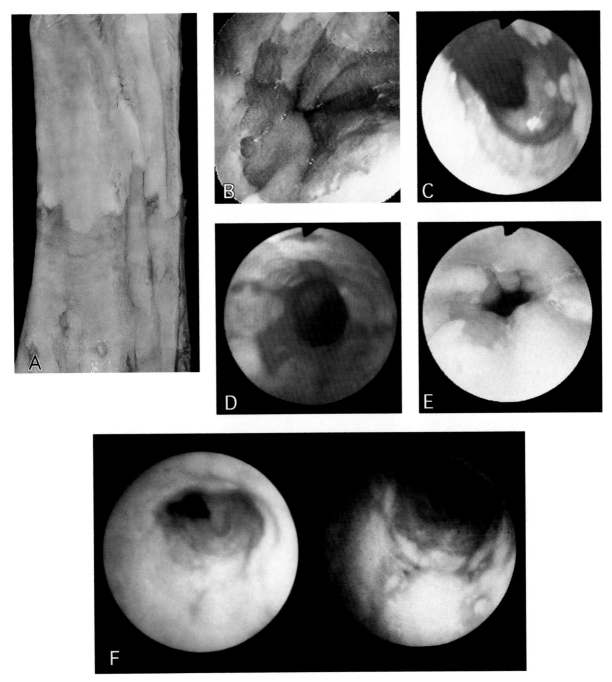

Figure 5-4
ENDOSCOPIC AND GROSS APPEARANCE OF NORMAL ESOPHAGUS
AT THE LOWER ESOPHAGEAL SPHINCTER AND BARRETT'S ESOPHAGUS

A: Esophagectomy specimen shows high-grade dysplasia unassociated with any gross lesions. There is circumferential replacement of the normal squamous epithelium by salmon-pink mucosa extending proximally from its usual location at the esophageal sphincter.

B: Endoscopic appearance of the normal esophagogastric junction (z-line).

C: Endoscopic appearance of Barrett's mucosa from the mid-esophagus showing circumferential involvement with residual whitish squamous islands.

D: Endoscopic appearance showing four mucosal tongues extending proximally from the esophagogastric junction.

E: Endoscopic appearance of a short segment showing short tongues of Barrett's mucosa extending upward from the gastroesophageal sphincter.

F: Endoscopic appearance showing circumferential involvement as well as mucosal tongues extending proximally.

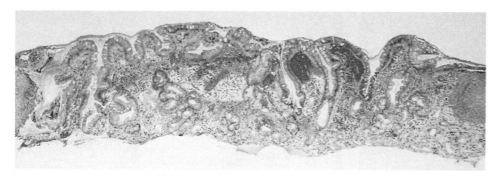

Figure 5-5
HISTOLOGY OF BARRETT'S ESOPHAGUS
Low-power view of a tongue of Barrett's mucosa with squamous epithelium on either side.

the underlying glands (fig. 5-6). Additionally, it has been shown that there may be reduplication of the muscularis mucosae with interposition of lamina propria between the two muscular layers. This may have clinical implications if invasion of the first layer of muscularis mucosae does not involve the submucosa because of new layers of lamina propria and muscularis mucosae. However, this remains to be confirmed (127).

**Histologic Findings.** The mucosal surface is usually flat and composed of pits or crypt-like structures as in the stomach but can be villiform especially if inflamed (fig. 5-7). The epithelium covering the surface and the pits is lined by a blend of goblet cells and columnar cells (fig. 5-6). The goblet cells characteristically contain acidic mucins, usually consisting of admixtures of sialomucins and lesser amounts of sulfomucins, which stain positively with Alcian blue at a low pH (2.5) (fig. 5-11A,B). The columnar cells are often heterogeneous: some resemble normal gastric foveolar epithelium, intestinal absorptive cells, or gastric mucous neck cells, whereas others are atypical (fig. 5-11C–E). For example, some of gastric-type columnar cells have an eosinophilic rather than clear cytoplasm. A significant number of these cells stain for acid mucins with Alcian blue at low pH (77a). A number of intestinal-type columnar absorptive cells have only a partially developed brush border. The mucous cell metaplasia of Barrett's esophagus may also include colon-like acid-sulfated mucins, demonstrable with the high iron diamine stain (fig. 5-11E) (28). Approximately half or more of biopsy specimens from Barrett's esophagus have scattered cells containing these mucins (59,143).

The question is frequently raised as to whether the Alcian blue stain is required for the diagnosis of Barrett's esophagus. In most instances goblet cells are numerous and easily found and therefore the special stain is unnecessary. However, Alcian blue stain is useful in detecting isolated goblet cells when histologically differentiating a short-segment Barrett's esophagus and an eccentric gastroesophageal junction.

**Glandular Component of Barrett's Esophagus.** In addition to metaplasia of surface and pit epithelium, there is metaplasia of mucous glands (figs. 5-5, 5-6). These glands are usually present as a thin band overlying the muscularis mucosae, but often they are sparse or even absent. They are usually composed of pure mucous glands but occasionally contain scattered parietal cells and resemble cardiac-type glands. As previously mentioned, we believe that if fundic-type mucosa is found in the esophagus, it almost always represents a hiatus hernia rather than Barrett's esophagus. In addition, Barrett's esophagus should not be confused with congenital islands of ectopic gastric mucosa, usually of fundic type. These occur mainly in the cervical esophagus (the inlet patches) and are characteristically separated from the stomach by a zone of intact squamous epithelium (see Heterotopic Gastric Mucosa at the end of this chapter).

Sometimes the glands become cystically dilated and may insinuate themselves between the muscle fibers of the muscularis mucosae and thus mimic early adenocarcinoma, especially if there is dysplasia. Differentiation between benign, dysplastic, and malignant cysts depends upon a careful examination of the cytology of the cells lining the cysts.

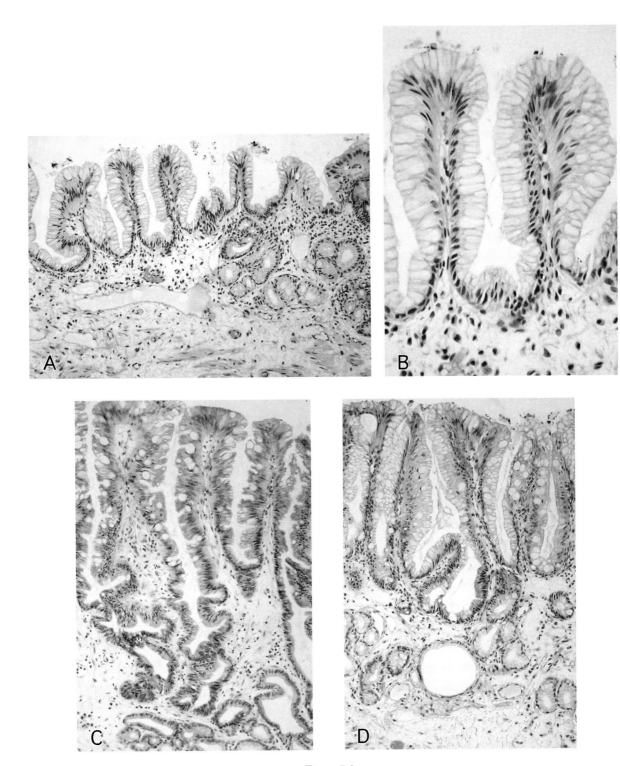

Figure 5-6
HISTOLOGY OF BARRETT'S ESOPHAGUS

A: Low-power view showing a predominantly columnar-lined surface epithelium, pits of gastric type, and underlying mucous glands with occasional intestinalized crypts.
B: High-power magnification of A showing columnar-lined epithelium.
C: Esophageal mucosa showing a predominantly intestinalized epithelium.
D: Barrett's mucosa showing a mixture of goblet cells and gastric-type columnar cells containing apical mucus droplets.

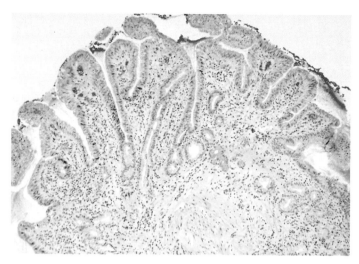

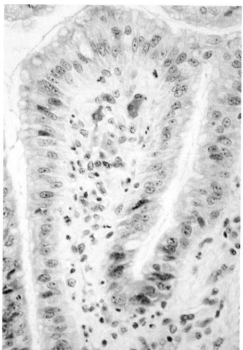

Figure 5-7
HISTOLOGY OF BARRETT'S ESOPHAGUS

Above: Low-power view of the mucosa showing the villous pattern typically seen in areas of erosion with regeneration.

Right: Higher magnification shows one of the villous proliferations lined by nondysplastic regenerative epithelium.

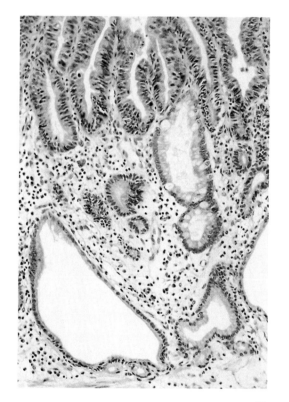

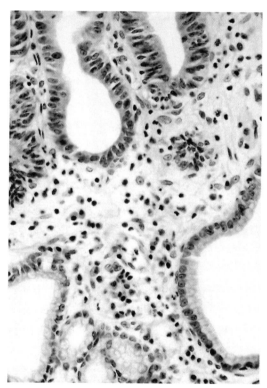

Figure 5-8
HISTOLOGY OF BARRETT'S ESOPHAGUS

Left: There is dysplasia of the surface, foveolar epithelium, and cystic dilatation of the mucous glands.

Right: Higher magnification shows the dysplastic foveolar epithelium and the underlying cystic mucous glands lined by nondysplastic epithelium.

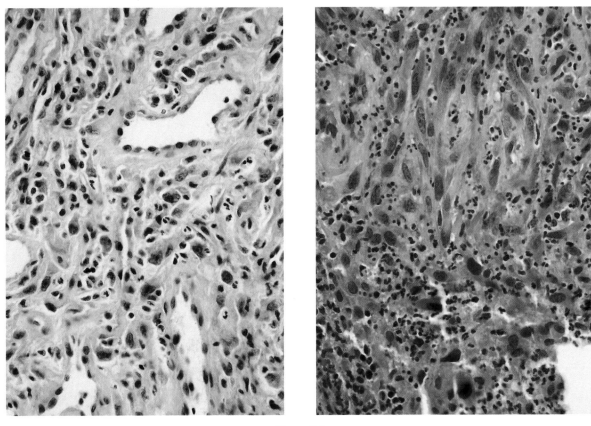

Figure 5-9
HISTOLOGY OF BARRETT'S ESOPHAGUS WITH MUCOSAL EROSION AND BIZARRE STROMAL CELLS
Left: Granulation tissue with an inflammatory infiltrate containing enlarged atypical macrophages.
Right: Acutely inflamed lamina propria with numerous enlarged, atypical stromal cells.

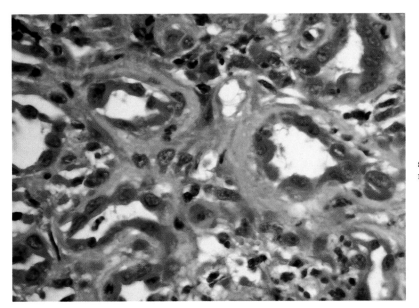

Figure 5-10
BARRETT'S ESOPHAGUS
WITH EROSION MIMICKING
ADENOCARCINOMA
Note the exuberant granulation tissue in which the prominent vessels may mimic adenocarcinoma.

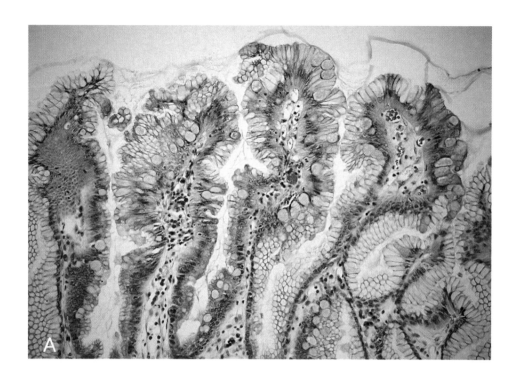

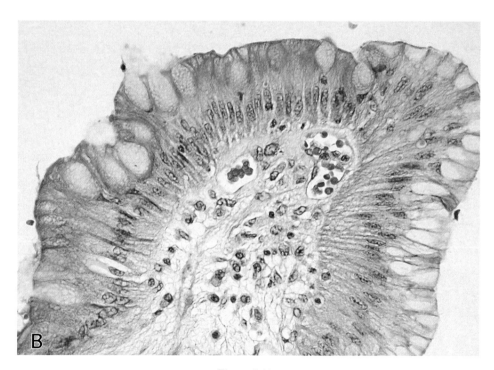

Figure 5-11
MUCIN STAINS OF BARRETT'S MUCOSA

A: Alcian blue stain of Barrett's mucosa shows the blue-staining goblet cells, a few specialized columnar cells, and the clear-staining gastric-type surface columnar cells.

B: Higher magnification of A shows the three cell types.

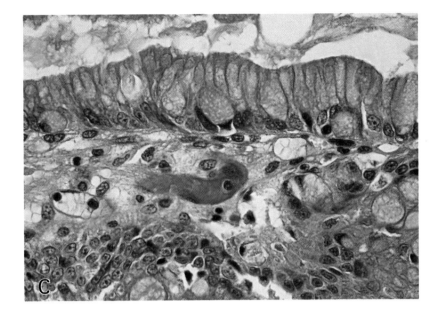

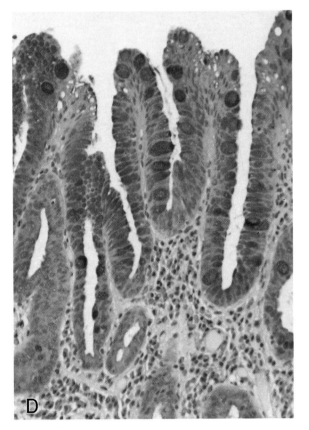

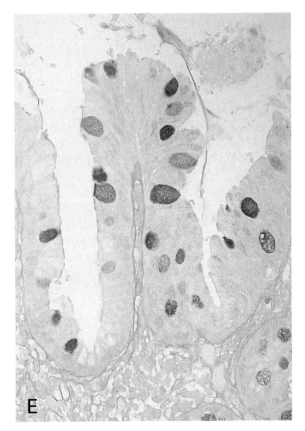

Figure 5-11 (Continued)

C: High-power magnification shows the blue-staining goblet and columnar cells.

D: PAS/Alcian blue stains demonstrate acid (blue) and neutral mucins (reddish-purple).

E: High iron diamine stains for sulfated (brown) and nonsulfated (blue) mucins.

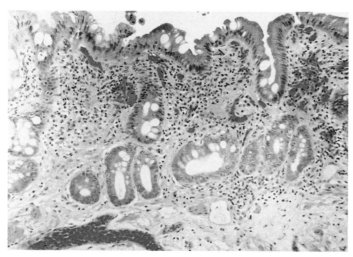

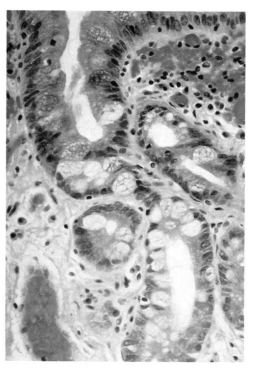

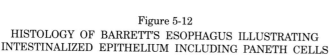

**Figure 5-12**
HISTOLOGY OF BARRETT'S ESOPHAGUS ILLUSTRATING
INTESTINALIZED EPITHELIUM INCLUDING PANETH CELLS

Above: Low-power view showing intestinalized mucosa.
Right: High-power view of an intestinal crypt with numerous Paneth cells at the base and side and numerous goblet cells in the upper half of the mucosa. (Hematoxylin and eosin/Alcian blue stain)

In the case of Barrett's esophagus, the cells lack features of dysplasia and carcinoma.

Other gastrointestinal elements may be present within the glands. These include Paneth cells (fig. 5-12) (39,56,98,112), endocrine cells, and pancreatic acini. Pepsinogen I, normally found in chief cells, and pepsinogen II, also found in chief cells and in antral and cardiac glands, have been demonstrated immunohistochemically in Barrett's mucosa (72).

There is usually only a mild accompanying inflammatory infiltrate of mononuclear cells in the lamina propria of Barrett's esophagus. However, sometimes the inflammation is intense, with heavy neutrophilic infiltration and erosions. *H. pylori* may be found in the esophagus of some patients with Barrett's mucosa, primarily in the cardiac-type mucosa, especially in mucosa that is actually inflamed (65,81,128,129). The organisms are present only in the distal 4 cm of the esophagus and only when they occur in the stomach as well (81,129). Thus, their presence appears to represent a consequence of reflux rather than a primary infection.

Biopsies from eroded or ulcerated areas reveal a superficial fibrino-purulent exudate, underly-

ing granulation tissue, and occasionally, bizarre stromal cells (fig. 5-9). Sometimes biopsies from what appears to be an ordinary Barrett's mucosa show large foci of granulation tissue when an erosion is not apparent endoscopically. Exuberant granulation tissue may on occasion mimic glandular epithelium and be confused with adenocarcinoma (fig. 5-10), particularly at frozen section; serial sections help differentiate the microvessels of granulation tissue from malignant glandular formation and factor VIII immunostaining helps confirm the vascular nature of the lesion. The bizarre stromal cells can sometimes be confused with sarcoma.

Biopsy specimens sometimes show squamous epithelium overlying specialized columnar epithelium (110), especially from the proximal zone of Barrett's esophagus. This change has been designated as "pseudoregression" or squamous metaplasia of the columnar epithelium (fig. 5-13). Presumably this represents an attempt to reverse the metaplastic process. This finding may be seen in cases of partial regression of Barrett's mucosa after antireflux medication or antireflux surgery (fundoplication) (16a,43,55,107,113–115,125).

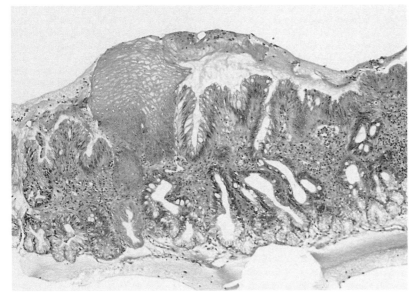

Figure 5-13
HISTOLOGY OF
BARRETT'S ESOPHAGUS
This section shows a small island of squamous epithelium replacing the surface columnar cells.

Figure 5-14
HISTOLOGIC MAP OF A PATIENT WITH DYSPLASIA AND INTRAMUCOSAL CARCINOMA IN BARRETT'S ESOPHAGUS
(Fig. 4 from Reid BJ, Weinstein WM, Lewin KJ, et al. Endoscopic biopsy can detect high-grade dysplasia or early adenocarcinoma in Barrett's esophagus without grossly recognizable neoplastic lesions. Gastroenterology 1988;94:81–90.)

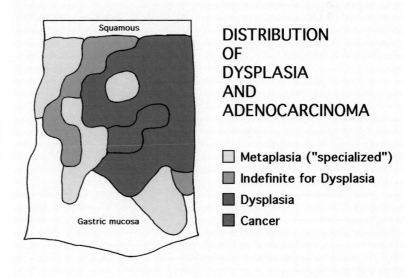

DISTRIBUTION OF DYSPLASIA AND ADENOCARCINOMA

☐ Metaplasia ("specialized")
☐ Indefinite for Dysplasia
☐ Dysplasia
☐ Cancer

## BARRETT'S DYSPLASIA

**Definition.** Dysplasia is defined as a benign neoplastic change of the epithelium confined to the basement membrane of the glands, that is, showing no evidence of invasion. High-grade dysplasia includes carcinoma in situ which is not reported separately as such. In assessing biopsies from patients with Barrett's esophagus, the main role of the pathologist is to be on the alert for histologic features of dysplasia and early adenocarcinoma because these are rarely visible endoscopically. Occasionally, however, the dysplastic epithelium proliferates in the form of a mass and is termed adenoma (57,68,96).

**Microscopic Findings.** Dysplasia invariably develops in a background of specialized (intestinalized) epithelium (fig. 5-14). We have found it in all parts of Barrett's esophagus, unrelated to the duration of disease (68,96). Microscopically, there is a combination of cytologic and architectural abnormalities which usually involve the full thickness of the mucosa or predominantly the surface and upper portion of the glandular crypt.

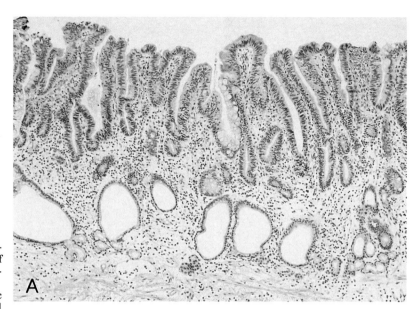

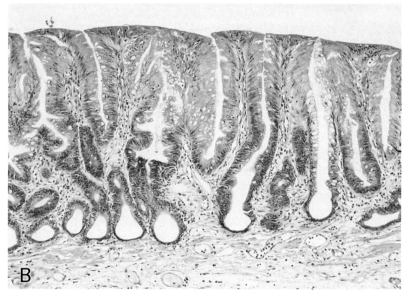

Figure 5-15
BARRETT'S ESOPHAGUS WITH
DYSPLASIA ILLUSTRATING
DISTRIBUTION OF
DYSPLASTIC EPITHELIUM

The dysplastic changes are commonly seen in the superficial portions of the mucosa but may sometimes be localized to the lower portions of the crypts.

A: In this section the dysplastic changes are present in the superficial portions of the mucosa. Note the underlying nondysplastic mucous glands, some of which are cystically dilated, in the lower portion of the mucosa.

B: Dysplastic epithelium occupies the lower half of the glands.

However, there are frequent exceptions to this "top-half" phenomenon, with predominant involvement of the lower portion of the gland crypts and surface maturation (fig. 5-15).

The dysplastic gland, may retain their normal configuration but more commonly they display architectural changes: budding, branching, crowding, and irregular shapes with papillary extensions into the lumina (fig. 5-15). An exaggerated villous configuration may be present. Cystic dilatation of the dysplastic mucosal glands may develop (fig. 5-15D), and may cause difficulty in differentiating dysplastic esopha-geal glands "trapped" in collagen-rich lamina propria and true invasive adenocarcinoma, especially in biopsy specimens (fig. 5-15D). The histogenesis of these cysts has been ascribed to a combination of two main factors: compression of the glandular outlets by fibrosis of the lamina propria, with proliferation of the muscularis mucosae and occlusion of the glands by proliferating dysplastic cells (106). In our experience, cystically dilated glands in Barrett's esophagus usually occur in the absence of significant fibrosis, so there appears to be still other causes for the cystic dilation.

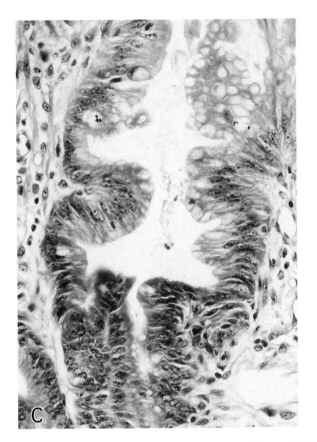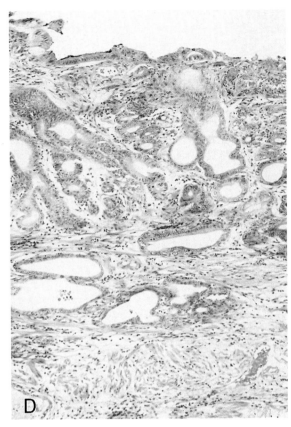

Figure 5-15 (Continued)

C: Higher magnification of the dysplastic epithelium in B showing marked crowding and pseudostratification of the enlarged hyperchromatic nuclei and sparsity of cytoplasm.

D: High-grade dysplasia with cystic dilatation of dysplastic glands. The glands in the lower portion of the mucosa appear to infiltrate the muscularis mucosae suggesting an early carcinoma.

**Cytologic Findings.** Dysplasia almost always shows both mucus depletion and prominent cytoplasmic basophilia, features that are easily recognized at low-power magnification (fig. 5-16). Cytologically, two types of dysplasia have been described (110). In our experience, these represent different grades of dysplasia. One type of dysplasia mimics adenomatous change elsewhere in the gastrointestinal tract, with nuclear crowding; stratification; enlarged, elongated hyperchromatic nuclei, often with small inconspicuous nucleoli; and increased numbers of abnormally shaped mitoses. This type of dysplasia is closely associated with intestinal metaplasia and typically gives rise to "intestinal types" of invasive carcinoma (fig. 5-17B). The second type consists of cells that have lost their nuclear polarity but are not stratified. The nuclei occupy the basal half of each cell and are round, enlarged, pleomorphic, and vesiculated, with a dense chromatin margin and one or more prominent nucleoli (figs. 5-18, 5-19) (44,58,93). This dysplasia is frequently associated with incomplete intestinal metaplasia characterized by epithelium with gastric-type mucin production. When carcinoma supervenes, it is usually of the poorly differentiated type. Both types of dysplasia are often found together. When carcinoma occurs in these cytologically mixed cases, it usually arises from the second type of dysplasia.

**Grading of Dysplasia.** A grading system for the dysplasia associated with Barrett's esophagus is now well accepted, and is similar to that employed for dysplasia in ulcerative colitis: high grade, low grade, and indefinite for dysplasia. Intramucosal carcinoma refers to neoplastic change that has invaded the lamina propria. The diagnosis of dysplasia is based on both architectural

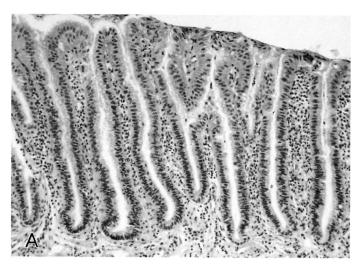

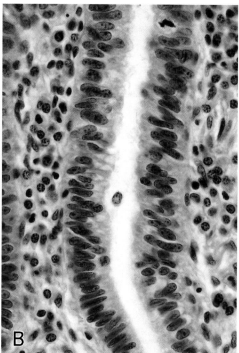

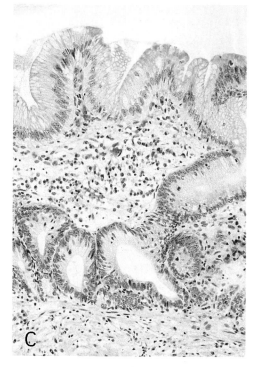

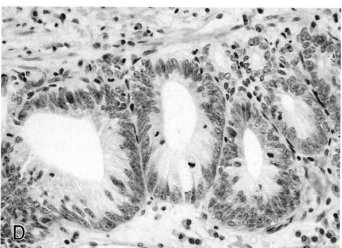

Figure 5-16

BARRETT'S ESOPHAGUS WITH LOW-GRADE DYSPLASIA

A: Low-power magnification of the mucosa showing simple straight but elongated tubules lined by dysplastic cells.

B: High-power magnification of the dysplastic tubules in A. The tubules are lined by pseudostratified epithelium, with hyperchromatic elongated nuclei occupying much of the cells.

C: Low-power view of the mucosa showing dysplasia confined to the lower half of the gland. The surface epithelium is nondysplastic.

D: High-power magnification of the dysplastic epithelium in C showing nuclear enlargement but retention of the basal orientation and some pseudostratification.

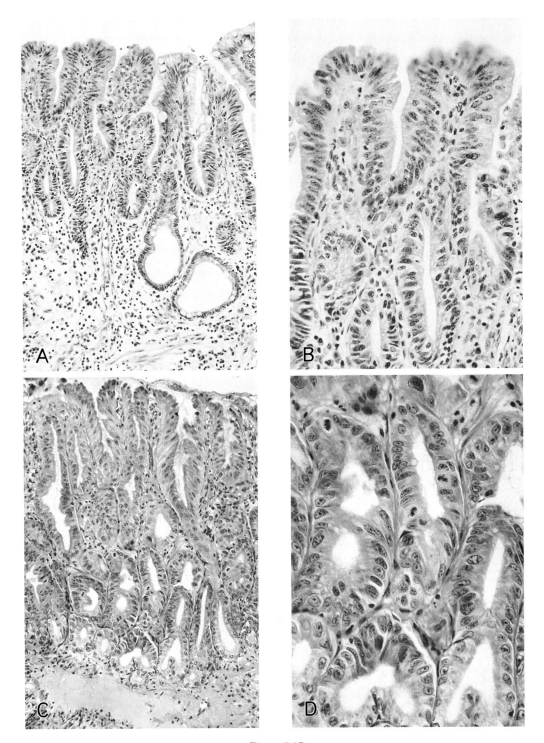

Figure 5-17
BARRETT'S ESOPHAGUS WITH LOW-GRADE DYSPLASIA

A: In this mucosal biopsy the dysplasia occupies the upper half of the mucosa. The lower half is nondysplastic and extensively cystic. There is marked cytologic atypia and focal budding and branching of the pits.

B: High-power magnification of the dysplastic surface epithelium illustrates the enlarged, elongated and stratified nuclei. Nucleoli are frequently small and indistinct.

C: Low-power view of the mucosa showing straight but elongated tubules crowded together.

D: High-power magnification showing the crowded glandular profiles lined by atypical cuboidal cells. These contain basally oriented, enlarged vesicular nuclei and prominent nucleoli.

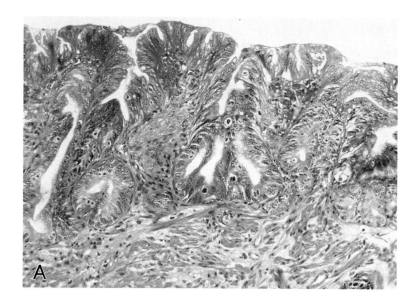

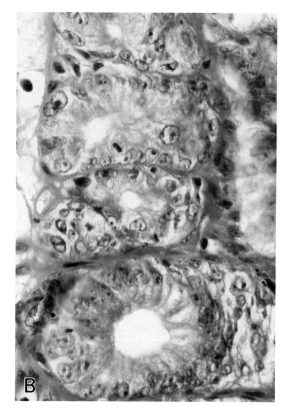

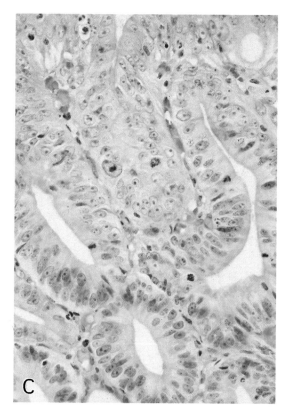

Figure 5-18

BARRETT'S ESOPHAGUS WITH HIGH-GRADE DYSPLASIA: HISTOLOGIC SPECTRUM

A: Low-power view showing marked distortion of the glandular architecture making it difficult to exclude intramucosal carcinoma with invasion into the lamina propria.

B: High-power magnification of the dysplastic cells. The cells are cuboidal and the nuclei have lost their normal basal polarity. The nuclei are greatly enlarged, rounded, and vesicular and contain one or more prominent nucleoli.

C: Another example of high-grade dysplasia demonstrating highly dysplastic cells similar to those described in B, occupying the upper two thirds of the picture. In contrast, the lower third contains low-grade dysplastic cells with small, elongated, basally oriented nuclei.

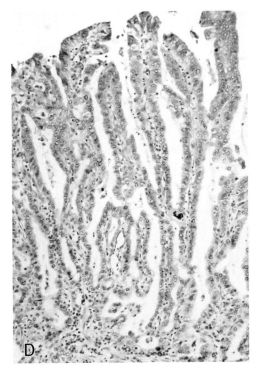

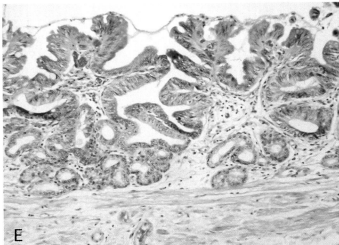

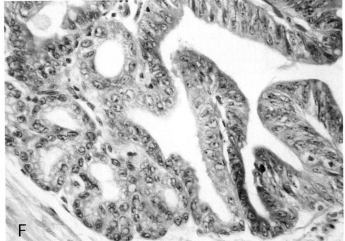

Figure 5-18 (Continued)

D: In this example the high-grade dysplasia has a villous pattern.

E: Another example of high-grade dysplasia demonstrating a complex villoglandular pattern.

F: Higher magnification of E demonstrates marked cytologic atypia. The dysplastic cells are cuboidal and the nuclei are large, vesicular and contain prominent nucleoli.

and cytologic changes that suggest neoplastic transformation; both may be present or only one may predominate.

*Low-Grade Dysplasia.* In low-grade dysplasia architectural changes tend to be mild, with little glandular distortion but some degree of crypt branching. The changes often involve the full length of the crypts but may be confined to the top or bottom halves (figs. 5-16, 5-17). The cytologic changes are also less severe, with smaller and less hyperchromatic nuclei. The basal nuclear polarity is better preserved, even when stratification is present.

*High-Grade Dysplasia.* The architectural changes in high-grade dysplasia are usually pronounced with branching, complex budding, a cribriform gland pattern (back-to-back and la-

beled as carcinoma in situ by some) in severe cases (figs. 5-18, 5-19), and villiform surface changes. The nuclear abnormalities include pronounced pseudostratification, with nuclei reaching the crypt luminal surface, or loss of basal polarity with markedly enlarged abnormal nuclei and nucleoli that vary greatly in size and shape and often exhibit bizarre chromatin patterns. Histologically, high-grade dysplasia may resemble a colonic tubular or sometimes villous adenoma. Raised sessile or pedunculated lesions are distinctly uncommon but can occur (fig. 5-20). The histologic features of high-grade dysplasia are sometimes difficult to differentiate from intramucosal and well-differentiated adenocarcinoma on biopsy. For a discussion of these problems see Differential Diagnosis of Biopsies and

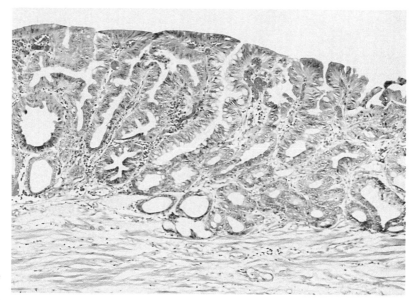

Figure 5-19
BARRETT'S ESOPHAGUS WITH
HIGH-GRADE DYSPLASIA
Top: Barrett's mucosa is completely replaced by dysplastic epithelium.
Bottom: High-power magnification showing dilated glandular profiles, which are tangentially cut, lined by highly atypical cuboidal cells containing enlarged vesicular nuclei and prominent nucleoli.

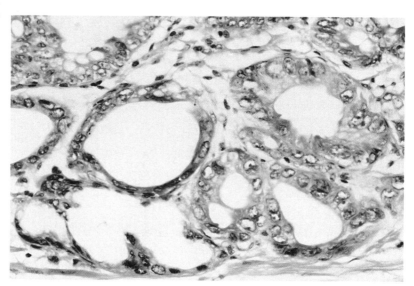

Associated Problems in the section on Adenocarcinoma of the Esophagus.

*Indefinite for Dysplasia.* This refers to changes that are perceived to be too severe for ordinary Barrett's metaplasia (i.e., reactive changes due to inflammation, erosion, or regeneration), but are not sufficient for the diagnosis of low-grade dysplasia. These include moderately distorted architecture, numerous dystrophic goblet cells, diminished or absent mucus production, increased cytoplasmic basophilia, nuclear abnormalities such as nuclear stratification, and increased but normal mitoses (fig. 5-21). Dystrophic goblet cells, which are goblet cells in which the nuclei are displaced from their usual basal orientation towards the lumen and the mucin lies on the basal rather than the luminal side, occur in Barrett's esophagus both with and without dysplasia, and thus are not helpful for diagnosing dysplasia (fig. 5-21F).

The major challenge in the diagnosis of dysplasia is in differentiating it from reactive or regenerative epithelial change. This is particularly difficult, if not impossible, in areas adjacent to erosions or ulcerations; in these cases the term

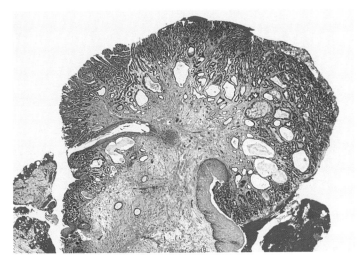

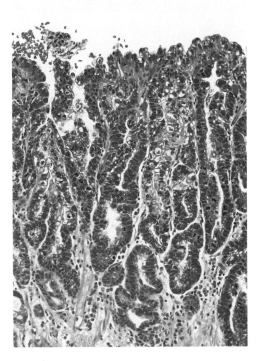

Figure 5-20

TUBULAR ADENOMA OF THE ESOPHAGUS

Above: Low-power view showing a typical pedunculated adenoma. These lesions, which are rare in the esophagus, are usually found in association with Barrett's esophagus. They are essentially similar to the usual forms of dysplasia associated with Barrett's esophagus except that they are pedunculated.

Right: High-power magnification shows the typical architectural features of a tubular adenoma.

"indefinite for dysplasia" should be applied (fig. 5-21). Areas adjacent to ulcers or erosions can also exhibit a megavillous appearance (see fig. 5-7), with an associated neutrophilic infiltrate. In general, the nuclei and nucleoli in reactive or regenerative change are not as large or irregular as those seen in dysplasia, are basally oriented, and are often infiltrated with inflammatory cells. These are interpretive findings and may be unreliable. Sometimes crypt branching may be present in reactive change; however, low-grade dysplasia should not be diagnosed unless cytologic changes are also present. Inflammation is not nearly as frequent or prominent in Barrett's esophagus as in ulcerative colitis, so it is usually not a problem in the diagnosis of dysplasia.

The issue of a second opinion on the grade of dysplasia has great clinical relevance since the management of patients varies with the assessment: simple Barrett's esophagus, low-grade dysplasia, or high-grade dysplasia. Patients with low-grade dysplasia have more frequent surveillance endoscopies and biopsies; esophagectomy is indicated for most patients with high-grade dysplasia.

The criteria for grading dysplasia described above were tested in a prospective study of inter-observer variation among eight morphologists (93). This study demonstrated that experienced gastrointestinal morphologists can diagnose high-grade dysplasia and intramucosal carcinoma with a high degree of agreement (in the range of 85 percent), and can thus detect most patients who need immediate rebiopsy or esophageal resection. However, interobserver agreement was significantly lower for lesser grades of dysplasia: there was only 72 percent agreement in the diagnosis of biopsies negative for dysplasia, and lower in the diagnosis of indefinite dysplasia or low-grade dysplasia. It is probable that these discrepancies in interobserver agreement are even greater among pathologists who rarely see cases of Barrett's esophagus with dysplasia. In our experience and that of others, obtaining additional biopsies frequently resolves histologic problems in diagnosis (60,104). It should be stressed that it is critical to adequately sample the esophagus, starting at the cardia and proceeding proximally until the normal squamous epithelium is reached. Consultation with a pathologist who has experience with cases of dysplasia in Barrett's esophagus can also minimize grading error.

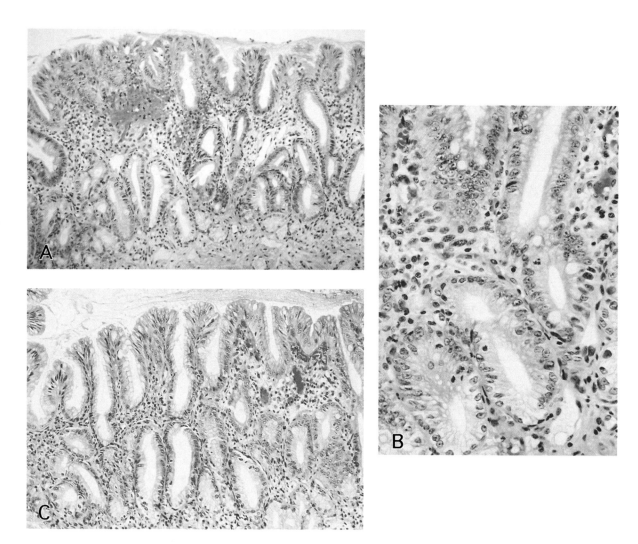

Figure 5-21
BARRETT'S ESOPHAGUS: LOW-POWER VIEWS OF MUCOSA COMPARING
REACTIVE CHANGES WITH INDEFINITE FOR DYSPLASIA

A: Specialized metaplastic epithelium. At low power the lower portions of the glands stand out because of increased basophilia due to their enlarged nuclei.

B: Higher magnification of A showing enlargement and crowding of nuclei at the base of the glands and a few scattered goblet cells. The nuclei still maintain their basal polarity and contain ample cytoplasm. There is also a moderate degree of inflammation.

C: Another example of reactive changes showing regular pits without branching.

**Ancillary Techniques in the Diagnosis of Dysplasia.** Some studies have indicated that certain population subgroups deserve closer follow-up than others. Currently the gold standard of prognostic indicators for the likelihood of cancer development in Barrett's esophagus is histology, specifically the demonstration of dysplasia. While there is good evidence for the concurrent association of high-grade dysplasia and carcinoma, only a few patients with high-grade dysplasia alone have developed subsequent carcinoma (68,79,96). Because of the diagnostic problems at the lower end of the spectrum of dysplasia enumerated above, namely the histologic differentiation of dysplasia from reactive atypia, the consistency of diagnosis, and the question of regression of dysplasia, investigators have looked at other markers, such as mucins, cytology, and flow cytometry, to identify subgroups that would benefit from closer surveillance.

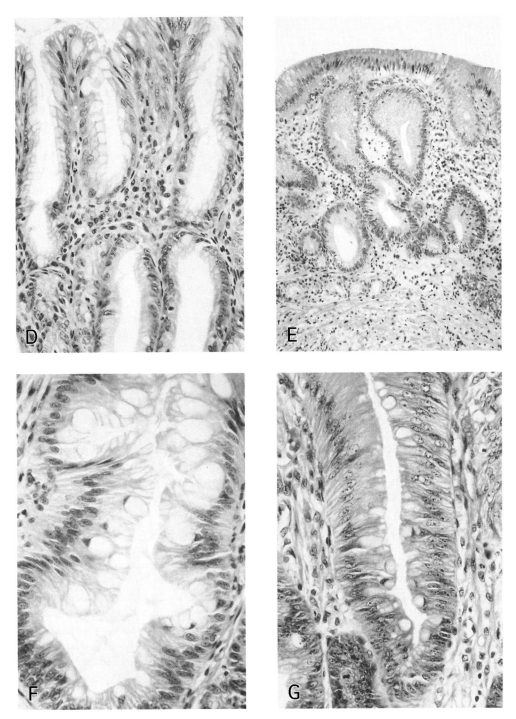

Figure 5-21 (Continued)

D: Higher magnification of C shows epithelial cells with clear cytoplasm and basally oriented nuclei that are slightly enlarged but regular. There is a chronic inflammation of the lamina propria.

E: Barrett's mucosa indefinite for dysplasia. The mucosa is characterized by crowding of the lower portions of the glands. There is epithelial maturation toward the surface although there is still some stratification and enlargement of the nuclei.

F: Higher magnification of an atypical gland shows somewhat enlarged, hyperchromatic, spindle-shaped, stratified nuclei. Note the presence of scattered dystrophic goblet cells, in the center of the field, characterized by the displacement of their nuclei towards the luminal surface of the cell.

G: Specialized epithelium indefinite for dysplasia. The nuclei are enlarged, pseudostratified, and crowded together in the lower half of the crypt. The nuclear changes are much less pronounced as the cells migrate towards the surface. Although surface maturation suggests a reactive process, it cannot be relied upon.

*Epithelial Mucins.* The epithelial cells in the Barrett mucosa contain a heterogeneous mixture of mucins consisting of neutral mucins, present mainly in the clear gastric columnar cells, and acid mucins. The acid mucins consist of two types, sialomucins and sulfomucins, and are found singly or mixed in the goblet and intermediate cells. In 1981, Jass (51) noted that sulfomucins were very common in the Barrett epithelium adjacent to well-differentiated Barrett-associated carcinomas. He therefore proposed that the finding of this mucin in biopsy specimens from patients with Barrett's esophagus might indicate a subset of patients requiring closer surveillance for impending cancer. Later, Peuchmaur (83) went a step further, suggesting that the presence of sulfomucins indicates mild dysplasia. However, subsequent studies have shown that up to 70 percent of patients with Barrett's esophagus without dysplasia can have sulfomucins distributed either focally or diffusely in esophageal biopsies (41,59). Currently, neither the presence nor the predominance of sulfated mucin in the specialized metaplastic epithelium of Barrett's esophagus has sufficiently high sensitivity or specificity for dysplasia or carcinoma to be of value in managing patients.

*Cytology.* The place of cytology in the diagnosis of dysplasia remains uncertain because of limited data (34,100,138). In one study, cytologic specimens obtained from three patients with histologically proven low- or high-grade dysplastic lesions were characterized by tightly cohesive, three-dimensional clusters of cells, with uniformly enlarged nuclei arranged in a crowded but orderly fashion. Molding and overlapping were present, with some degree of regularity. Lack of cohesion of cells appeared to be the most useful feature for discriminating between pure dysplasia and adenocarcinoma. Despite this demonstration of a correlation between cytology and histology in some dysplastic lesions in Barrett's esophagus, a definitive study showing whether cytology can discriminate between reactive atypia, indeterminate dysplasia, and low- and high-grade dysplasia has not yet been done.

*Flow Cytometry.* Analysis of the DNA content in Barrett's esophagus with dysplasia by flow cytometry has been proposed as an objective test for identifying patients at high risk for malignancy. This technique can be used to estimate the rate of cellular proliferation and to detect aneuploid populations of cells (cells that contain an abnormal number of chromosomes) (118). Current studies of flow cytometry in Barrett's esophagus have been encouraging, with some investigators describing excellent agreement between dysplasia and flow cytometric abnormalities (27,94). As genomic instability continues, multiple aneuploid subclones develop, one of which acquires the capacity for invasion and becomes an early carcinoma; in some cases, genomic instability continues after the development of cancer, leading to further aneuploid subclones and tumor cell heterogeneity (90–92). However not all investigators have had such success with cytometry (27,31,94). There are many methodologic differences between the reported studies which may account for differences in the results: some investigators used fresh tissue obtained at endoscopic biopsies, others used paraffin-fixed sections from surgical specimens, and yet others included patients with coexistent Barrett-associated adenocarcinoma. Furthermore, the presence of aneuploidy does not always mean cancer or dysplasia (26,71).

Flow cytometry and DNA image analysis cytometry potentially have several important roles in the management of dysplasia and cancer in patients with Barrett's esophagus. At least one study suggests that Barrett-associated carcinoma with aneuploidy has a worse prognosis than diploid tumors (29,31). For biopsies that are non-neoplastic, low-grade dysplasia, or indefinite for dysplasia, a normal DNA pattern provides a measure of reassurance, whereas an abnormal pattern might prompt rebiopsy or more frequent endoscopic biopsy surveillance. Current data show that repeated demonstration of aneuploidy in follow-up endoscopies may be associated with high-grade dysplasia and adenocarcinoma, defining a group requiring closer surveillance (29,87,91). Conversely, a finding of aneuploidy on a single occasion may not have the same implications. An even more untested role for cytometry is for predicting heightened cancer risk in a subset of patients whose biopsies show Barrett's esophagus with DNA aneuploidy but who do not currently have any histologic evidence of dysplasia; patients repeatedly free of aneuploidy or dysplasia may be in a low-risk group for whom surveillance frequency may eventually be decreased. Because dysplasia and carcinoma are not common in unselected patients with Barrett's esophagus, longitudinal studies of larger numbers of patients are required to determine the benefit of these techniques. Flow cytometry remains in the research arena rather than a tool that should be presently applied in routine clinical practice.

Other diagnostic methods, such as counts of nucleolar organizer regions by silver staining technique and ornithine decarboxylase activity, and oncogene markers such as P53 (see section on DNA and oncogene markers) have been evaluated for their usefulness in distinguishing reactive from dysplastic changes in Barrett's esophagus. At present they have not been shown to be of practical value (14,32,33).

**Treatment.** Because the endoscopic appearance of Barrett's esophagus with or without dysplasia and early carcinoma are indistinguishable, multiple endoscopic biopsies are required in order to confirm a diagnosis (24). The value of screening for dysplasia and curable adenocarcinoma is not universally accepted (1,134). Those against screening for dysplasia believe that carcinoma is usually far advanced by the time dysplasia is first discovered; dysplasia is not commonly encountered; and long-term survival is not improved. The latter was the conclusion of one study from Holland, which found that the long-term survival of patients with Barrett's esophagus who develop carcinoma was no different from an age- and sex-matched control of the general population without Barrett's esophagus. The authors concluded that systematic endoscopic surveillance with biopsies of patients with Barrett's esophagus was not indicated (134). Such pessimism appears premature if biopsy screening is properly done. However, if the endoscopist takes nonsystematic tiny biopsies and does not orient and process them optimally, the cure rate for neoplasia is likely to be greatly reduced.

The current suggestions for the management of patients with Barrett's esophagus and dysplasia are as follows, although it should be noted that these recommendations are in large part arbitrary and vary from center to center (18a,54,63, 79,84,95,96,106,119). At UCLA, two biopsies are taken from each level (from opposite walls), every 2 cm and from all target lesions, such as ulcers, bumps, masses, and strictures, preferably with

jumbo (9 mm) forceps, starting at the gastric cardia and progressing proximally (fig. 5-22). The final specimen is taken in what is considered to be squamous epithelium to verify the upper zone of the Barrett mucosa. Biopsies are taken from the cardia to ensure that the most distal part of the Barrett mucosa is sampled to rule out dysplasia; to define exactly where the lower esophageal sphincter zone is located; and to exclude proximal gastric intestinal metaplasia when the question of short-segment Barrett's esophagus arises. In addition, it is recommended that for most cases a second histologic opinion be obtained for all biopsies with any evidence of dysplasia from an experienced pathologist.

Unfortunately, some endoscopists fail to provide sufficient site information to allow the pathologist to determine whether Barrett's esophagus exists and how extensive it is. This problem arises when biopsy specimens are submitted with no indication of the specific location in the esophagus, the number of centimeters from the incisors, and the location of the lower esophageal sphincter region. In such instances, the pathologist is left to guess. Endoscopic surveillance every 1 to 2 years is sufficient if dysplasia is absent on an adequate initial biopsy evaluation as described above.

For cases that exhibit changes that are indefinite for dysplasia, a second opinion and rebiopsy are recommended. In our experience rebiopsy material often resolves the issue of indefinite for dysplasia. If it does not, rebiopsy at yearly intervals is recommended.

If low-grade dysplasia is detected and agreed upon by several observers, it is usually treated medically with antireflux measures and increased surveillance. This entails rebiopsy at 6-month intervals. It is uncertain how long to continue this more intensive surveillance: for now it is recommended that the 6-month reevaluation be continued for at least 2 years before considering reducing the frequency, especially if two consecutive biopsies are negative for dysplasia (63,84). For high-grade dysplasia there should be immediate rebiopsy to see if a coexistent carcinoma was missed. Intramucosal carcinoma or carcinoma superficially invasive into submucosa can occur in Barrett's esophagus without any associated grossly visible target lesions. If intramucosal carcinoma is found on

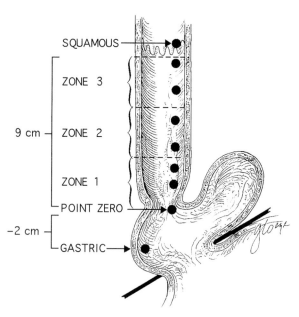

SQUAMOUS

ZONE 3

ZONE 2

9 cm

ZONE 1

POINT ZERO

−2 cm

GASTRIC

Figure 5-22
ESOPHAGEAL BIOPSY PROTOCOL FOR
BARRETT'S ESOPHAGUS SURVEILLANCE
(Courtesy of Dr. W.M. Weinstein, Los Angeles, CA.)

rebiopsy, then surgery is recommended, since at this stage there is already a low, but significant, potential to metastasize (81a). If only high-grade dysplasia is detected on rebiopsy, then the decision concerning esophagectomy has to be individualized. Whenever high-grade dysplasia without associated carcinoma is detected, it is useful to get a second opinion from a pathologist who has considerable experience with dysplasia in Barrett's esophagus.

Esophagectomy in the setting of high-grade dysplasia usually entails a near total resection with proximal mobilization of the stomach and anastomosis to the remaining esophagus in the neck. Colon interpositions are now less commonly done. In centers with experience with esophagectomy, surgical mortality for nonadvanced esophageal malignancy is 5 percent or less. In younger patients without other conditions that markedly enhance operative risk, esophagectomy for multifocal high-grade dysplasia is recommended. The alternative is not just the risk of developing carcinoma but the attendant chronic worry and need for rebiopsy every 3 to 6 months for the rest of the person's life. For patients who are frail, follow-up is indicated. Endoscopic sur-

veillance is not performed for those patients who decline surgery no matter what the findings in follow-up, or for those who are prohibitive operative risks because of other medical conditions.

Occasionally, patients have only a small zone of high-grade dysplasia. The practice of the future in some of these instances may be to use local endoscopic treatment such as snare resection, laser, or electrocoagulation.

## ADENOCARCINOMA OF THE ESOPHAGUS

Primary adenocarcinoma of the esophagus is a relatively uncommon tumor, accounting for between 1 to 50 percent of all malignant esophageal tumors depending on the geographical location. In areas with a high incidence of esophageal squamous cell carcinoma, such as China, almost no esophageal adenocarcinomas are seen.

In the United States, primary adenocarcinoma of the esophagus was uncommon in the past, with an incidence of 10 percent of all esophageal cancers. However, over the past decade there has been a striking increase in incidence of Barrett-associated adenocarcinoma: 9 percent increase per year in males and 5 percent in females (8,82). This tumor now accounts for approximately 34 percent of all primary esophageal malignancies and 80 percent of all carcinomas of the lower third of the esophagus (the remainder are mainly squamous cell carcinomas). The cause of this dramatic increase in frequency is unclear, although improved diagnostic techniques may be partially responsible (8,16a,40,48,61,67,137,141).

Recent studies have shown a marked similarity in age distribution, sex ratio, race, clinical presentation, and pathologic features between adenocarcinoma in Barrett's esophagus and adenocarcinoma of the cardia. It has been suggested that these findings indicate common etiologic factors between these two conditions, such as reflux and increased alcohol and tobacco consumption (8,16,40,53,66,81a,116,130,137).

**Etiology and Pathogenesis.** See Barrett's Esophagus.

**Clinical Features.** In the United States, as for Barrett's esophagus, there is a heavy predominance in males, with male to female ratios in the range of 3:1 to 7:1, and whites (over 80 percent) in contrast to squamous cell carcinoma which has a predominance in blacks (6 to 1) (8,42,45,50, 53,55,66,101,115,117,130,137). The age range is 20 to 90 years, with a mean of 60 years (23). The median age of patients with Barrett's esophagus and carcinoma is about 5 years higher than for those without carcinoma (21,47,115).

There are no unique clinical features of early cancer beyond those of Barrett's esophagus, that is, patients may be asymptomatic or have symptoms of gastroesophageal reflux disease. A change in symptoms, such as progressive dysphagia, is indicative of advanced esophageal cancer (22). Since staging is critical in determining both operability and prognosis, it is important to stage the patient as accurately as possible prior to surgery, as well as at the time of surgery. Ultrasound, computerized tomography (CT), and magnetic resonance (MRI) scans have been shown to be highly predictive in detecting nonpalpable supraclavicular lymph node metastases and in determining the resectability of esophageal carcinomas (adenocarcinoma and squamous cell carcinoma). In one study the preoperative assessment of supraclavicular lymph node metastases was prospectively studied in 100 patients with esophageal carcinoma (adenocarcinoma and squamous cell carcinoma). Findings at CT and palpation were compared and confirmed by ultrasound-guided fine-needle aspiration biopsy. Supraclavicular metastases were detected by CT in 11 of 13 patients (predictive value, 0.85) but were palpable in only 3 cases (126,135).

Endoscopic ultrasound, a technique that is still in an early stage of development, is promising for accurately determining the depth of tumor invasion and for identifying local lymph node metastases. Early results compare favorably with other forms of examination such as CT, conventional radiography, endoscopy, and external ultrasound. Endoscopic ultrasound instruments are undergoing further refinements, and more extensive prospective investigations are necessary before this diagnostic method can be considered routine for diagnostic purposes (64,131,136).

**Gross and Endoscopic Findings.** Almost 80 percent of esophageal adenocarcinomas are located in the lower third of the esophagus; half extend into the proximal stomach. Endoscopically, high-grade dysplasia and intramucosal carcinoma are not distinguishable from Barrett's esophagus. Once the tumor has progressed be-

yond the early stages, the gross appearance varies from slight mucosal irregularities or plaques measuring a few millimeters in diameter (65 percent of cases), to large, exophytic, fungating, or deeply ulcerated masses which may measure up to 10 cm and may occlude the lumen (35 percent of cases) (fig. 5-23) (40,116,130,137). Most tumors are advanced at the time of diagnosis and have extended to the adventitial tissues. Most lesions are flat and ulcerated and about a third are polypoid or fungating. Diffusely infiltrative lesions are rare (fig. 5-23I) (62,74). Occasionally, tumors are multifocal and there is one report of an esophageal adenocarcinoma that resembled esophageal varices on radiologic and endoscopic examination (77,116,140). The salmon-pink mucosa of Barrett's esophagus may be obvious in adjacent mucosa (fig. 5-23G). However if the tumor occurs in the lower esophagus at the upper end of the columnar epithelium or in a tongue of epithelium, it may not be possible to confirm that it arose in the Barrett epithelium until histologically confirmed, and even then it may sometimes be impossible to distinguish from a tumor arising in the gastric cardia and extending up into the esophagus.

**Histologic Findings.** Most adenocarcinomas are accompanied by and arise from typical dysplasia (fig. 5-24) (12,102,116). The amount of residual Barrett's epithelium is variable and is sometimes absent, presumably because it has been replaced by the advancing carcinoma. The tumors show a histologic spectrum virtually identical to that found in the stomach. In rare instances, primarily in those patients with Barrett's esophagus in surveillance programs, early adenocarcinoma confined to the mucosa (intramucosal carcinoma) or submucosa, may be found (fig. 5-24A,C,D). As the tumor progresses there is infiltration into the muscularis propria and the adventitial tissue of the mediastinum. Lymph node metastases are common and occur in three quarters of cases. A few tumors are adenosquamous carcinomas in which the squamous component predominates (see Adenosquamous Carcinoma).

The majority of adenocarcinomas are of the intestinal type, but some are diffuse or a combination of types. Differentiation may include virtually all mature and immature cell types found in the normal esophagus, stomach, or intestine, including endocrine cells, Paneth cells, and

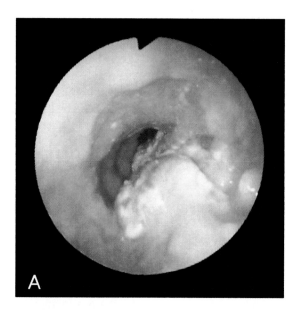

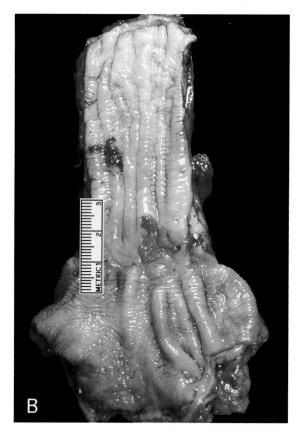

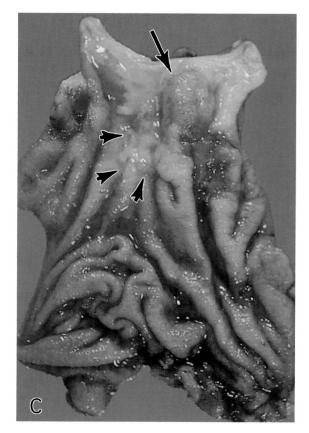

Figure 5-23

GROSS APPEARANCES OF ADENOCARCINOMA IN BARRETT'S ESOPHAGUS

A: Endoscopic section showing nodular plaques.

B: A tiny adenocarcinoma consisting of a small pinkish plaque just above the esophagogastric junction.

C: Carcinoma in short-segment Barrett's esophagus. The squamocolumnar junction is highly irregular (arrowheads) with the gastric mucosa extending well into the squamous mucosa on the left. On the right is a small nodular carcinoma (arrow). (Fig. 12-26 from Lewin KJ, Riddell RH, Weinstein WM. Gastrointestinal pathology and its clinical implications. New York: Igaku Shoin, 1992:475.)

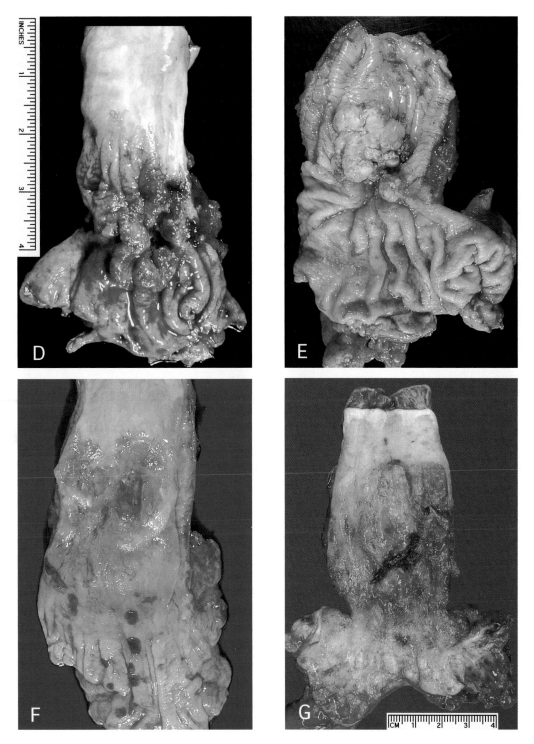

Figure 5-23 (Continued)

D: Adenocarcinoma in short-segment Barrett's esophagus. The tumor straddles the esophagogastric junction, and consists of thickened mucosal folds.

E: Nodular adenocarcinoma situated in the lowermost portion of the esophagus.

F: Ulcerated nodular adenocarcinoma. This is a relatively small, centrally ulcerated, nodular carcinoma present near the upper squamocolumnar margin.

G: Large exophytic adenocarcinoma occupying much of the distal esophagus. The Barrett's esophagus is visible as a tan mucosa above and to one side of the tumor.

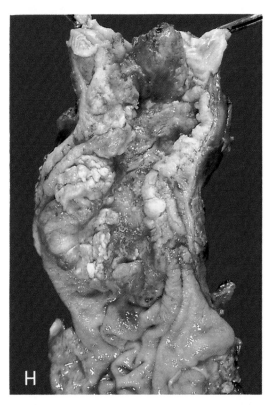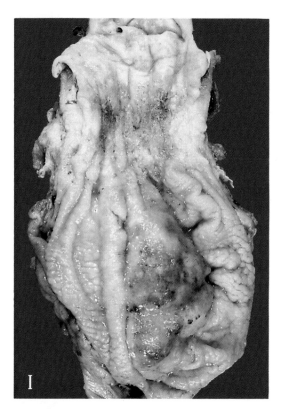

Figure 5-23 (Continued)
GROSS APPEARANCES OF ADENOCARCINOMA IN BARRETT'S ESOPHAGUS
H: Large, exophytic, fungating adenocarcinoma of the esophagus occupying the full circumference of the lumen.
I: Diffusely infiltrative adenocarcinoma occupying the distal esophagus.

squamous epithelium (fig. 5-24) (6,40,53,116). Most adenocarcinomas are well to moderately differentiated. Well-differentiated tumors may pose a diagnostic problem on biopsy because the infiltrating component may be unrecognizable as invasive and be reported as high-grade dysplasia or carcinoma in situ. Some carcinomas have a prominent component of cystically dilated neoplastic glands. At low power these may look deceptively bland, especially when lined by low cuboidal tumor cells, and they may be confused with Barrett's esophagus in biopsies (fig. 5-24F,G) (see Differential Diagnosis).

Poorly differentiated carcinomas are often diffusely infiltrative. They are comprised of poorly formed tubules (fig. 5-24K–O) or sometimes, signet ring cells, and are often accompanied by a desmoplastic reaction similar to linitis plastica in the stomach. Vascular and perineural invasion are common. The amount of mucus secreted is also variable, ranging from intracellular mucin production, to mucus secretion within glands, to extracellular pools of mucin.

**Differential Diagnosis.** In most instances biopsies present few problems and the histologic findings are both accurate and sensitive (38). In a small proportion of tumors, however, diagnosis may be more difficult, especially in tumors associated with strictures or widespread inflammation. When tight strictures are present, vigorous brushing and subsequent cytology may allow diagnosis when biopsies fail. Occasionally, erosions with granulation tissue may pose a problem, primarily in frozen sections. Plump endothelial cells sometimes mimic adenocarcinoma, if the endothelial cells lining the vascular spaces are not recognized as such (see fig. 5-10). Serial sections usually reveal the vascular nature of the pseudoglandular structures. Immunohistochemistry with factor VIII and cytokeratin antibodies readily differentiates the two types of cells, although this is rarely necessary.

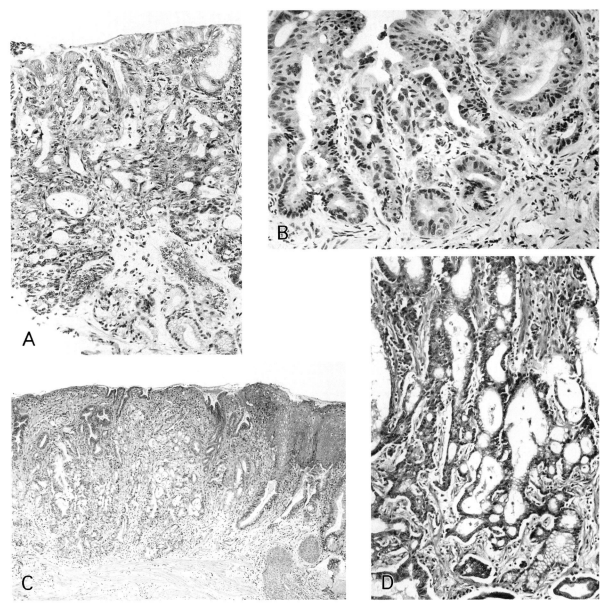

Figure 5-24
HISTOLOGIC SPECTRUM OF ESOPHAGEAL ADENOCARCINOMAS
ASSOCIATED WITH BARRETT'S ESOPHAGUS

A: High-grade dysplasia with early intramucosal carcinoma. The lesion is confined to the mucosa and shows high-grade dysplasia and a few clumps of cytologically malignant cells that appear to be infiltrating the lamina propria.

B: High-power view of high-grade dysplasia and early intramucosal carcinoma shows atypical clusters of cells and glands infiltrating the lamina propria.

C: Low-power view of an infiltrating carcinoma confined to the mucosa adjacent to the squamocolumnar junction.

D. High-power view of C shows moderately differentiated glands, some of which have a cribriform pattern.

The differential diagnosis of cysts, especially in esophageal biopsies, includes cystic dilatation of mucosal and submucosal esophageal glands and ducts, Barrett's esophagus, dysplastic glands, and carcinoma. The major difference between neoplastic (dysplasia and carcinoma) cysts and non-neoplastic cysts is the presence of dysplastic epithelial cells lining the dilated glands. At low power these cells may look deceptively bland in dysplasia and carcinoma because

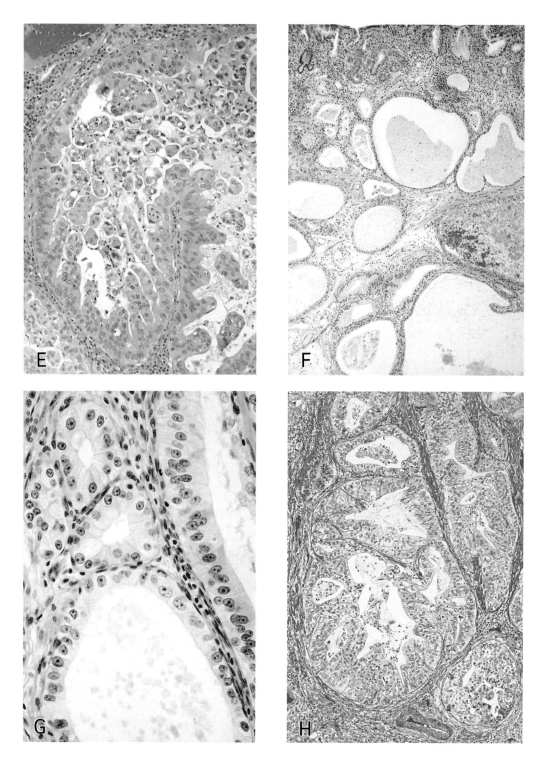

Figure 5-24 (Continued)
HISTOLOGIC SPECTRUM OF ESOPHAGEAL ADENOCARCINOMAS
ASSOCIATED WITH BARRETT'S ESOPHAGUS

E: Well-differentiated papillary adenocarcinoma.

F: This tumor is composed of cystically dilated glandular profiles infiltrating the mucosa and submucosa.

G: Higher magnification of F shows that the epithelium lining the dilated glands is composed of low cuboidal cells with vesicular nuclei and prominent nucleoli.

H: Moderately differentiated adenocarcinoma.

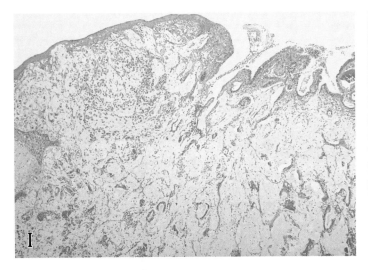

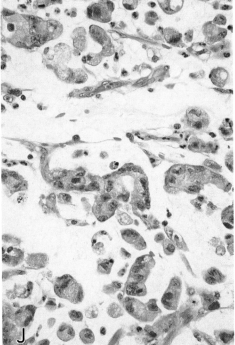

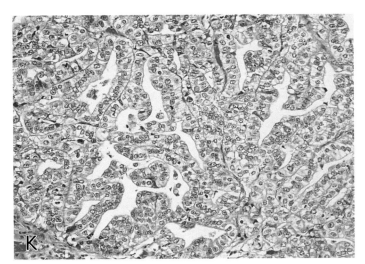

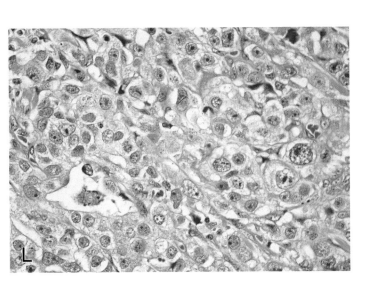

Figure 5-24 (Continued)

I: Mucinous adenocarcinoma, low-power magnification. Most of this section is covered by squamous epithelium. There is diffuse mucinous infiltration of the tissue.

J: Higher magnification of I shows goblet cells and atypical glandular profiles floating in pools of mucin.

K: Poorly differentiated adenocarcinoma with a clear cell pattern.

L: Poorly differentiated adenocarcinoma composed of sheets of uniform epithelial cells containing large vesicular nuclei and prominent nucleoli. Just to the left of center is a poorly formed gland lumen.

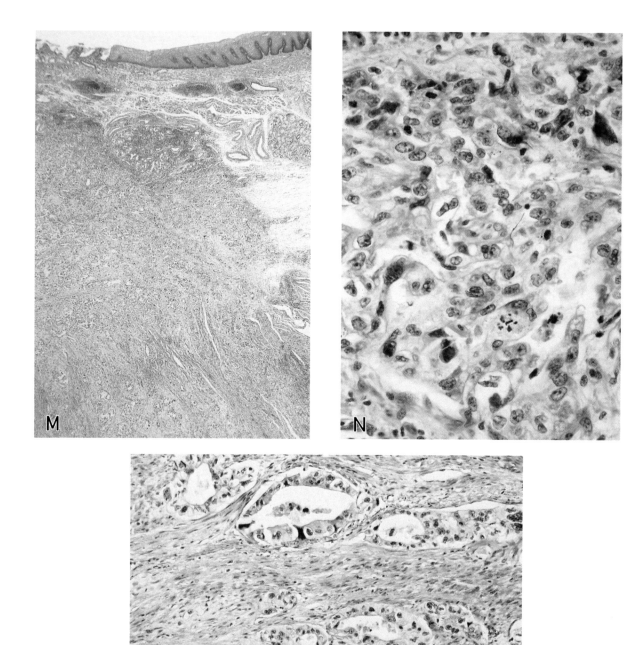

Figure 5-24 (Continued)
HISTOLOGIC SPECTRUM OF ESOPHAGEAL ADENOCARCINOMAS
ASSOCIATED WITH BARRETT'S ESOPHAGUS

M: Poorly differentiated adenocarcinoma consisting of sheets of malignant cells diffusely infiltrating the submucosa and muscularis propria.

N: Higher magnification of M showing marked anaplasia and little glandular differentiation.

O: Higher magnification of another area of M showing poorly differentiated adenocarcinoma with poorly formed tubules diffusely infiltrating the esophageal wall. There is a marked accompanying desmoplasia.

they are often low cuboidal in configuration. However, at higher magnification the typical features of dysplasia are seen, namely, enlarged hyperchromatic nuclei and reduced cytoplasm, which is often basophilic.

Differentiating between high-grade dysplasia and carcinoma on biopsy is difficult, if not impossible in some cases. This is especially true for cases in which it is difficult to determine whether the glands are invading the lamina propria: small distorted or abortive glands within the lamina propria, glands that are closely packed together, or glands that grow in a cribriform pattern (fig. 5-24D). Cytologic features may be identical in both situations, so invasion in carcinoma must be demonstrated. However, as already noted, invasion is mimicked in some cases of dysplasia in which elongated dysplastic glands abut or even insinuate between the muscle bundles of the muscularis mucosae. If the muscularis mucosae has been destroyed by previous ulceration, the mucosal/submucosal border may be obscured. In these cases, other criteria of invasion are sought, such as the presence of single or small clumps of cells infiltrating the lamina propria, muscularis mucosae, or submucosa (fig. 5-24A–C). In difficult cases, examination of serial cuts to follow tiny cell clusters or single cells is needed, and sometimes further biopsies are necessary. The question of separating high-grade dysplasia from carcinoma is more than of theoretical importance since in many institutions the treatment is radically different.

Another problem occurs in well-differentiated dysplastic lesions in which the only way to make a diagnosis of carcinoma is by demonstrating invasion through the muscularis mucosae. If one biopsy is taken and is superficial, a diagnosis of carcinoma is impossible. This problem is circumvented by the multiple biopsies advocated in surveillance protocols. In the future, endoscopic ultrasound examination by the endoscopist may alert the clinician to the possibility of invasive tumor.

Sometimes tumors are so poorly differentiated that it is difficult to determine whether they are of squamous or glandular type. If Barrett's esophagus, with or without dysplasia, is present, then it is more than likely that the tumor is a poorly differentiated adenocarcinoma. Differentiating Barrett-associated adenocarcinoma from adenocarcinoma of the gastric cardia is discussed under Carcinoma of the Gastric Cardia in chapter 11.

**Tumor Spread and Metastasis.** There is little accurate information regarding the spread and complications of esophageal adenocarcinoma because the few autopsy studies that have been done have lumped adenocarcinoma with squamous cell carcinoma of the esophagus and adenocarcinomas are a small portion of the total cases (2,4,10). Nevertheless, it does appear that most esophageal adenocarcinomas behave somewhat the same as squamous carcinomas. They tend to spread primarily locally, and usually cause death from local complications. Distant metastases occur late. About 80 percent of tumors spread by direct extension through the muscularis propria to the periadventitial tissues and then into adjacent tissues and organs. Lymph node involvement appears to be frequent once the tumor extends to the periadventitial tissues, occurring in up to 70 percent of cases. Angioinvasion occurs in half the cases (40,53, 108). The most common site of invasion is the tracheobronchial tree, frequently resulting in esophagotracheal or esophagobronchial fistulae. The mediastinum and lung are the next most common sites of involvement, often resulting in pneumonia, mediastinitis, and abscess formation. Other organs that can be involved include aorta, heart, liver, and spine.

**Staging and Prognosis.** Although resectability rates are high, long-term survival of patients with esophageal adenocarcinoma is very poor. Early detection is mandatory for long-term survival (81a,124).

As with squamous cell carcinoma, the most important overall factor influencing the prognosis of esophageal adenocarcinoma is tumor stage at the time of resection. The most important individual factors for prognosis are the depth of invasion through the esophageal wall, the presence of involved lymph nodes, and the size of the tumor. These factors are reflected in staging and grouping systems such as the TNM (clinical) and pTNM (pathologic) systems. The most recent and widely used classification is that of the American Joint Committee on Cancer (AJCC) and the international counterpart the International Union Against Cancer (UICC) (see TNM Classification in chapter 1) (133). This classification scheme has been validated for squamous cell esophageal cancers in Japan (49).

Very few reports of esophageal adenocarcinoma are large enough to provide valid survival figures when stratified for both depth of invasion and nodal metastases. The largest study consisted of 65 cases of adenocarcinoma in patients with Barrett's esophagus. The overall adjusted actuarial 5-year survival rate was 25 percent. The 3-year survival rates were 100 percent for patients with stage 0 carcinoma, 85.7 percent for patients with stage I, 53.6 percent for patients with stage IIa, 45 percent for patients with stage IIb, 25 percent for patients with stage III, and 0 percent for patients with stage IV carcinoma. In most instances, patients with tumor limited to the lamina propria (intramucosal carcinoma), the submucosa, and even into, but not through, the muscularis propria have an excellent prognosis of probably between 90 and 100 percent. The prognosis is about 45 percent when the muscularis propria is just penetrated (stage IIa), 15 to 25 percent with moderate extension beyond it, and virtually 0 percent when adjacent organs are involved (142)

Esophageal adenocarcinomas tend to spread proximally in the submucosal lymphatics and have been reported at the resection margin in about one third of cases (116). Thus, it is wise to obtain frozen sections from the proximal resected margin in order to detect tumor in patients in whom further proximal resection can be carried out. Adenocarcinoma of the lower third of the esophagus is particularly likely to be accompanied by intra-abdominal nodal secondaries and so it might be helpful to request samples of these nodes for permanent sections.

**Treatment.** The management of invasive adenocarcinoma of the esophagus is surgical. Surgery has also been advocated as a palliative procedure to allow oral intake of food and control of saliva during the final months of the patient's life. However, since many patients are elderly, some may not be fit enough to endure this extensive operation, even though the operative mortality rate has dropped to 5 to 10 percent (75). The operation includes resection of the lesion and all existing Barrett's epithelium in appropriate surgical candidates because a second carcinoma may develop in residual columnar epithelium (79,124). Surgical resectability depends upon whether the tumor extends to the adjacent organs. The type of operation should depend on stage of disease: esophagectomy for intramucosal disease; en bloc esophagectomy with splenic preservation for in-

tramural and transmural disease. There are two approaches to esophageal resection: a transhiatal or a transthoracic esophagectomy. Some reports suggest that transhiatal esophagectomy has a lower morbidity and mortality rate than transthoracic esophagectomy, while others suggest an increased long-term survival with the latter operation. However, in one report no difference in survival was found between both methods (75). Serum carcinoembryonic antigen (CEA) is useful for the postoperative diagnosis of recurrent disease in those cases in which the primary tumor stained for CEA (22).

Various combinations of surgery, chemotherapy, and radiation therapy have been tried in advanced cases of adenocarcinoma of the esophagus. However, to date the results of surgery with adjuvant chemotherapy and radiation have not been any better than with surgery alone (30,123).

## ADENOSQUAMOUS CARCINOMA OF THE ESOPHAGUS AND ADENOACANTHOMA

Adenosquamous carcinoma of the esophagus is a rare aggressive tumor containing coexisting infiltrating adenocarcinoma and squamous cell carcinoma (fig. 5-25) (144,144a,146). The literature on the histogenesis of this tumor is confusing, probably because of its heterogeneity. Some have been ascribed to squamous differentiation in Barrett's esophagus, others from glandular metaplasia in squamous cell carcinomas (145), and yet others to an origin from the submucosal glands (144a,147). These tumors may be confused histologically with mucoepidermoid carcinoma. In the upper aerodigestive tract, adenosquamous carcinomas are more aggressive than mucoepidermoid tumors and by extension this may also be true for the esophagus (144a). In mucoepidermoid carcinomas, the mucus-secreting cells occur within islands of squamous carcinoma, whereas in true adenosquamous carcinoma both elements may coexist, but are infrequently admixed. Other differential features include the presence of keratinization, metastasizing glandular profiles with extensive mucin production, and marked nuclear pleomorphism, features not observed in mucoepidermoid carcinoma (144a). When mature squamous epithelium is present in adenocarcinoma, it is referred to by some as adenoacanthoma.

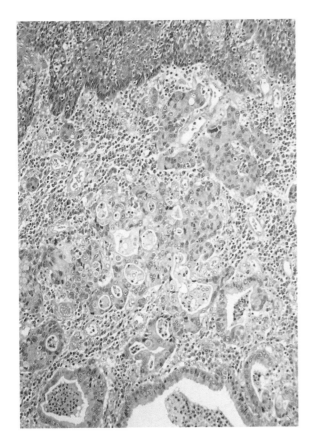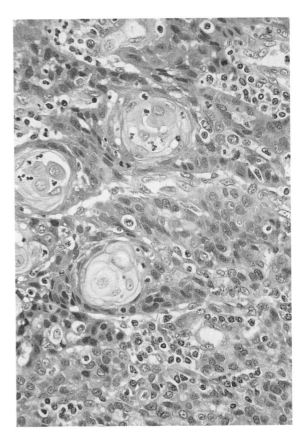

Figure 5-25
ADENOSQUAMOUS CARCINOMA OF THE ESOPHAGUS
Left: Low-power view of mucosa and submucosa showing dysplastic surface squamous epithelium and underlying adenosquamous carcinoma.
Right: High-power magnification shows the keratinizing squamous carcinoma.

## ADENOCARCINOMA OF THE ESOPHAGUS UNASSOCIATED WITH BARRETT'S ESOPHAGUS

Rare esophageal adenocarcinomas arise from glandular epithelium unassociated with Barrett's esophagus. These include adenocarcinomas arising from heterotopic gastric mucosa and carcinomas of the mucosal and submucosal glands and ducts.

### Adenocarcinoma Arising from Heterotopic Gastric Mucosa of the Esophagus (the Inlet Patch)

Heterotopic gastric mucosa of the upper esophagus is a congenital condition that results from rests of gastric precursor cells that are thought to remain after an incomplete replacement of the original esophageal mucosa by stratified squamous epithelium. A grossly visible focus of the ectopic mucosa, also known as an "inlet patch," is not uncommon and is found in 2.5 to 4 percent of patients undergoing upper endoscopy (152,154a). Microscopic foci of gastric mucosa are thought to be even more common (156). In most instances heterotopic gastric mucosa of the esophagus is benign, but in rare cases the mucosa may undergo peptic ulceration, incomplete or complete intestinal metaplasia, or dysplasia, and carcinoma may occur (155,156a). Although carcinoma arising from heterotopic rests in the upper esophagus is frequently mentioned in the literature, the number of actual cases reported is in the single digits (151). The tumor is seen in middle-aged patients who present with dysphagia. Endoscopy reveals a friable ulcerated tumor in the proximal esophagus. Grossly and microscopically, the tumors resemble gastric and esophageal adenocarcinomas (fig. 5-26). They commonly extend

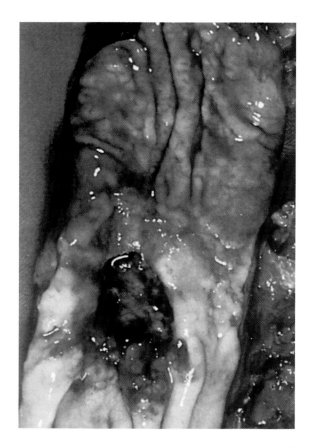
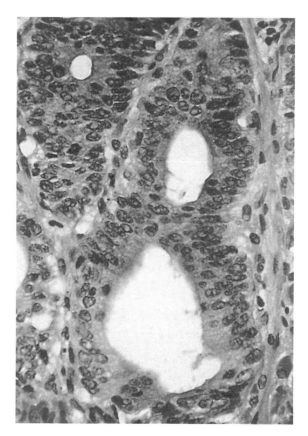

Figure 5-26
ADENOCARCINOMA ARISING IN HETEROTOPIC GASTRIC MUCOSA IN THE CERVICAL ESOPHAGUS

Left: Cervical esophagus with circumferential heterotopic gastric mucosa extending to the upper margin. At the lower margin is a deep peptic ulcer, the distal edge of which had a focus of intestinal metaplasia, dysplasia, and well-differentiated adenocarcinoma.

Right: Part of the invasive adenocarcinoma. (Fig. 12-27A,C from Lewin KJ, Riddell RH, Weinstein WM. Gastrointestinal pathology and its clinical implications, New York: Igaku Shoin, 1992:476 .)

through the esophageal wall at the time of diagnosis and often metastasize to local lymph nodes. Microscopically they are adenocarcinomas with varying degrees of differentiation, and sometimes with papillary features. Ectopic gastric fundic gland mucosa must be demonstrated adjacent to the carcinoma in order to corroborate the diagnosis, although any proximal esophageal adenocarcinoma probably started in an inlet patch.

Adenocarcinoma of the esophagus arising from heterotopic gastric mucosa must be distinguished from carcinoma arising from Barrett's esophagus. The latter usually occurs in the lower esophagus, and the adjacent Barrett's esophagus (which for all practical purposes never contains fundic-type mucosal glands) extends distally to the stomach. In contrast, carcinomas arising in heterotopic gastric mucosa are almost exclusively found in the upper third of the esophagus and are separated from the gastric cardia by intervening normal squamous epithelium. Rarely, adenocarcinomas can arise from esophageal mucosal and submucosal glands (see below). Unless Barrett's esophagus is excluded and an intact overlying mucosa and origin of the carcinoma from the mucosal or submucosal ducts or glands demonstrated, the diagnosis is impossible to substantiate.

## Adenocarcinoma of Submucosal Glands

These are rare salivary gland–type tumors arising from the submucosal glands and their ducts (148–150,153,154,157). Most are adenoid cystic carcinomas, and are frequently aggressive and rapidly fatal. For a detailed description see chapter 3.

## Choriocarcinoma of the Esophagus

Choriocarcinoma is a malignant neoplasm that produces trophoblastic tissue and usually occurs in the genital system. The tumor has also been documented in extragenital sites such as the retroperitoneum, mediastinum, urinary bladder, and prostate, and infrequently in other organs. In the gastrointestinal tract, choriocarcinomas are exceedingly rare: only 54 cases were reported in the world literature by 1988, of which only 4 occurred in the esophagus (158–160).

The histogenesis of extragonadal choriocarcinoma probably varies depending on the site (158,159). Tumors originating in the retroperitoneum, mediastinum, bladder, prostate, and pineal gland probably arise from displaced gonadal anlage or in rests of primordial germ cells which fail to complete their normal migration from the developing urogenital ridge to the adult gonad. Choriocarcinomas of the gastrointestinal tract are thought to arise from retrodifferentiation of adenocarcinomas (159). This hypothesis is based on the fact that the majority of choriocarcinomas of the gastrointestinal tract (33 of 54), including two in the esophagus, were admixed with adenocarcinomas (158). It is postulated that in cases of pure choriocarcinoma, in which no adenocarcinomatous elements are found, the carcinoma was destroyed by the more aggressive choriocarcinoma. This idea is supported by patient age at presentation of gastrointestinal choriocarcinoma, which is similar to that of adenocarcinoma rather than genital choriocarcinoma, which occurs in a younger age group. An alternative possibility is that pure choriocarcinoma of the gastrointestinal tract represents long-delayed metastasis of primary gonadal tumors, but there is no evidence for this.

Clinically, all four patients with esophageal choriocarcinoma reported to date were in their early forties. They presented either with severe gastrointestinal hemorrhage or widespread metastatic disease, and all were dead within 3 months. The patients had markedly elevated serum gonadotrophins and gynecomastia. Diagnosis was made by endoscopic biopsy in three cases and by brush cytology in one (160).

On gross examination, choriocarcinomas are large, exophytic, fungating tumors that may encircle the esophagus. There is marked necrosis and hemorrhage, often with little evidence of grossly viable tumor.

Microscopic examination reveals the typical features of choriocarcinoma, with an admixture of syncytiotrophoblasts and cytotrophoblasts. All cases had extensive necrosis and hemorrhage of tumor gith extension usually through the muscularis propria. Viable tumor cells were present only at the periphery. A careful search of the tumor often revealed foci of adenocarcinoma. The cytotrophoblastic component of the tumor was composed of small cells with relatively little cytoplasm arranged in cords and clusters. The syncytiotrophoblasts were characterized by large irregularly shaped cells with vacuolated cytoplasm and indistinct cell borders. They were multinucleated, with numerous clusters or rows of large pleomorphic hyperchromatic nuclei; large irregularly shaped nucleoli were often surrounded by a clear halo.

In one case cytologic brushings showed both syncytiotrophoblastic and cytotrophoblastic cells (160). These were characterized by clustered and single malignant cells with ample cytoplasm, large bizarre nuclei, and prominent irregular nucleoli. The nuclear chromatin was irregular, with clumping at the borders. There were numerous giant multinucleated cells, with nuclear molding and abundant amphophilic cytoplasm.

For further details see Choriocarcinomas of the Stomach, chapter 12.

## REFERENCES

### Barrett Esophagus, Barrett's Dysplasia, and Adenocarcinoma

1. Agha FP, Keren DF. Barrett's esophagus complicating achalasia after esophagomyotomy. A clinical, radiologic, and pathologic study of 70 patients with achalasia and related motor disorders. J Clin Gastroenterol 1987;9:232–7.

2. Appelqvist P. Carcinoma of the oesophagus and gastric cardia at autopsy in Finland. Ann Clin Res 1975;7:334–40.

3. Atkinson M. Barrett's oesophagus—to screen or not to screen? Gut 1989;30:2–5.

4. Attah EB, Hajdu SI. Benign and malignant tumors of the esophagus at autopsy. J Thorac Cardiovasc Surg 1968;55:396–404.

5. Attwood SE, DeMeester RR, Bremner CG, Barlow AP, Hinder RA. Alkaline gastroesophageal reflux: implications in the development of complications in Barrett's columnar-lined esophagus. Surgery 1989;106:764–70.

6. Banner BF, Memoli VA, Warren WH, Gould VE. Carcinoma with multidirectional differentiation arising in Barrett's esophagus. Ultrastruct Pathol 1983;4:205–17.

7. Blaser MJ, Perez-Perez GI, Lindenbaum J, et al. Association of infection due to Helicobacter pylori with specific upper gastrointestinal pathology. Rev Infect Dis 1991;13:704–8.

8. Blot WJ, Devesa SS, Fraumeni JF Jr. Continuing climb in rates of esophageal adenocarcinoma: an update [Letter]. JAMA 1993;270:1320.

9. Blount PL, Ramel S, Raskind WH, et al. 17p allelic deletions and p53 protein overexpression in Barrett's adenocarcinoma. Cancer Res 1991;15:5482–6.

10. Bosch A, Frias Z, Caldwell WL, Jaeschke WH. Autopsy findings in carcinoma of the esophagus. Acta Radiol Oncol 1979;18:103–12.

11. Boynton RF, Blount PL, Yin J, et al. Loss of heterozygosity involving the APC and MCC genetic loci occurs in the majority of human esophageal cancers. Proc Nat Acad Sci 1992;99:3385–8.

12. Bremner CG, Lynch VP, Ellis FH, Jr. Barrett's esophagus: congenital or acquired? An experimental study of esophageal mucosal regeneration in the dog. Surgery 1970;68:209–16.

13. Burgess JN, Payne WS, Andersen HA, et al. Barrett esophagus. The columnar-epithelial-lined lower esophagus. Mayo Clin Proc 1971;46:728–34.

14. Burke AP, Sobin LH, Shekitka KM, Avallone FA. Correlation of nucleolar organizer regions and glandular dysplasia of the stomach and esophagus. Mod Pathol 1990;3:357–60.

15. Burke AP, Sobin LH, Shekitka KM, Helvig EB. Dysplasia of the stomach and Barrett esophagus: a follow-up study. Mod Pathol 1991;4:336–41.

16. Cameron AJ, Lomboy CT, Pera M, Carpenter HA. Adenocarcinoma of the esophagogastric junction and Barrett's esophagus. Gastroenterology 1995;109:1541–6.

16a. Cameron AJ, Ott BJ, Payne WS. The incidence of adenocarcinoma in columnar-lined (Barrett's) esophagus. N Engl J Med 1985;313:857–9.

17. Cameron AJ, Zinsmeister AR, Ballard DJ, Carney JA. Prevalence of columnar-lined (Barrett's) esophagus. Comparison of population-based clinical and autopsy findings. Gastroenterology 1990;99:918–22.

18. Casson AG, Mukhopadhyay R, Cleary KR, Ro JY, Levin B, Roth JA. P53 gene mutations in Barrett's epithelium and esophageal cancers. Cancer Res 1991;51:4495–9.

18a. Chow WH, Finkle WD, McLaughlin JK, Frankl H, Ziel HK, Fraumeni JF Jr. The relation of gastroesophageal reflux disease and its treatment to adenocarcinomas of the esophagus and gastric cardia. JAMA 1995;274:474–7.

19. Cooper BT, Barbezat GO. Barrett's oesophagus: a clinical study of 52 patients. Q J Med 1987;238:97–108.

20. Crabb DW, Berk MA, Hall TR, Conneally PM, Biegel AA, Lehman GA. Familial gastroesophageal reflux and development of Barrett's esophagus. Ann Intern Med 1985;103:52–4.

21. Dahms BB, Rothstein FC. Barrett's esophagus in children: A consequence of chronic gastroesophageal reflux. Gastroenterology 1984;86:318–23.

22. DeMeester TR, Attwood SE, Smyrk TC, Therkildsen DH, Hinder RA. Surgical therapy in Barrett's esophagus. Ann Surg 1990;212:528–40.

23. Duhaylongsod FG, Wolfe WG. Barrett's esophagus and adenocarcinoma of the esophagus and gastroesophageal junction. J Thorac Cardiovasc Surg 1991;102:36–41.

24. Ellis FH Jr. Barrett's esophagus, a continuing conundrum. Postgrad Med 1991;90:135–8, 143–6.

25. Emery JL, Haddadin AJ. Gastric type epithelium in the upper esophageal pouch in children with tracheo-esophageal fistula. J Pediatr Surg 1971;6:449–53.

26. Fennerty MB, Sampliner RE, Way D, Riddell R, Steinbronn K, Garewal HS. Discordance between flow cytometric abnormalities and dysplasia in Barrett's esophagus. Gastroenterology 1989;97:815–20.

27. Fennerty MB, Way D, Sampliner RE, Riddell RH, Sloan D, Garewal H. Discordance between flow cytometry and dysplasia in patients with Barrett's esophagus [Abstract]. Gastroenterology 1988;94:125.

28. Filipe MI. Mucins in the human gastrointestinal epithelium: A review. Invest Cell Pathol 1979;2:195–216.

29. Flejou JF, Boublet B, Metayer J, Hemet J, Potet F. Flow cytometric study of adenocarcinoma in Barrett esophagus: prognostic implications [Abstract]. Gastroenterology 1989;96:153

30. Forastiere AA, Gennis M, Orringer MV, Agha FP. Cisplatin, vinblastine and mitoquazone chemotherapy for epidermoid and adenocarcinoma of the esophagus. Clin Oncol 1987;5:1143–9.

31. Garewal HS, Sampliner RE, Fennerty MB. Flow cytometry in Barrett's esophagus. What have we learned so far? Dig Dis Sci 1991;36:548–51.

32. Garewal HS, Sampliner R, Gerner E, et al. Ornithine decarboxylase activity in Barrett's esophagus: a potential marker for dysplasia. Gastroenterology 1988;94:819–21.

33. Garewal HS, Sampliner R, Liu Y, Trent JM. Chromosomal rearrangements in Barrett's esophagus. A premalignant lesion of esophageal adenocarcinoma. Cancer Genet Cytogenet 1989;42:281–6.

34. Geisinger KR, Teot LA, Richter JE. A comparative cytopathologic and histologic study of atypia, dysplasia, and adenocarcinoma in Barrett's esophagus. Cancer 1992;69:8–16.

35. Gillen P, Keeling P, Byrne PJ, Hennessy TP. Barrett's oesophagus: pH profile. Br J Surg 1987;74:774–6.

36. Goldstein N, Weinstein WM, Marin-Sorenson M, et al. Short segment Barrett's esophagus (BE) and the cardia mucosa in gastroesophageal reflux disease (GERD) have a similar prevalence of specialized epithelium. Gastroenterology 1991;100:A72.

37. Gottfried MR, McClave SA, Boyce HW. Incomplete intestinal metaplasia in the diagnosis of columnar lined esophagus (Barrett's esophagus). Am J Clin Pathol 1989;92:741–6.

38. Graham DY, Schwartz JT, Cain GD, Gyorkey F. Prospective evaluation of biopsy number in the diagnosis of esophageal and gastric carcinoma. Gastroenterology 1982;82:228–31.

39. Griffin M, Sweeney EC. The relationship of endocrine cells, dysplasia and carcinoembryonic antigen in Barrett's mucosa to adenocarcinoma of the oesophagus. Histopathology 1987;11:53–62.

40. Haggitt RC, Barrett's esophagus, dysplasia and adenocarcinoma. Hum Pathol 1994;25:982–93.

41. Haggitt RC, Reid BJ, Rabinovitch PS, Rubin CE. Barrett's esophagus. Correlation between mucin histochemistry, flow cytometry, and histologic diagnosis for predicting increased cancer risk. Am J Pathol 1988;131:53–61.

42. Hameeteman W, Tytgat GN, Houthoff HJ, van den Tweel JG. Barrett's esophagus: development of dysplasia and adenocarcinoma. Gastroenterology 1989;96:1249–56.

43. Hamilton SR, Hutcheon DF, Ravich WJ, Cameron JL, Paulson M. Adenocarcinoma in Barrett's esophagus after elimination of gastroesophageal reflux. Gastroenterology 1984;86:356–60.

44. Hamilton SR, Smith RR. The relationship between columnar epithelial dysplasia and invasive adenocarcinoma arising in Barrett's esophagus. Am J Clin Pathol 1987;87:301–12.

45. Hamilton SR, Smith RR, Cameron JL. Prevalence and characteristics of Barrett esophagus in patients with adenocarcinoma of the esophagus or esophagogastric junction. Hum Pathol 1988;19:942–8.

46. Hamilton SR, Yardley JH. Regeneration of cardiac-type mucosa and acquisition of Barrett mucosa after esophagogastrostomy. Gastroenterology 1977;72:669–75.

47. Hassall E, Weinstein WM, Ament ME. Barrett's esophagus in childhood. Gastroenterology 1985;89:1331–7.

48. Hesketh PJ, Clapp RW, Doos WG, Spechler SJ. The increasing frequency of adenocarcinoma of the esophagus. Cancer 1989;64:526–30.

49. Iizuka T, Isono K, Kakegawa T, Watanabe H. Parameters linked to ten-year survival in Japan of resected esophageal carcinoma. Japanese Committee for Registration of Esophageal Carcinoma Cases. Chest 1989;96:1005–11.

50. James PD, Atkinson M. Value of DNA image cytometry in the prediction of malignant change in Barrett's oesophagus. Gut 1989;30:899–905.

51. Jass JR. Mucin histochemistry of the columnar epithelium of the oesophagus: a retrospective study. J Clin Pathol 1981;34:866–70.

52. Johnson DA, Winters C, Spurling TJ, Chobanian SJ, Cattau EL Jr. Esophageal acid sensitivity in Barrett's esophagus. J Clin Gastroenterol 1987;9:23–7.

53. Kalish RJ, Clancy PE, Orringer MB, Appelman HD. Clinical, epidemiologic, and morphologic comparison between adenocarcinomas arising in Barrett's esophageal mucosa

and in the gastric cardia. Gastroenterology 1984;86:461–7.

54. Katzka DA. Barrett's esophagus: detection and management. Gastroenterol Clin North Am 1989;18:339–57.

55. Katzka DA, Reynolds JC, Saul SH, Plotkin A, et al. Barrett's metaplasia and adenocarcinoma of the esophagus in scleroderma. Am J Med 1987;82:46–52.

55a. Krishnadath KK, Tilanus HW, van Blankenstein M, Bosman FT, Mulder AH. Accumulation of p53 protein in normal, dysplastic, and neoplastic Barrett's oesophagus. J Pathol 1995;175:175–80.

55b. Krishnamurthy S, Dayal Y. Pancreatic metaplasia in Barrett's esophagus. An immunohistochemical study. Amer J Surg Pathol 1995;19:1172–80.

56. Layfield LJ, Weinstein WM, Ulich TR, Cheng L, Lewin KJ. Serotonin and polypeptide hormone production in Barrett's esophagus. Surg Pathol 1988;1:131–6.

57. Lee RG. Adenomas arising in Barrett's esophagus. Am J Clin Pathol 1986;83:629–32.

58. Lee RG. Dysplasia in Barrett's esophagus. A clinical pathologic study of six patients. Am J Surg Pathol 1985;9:845–52.

59. Lee RG. Mucins in Barrett's esophagus: a histochemical study. Am J Clin Pathol 1984;81:500–3.

59a. Levine DS. Barrett's oesophagus and p53. Lancet 1994;344:212–3.

60. Levine DS, Haggitt RC, Blount PL, Rabinovitch PS, Rusch VW, Reid BJ. An endoscopic biopsy protocol can differentiate high-grade dysplasia from early adenocarcinoma in Barrett's esophagus. Gastroenterology 1993;105:40–50.

61. Levine DS, Rubin CE, Reid BJ, Haggitt RC. Specialized metaplastic columnar epithelium in Barrett's esophagus. A comparative transmission electron microscopic study. Lab Invest 1989;60:418–32.

62. Levine MS, Dillon EC, Saul SH, Laufer I. Early esophageal cancer. AJR Am J Roentgenol 1986;146:507–12.

63. Lewin KJ, Riddell RH, Weinstein WM. Inflammatory disorders of the esophagus: reflux and nonreflux types. In: Lewin KJ, Riddell RH, Weinstein WM., eds. Gastrointestinal pathology and its clinical implications. Igaku-Shoin: New York, 1992:401–39.

64. Lightdale CJ, Botet JF, Kelsen DP, Turnbull AD, Brennan MF. Diagnosis of recurrent upper gastrointestinal cancer at the surgical anastomosis by endoscopic ultrasound. Gastrointest Endosc 1989;35:407–13.

65. Loffeld RL, Ten Tije BJ, Arends JW. Prevalence and significance of Helicobacter pylori in patients with Barrett's esophagus. Am J Gastroenterol 1992;87:1598–600.

66. MacDonald WC, MacDonald JB. Adenocarcinoma of the esophagus and/or gastric cardia. Cancer 1987;60:1094–8.

67. Mandard AM, Marnay J, Gignoux M, et al. Cancer of the esophagus and associated lesions: detailed pathologic study of 100 esophagectomy specimens. Hum Pathol 1984;15:660–9.

68. McArdle JE, Lewin KJ, Randall G, Weinstein W. Distribution of dysplasias and early invasive carcinoma in Barrett's esophagus. Hum Pathol 1992;23:479–82.

69. McClave SA, Boyce HW, Gottfried MR. Early diagnosis of columnar-lined esophagus: a new endoscopic diagnostic criterion. Gastrointest Endosc 1987;33:413–6.

70. McDonald GB, Brand DL, Thorning DR. Multiple adenomatous neoplasms arising in columnar-lined (Barrett's) esophagus. Gastroenterology 1977;72:1317–21.

71. McKinley MJ, Budman DR, Grueneberg D, Bronzo RL, Weissman GS, Kahn E. DNA content in Barrett's esophagus and esophageal malignancy. Am J Gastroenterol 1987;82:1012–5.

71a. Menke-Pluymers MB, Mulder AH, Hop WC, van Blankenstein M, Tilanus HW. Dysplasia and aneuploidy as markers of malignant degeneration in Barrett's esophagus. The Rotterdam Oesophageal Tumor Study. Gut 1994;35:1348–51.

72. Meuwissen SG, Bosma A, van Donk E, et al. Immunohistochemical localization of pepsinogen A and C containing cells in Barrett's oesophagus. Virchows Arch [A] 1988;413:11–6.

73. Meyer W, Vollmar F, Bar W. Barrett-esophagus following total gastrectomy. A contribution to its pathogenesis. Endoscopy 1979;2:121–6.

74. Ming SC, Bullough PG. Coexisting adenocarcinomas of the esophagus and of the esophagogastric junction. Sm J Dig Dis 1963;8:439–43.

75. Moon MR, Schulte WJ, Haasler GB, Condon RE. Transhiatal and transthoracic esophagectomy for adenocarcinoma of the esophagus. Arch Surg 1992;127:951–5.

76. Naef AP, Savary M, Ozzello. Columnar-lined lower esophagus: an acquired lesion with malignant predisposition. Report on 140 cases of Barret's esophagus with 12 adenocarcinomas. J Thorac Cardiovasc Surg 1975;70:826–935.

77. Odes HS, Maor E, Barki Y, Charuzi I, Krawiec J, Bar-ziv J. Varicoid carcinoma of the esophagus. Report of a patient with adenocarcinoma and review of the literature. Am J Gastroenterol 1980;73:141–5.

77a. Offner FA, Weinstein WM, Lewin KJ. Columnar, non-goblet cell metaplasia: a neglected feature in the diagnosis of Barrett's esophagus [Abstract]. Gastroenterology 1995;108:180.

78. Osama M, Abdelatif A, Chandler FW. Differential expression of c-myc and H-ras oncogenes in Barrett's epithelium. Arch Pathol Lab Med 1991;115:880–5.

79. Palley SL, Sampliner RE, Garewal HS. Management of high-grade dysplasia in Barrett's esophagus. J Clin Gastroenterol 1989;11:369–72.

80. Paull A, Trier JS, Dalton MD, Camp RC, Loeb P, Goyal RK. The histologic spectrum of Barrett's esophagus. N Engl J Med 1976;295:476–80.

81. Paull G, Yardley JH. Gastric and esophageal Campylobacter pylori in patients with Barrett's esophagus. N Engl J Med 1988;95:216–8.

81a. Paraf F, Flejou JF, Pignon JP, Fekete F, Potet F. Surgical pathology of adenocarcinoma arising in Barrett's esophagus. Analysis of 67 cases. Am J Surg Pathol 1995;19:183–91.

82. Pera M, Cameron AJ, Trastek VF, Carpenter HA, Zineister AR. Increasing incidence of adenocarcinoma of the esophagus and esophagogastric junction. Gastroenterology 1993;104:510–3.

83. Peuchmaur M, Potet F, Goldfain D. Mucin histochemistry of the columnar epithelium of the oesophagus (Barrett's oesophagus): a prospective biopsy study. J Clin Pathol 1984;37:607–10.

84. Polepalle SC, McCallum RW. Barrett's esophagus. Current assessment and future perspectives. Gastroenterol Clin North Am 1990;19:733–44.

85. Rabinovitch PS, Reid BJ, Haggitt RC, Norwood TH, Rubin CE. Progression to cancer in Barrett's esophagus is associated with genomic instability. Lab Invest 1989;60:65–71.

86. Ramage JK, Hall J, Williams JC. Barrett's oesophagus [Letter]. Lancet 1987;2:851

87. Raskind WH, Norwood T, Levine DS, et al. Persistent clonal areas and clonal expansion in Barrett's esophagus. Cancer Res 1992;52:2946–50.

88. Recht MP, Levine MS, Katzka DA, Reynolds JC, Saul SH. Barrett's esophagus in scleroderma: increased prevalence and radiographic findings. Gastrointest Radiol 1988;13:1–5.

89. Rector LE, Connerley ML. Aberrant mucosa in the esophagus in infants and children. Arch Pathol 1941;31:285–94.

90. Reid BJ. Barrett's esophagus and esophageal adenocarcinoma. Gastroenterol Clin North Am 1991;20:817–34.

91. Reid BJ, Blount PL, Levine DS, et al. Flow-cytometric and histological progression to malignancy in Barrett's esophagus: prospective endoscopic surveillance of a cohort. Gastroenterology 1992;102:1421–4.

92. Reid BJ, Blount PL, Rubin CE, Levine DS, Haggitt RC, Rabinovitch PS. Predictors of progression to malignancy in Barrett's esophagus: endoscopic, histologic and flow cytometric followup of a cohort. Gastroenterology 1992;102:1212–9.

93. Reid BJ, Haggitt RC, Rubin CE, et al. Observer variation in the diagnosis of dysplasia in Barrett's esophagus. Human Pathology 1988;19:166–78.

94. Reid BJ, Haggitt RL, Rubin LE, Rabinovitch PS. Barrett's esophagus: Correlation between flow cytometry and histology in detection of patients at risk for adenocarcinoma. Gastroenterology 1987;93:1–11.

95. Reid BJ, Weinstein WM. Barrett's esophagus and adenocarcinoma. Ann Rev Med 1987;38:477–92.

96. Reid BJ, Weinstein WM, Lewin KJ, et al. Endoscopic biopsy can detect high-grade dysplasia or early adenocarcinoma in Barrett's esophagus without grossly recognizable neoplastic lesions. Gastroenterology 1988;94:81–90.

97. Riddell RH. Dysplasia and regression in Barrett's esophagus. In: Spechler SJ, Goyal RK., eds. Barrett's esophagus. Pathophysiology, diagnosis and management. Elsevier: New York, 1984: 143–52.

98. Rindi G, Bishop AE, Daly MJ, Isaacs P, Lee FI, Polak JM. A mixed pattern of endocrine cells in metaplastic Barrett's oesophagus. Evidence that the epithelium derives from a pluripotential stem cell. Histochemistry 1987; 87:377–83.

99. Robertson DA, Ayres RC, Smith CL. Screening for colonic cancer in patients with Barrett's oesophagus. BMJ 1989; 298:650

100. Robey SS, Hamilton SR, Gupta PK, Erozan YS. Diagnostic value of Cytopathology in Barrett esophagus and associated carcinoma. Am J Clin Pathol 1988;89:493–8.

101. Rogers EL, Goldkind S., Iseri OA, et al. Adenocarcinoma of the lower esophagus: A disease primarily of white men with Barrett's esophagus. J Clin Gastroenterol 1986;8:613–518.

102. Rosenberg C, Budev H, Edwards RC, Singal S, Steiger Z, Sundareson AS. Analysis of adenocarcinoma in Barrett's esophagus utilizing a staging system. Cancer 1985;55:1353–60.

103. Rosengard AM, Hamilton SR. Squamous carcinoma of the esophagus in patients with Barrett esophagus. Mod Pathol 1989;2:2–7.

104. Rubin CE, Haggitt RC, Levine DS. Endoscopic mucosal biopsy. In: Yamada T, Alpers DH, Owyang C, Silverstein FE, eds. Textbook of gastroenterology. Philadelphia: Lippincott, 1991:2479–523.

105. Rubio CA, Aberg B. Barrett's mucosa in conjunction with squamous carcinoma of the esophagus. Cancer 1991;68:583–6.

106. Rubio CA, Riddell R. Musculo-fibrous anomaly in Barrett's mucosa with dysplasia. Am J Surg Pathol 1988;12:885–9.

106a. Rusch VW, Levine DS, Haggitt RC, Reid BJ. The management of high-grade dysplasia and early cancer in Barrett's esophagus. A multidisciplinary problem. Cancer 1994;74:1225–9.

107. Sampliner RE, Steinbronn K, Garewal HS, Riddell RH. Squamous mucosa overlying columnar epithelium in Barrett's esophagus in absence of anti-refux surgery. Am J Gastroenterol 1988;83:510–2.

108. Sanfey H, Hamilton SR, Smith RR, Cameron JL. Carcinoma arising in Barrett's esophagus. Surg Gynecol Obstet 1985;161:570–4.

109. Sasano H, Miyazaki S, Gooukon Y, Nishihihira T, Sawai T, Hagura H. Expression of p53 in human esophageal carcinoma: an immunohistochemical study with correlation to proliferating cell nuclear antigen expression. Hum Pathol 1992;23:1238–43.

110. Schmidt HG, Riddell RH, Walther B, Skinner DB, Riemann JF. Dysplasia in Barrett's esophagus. J Cancer Res Clin Oncol 1985;110:145–52.

111. Schnell T, Sontag G, Chejfec G, et al. Does length of Barrett's esophagus correlate with age, cigarette or alcohol consumption, or risk of adenocarcinoma [Abstract]. Gastroenterology 1990;98:A120

112. Schreiber DS, Apstein M, Hermos JA. Paneth cells in Barrett's esophagus. Gastroenterology 1978;74:1302–4.

113. Segel MC, Campbell WL, Medsger TA Jr, Roumm AD. Systemic sclerosis (scleroderma) and esophageal adenocarcinoma: is increased patient screening necessary? Gastroenterology 1985;89:485–9.

114. Shah AN, Gunby TC. Adenocarcinoma and Barrett's esophagus following surgically treated achalasia. Gastrointest Endosc 1984;30:294–6.

115. Skinner DB, Walther BC, Riddell RH, Schmidt H, Iascone C, De Meester TR. Barrett's esophagus: comparison of benign and malignant cases. Ann Surg 1983;198:554–66.

116. Smith RR, Hamilton SR, Boitnott JK, Rogers EL. The spectrum of carcinoma arising in Barrett's esophagus. A clinicopathologic study of 26 patients. Am J Surg Pathol 1984;8:563–73.

117. Sontag SJ, Schnell TG, Chejfec G, et al. Barrett's oesophagus and colonic tumours. Lancet 1985;1:946–9.

118. Spechler SJ. Barrett's esophagus: what's new and what to do. Am J Gastroenterol 1989;84:220–3.

119. Spechler SJ. Endoscopic surveillance for patients with Barrett's esophagus: does the cancer risk justify the practice? Ann Intern Med 1987;106:902–4.

120. Spechler SJ, Goyal RK. Barrett's esophagus. N Engl J Med 1986;315:362–71.

121. Spechler SJ, Robbins AH, Rubins HB, et al. Adenocarcinoma and Barrett's esophagus. An overrated risk?. Gastroenterology 1984;87:927–33.

122. Spechler SJ, Schimmel EM, Dalton JW, et al. Barrett's epithelium complicating lye ingestion with sparing of the distal esophagus. Gastroenterology 1981;81:580–3.

122a. Spechler SJ, Zeroogian JM, Antonioli DA, Wang HH, Goyal RK. Prevalence of metaplsia at the gastro-oesophageal junction. Lancet 1994;344:1533–6.

123. Steiger Z, Wilson RF, Leichman L, Busuito MJ, Rosenberg JC. Primary adenocarcinoma of the esophagus. J Surg Oncol 1987;36:68–70.

124. Streitz JM Jr, Ellis FH Jr, Gibb SP, Balogh K, Watkins E Jr. Adenocarcinoma in Barrett's esophagus. A clinicopathologic study of 65 cases. Ann Surg 1991;213:122–5.

125. Symonds DA, Ramsey HE. Adenocarcinoma arising in Barrett's esophagus with Zollinger-Ellison syndrome. Am J Clin Pathol 1980;73:823–6.

126. Takashima S, Takeuchi N, Shiozaki H, et al. Carcinoma of the esophagus; CT vs MR imaging in determining resectability. AJR Am J Roentgenol 1991;156:297–302.

127. Takubo K, Sasajima K, Yamashita K, Tanaka Y, Fujita K. Double muscularis mucosae in Barrett's esophagus. Hum Pathol 1991;22:1158–61.

128. Talley NJ, Cameron AJ, Shorter RG, Zinsmeister AR, Phillips SF. Campylobacter pylori and Barrett's esophagus. Mayo Clin Proc 1988;63:1176–80.

129. Tally R, Weinstein WM, Marin-Sorensen M, Schneidman D, Reedy TJ, Van Deventer G. Campylobacter pylori colonization of Barrett's esophagus [Abstract]. Gastroenterology 1988;94:454.

130. Thompson JJ, Zinsser KR, Enterline HT. Barrett's metaplasia and adenocarcinoma of the esophagus and gastroesophageal junction. Hum Pathol 1983;14:42–61.

131. Tio TL, den Hartog Jager FC, Tytgat GN. The role of endoscopic ultrasonography in assessing local resectability of oesophagogastric malignancies. Accuracy, pitfalls and predictability. Scand J Gastroenterol 1986;123(Suppl):78–86.

132. TNM classification of malignant tumours. Spiessl B, Beahrs OH, Hermanek P, et al. eds. UICC International Union Against Cancer. 4th ed. Berlin: Springer Verlag, 1992.

133. Tripp MR, Sampliner RE, Kogan FJ, Morgan TR. Colorectal neoplasms and Barrett's esophagus. Am J Gastroenterol 1986;81:1063–4.

133a. Vaezi MF, Richter JE. Synergism of acid and duodenogastroesophageal reflux in complicated Barrett's esophagus. Surgery 1995;117:699–704.

134. Van der Veen AH, Dees J, Blankensteijn JD, Van Blankenstein M. Adenocarcinoma in Barrett's oesophagus: an overrated risk. Gut 1989;30:14–8.

135. Van Overhagen H, Lameris JS, Berger MY, et al. Supraclavicular lymph node metastases in carcinoma of the esophagus and gastroesophageal junction: assessment with CT, US, and US-guided fine-needle aspiration biopsy. Radiology 1991;179:155–8.

136. Vilmann P, Hancke S. Endoscopic ultrasound scanning of the upper gastrointestinal canal. Ugeskr Laeger 1991;153:414–7.

137. Wang HH, Antonioli DA, Goldman H. Comparative features of esophageal and gastric adenocarcinomas: recent changes in type and frequency. Hum Pathol 1986;17:482–7.

138. Wang HH, Ducatman BS, Thibault S. Cytologic features of premalignant glandular lesions in the upper gastrointestinal tract. Acta Cytol 1991;35:199–203.

139. Winters C Jr, Spurling TJ, Chobanian SJ, et al. Barrett's esophagus. A prevalent, occult complication of gastroesophageal reflux disease. Gastroenterology 1987;92:118–24.

140. Witt TR, Bains MS, Zaman MB, Martini N. Adenocarcinoma in Barrett's esophagus. J Thorac Cardiovasc Surg 1983;85:337–45.
141. Yang PC, Davis S. Incidence of cancer of the esophagus in the U.S. by histologic type. Cancer 1988;61:612–7.

142. Yoshida M, Ide H, Yamada A, Endo M. Early detection of adenocarcinoma of the esophagus. Endoscopy 1986;18:44–8.
143. Zwas F, Shields HM, Doos WG, et al. Scanning electron microscopy of Barrett's epithelium and its correlation with light microscopy and mucin stains. Gastroenterology 1986;90:1932–41.

### Adenosquamous Carcinoma and Adenoacanthoma

144. Banner BF, Memoli VA, Warren WH, Gould VE. Carcinoma with multidirectional differentiation arising in Barrett's esophagus. Ultrastruct Pathol 1983;4:205–17.
144a. Bombi JA, Riverola A, Bordas JM, Cardesa A. Adenosquamous carcinoma of the esophagus. A case report. Pathol Res Pract 1991;187:514–9.
145. Kuwano H, Nagamatsu M, Matsuda H, Mori M, Sugimachi K. Coexistence of intraepithelial carcinoma and

glandular differentiation in esophageal squamous cell carcinoma. Cancer 1988;62:1568–72.
146. Pascal RR, Clearfield HR. Mucoepidermoid (adenosquamous) carcinoma arising in Barrett's esophagus. Dig Dis Sci 1987;32:428–32.
147. Raphael HA, Ellis FH Jr, Dockerty MB. Primary adenocarcinoma of the esophagus: 18-year review and review of literature. Ann Surg 1966;164:785–96.

### Adenocarcinoma Unassociated with Barrett Esophagus

148. Azzopardi JG, Menzies T. Primary oesophageal adenocarcinoma: confirmation of its existence by the finding of mucous gland tumors. Br J Surg 1961;49:497–506.
149. Blaauwgeers JL, Allema JH, Bosma A, Brummelkamp WH. Early adenoid cystic carcinoma of the upper esophagus. Eur J Surg Oncol 1990;16:77–81.
150. Cerar A, Jutersek A, Vidmar S. Adenoid cystic carcinoma of the esophagus. A clinicopathologic study of three cases. Cancer 1991;67:2159–64.
151. Christensen WN, Sternberg SS. Adenocarcinoma of the upper esophagus arising in ectopic gastric mucosa. Two case reports and review of the literature. Am J Surg Pathol 1987;11:397–402.
152. Feller SC, Weaver GA. Heterotopic gastric mucosa in the upper esophagus [Letter]. Gastroenterology 1986;90:257–8.
153. Goldfarb TG. Esophageal gland adenocarcinoma of the mid-esophagus. Report of a case. Am J Clin Pathol 1967;48:281–5.
154. Kim JH, Lee MS, Cho SW, Shim CS. Primary adenoid cystic carcinoma of the esophagus: a case report. Endoscopy 1991;23:38–41.

154a. Rector LE, Connerley ML. Aberrant mucosa in the esophagus in infants and children. Arch Pathol 1941;31:285–94.
155. Schmidt H, Riddell RH, Walther B, Skinner DB, Riemann JF, Groitl H. Adnokarzinome in heterotoper Magenschleimhaut des proximalen Oesophagus. (Adenocarcinoma of heterotopic gastric mucosa in the proximal esophagus). Leber Magen Darm 1985;15:144–7.
156. Schridde H. Uber Magenschleimhaut-Inseln von Bau der Cardialdrusenregion und den unteren, oesophagelin Cardialdrusen gleichende Druksen in obersten Oesophagusabschnitt. Virchows Arch [A] 1904;175:1–16.
156a. Takagi A, Ema Y, Horii S, Morishita M, Miyaishi O, Kino I. Early adenocarcinoma arising from ectopic gastric mucosa in the cervical esophagus. Gastrointest Endosc 1995;41:167–70.
157. Woodard BH, Shelburne JD, Vollmer RT, Postlethwait RW. Mucoepidermoid carcinoma of the esophagus: a case report. Hum Pathol 1978;9:352–4.

### Choriocarcinoma of the Esophagus

158. Kikuchi Y, Tsuneta Y, Kawai T, Aizawa M. Choriocarcinoma of the esophagus producing chorionic gonadotropin. Acta Pathol Jpn 1988;38:489–99.
159. McKechnie JC, Fechner RE. Choriocarcinoma and adenocarcinoma of the esophagus with gonadotropin secretion. Cancer 1971;27:694–702.

160. Trillo AA, Accettullo LM, Yeiter TL. Choriocarcinoma of the esophagus: histologic and cytologic findings. A case report. Acta Cytol 1979;23:69–74.

# 6

# MESENCHYMAL TUMORS AND
# TUMOR-LIKE PROLIFERATIONS OF THE ESOPHAGUS

Compared to the stomach, where stromal tumors are relatively common, few stromal tumors of clinical significance arise within the esophagus. Leiomyomas are the most common, followed by granular cell tumors. After that, all the rest are so rare that only skimpy clinical, radiologic, endoscopic, and morphologic data are available. It is likely that at least one of every type of stromal tumor, both benign and malignant, has occurred in the esophagus. In this chapter, only the more common of these rare tumors are discussed.

## LEIOMYOMA

**General Considerations.** In contrast to the stomach, where typical, well-differentiated smooth muscle tumors are unusual and stromal tumors of questionable differentiation are the rule, the most common stromal tumors by far in the esophagus are classic leiomyomas, composed of mature smooth muscle cells. They are identical to the leiomyomas that arise in the myometrium. Gastric-type stromal tumors composed of undifferentiated and poorly differentiated cells are so rare in the esophagus that there is no literature that describes and analyzes them.

Most esophageal leiomyomas are tiny, a few millimeters in diameter at most, so that they are usually not apparent upon gross inspection. Instead, they are discovered by accident during light microscopic examination. They arise mostly within the inner circular layer of the muscularis propria but also in the muscularis mucosae (figs. 6-1–6-4) (56). Tiny leiomyomas are called *seedling leiomyomas,* and they presumably are the forerunners (seedlings) of the large symptomatic ones (56). About two thirds of these tiny tumors arise in and around the esophagogastric junction, the area of the lower esophageal sphincter (see Gastric Mesenchymal Tumors).

**Clinical Features.** Clinically significant leiomyomas are those that are large and cause symptoms of obstruction, such as dysphagia. However, some large tumors are asymptomatic and are found by accident as a result of chest X rays or endoscopy for other diseases. In the exhaustive review of the leiomyoma literature by Seremetis et al. (54), covering cases from the sixteenth century to the early 1970s, dysphagia; retrosternal, epigastric, or noncardiac chest pain; and pyrosis were the most common symptoms,

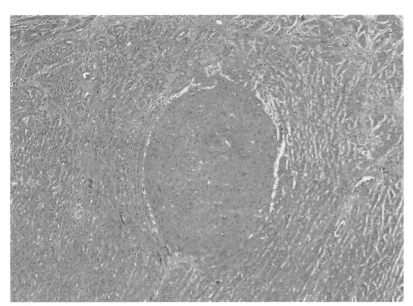

Figure 6-1
SMALL (SEEDLING) LEIOMYOMA OF THE INNER LAYER OF THE MUSCULARIS PROPRIA

The tumor is well circumscribed and distinctly different from the surrounding muscularis, although it and the muscularis are composed of the same cells.

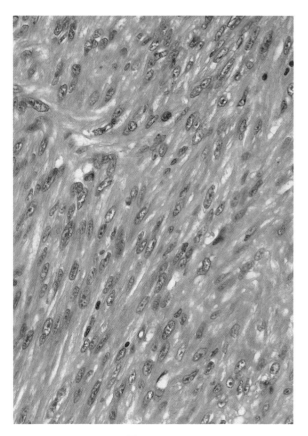

Figure 6-2
SEEDLING LEIOMYOMAS
All leiomyomas of the esophagus are composed of mature, hypertrophied smooth muscle cells, such as these, with elongated nuclei and abundant, longitudinally fibrillar cytoplasm.

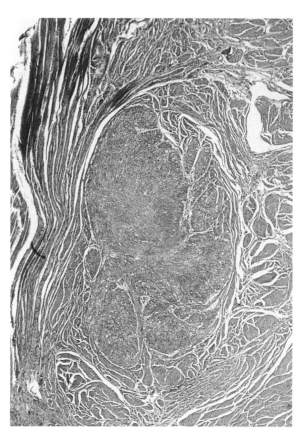

Figure 6-3
SEEDLING LEIOMYOMAS
A cluster of seedling leiomyomas within the muscularis propria, forming a single multilobular mass.

occurring in 80 to 90 percent of symptomatic patients; weight loss occurred in half. This has been substantiated by other reports (51,55). Which symptoms are due to the leiomyoma or to other diseases of the esophagus is not known. The duration of symptoms is usually long, 2 years or more, mimicking chronic gastroesophageal reflux clinically. There is no predictable patient profile. In four studies (11, 26, 20, and 19 patients) the male to female ratio was about 2 to 1, and the mean age was in the mid to late fifth decade (25,37,49,53). The location of the leiomyoma within the esophagus varies but in general, about 90 percent are in the lower and middle thirds.

The diagnosis is unlikely to be made by endoscopic biopsy, since the large, symptomatic tumors are deep within the muscularis propria and the overlying mucosa is usually intact. The tumors hardly ever ulcerate the mucosa. Instead, the mucosa often seems to slide over the tumor (49). On rare occasions, when the leiomyoma is large and compresses the mucosa, a deep endoscopic biopsy can capture a big chunk of smooth muscle (fig. 6-5). The tumors can be detected by radiographic imaging studies, which identify them as intramural with smooth round contours and sharp edges. Since leiomyomas are the most common intramural tumor, these features are almost specific. The finding of a mass in the posterior mediastinum on chest X ray identifies half of the large tumors. Endoscopic ultrasonography helps to determine the extent of the tumor (21).

**Morphologic Findings.** Most leiomyomas are intramural sessile lumps, but a few are polypoid masses projecting into the lumen. Their sizes vary from a few centimeters to huge tumors, the largest of which weighed 5 kg (27,38). There have been reports of circumferential leiomyomas

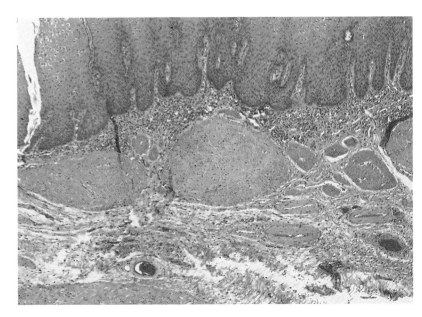

Figure 6-4
SEEDLING LEIOMYOMAS
Multiple seedling leiomyomas of the
muscularis mucosae in a patient with
leiomyomatosis.

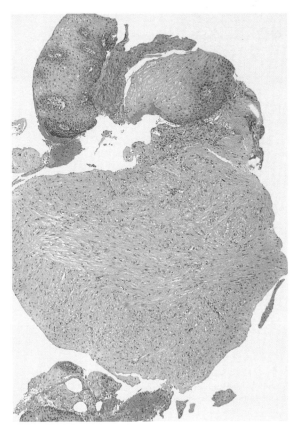

Figure 6-5
LEIOMYOMA
The large lump of spindle cells is the superficial part of
a leiomyoma that was captured by endoscopic biopsy. The
overlying mucosa is at the top.

and recurrent leiomyomas, but their descriptions overlap the descriptions of leiomyomatosis, and they may be manifestations of that condition (39). Most clinically important leiomyomas are single, but there are a few reports of multiple tumors (31). Grossly, leiomyomas are well circumscribed and pale, occasionally lobulated, and usually pink to white, depending upon whether they are described previous to, during, or after fixation (fig. 6-6). They are firm, gristly, and on cut section, have a whorled appearance, much like their myometrial counterparts. Except for a rare clinically obvious tumor in the muscularis mucosae, almost all significant leiomyomas are situated in the muscularis propria, mostly in the inner layer (63). Microscopically, they contain mature-appearing smooth muscle cells arranged in fascicles and whorls (figs. 6-7, 6-8). In most tumors, the muscle cells are hypertrophied, with unusually large amounts of cytoplasm. Thus esophageal leiomyomas differ somewhat from uterine leiomyomas in which the smooth muscle cells are usually smaller and more closely packed. Mitotic figures are rare, and very cellular tumors do not occur. There is no literature that describes atypical variants, such as occur in the uterus. Hyalinization with deposition of dense collagen is common in the center of large leiomyomas. In a few cases, such collagenized foci become calcified.

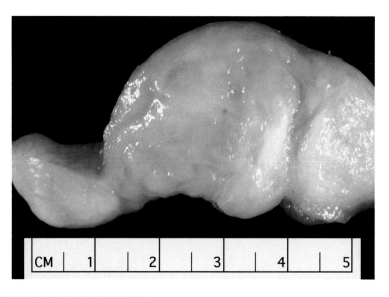

Figure 6-6
LOBULATED LEIOMYOMA

This is the cut surface of a lobulated leiomyoma, about 5 cm in greatest diameter. It is white and whorled, and it bulges above the cut surface.

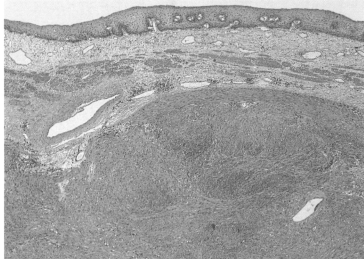

Figure 6-7
LEIOMYOMA IN MUSCULARIS PROPRIA

A large leiomyoma in the muscularis propria compresses the submucosa. The dark muscle layer beneath the mucosa is the muscularis mucosae.

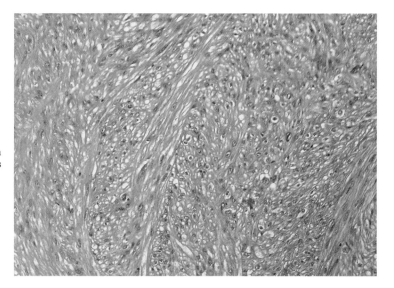

Figure 6-8
ESOPHAGEAL LEIOMYOMA: GROWTH PATTERN

This is a characteristic pattern of growth for esophageal leiomyomas. The muscle cells are arranged in broad sweeping fascicles.

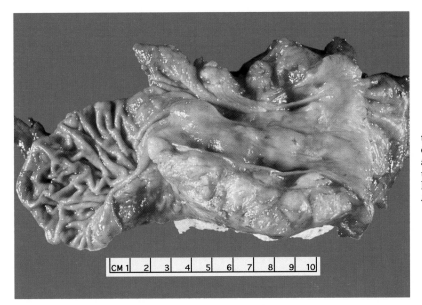

Figure 6-9
LEIOMYOMATOSIS
In this illustration, the stomach is to the left. The muscularis propria of the distal esophagus is massively thickened and appears to be composed of a continuous line of nodules, each of which looks like a leiomyoma. (Courtesy of Dr. R. M. Abellera, LaCrosse, WI.)

**Treatment.** The treatment depends upon the clinical importance of the tumor. If the tumor causes significant symptoms, then it must be resected. Most such leiomyomas are treated by transthoracic enucleation, while others have been removed endoscopically, sometimes after ethanol injection to induce necrosis (8,21,51).

## LEIOMYOMATOSIS

Leiomyomatosis is an uncommon condition, mainly of the distal esophagus, in which the muscularis propria becomes diffusely nodular, hypertrophied, and disorganized, so that it resembles a continuous cluster of leiomyomas. The literature is confusing in that some cases reported to be leiomyomatosis may be diffuse hypertrophy of the muscularis propria, also known as idiopathic muscular hypertrophy, a rare condition in which the entire muscularis propria is uniformly thick, without the formation of nodules (22). Furthermore, multiple esophageal leiomyomas, each of which is discrete and separate, do not qualify as diffuse leiomyomatosis, a disease characterized by confluent muscle masses (36).

Leiomyomatosis is so rare that the world literature contains fewer than 100 cases, mostly in the form of single case reports (10,24,33,36). The largest series, from Mexico, only described six cases, four of which belonged to one family, indi-

cating that heredity may have a role in pathogenesis (30). The patients are often children and young adults, and females may be affected more often than males (22). Some patients have dysphagia, but peculiarly, considering the extent of involvement of the esophageal musculature, some patients have no symptoms (33,36). Several associated lesions have been described, including multiple vulvar or uterine leiomyomas, leiomyomas of the respiratory tract, and a hereditary nephropathy resembling Alport's syndrome (10,30,54).

Although most of the esophagus is involved, dominant masses may only involve a segment, mostly the distal part. As is true for seedling leiomyomas, the inner circular muscularis propria is the major site, but the outer muscle and the muscularis mucosae may also contain nodules. The muscle nodules are continuous with each other, much as are the bundles of muscle in the normal muscularis (figs. 6-9, 6-10). These nodules, however, are indistinguishable from leiomyomas. They are composed of hypertrophied smooth muscle cells that have lost their usual parallel orientation and have formed fascicles and whorls. The nodules contain variable amounts of collagen, much like typical isolated leiomyomas. Additional findings in the esophagus in various case reports include localized thickening of the muscle of small submucosal blood vessels; proliferation of smooth

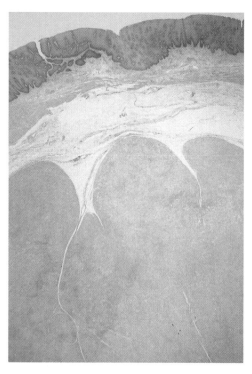

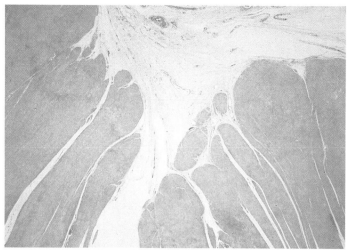

Figure 6-10
LEIOMYOMATOSIS

Left: In this low-power view, the smooth muscle bundles of the inner muscularis propria are enlarged, rounded, and separated, so that they seem to have converted to a series of confluent leiomyomas of different sizes.

Above: Another view of the muscularis propria with large, discrete bundles of hypertrophic smooth muscle.

muscle in the submucosa; unusual prominence, possibly hypertrophy, of the myenteric nerve plexus; and lymphocyte, plasma cell, and eosinophil infiltrates in the muscle nodules (24,33).

Treatment has consisted of either resection or a Heller-type myotomy with a longitudinal slit through the muscularis propria.

## MALIGNANT MESENCHYMAL TUMORS: SARCOMAS

**General Considerations.** Although small typical leiomyomas are common in the esophagus, sarcomas are so rare that there is little data about their appearance and natural history. In a massive review of the world literature through the end of 1971, Seremetis et al. (54) found no more than 40 reported esophageal leiomyosarcomas. In another review of the literature through early 1990, the authors found 82 reported cases of esophageal leiomyosarcoma, 2 cases per year above the 40 accumulated by Seremetis et al. (47). These cases often do not have convincing histologic illustrations, so that the diagnosis of sarcoma of any kind is in doubt. In the English language literature, the largest published series of primary esophageal sarcomas from a singe institution included only 13 cases accumulated between 1946 and

1988 (14): 11 tumors were designated as leiomyosarcoma, 1 as malignant neurilemoma, and 1 as synovial sarcoma. However, in this series, the diagnoses were based upon review of records only, and there was no attempt to review the tumors morphologically. As a result, the diagnoses of all these tumors as sarcomas are in doubt, pending histologic review.

The peculiar polypoid squamous cell carcinomas with sarcomatous metaplasia (pseudosarcomatous squamous cell carcinomas) occur in the esophagus far more often than sarcomas (see chapter 4). Some of these have very little residual carcinoma, and have the same gross polypoid appearance and distribution along the esophagus as do the reported sarcomas. Therefore, any diagnosis of sarcoma of the esophagus must be questioned unless pseudosarcomatous carcinoma has been excluded by the confident demonstration of no carcinomatous component after examination of multiple sections of both the tumor and the marginal mucosa. One report of three leiomyosarcomas included one tumor that had an area of squamous cell carcinoma; in another report, one of two cases of sarcoma also had squamous carcinoma (26,50). These tumors were probably pseudosarcomatous carcinomas and

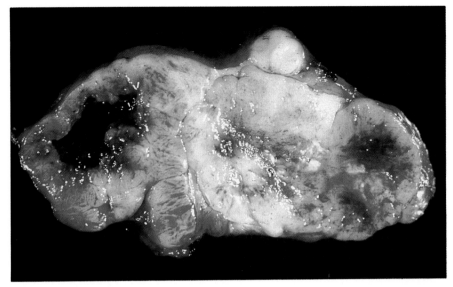

Figure 6-11
INTRAMURAL
ESOPHAGEAL SARCOMA
This large tumor has foci of
hemorrhage and necrosis and
thus looks different than a typical leiomyoma.

not leiomyosarcomas. The distinction between sarcoma and pseudosarcomatous carcinoma becomes further blurred in papers that describe them both as sarcomas (47).

Nevertheless, to obtain any data about esophageal sarcomas, most of the reported sarcomas have to be accepted as bona fide. Those sarcomas reported to be intramural, rather than polypoid, are most likely to be real sarcomas and not sarcomatoid carcinomas. Tumors designated as leiomyosarcomas account for 90 percent of esophageal sarcomas. Small numbers of rhabdomyosarcomas, synovial sarcomas, and malignant nerve sheath tumors, one of which was a triton tumor with rhabdomyoblastic differentiation, also have been reported (3,9,17,47,61). At least one of every other type of sarcoma probably has been reported by now, including osteosarcoma, chondrosarcoma, fibrosarcoma, malignant fibrous histiocytoma, and liposarcoma (1,47).

**Clinical Features.** The clinical characteristics of esophageal sarcomas are identical to those of carcinomas, namely, dysphagia and weight loss, generally for only a few months. Some patients have epigastric or substernal pain. Endoscopically, many appear as polypoid intraluminal masses, sometimes with overlying ulcers. Some patients have evidence of metastases, such as hepatomegaly, at the time of presentation.

**Morphologic Findings.** Grossly, some sarcomas are polypoid with large intraluminal and smaller intramural components, others are pre-

dominantly intramural, and a few are mostly extramural with the main mass in the posterior mediastinum. They may have areas of necrosis and hemorrhage, and they are generally not as whorled and gristly as leiomyomas (fig. 6-11).

Microscopically, the sarcomas are generally composed of spindle cells with varying degrees of pleomorphism, mitoses, necrosis, calcification, and differentiation along specialized cell lines including smooth muscle, rhabdomyoblastic, synovial, chondroid, and osteoid. Since there are so few cases available for analysis, there are no published criteria for malignancy if there are no obvious malignant features. Furthermore, it is not clear whether there is a group of unique malignant stromal tumors of the esophagus as there is in the stomach. Therefore, the only criteria that we can recommend are those that are used for sarcomas in other sites, particularly leiomyosarcomas in the somatic soft tissues, and for sarcomas of other gastrointestinal organs, such as the stomach (see chapter 14) (4,23). Such criteria include dense cellularity, far greater than that found in typical leiomyomas; unusual spindle or epithelioid cells; easily found mitotic figures; and infiltrating edges (fig. 6-12).

One sarcoma mimic frequently encountered in mucosal biopsies is the bizarre stromal proliferation that occurs in the beds of chronic ulcers. These also may be confused with undifferentiated carcinoma cells (figs. 6-13, 6-14). The cells are fibroblasts or myofibroblasts, and they are

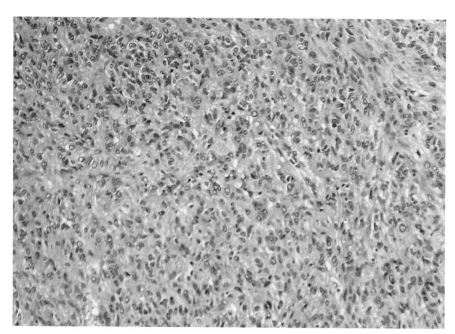

Figure 6-12
ESOPHAGEAL SARCOMA
Top: Low magnification view of a densely cellular neoplasm. The cells are smaller than leiomyoma cells; the nuclei are larger, rounder, and more hyperchromatic; and there are scattered mitoses.
Bottom: High magnification view.

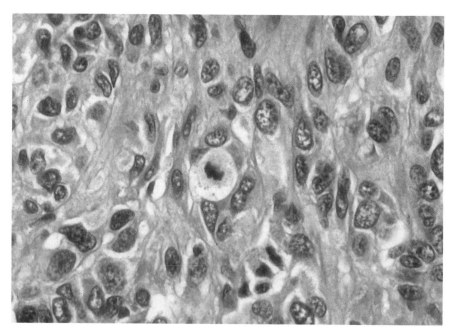

most prominent close to the surface of the ulcer, where the granulation tissue is most proliferative. They are spindled, stellate, epithelioid, and occasionally multinucleated. The nuclei are large, often hyperchromatic, and sometimes peculiarly shaped. Mitoses are occasional. The cells are mixed with other granulation tissue elements, including capillary buds and inflammatory cells. A useful rule is that the diagnosis of malignancy, especially sarcoma, in an esophageal biopsy, should not be made based upon bizarre cells in the granulation tissue from the base of an ulcer.

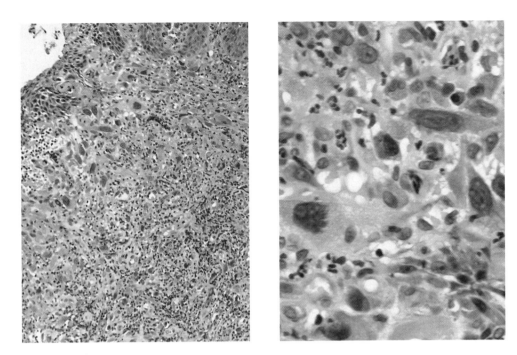

Figure 6-13
BIZARRE STROMAL REACTION IN AN ULCER BED

Left: At the top is the surface of a healing ulcer with the long prongs of primitive squamous cells penetrating the granulation tissue that contains large cells with dark, pleomorphic nuclei. These cells are mixed with inflammatory cells.

Right: High magnification view.

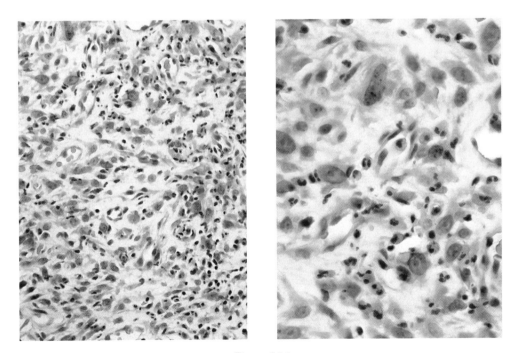

Figure 6-14
BIZARRE STROMAL REACTION

Left: Another example of a bizarre stromal reaction at the base of an ulcer. In this lesion, the large abnormal spindle cells appear to stream in parallel.

Right: In the high-power view, their association with capillary buds is evident.

## GRANULAR CELL TUMOR

The most common esophageal stromal tumor, after leiomyoma, is the granular cell tumor. Other neural tumors, including neurofibromas and schwannomas, histologically identical to those that occur in the soft tissues, are curiosities, the subjects of rare case reports (19,20,52, 60). Some reported cases were actually large schwannomas of the vagus nerve outside the esophagus causing esophageal symptoms by compression. A few granular cell tumors occurred in patients with neurofibromatosis; one even presented as a large intralumenal polypoid mass, mimicking a giant fibrovascular polyp.

**Clinical Features.** In some series, the esophagus is the most common gut site for granular cell tumors (35). They usually do not produce symptoms because they are too small, although rare large tumors producing obstructive symptoms have been reported. In fact, increasing size is proportional to increasing likelihood of symptoms. In an extensive review of the literature, almost three fourths of tumors were 2 cm or less in maximal diameter (18). Most are found incidentally during upper endoscopy performed for other reasons. About 60 percent occur in the lower esophagus with the remainder split evenly between the upper and middle. Occasional cases of multiple tumors have been reported. Most of the patients are in their 40s at the time the tumors are detected, and men and blacks seem to be at risk. A set of highly suggestive endoscopic features has been identified: the tumors are sessile, yellow or yellow-white, and firm to palpation with the biopsy forceps; the overlying epithelium is intact (12).

**Morphologic Findings.** Granular cell tumors of the esophagus are identical to those that arise elsewhere. They contain plump spindled or epithelioid cells with small nuclei. The abundant cytoplasm is filled with coarse red granules, presumably irregular lysosomes, that stain intensely with periodic acid–Schiff stain (fig. 6-15). The nuclei and cytoplasm also stain with antibodies to S-100 protein. The cells are arranged in packets of short fascicles, sometimes separated by collagen fibers, and they commonly involve, at least in part, the most superficial lamina propria where the nests interdigitate with prongs of squamous epithelium. In occasional cases, the squamous epithelium undergoes pseudoepithe-

liomatous hyperplasia that may be confused with well-differentiated squamous carcinoma. Since they usually hug the base of the squamous epithelium, they are often detected by biopsy as long as superficial lamina propria is obtained. Unfortunately, many esophageal biopsies do not include lamina propria, and the tumor is not detected, no matter how superficial it is.

Not all granular cell tumors are located superficially. Many also involve the submucosa, sometimes extending into the muscularis propria. A few tumors have been confined to the muscularis propria or to the adventitia (35).

**Prognosis.** Although the natural history of esophageal granular cell tumors is not known, a few small tumors have been followed after biopsy for several years with no change in size, suggesting that once they are found, they are stable and have little growth potential (12). This is a bit peculiar, considering the fact that large granular cell tumors do occur in the esophagus, and they presumably started as small tumors. Based upon such cases, small granular cell tumors may be biopsied for diagnosis and then followed by periodic esophagoscopy or removed endoscopically. Large, symptomatic tumors require resection to relieve the symptoms.

A few malignant granular cell tumors have been reported in the esophagus (42). The diagnosis of malignancy was usually not based upon metastasis, but upon other parameters, including infiltrative growth into adjacent structures (18).

## FIBROVASCULAR POLYPS (GIANT FIBROVASCULAR POLYPS, FIBROLIPOMAS) AND LIPOMAS

The literature covering esophageal lipomas and giant fibrovascular polyps includes mostly single case reports. The largest series only contains four cases (7,15,34,44,45,46,48,62). Lipomas of the esophagus are so rare that in a 1984 review of over 1,400 published cases of lipomas of the entire gastrointestinal tract, only 1.5 percent, or about 20 cases, were esophageal (13). So many reported cases of these two supposedly distinct tumors have overlapping clinical and histologic features that it is impossible to separate them. They both present as large, elongated intralumenal masses, originating in the upper esophagus,

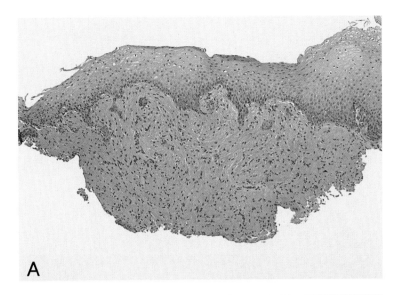

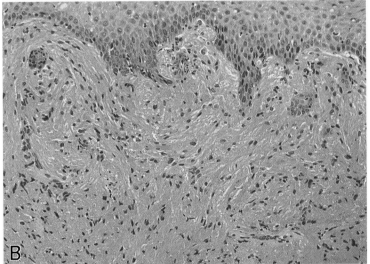

Figure 6-15
GRANULAR CELL TUMOR
The tumor fills the lamina propria, extending up to the base of the squamous epithelium that has spike-like or saw-tooth–like rete poking downward into the tumor. At high power, the spindled tumor cells are full of fine cytoplasmic granules. (A: low magnification; B: medium magnification; C: high magnification.)

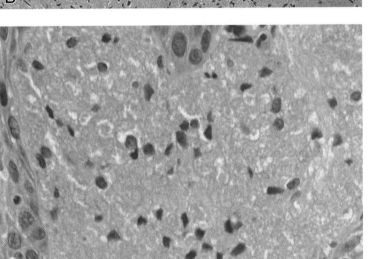

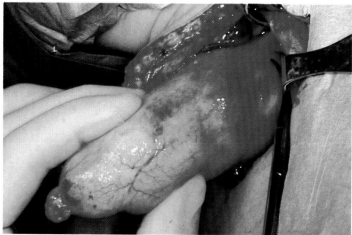

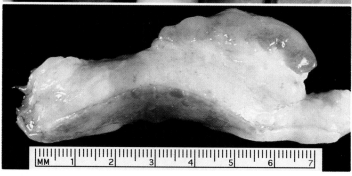

Figure 6-16
GIANT FIBROVASCULAR POLYP

Top: The tumor has been mobilized through an esophagotomy incision in the neck. Its narrow pedicle attachment to the esophageal mucosa is being cut.

Bottom: The mass is seen in cross section. It is composed of white glistening tissues, covered top and bottom by mucosa. (Courtesy of Dr. Mark Orringer, Ann Arbor, MI.)

to which they are attached by pedicles. Therefore, these two lesions are discussed together.

**Clinical Features.** Although fibrovascular polyps are rare, they are undoubtedly the most spectacular of all esophageal stromal proliferations from a clinical standpoint. The fact that many of the case reports refer to them as "giant," indicates that they are unique. Most have been described as large, pedunculated tumors that arise in the proximal esophagus behind the cricoid cartilage and fill the lumen, extending distally, sometimes all the way to the esophagogastric junction. The proximal location of their attachment to the mucosa explains why many fibrovascular polyps have presented as regurgitated masses in the mouth. Others have led to airway obstruction as the mass impacted on the larynx, also following regurgitation, and this has been fatal in a few cases (2,62). Other symptoms include those of most esophageal lesions, dysphagia, chest pain, or both. Weight loss of about 11 kg is common, presumably secondary to the dysphagia. Peculiarly, the duration of symptoms is unusually short, considering the large size of the

polyps; in other words, these lesions seem to reach very large sizes before they become symptomatic. This dichotomy between duration of symptoms and tumor size is undoubtedly because the tumors are soft and pliable and allow intralumenal contents to pass with little impedance; in addition, the esophagus around them is commonly dilated (40). In fact, the dilatation is so prominent that some cases resemble the dilated esophagus of achalasia. Men are affected about three times as often as women, and all the patients are adults. Radiographically, the typical findings are a long, smooth, mobile, intralumenal mass within a dilated lumen. Endoscopically, the large, long polyp is apparent, but in some cases, the polyp is missed because the lumen is dilated and the normal mucosa covering the polyps makes them appear as part of the esophageal wall.

**Morphologic Findings.** Grossly, fibrovascular polyps are soft, long, slender projections usually covered by normal mucosa, sometimes with a bulbous expansion of the tip (fig. 6-16). Some are lobulated (48). Erosions or ulcers are rare, and when present, tend to involve the tip. They

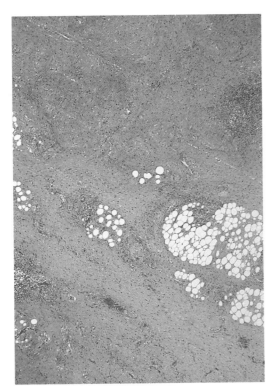 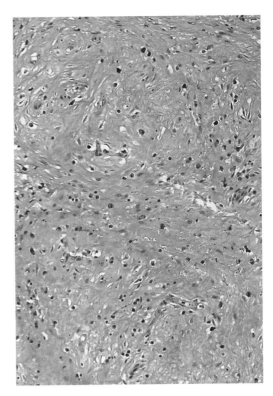

Figure 6-17
GIANT FIBROVASCULAR POLYP

Left: The tumor has a mixture of tissues and the adipocytes form lobules of different sizes. Tumors that are dominated by adipocytes are likely to be reported as lipomas. The pale blue areas are myxoid, while the darker red areas are densely collagenized.

Right: A higher power view of one of the myxoid areas, containing spindle cells and vessels. This mix, especially when a few adipocytes are included, might be confused with a myxoid liposarcoma.

have a narrow point of attachment to the wall in the cervical esophagus. On cross section, they usually have a loose, edematous or myxoid look, with white fibrous tissue areas mixed with yellow adipose tissue lobules. Microscopically, they are expansions of the lamina propria composed of a mixture of loose, collagenized, highly vascularized tissue, often rich in mucopolysaccharides. There are scattered lymphoid aggregates and lobules of adipose tissue, scattered individual adipocytes, or small clusters of adipocytes in unpredictable proportions (fig. 6-17). It is presumably this variability that has led to misdiagnosis as lipoma or fibrolipoma. Others have so little adipose tissue that the term fibrovascular polyp is appropriate. Inflammatory cells, including plasma cells, may be scattered throughout, and mast cells may be prominent. The vessels are a mixture of muscular arteries, thin-walled veins, and capillaries. The myxoid zones sometimes contain spindle cells, and if these areas are

the most prominent, the tumor may resemble a myxoid neurofibroma. The surface is covered by non-neoplastic squamous epithelium that may be normal, hyperplastic, atrophic, ulcerated, or any mixture. Recently, we saw two cases that contained foci of highly proliferative small spindle cells, which suggested that a sarcoma was developing within the giant polyp, but we have no long-term follow-up for these cases.

This peculiar composition of a mixture of normal or near-normal stromal tissues suggests that the fibrovascular polyp is not a neoplasm. It may be an acquired malformation or hamartoma of lamina propria, or it may be some unusual form of inflammatory polyp or post-injury phenomenon, although preceding inflammations and injuries have not been described. It is unique to the esophagus. The only lesions in other parts of the body that even remotely resemble it are skin and anal tags that contain adipose tissue, and they are small polyps.

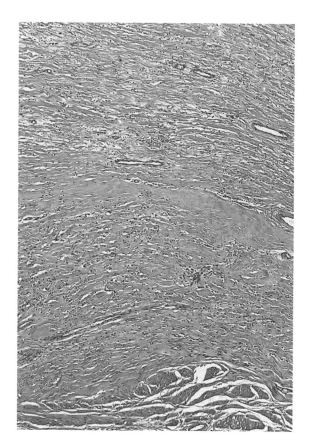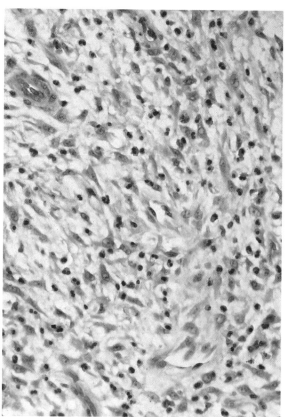

Figure 6-18
INFLAMMATORY FIBROID POLYP

Left: The muscularis propria (at the bottom) is partly replaced by the very vascular tumor.

Right: At high power, the tumor constituents are seen to be a mix of inflammatory cells, plump stromal cells, blood vessels, and collagen fibers.

Resection is the treatment of choice and is curative, although there is at least one report of a recurrent polyp after resection (58). Since these masses are attached by a pedicle to the upper esophagus, usually they can be removed by an incision in the cervical esophagus, followed by delivery of the mass through the incision and amputation (5). In one report, the dilated esophageal lumen returned to normal size after the mass was removed (46). There is a report of one tumor diagnosed as a giant lipomatous polyp that contained what was described as focal liposarcomatous change (6).

The few lipomas that have not been variants of the fibrovascular polyp type have been round, smooth intramural tumors that resemble leiomyomas radiographically and endoscopically. However, some are pliable, so that they may change shape during radiologic examinations (59).

## INFLAMMATORY FIBROID POLYPS (INFLAMMATORY PSEUDOTUMORS)

A few inflammatory fibroid polyps of the esophagus have been reported, but not enough data exists to formulate a profile for either the tumors or the patients who have them (41,64). The patients have all been adults with either dysphagia or melena from bleeding ulcers over the tumors. The tumors are composed of a loose, edematous stroma, apparently lamina propria, that contains thin-walled blood vessels, inflammatory cells including plasma cells, lymphocytes, mast cells, eosinophils, and stellate and spindle stromal cells that are fibroblasts or myofibroblasts. In our experience, esophageal inflammatory fibroid polyps resemble those in the small intestine: they look like excessive granulation tissue with areas of spindle cells that resemble those in tissue cultures of fibroblasts (fig. 6-18).

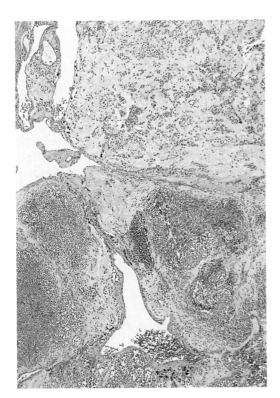 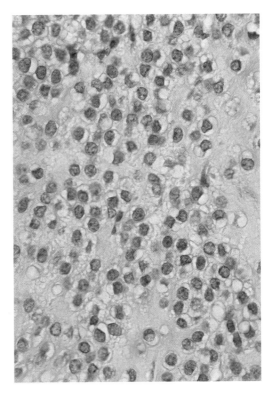

Figure 6-19
GLOMUS TUMOR

Left: The round glomus cells with clear cytoplasm are arranged in sheets and strands mixed with an extensively liquefied and hyalinized stroma that contains dilated vascular spaces.

Right: High-magnification view.

In contrast, inflammatory fibroid polyps in the stomach have a more organized appearance, with perivascular orientation of the spindle and inflammatory cells (see chapter 9).

## VASCULAR TUMORS

*Esophageal hemangiomas* do occur, and some of them have been reported. In a review of the literature published prior to 1992, the author found 56 cases in 45 reports (28,29,43). Some of these presented with severe bleeding, others with dysphagia. They have been distributed evenly throughout all levels of the esophagus (32). In some cases, the diagnosis was made after excision of the tumor, but in other cases, it was based upon biopsy. A diagnosis of hemangioma based only upon biopsies of bleeding gastrointestinal lesions is uncertain, since other masses induce dilatation of vessels at their edges. Some of the hemangiomas have cavernous channels; others are pyogenic granulomas with lobular clusters of small capillary channels.

A few *lymphangiomas*, probably less than 10 total, have also been reported (11,16,57). These are generally superficial, and some appear to contain cysts when viewed endoscopically.

We have seen two typical *glomus tumors* in the esophagus. In one patient, the glomus tumor was in the upper esophagus. Biopsies were not diagnostic, and the diagnosis only was made on examination of the resected tumor (fig. 6-19). While glomus tumors are well known to occur in the stomach, only two others have been reported in the esophagus. They contain typical round glomus cells with pale to clear cytoplasm. These cells are arranged about vascular spaces of various sizes, and there is often considerable stromal liquefaction and hyalinization.

There was a single case report of a *submucosal hemangiopericytoma* of the esophagus in a 32-year-old man. The authors were able to find only one other reported case of this unusual vascular tumor in the esophagus (13a).

## REFERENCES

1. Aagaard MT, Kristensen IB, Lund O, Hasenkam JM, Kimose HH. Primary malignant non-epithelial tumours of the thoracic oesophagus and cardia in a 25-year surgical material. Scand J Gastroenterol 1990;25:876–82.

2. Allen MS Jr, Talbot WH. Sudden death due to regurgitation of a pedunculated esophageal lipoma. J Thorac Cardiovasc Surg 1967;54:756–8.

3. Amr SS, Shihabi NK, Hajj HA. Synovial sarcoma of the esophagus. Am J Otolaryngol 1984;5:266–9

4. Appelman HD. Stromal tumors of the esophagus, stomach and duodenum. In: Appelman HD, ed. Pathology of the esophagus, stomach, and duodenum. New York: Churchill Livingstone, 1984:195–8.

5. Avezzano EA, Fleischer DE, Merida MA, Anderson DL. Giant fibrovascular polyps of the esophagus. Am J Gastroenterol 1990;85:299–302.

6. Bak YT, Kim JH, Kim JG, et al. Liposarcoma arising in a giant lipomatous polyp of the esophagus. Korean J Intern Med 1989;4:86–9.

7. Barki Y, Elias H, Tovi F, Bar-Ziv J. A fibrovascular polyp of the oesophagus. Br J Radiol 1981;54:142–4.

8. Benedetti G, Sablich R, Bonea M, Mariuz S. Fiberoptic endoscopic resection of symptomatic leiomyoma of the upper esophagus. Acta Chir Scand 1990;156:807–8.

9. Bloch MJ, Iozzo RV, Edmunds H Jr, Brooks JJ. Polypoid synovial sarcoma of the esophagus. Gastroenterol 1987;92:229–33.

10. Bloch P, Quijada J. Diffuse leiomyomatosis of the esophagus. Analysis of a case and review of the literature. Gastroenterol Clin Biol 1992;16:890–3.

11. Brady PG, Milligan FD. Lymphangioma of the esophagus—diagnosis by endoscopic biopsy. Am J Dig Dis 1973;18:423–5.

12. Brady PG, Nord HJ, Connar RG. Granular cell tumor of the esophagus: natural history, diagnosis, and therapy. Dig Dis Sci 1988;33:1329–33.

13. Bruneton JN, Quoy AM, Dageville X, Lecomte P. Lipomas of the digestive tract. Ann Gastroenterol Hepatol 1984;20:27–32.

13a. Burke JS, Ranchod M. Hemangiopericytoma of the esophagus. Hum Pathol 1981;12:96–100.

14. Caldwell CB, Bains MS, Burt M. Unusual malignant neoplasms of the esophagus. Oat cell carcinoma, melanoma, and sarcoma. J Thoracic Surg 1991;101:100–7.

15. Carter MM, Kulkarni MV. Giant fibrovascular polyp of the esophagus. Gastrointest Radiol 1984;9:301–3.

16. Castellanos D, Sebastian JJ, Larrad A, et al. Esophageal lymphangioma: case report and review of the literature. Surgery 1990;108:593–4.

17. Chetty R, Learmonth GM, Price SK, Taylor DA. Primary oesophageal rhabdomyosarcoma. Cytopathol 1991;2:103–8.

18. Coutinho DS, Soga J, Yoshikawa T, et al. Granular cell tumors of the esophagus: a report of two cases and review of the literature. Am J Gastroenterology 1985;80:758–62.

19. DeVault KR, Miller LS, Yaghsezian H, et al. Acute esophageal hemorrhage from a vagal neurilemoma. Gastroenterology 1992;102:1059–61.

20. Eberlein TJ, Hannan R, Josa M, Sugarbaker, DJ. Benign schwannoma of the esophagus presenting as a giant fibrovascular polyp. Ann Thorac Surg 1992;53:343–5.

21. Eda Y, Asaki S, Yamagata L, Ohara S, Shibuya D, Toyota T. Endoscopic treatment for submucosal tumors of the esophagus: studies in 25 patients. Gastroenterol Jpn 1990;25:411–6.

22. Enterline H, Thompson J. Pathology of the esophagus. New York: Springer-Verlag, 1984:165–80.

23. Enzinger FM, Weiss SW. Soft tissue tumors. 2nd ed. St Louis: CV Mosby, 1988:402–32.

24. Fernandes JP, Mascarenhas MJ, da Costa JC, Correia JP. Diffuse leiomyomatosis of the esophagus: a case report and review of the literature. Dig Dis Sci 1975;20:684–90.

25. Fountain SW. Leiomyoma of the esophagus. Thorac Cardiovasc Surg 1986:34:194–5.

26. Gaede JT, Postlethwait RW, Shelburne JD, Cox JL, Hamilton WF. Leiomyosarcoma of the esophagus. Report of two cases, one with associated squamous cell carcinoma. J Thorac Cardiovasc Surg 1978;75:740–6.

27. Gallinger S, Steinhardt MI, Goldberg M. Giant leiomyoma of the esophagus. Am J Gastroenterol 1983;78:708–11.

28. Gilbert HW, Weston MJ, Thompson MH. Cavernous haemangioma of the oesophagus. Br J Surg 1990;77:106.

29. Govoni AF. Hemangiomas of the esophagus. Gastrointest Radiol 1982;7:113–7.

30. Guarner V, Garcia Torres R. Diffuse leiomyomatosis of the esophagus, tracheobronchial, genital, and renal insufficiency. In: DeMeester TR, Skinner DB, eds. Esophageal disorders: pathophysiology and therapy. New York: Raven Press, 1985:447–57.

31. Haber K, Winfield AC. Multiple leiomyomas of the esophagus. Am J Dig Dis 1974;19:678–80.

32. Hanel K, Talley NA, Hunt DR. Hemangioma of the esophagus: an unusual cause of upper gastrointestinal bleeding. Dig Dis Sci 1981;26:257–63.

33. Heald J, Moussalli H, Hasleton PS. Diffuse leiomyomatosis of the oesophagus. Histopathology 1986;10:755–9.

34. Jang GC, Clouse ME, Fleischner FG. Fibrovascular polyp: a benign intralumenal tumor of the esophagus. Radiology 1969;92:1196–200.

35. Johnston J, Helwig EB. Granular cell tumors of the gastrointestinal tract and perianal region: a study of 74 cases. Dig Dis Sci 1981;26:807–16.

36. Kabuto T, Taniguchi K, Iwanaga T, Terasawa T, Tateishi R, Taniguchi H. Diffuse leiomyomatosis of the esophagus. Dig Dis Sci 1980;25:388–91.

37. Kostianen S, Virkkula L, Teppo L. Smooth-muscle tumours of the oesophagus. Scand J Thor Cardiovasc Surg 1973;7:98–103.

38. Kramer MD, Gibb SP, Ellis FH Jr. Giant leiomyoma of the esophagus. J Surg Oncol 1986;33:166–9.

39. Lee ME, Overholt RH. Esophageal myomectomy for recurrent multiple leiomyomas of the esophagus: manometric and cineradiographic documentation. Ann Thorac Surg 1977;23:68–72.

40. Lewis BS, Waye JD, Khilmani MT, Biller HF. Fibrovascular polyp of the esophagus. Mt Sinai J Med 1988;55:324–5.

41. LiVolsi VA, Perzin KH. Inflammatory pseudotumors (inflammatory fibrous polyps) of the esophagus. A clinicopathologic study. Am J Dig Dis 1975;20:475–81.

42. Ohmori T, Arita N, Uraga N, Tabei R, Tani M, Okamura H. Malignant granular cell tumor of the esophagus. A case report with light and electron microscopic, histochemical, and immunohistochemical study. Acta Pathol Jpn 1987;37:775–83.

43. Okumura T, Tanoue S, Chiba K, Tanaka S. Lobular capillary hemangioma of the esophagus. A case report and review of the literature. Acta Pathol Jpn 1983;33:1303–8.

44. Patel J, Kieffer RW, Martin M, Avant GR. Giant fibrovascular polyp of the esophagus. Gastroenterology 1984;87:953–6.

45. Peiser J, Ovnat A, Herz A, Hirsch M, Charuzi I. Lipoma of the esophagus. 1984;20:1068–70.

46. Penagini R, Ranzi T, Velio P, et al. Giant fibrovascular polyp of the oesophagus: report of a case and effects on oesophageal function. Gut 1989;30:1624–29.

47. Perch SJ, Soffen EM, Whittington R, Brooks JJ. Esophageal sarcomas. J Surg Oncol 1991;48:194–8.

48. Petras R, Whitman G, Winkelman E, Falk G, Rice T. Fibrovascular polyp of the esophagus: a report of 4 cases and a review of the literature [Abstract]. Mod Pathol 1990;3:79A.

49. Preda F, Alloisio M, Lequaglie C, Ongari M, Ravasi G. Leiomyoma of the esophagus. Tumori 1986;72:503–6.

50. Rainer WG, Brus R. Leiomyosarcoma of the esophagus; review of the literature and report of 3 cases. Surgery 1965;58:343–50.

51. Rendina EA, Venuta F, Pescarmona EO, et al. Leiomyoma of the esophagus. Scand J Thorac Cardiovasc Surg 1990;24:79–82.

52. Saitoh K, Nasu M, Kamiyama R, et al. Solitary neurofibroma of the esophagus. Acta Pathol Jpn 1985:527–31.

53. Seremetis MG, DeGuzman VC, Lyons WS, Peabody JW Jr. Leiomyoma of the esophagus. A report of 19 surgical cases. Ann Thorac Surg 1973;16:308–16.

54. Seremetis MG, Lyons WS, DeGuzman VC, Peabody JW Jr. Leiomyomata of the esophagus. An analysis of 838 cases. Cancer 1976;38:2166–77.

55. Solomon MP, Rosenblum H, Rosato FE. Leiomyoma of the esophagus. Ann Surg 1984;199:246–8.

56. Takubo K, Nakagawa H, Tsuchiya S, Mitomo Y, Sasajima K, Shirota A. Seedling leiomyoma of the esophagus and esophagogastric junction zone. Hum Pathol 1981;12:1006–10.

57. Tamada R, Sugimachi K, Yaita A, Inokuchi K, Watanabe H. Lymphangioma of the esophagus presenting symptoms of achalasia—a case report. Jpn J Surg 1980;10:59–62.

58. Timmons B, Sedwitz JL, Oller DW. Benign fibrovascular polyp of the esophagus. South Med J 1991;84:1370–2.

59. Tolis GA, Shields TW. Intramural lipoma of the esophagus. Ann Thorac Surg 1967;3:60–2.

60. Vaghei R, Yost NI. Vagal schwannoma involving esophagus. Ann Thorac Surg 1991;52:1334–6.

61. Vartio T, Nickels J, Hockerstedt K, Scheinin TM. Rhabdomyosarcoma of the oesophagus. Light and electron microscopic study of a rare tumor. Virchows Arch [A] 1980;386:357–61.

62. Vrabec DP, Colley AT. Giant intralumenal polyps of the esophagus. Ann Otol Rhinol Laryngol 1983;92:344–8.

63. Watanabe M, Baba T, Hotchi M. A case of leiomyoma of the lamina muscularis mucosae of the esophagus with a complication of carcinoma in situ of the overlying mucosa. Acta Pathol Jpn 1987;37:1845–51.

64. Wolf BC, Khettry U, Leonardi HK, Neptune WB, Bhattacharyya AK, Legg MA. Benign lesions mimicking malignant tumors of the esophagus. Hum Pathol 1988;19:148–54.

# 7

# MISCELLANEOUS TUMORS OF THE ESOPHAGUS

The esophagus is the uncommon site of origin of several unusual unrelated neoplasms. Some of these, such as endocrine and lymphoid tumors, are common in the stomach, but rare in the esophagus. Others, such as melanomas, are more common in the esophagus than in the stomach. Because these tumors have morphologic characteristics that they share with other more common tumors, there are likely to be problems in diagnosis. The following descriptions stress the differential diagnostic issues.

## ENDOCRINE TUMORS

Primary endocrine cell tumors of the esophagus presumably arise from endocrine cells scattered among the squamous epithelial cells (24). The endocrine cells are most prominent in the lower end of the esophagus, which is also the most common site of these tumors (1). Three types of tumors have been described: carcinoid tumor, small cell carcinoma (oat cell carcinoma), and combined tumors (mixtures of carcinomas and endocrine cell tumors).

### Carcinoid Tumor

These are extremely rare: only five pure cases and one associated with adenocarcinoma in Barrett's esophagus have been reported in the English literature up to 1993 (3,5,7–9,22). One tumor was located in the submucosa and caused esophageal obstruction (13). Histologically, they are similar to gastrointestinal carcinoid tumors, although variable patterns, such as the trabecular pattern typical of foregut carcinoids and solid nests, with or without rosettes, typical of midgut carcinoids, have been described (7,22).

### Small Cell Carcinoma (Small Cell Undifferentiated Carcinoma, Oat Cell Carcinoma)

**Clinical Features.** This tumor is twice as common in males as females; it occurs in adults, mostly in the sixth decade of life (1). Patients usually present at an advanced stage of tumor growth with severe weight loss, dysphagia, and

sometimes chest pain (18,19). There is often a history of heavy smoking of more than 50 pack years, and one reported case was associated with longstanding achalasia (1,21). Although these tumors have endocrine cell differentiation and may contain variable amounts of peptide hormones, endocrinopathies have not been reported. The prognosis is poor, with a survival period in most cases of less than 6 months (2,6). However, there are a few reported cases of longer survival: one patient treated with combination chemotherapy (cyclophosphamide, vincristine, and VP-16) and local radiotherapy was in remission 22 months after diagnosis (14).

**Morphologic Findings.** Almost all small cell carcinomas occur in the distal half of the esophagus and usually appear as large, polypoid, fungating masses or ulcerating stenotic lesions, measuring anywhere from 4 to 14 cm in greatest diameter (fig. 7-1). Sometimes they are associated with fistulae into the trachea or bronchi (1,17,19).

Histologically, these tumors resemble small cell carcinomas of the lung. They form diffusely infiltrating masses composed of solid sheets, nests, or ribbons (fig. 7-2), often with a streaming pattern; they sometimes form rosettes containing mucin within their lumens (1). Occasionally,

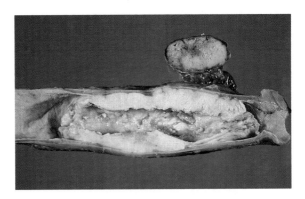

Figure 7-1
SMALL CELL CARCINOMA OF THE ESOPHAGUS: GROSS APPEARANCE

The tumor consists of a large, bulky, ulcerated, infiltrative lesion occupying most of the distal half of the esophagus. It has a raised everted margin and has caused marked narrowing of the lumen.

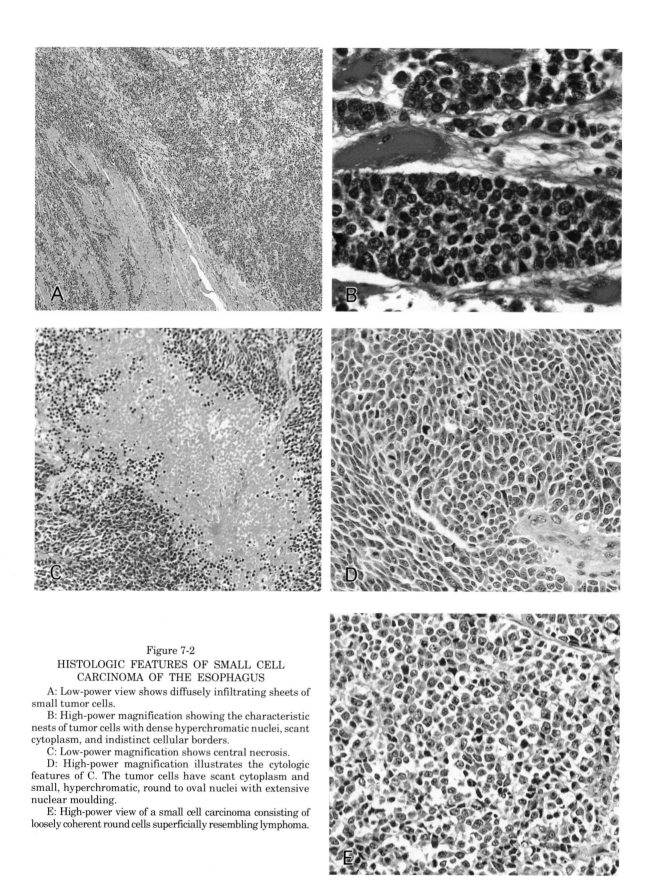

Figure 7-2
HISTOLOGIC FEATURES OF SMALL CELL
CARCINOMA OF THE ESOPHAGUS

A: Low-power view shows diffusely infiltrating sheets of small tumor cells.

B: High-power magnification showing the characteristic nests of tumor cells with dense hyperchromatic nuclei, scant cytoplasm, and indistinct cellular borders.

C: Low-power magnification shows central necrosis.

D: High-power magnification illustrates the cytologic features of C. The tumor cells have scant cytoplasm and small, hyperchromatic, round to oval nuclei with extensive nuclear moulding.

E: High-power view of a small cell carcinoma consisting of loosely coherent round cells superficially resembling lymphoma.

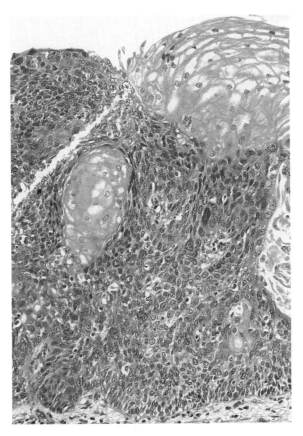

Figure 7-3
SMALL CELL CARCINOMA OF THE
ESOPHAGUS: IN SITU COMPONENT

The small cell carcinoma appears to be arising in the basal half of the squamous epithelium and occupying the full thickness of the epithelium on the extreme left of the field. It resembles a very poorly differentiated in situ squamous cell carcinoma.

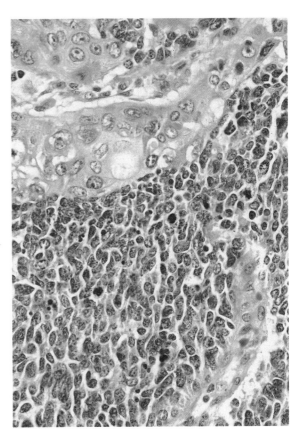

Figure 7-4
SMALL CELL CARCINOMA OF THE ESOPHAGUS

High-power magnification shows squamous cell differentiation at the top of the figure.

in situ lesions are present in the adjacent squamous epithelium (fig. 7-3). They are sometimes admixed with foci of squamous carcinoma, adenocarcinoma, or both, with the former frequently consisting of mature-appearing balls of squamous cells (fig. 7-4) (1,2). The bulk of the tumor contains small, round or oval lymphocyte-like cells with hyperchromatic nuclei, scant cytoplasm, and frequent mitoses. Occasionally, intermediate-sized cells or even rare giant cells may be found. As in the lung, nuclear moulding is seen. There is one report describing the cytologic features of these tumors, which are characterized by small malignant cells in isolation with minimal cytoplasm. Cellular molding was present in two of the cases (11,12).

Silver stains show that these tumors contain some argyrophilic but not argentaffinic cells (1,23). Ultrastructurally, they contain dense core granules. Immunohistochemical analysis demonstrates endocrine cell markers such as neuron-specific enolase and chromogranin, and epithelial markers such as keratin and epithelial membrane antigen (11). In addition, peptides such as gastrin, serotonin, adrenocorticotrophic hormone (ACTH), and calcitonin have been demonstrated within some of these tumors; however, no patients have had clinical endocrinopathies (15,16,17,20).

**Differential Diagnosis**. Unfortunately not all small cell carcinomas have the histochemical, immunohistochemical, and ultrastructural markers of endocrine cell tumors (4). Thus, some small cell carcinomas may in fact be poorly differentiated squamous cell carcinomas or adenocarcinomas. Features that differentiate small cell carcinoma from poorly differentiated squamous cell carcinoma include the demonstration of argyrophilia or chromogranin immunoreactivity,

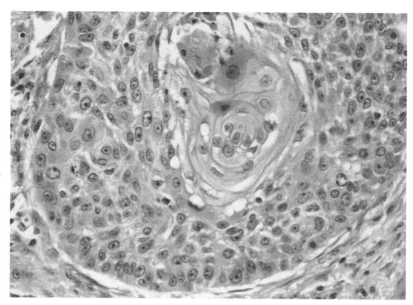

Figure 7-5
POORLY DIFFERENTIATED
SQUAMOUS CELL CARCINOMA
OF SMALL CELL TYPE
High-power magnification shows a tumor composed of cohesive, small, somewhat spindly cells and a central nest of squamous cells.

although this may be not be true of all tumors; ultrastructural demonstration of dense core granules; and the absence of tonofilaments and desmosomes (10). Squamous cell carcinomas demonstrate a general gradation of smaller to larger squamous cells with intercellular bridges and possible keratinization (figs. 7-4, 7-5).

## MALIGNANT LYMPHOMA AND PLASMACYTOMA

Lymphomas of the esophagus are rare. Most are secondary, resulting from local extension of hilar and gastric nodal disease (34,36). About a dozen primary cases of esophageal lymphoma have been reported to date, most of which, in the last few years, have occurred in patients with acquired immunodeficiency syndrome (AIDS) or in the immunosuppressed (25–39).

Clinically, the patients present with a variety of esophageal symptoms mimicking carcinoma, such as dysphagia. The endoscopic and gross appearances are similar to those of carcinoma, and include multiple polypoid masses, linear rugae, and ulcers or strictures with proximal dilatation (27,32,33,35,37). However, it has been suggested that multicentricity of tumor is more indicative of lymphoma than carcinoma (28).

Histologically, most primary esophageal lymphomas are large cell or immunoblastic B-cell lymphomas (fig. 7-6). However, other phenotypic types, such as T-cell lymphoma, large cell anaplastic Ki-1 lymphoma, Hodgkin's disease, and plasmacytoma have been described (29,35,37,38). For detailed histologic features of lymphoma, refer to the chapter on gastric lymphomas.

## MALIGNANT MELANOMA

As was noted in the discussion of normal anatomy in chapter 2, basal melanocytes are found in a small number of normal esophagi, so it is not surprising that melanomas arise within the esophagus. In a study from India, 21 pigmented melanocyte-containing patches were found in 1,000 consecutive routine esophagoscopies, mainly in the middle and lower esophagus where melanomas usually arise (50). Primary malignant melanoma of the esophagus is so rare that the largest reported series from the United States, from Memorial Hospital for Cancer and Allied Diseases in New York, includes only eight cases, most of which were reported twice (41,43). A study from Japan found only 16 melanomas among almost 12,000 primary esophageal malignancies (49). In a review of the literature up to early 1989, only 139 cases were found (49). It is estimated that melanoma accounts for 0.1 percent of primary esophageal malignancies (46); in the United States, there will be no more than about 10 new cases of esophageal melanoma per year.

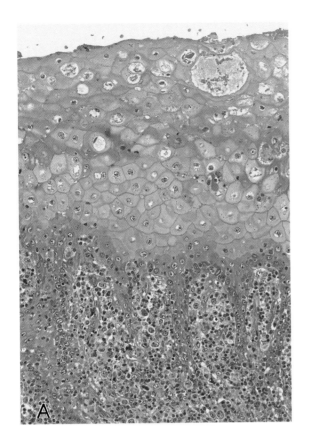

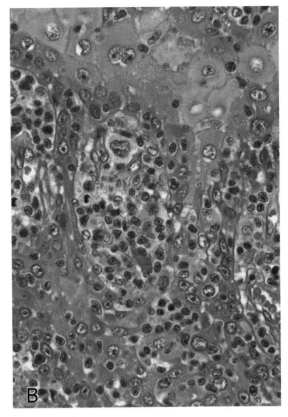

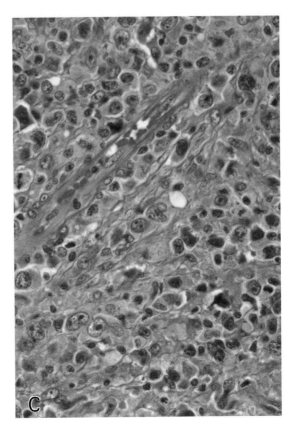

Figure 7-6
LARGE CELL LYMPHOMA OF THE ESOPHAGUS

A: Low-power magnification of a lymphomatous infiltrate extending to the squamous epithelium.

B: High-power magnification of the atypical large lymphocytes admixed with numerous smaller lymphocytes, many of which appear normal.

C: High-power view of a deeper area shows a fairly monomorphous infiltrate of large atypical lymphocytes.

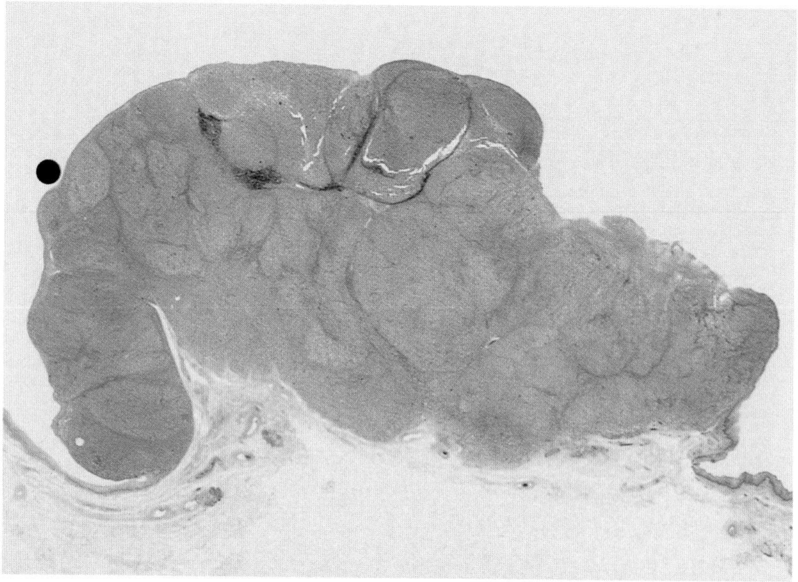

Figure 7-7
SESSILE POLYPOID MELANOMA
A large, sessile, polypoid melanoma
that invades no deeper than the superficial submucosa. The black dot marks
a spot in the squamous epithelium in
which there is a junctional component.

**Clinical Features.** Melanomas have the same clinical characteristics as carcinomas of the esophagus (41,48,49). Most of the patients are in the sixth and seventh decades, with a mean age of 60 years. One case was reported in a 7-year-old boy (40) Males develop melanomas about twice as often as females, a much lower male to female ratio than for carcinomas; in some series, females and males are equally affected (41). Dysphagia, heartburn or substernal or epigastric pain, and weight loss are the common symptoms, with a duration of 3 to 4 months prior to diagnosis. Endoscopically, esophageal melanomas are often polypoid and arise within the lower and middle parts of the tube. There are no consistent predisposing high-risk factors.

**Morphologic Findings.** Grossly, esophageal melanomas are usually polypoid and often ulcerated. These features are evident radiographically and endoscopically. Growth is largely radial or horizontal; vertical growth is limited. This sometimes results in large tumors that invade no deeper than the submucosa (fig. 7-7) (46). Nevertheless, large tumors commonly invade transmurally into the adventitia or even beyond. Tumor size varies, with the largest measuring over 17 cm in diameter. Satellite nodules, presumably intramural metastases, some appearing several centimeters from the primary, sometimes occur. The mucosa may be pigmented at the edges, an alteration often referred to as *melanosis,* which may extend

for many centimeters from the primary invasive tumor (42). Most tumors are pigmented or partly pigmented. A few cases with more than one melanoma have been reported (43).

Microscopically, the tumors usually arise within a field of atypical junctional melanocyte proliferation, with a lentiginous pattern in which there are single atypical melanocytes and small clusters within the basal layer (fig. 7-8). In these cases, the atypical melanocytes are often large, with clear or pale cytoplasm and large vesicular or hyperchromatic, occasionally bizarre nuclei. Some of these cells contain a few melanin granules. There is sometimes a thick layer of melanocytes in the basal epithelium (44). Usually, there is no pagetoid junctional component and larger clusters of atypical melanocytes occur higher up in the squamous epithelium than in the basal layer (52). Esophageal melanomas seem to belong to the same family of acrolentiginous melanomas to which other mucosal melanomas belong, including those in the upper aerodigestive tract and anus. In many cases, in addition to the atypical basal melanocytes, more benign-appearing melanocytes, comparable to nevus cells, are found in the basal layer (45).

The invasive component is usually epithelioid, but some tumors mainly are composed of spindle cells or a mixture (fig. 7-9). The cells are arranged in uniform nests or sheets. Pleomorphism with giant forms and mitoses are variable, and

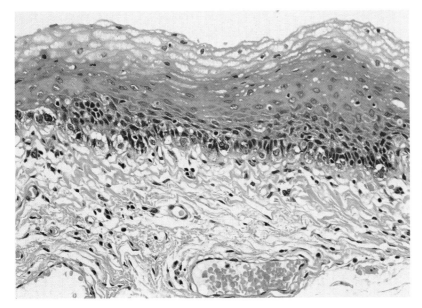

Figure 7-8
ATYPICAL JUNCTIONAL
MELANOCYTIC HYPERPLASIA
ADJACENT TO A MELANOMA
Bizarre melanocytic cells, most of
which are single with a few small clusters, obliterate the basal layer of the
squamous mucosa. This change defines
this tumor as primary in the esophagus,
rather than metastatic.

Figure 7-9
MELANOMA
This melanoma is composed of epi-
thelioid cells with pleomorphic nuclei.
Many of the cells have abundant pale
cytoplasm, and some contain melanin.

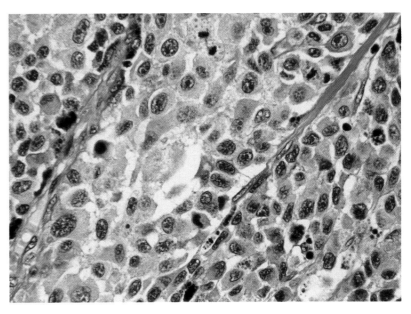

cytoplasmic pigmentation is common. Cytologically, the tumor cells are identical to cutaneous
melanoma cells. They have large vesicular or
hyperchromatic nuclei, some of which have
prominent eosinophilic nucleoli. Small cell, balloon cell, and signet ring cell variants have been
described (51). There is a tendency for the periphery to be circumscribed with an expansile,
rather than infiltrative, growth pattern. Ultrastructural studies in a few cases have shown that
the tumor cells have melanocytic characteristics
and typical melanosomes (43,44).

**Differential Diagnosis.** Because primary
melanoma is so rare, and because cutaneous
melanomas occasionally metastasize to the
esophagus, rigid criteria must be used to determine whether a melanoma is primary or metastatic to the esophagus. The major criterion for
primary melanoma is the presence of a junctional component in the overlying or adjacent
mucosa. However when the tumors are large,
bulky, and ulcerated, the overlying epithelium
may be totally destroyed, thereby obliterating
the junctional component.

Since some melanomas are not pigmented, and can be composed of virtually any cell type and size, they mimic many other malignancies. Melanomas composed of epithelioid cells resemble carcinomas; this is especially problematic when the cells have signet ring features. Those epithelioid melanomas with small cells mimic lymphoma or small cell carcinoma. Melanomas composed of spindle cells, particularly those that are desmoplastic, look like sarcomas. The differential diagnosis is resolved by the use of a simple panel of immunohistochemical antibodies, including those against cytokeratins, leukocyte common antigen (LCA), S-100 protein, and the melanoma marker HMB45. Carcinomas stain with antibodies to cytokeratins, but not to those for S-100, LCA, or HMB45. Lymphomas only stain with antibodies to LCA. Melanomas routinely express S-100 and most express HMB45 (51). Sarcomas, in general are negative for all these markers. Sometimes, however, these markers do not work as expected, so that the melanoma either does not stain at all or stains inappropriately, and the result is a diagnosis of "undifferentiated malignant neoplasm of unknown type." Electron microscopic detection of melanosomes may determine the tumor type in such cases. Also, since the esophagus is such an uncommon site for melanomas and such a common site for carcinomas, even typical melanomas, especially those that are not pigmented, may not be diagnosed unless the pathologist is aware of the possibility of melanoma. About a quarter of biopsied melanoma cases are not correctly diagnosed until the resected specimen is evaluated (47).

**Treatment and Prognosis.** Data are insufficient to relate stage characteristics, such as depth of invasion or size, to survival because these tumors are so rare. It has been stated that esophageal melanomas are biologically more aggressive than their cutaneous counterparts. However, it is likely that esophageal melanomas are detected at a time in their evolution when, as a group, they are larger and more advanced than cutaneous melanomas. In general, when esophageal melanomas are discovered, they are advanced lesions with frequent extra-esophageal spread, so that many are not resectable. The average survival time after esophagectomy is 1 year or less, with a 5-year survival of no more than 2 percent (41,49). Currently, resection is the

only recognized treatment, and it may be the best method for palliation of obstructing tumors, although local endoscopic laser treatment may eventually have a role in palliation. The value of adjuvant radiation or chemotherapy is currently unknown. There are obviously insufficient cases for controlled therapeutic trials. Common metastatic sites include regional lymph nodes, liver, mediastinal soft tissues, lung, and brain.

## NEOPLASMS METASTATIC TO THE ESOPHAGUS

The most common malignant tumors that metastasize to the esophagus are the same three that metastasize to the stomach: carcinomas of the lung and breast, and melanoma. They generally expand within the submucosa, secondarily invading the mucosa and the muscularis propria. Histologically, particularly on biopsy, they may be confused with primary esophageal melanoma, squamous cell carcinoma, or adenocarcinoma, so it is critical that the history of a primary tumor is conveyed to the pathologist who interprets the biopsy (fig. 7-10). The limited published information on carcinoma of lung and melanoma metastatic to the esophagus is summarized below.

### Metastatic Carcinoma of the Lung

In an autopsy study of 423 bronchogenic carcinomas over a 36-year period, the esophagus was the most common gastrointestinal site of metastasis by far (53). Thirty-three of these carcinomas metastasized to the esophagus: 27 only involved the esophagus, while the other 6 involved the esophagus in concert with another gut site that was anywhere from the stomach to the colon. Rare carcinomas of the lung involve the esophagus by direct extension through the pleura and into the posterior mediastinum.

### Metastatic Melanoma

Of patients dying with widely disseminated cutaneous malignant melanoma, 4 percent have metastases to the esophagus (55). These are usually intramural and small, and as a result, do not cause clinical symptoms. However, there have been a few reports of melanoma metastases that have been large enough to produce clinical esophageal disease, including one that occurred 11 years after a cutaneous melanoma was excised

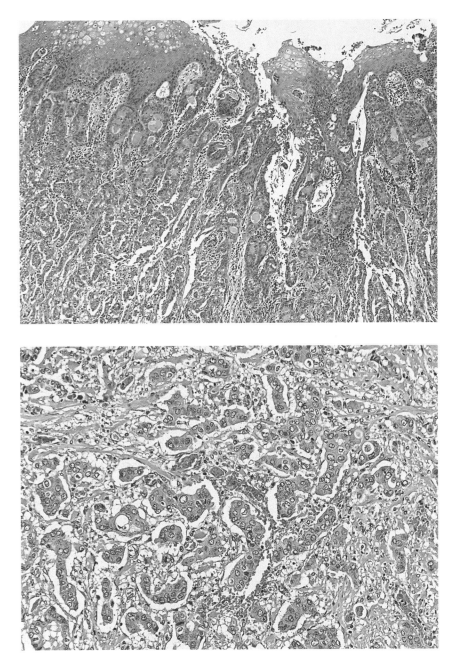

Figure 7-10
METASTATIC CARCINOMA FROM THE BREAST TO THE ESOPHAGUS

Top: Superficially, the squamous epithelium is intact except for a defect in the middle where the carcinoma has pushed through. Carcinomatous strands attach to and appear to invade the base of the epithelium.

Bottom: Deeper in the lesion, nests of carcinoma cells are embedded in a desmoplastic stroma, a common pattern in carcinoma of the breast.

(54). Differentiating metastatic, symptom-producing melanoma from a primary melanoma can be difficult. A history of a verified melanoma arising in an extra-esophageal site, usually the skin, and a lack of atypical intramucosal melanocytic proliferation at the edges of the tumor, are the most important hints that the tumor is metastatic.

# REFERENCES

## Endocrine Tumors

1. Attar BM, Lenvendoglu H, Rhee H. Small cell carcinoma of the esophagus. Report of three cases and review of the literature. Dig Dis Sci 1990;35:145–52.
2. Beyer KL, Marshall JB, Diaz-Arias AA, Loy TS. Primary small-cell carcinoma of the esophagus. Report of 11 cases and review of the literature. J Clin Gastroenterol 1991;13:135–41.
3. Brenner S, Heimlich H, Widman M. Carcinoid of the oesophagus. NY State J Med 1969;69:137–9.
4. Briggs JC, Ibrahim NB. Oat cell carcinoma of the oesophagus: a clinico-pathological study of 23 cases. Histopathology 1983;7:261–77.
5. Brodman HR, Pai BN. Malignant carcinoid of the stomach and distal oesophagus. Am J Dig Dis 1968;13:677–81.
6. Caldwell CB, Bains MS, Burt M. Unusual malignant neoplasms of the esophagus. Oat cell carcinoma, melanoma, and sarcoma. J Thorac Cardiovasc Surg 1991;101:100–7.
7. Cary NR, Barron DJ, McGoldrick JP, Wells FC. Combined oesophageal adenocarcinoma and carcinoid in Barrett's oesophagitis: potential role of enterochromaffin-like cells in oesophageal malignancy. Thorax 1993;48:404–5.
8. Chong FK, Graham JH, Madoff IM. Mucin producing carcinoid (composite tumour) of the upper third of the oesophagus: a variant of carcinoid tumour. Cancer 1979;44:1853–9.
9. Hirata M, Nakanishi M, Sasaki M, et al. Carcinoid of the esophagus. Jap J Gastroenterology 1989;86:1692–6.
10. Ho KJ, Herrera GA, Jones JM, Alexander CB. Small cell carcinoma of the esophagus: evidence for a unified histogenesis. Hum Pathol 1984;15:460–8.
11. Hoda SA, Hajdu SI. Small cell carcinoma of the esophagus. Cytology and immunohistology in four cases. Acta Cytol 1992;36:113–20.
12. Horai T, Kobayashi A, Tateishi R, et al. A cytologic study on small cell carcinoma of the esophagus. Cancer 1978;41:1890–6.
13. Horing E, Egner E, von Gaisberg U, Kieninger G. Carcinoid tumor of the esophagus. A rare differential diagnosis in submucosal esophageal tumor. Z Gastroenterologie 1990;28:10–3.
14. Hussein AM, Feun LG, Sridhar KS, Benedetto P, Waldman S, Otrakji CL. Combination chemotherapy and radiotherapy for small-cell carcinoma of the esophagus. A case report of long-term survival and review of the literature. Am J Clin Oncol 1990;13:369–73.
15. Imai T, Sonnohe Y, Okano H. Oat cell carcinoma (apudoma) of the esophagus: a case report. Cancer 1978;41:358–64.
16. Martin MR, Kahn LB. So-called pseudosarcoma of the esophagus. Nodal metastases of the spindle cell element. Arch Pathol Lab Med 1977;101:604–9.
17. Matsusaka T, Watanabe H, Enjoji M. Anaplastic carcinoma of the esophagus. Report of three cases and their histogenetic consideration. Cancer 1976;37:1352–8.
18. McFadden DW, Rudnicki M, Talamini MA. Primary small cell carcinoma of the esophagus. Ann Thor Surg 1989;47:477–80.
19. Mulder LD, Gardiner GA, Weeks DA. Primary small cell carcinoma of the esophagus: case presentation and review of the literature. Gastrointest Radiol 1991;16:5–10.
20. Nishimaki T, Suzuki T, Fukuda T, Aizawa K, Tanaka O, Muto T. Primary small cell carcinoma of the esophagus with ectopic gastrin production. Report of a case and review of the literature. Dig Dis Sci 1993;38:767–71.
21. Proctor DD, Fraser JL, Mangano MM, Calkins DR, Rosenberg SJ. Small cell carcinoma of the esophagus in a patient with longstanding primary achalasia. Am J Gastroenterol 1992;87:664–7.
22. Rankin R, Nirodi NS, Browne MK. Carcinoid tumour of the oesophagus. Case report. Scott Med J 1980;25:245–9.
23. Reid HA, Richardson WW, Corrin B. Oat cell carcinoma of the esophagus. Cancer 1980;45:2342–7.
24. Tateishi R, Taniguchi H, Wada A, Horai T, Taniguchi K. Argyrophil cells and melanocytes in esophageal mucosa. Arch Pathol 1974;98:87–9.

## Lymphoma

25. Ahmed N, Ramos S, Sika J, et al. Primary extramedullary esophageal plasmacytoma. First case report. Cancer 1976;38:943–7.
26. Benamouzig R, Tulliez M, Chaussade S, et al. Lymphome non hodgkinien primitif de l'oesophage chez un patient atteint d'un syndrome d'immunodeficience acquise (SIDA). Gastroenterol Clin Biol 1992;16:477–9.
27. Berman MD, Falchuk KR, Trey C, Gramm HF. Primary histiocytic lymphoma of the esophagus. Dig Dis Sci 1979;24:883–6.
28. Bernal A, del Junco GW. Endoscopic and pathologic features of esophageal lymphoma: a report of four cases in patients with acquired immune deficiency syndrome. Gastrointest Endosc 1986;32:96–9.
29. Bolondi L, De Giorgio R, Santi V, et al. Primary non-Hodgkin's T-cell lymphoma of the esophagus. A case with peculiar endoscopic ultrasonographic pattern. Dig Dis Sci 1990;35:1426–30.
30. Doki T, Hamada S, Murayama H, Suenaga H, Sannohe Y. Primary malignant lymphoma of the esophagus. A case report. Endoscopy 1984;16:189–92.
31. Matsuura H, Saito R, Nakajima S, Yoshihara W, Enomoto T. Non-Hodgkin's lymphoma of the esophagus. Am J Gastoenterol 1985;80:941–6.
32. Nagrani M, Lavigne BC, Siskind BN, Knisley RE, Traube M. Primary non-Hodgkin's lymphoma of the esophagus. Arch Intern Med 1989;149:193–5.
33. Nissan S, Bar-Moar JA, Levy E. Lymphosarcoma of the esophagus: a case report. Cancer 1974;34:1321–3.
34. Okerbloom JA, Armitage JO, Zetterman R, Linder J. Esophageal involvement by non-Hodgkin's lymphoma. Am J Med 1984;77:359–61.

35. Pearson JM, Borg-Grech A. Primary Ki-1(CD 30)-positive, large cell, anaplastic lymphoma of the esophagus. Cancer 1991;68:418–21.

36. Rosenberg SA, Diamond HD, Jaslowitz B, Craver LF. Lymphosarcoma: a review of 1,269 cases. Medicine (Baltimore) 1961;40:31–84.

37. Stein HA, Murray D, Warner HA. Primary Hodgkin's disease of the esophagus. Dig Dis Sci 1981;26:457–61.

38. Tsukada T, Ohno T, Kihira H, et al. Primary esophageal non-Hodgkins lymphoma. Intern Med 1992;31:569–72.

39. Williams MR, Chidambaram M, Salama FD, Ansell ID. Tracheo-esophageal fistula due to primary lymphoma of the esophagus. J R Coll Surg Edinb 1984;29:60–1.

## Melanoma

40. Basque GJ, Boline JE, Holyoke JB. Malignant melanoma of the esophagus: first reported case in a child. Am J Clin Pathol 1970;53:609–11.

41. Caldwell CB, Bains MS, Burt M. Unusual malignant neoplasms of the esophagus. Oat cell carcinoma, melanoma, and sarcoma. J Thorac Cardiovasc Surg 1991;101:100–7.

42. De Mik JI, Kooijman CD, Hoekstra JB, Tytgat GN. Primary malignant melanoma of the oesophagus. Histopathology 1992;20:77–9.

43. DiCostanzo DP, Urmacher C. Primary malignant melanoma of the esophagus. Am J Surg Pathol 1987;11:46–52.

44. Frable WJ, Kay S, Schatzki P. Primary malignant melanoma of the esophagus: an electron microscopic study. Am J Clin Pathol 1972;58:659–67.

45. Guzman RP, Wightman R, Ravinsky E, Unruh HW. Primary malignant melanoma of the esophagus with diffuse melanocytic atypia and melanoma in situ. Am J Clin Pathol 1989;92:802–4.

46. Ludwig ME, Shaw R, de Suto-Nagy G. Primary malignant melanoma of the esophagus. Cancer 1981;48:2528–34.

47. Mills SE, Cooper PH. Malignant melanoma of the digestive system. Pathol Annu 1983;18:1–26.

48. Sabanathan S, Eng J. Primary malignant melanoma of the esophagus. Scand J Thorac Cardiovasc Surg 1990;24:83–5.

49. Sabanathan S, Eng J, Pradhan GN. Primary malignant melanoma of the esophagus. Am J Gastroenterol 1989;84:1475–81.

50. Sharma SS, Venkateswaran S, Chacko A, Mathan M. Melanosis of the esophagus. An endoscopic, histochemical, and ultrastructural study. Gastroenterol 1991;100:13–6.

51. Symmans WF, Grimes MM. Malignant melanoma of the esophagus: histologic variants and immunohistochemical findings in four cases. Surg Pathol 1991;4:222–34.

52. Takubo K, Kanda Y, Ishii M. Primary malignant melanoma of the esophagus. Hum Pathol 1983;14:727–30.

## Metastastic Neoplasms

53. Antler AS, Ough Y, Pitchumoni CS, Davidian M, Thelmo W. Gastrointestinal metastases from malignant tumors of the lung. Cancer 1982;49:170–2.

54. Eng J, Pradhan GN, Sabanathan S, Mearns AJ. Malignant melanoma metastatic to the esophagus. Ann Thorac Surg 1989;48:287–8.

55. Ludwig ME, Shaw R, de Suto-Nagy G. Primary malignant melanoma of the esophagus. Cancer 1981; 48:2528–34.

**8**

# THE STOMACH: EMBRYOLOGY, NORMAL ANATOMY, AND TUMOR DERIVATION

## EMBRYOLOGY

The stomach is derived from the caudal or distal part of the foregut. It is seen first as a dilatation at about the fifth week of gestation, following which it rotates approximately 90° clockwise so that the left side faces anteriorly while the right side is posterior (5). As the rotation occurs, the part that was initially posterior grows faster than the part that was anterior, resulting in a short left side, the lesser curvature, and a long right side, the greater curvature. Eventually, the distal end of the embryonic stomach moves to the right and is pulled upward, resulting in the mature placement of the pylorus, while the proximal end moves to the left and slightly distally, leading to the normal position of the cardioesophageal junction.

## NORMAL ANATOMY

### Gross Anatomy

The normal stomach lies in the central and left anterior upper abdomen. It begins as the cardia, a narrow cuff, generally no more than 1 to 2 cm, immediately distal to the lower esophageal sphincter musculature, and then it expands

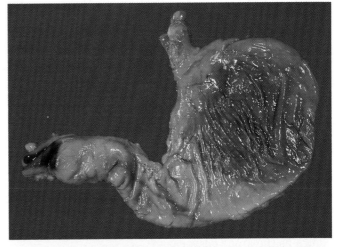

Figure 8-1
GROSS VIEWS OF THE NORMAL STOMACH
(AUTOPSY MATERIALS)

Top: External view.
Bottom: Internal view of the posterior wall. In both views, the distal esophagus is the short, narrow tube at the upper center. It enters the stomach at the first 1 to 2 cm of the cardia. The body extends distally from the cardia to the bend on the left, the angulus. Distal to the angulus is the antrum, which terminates at the pylorus. The bulge on the upper right is the fundus.

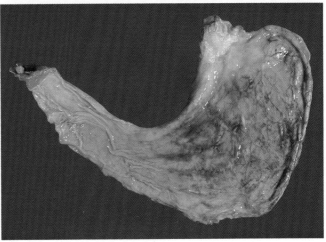

into the dilated body or corpus (fig. 8-1). To the left of the midline, the proximal part of the body extends cephalad into the diaphragmatic concavity as a bulge known as the fundus. From the fundus the body extends distally as a broad curve facing the left side, known as the greater curvature. On the right side, the body extends distally as a much shorter concavity, known as the lesser curvature. Distally, the body gradually tapers toward the point where the stomach takes a sharp angle turn to the right, the angulus, roughly the dividing line between the body and the antrum (10). The antrum, the distal third of the stomach, is narrower than the body. It also tapers to end at the pylorus, the last centimeter of stomach immediately overlying the muscular pyloric sphincter. This sphincter is a circumferential thickened ridge of the internal layer of the muscularis propria, and is the dividing line between the stomach and the duodenum.

The external surface is almost completely covered by smooth, shiny peritoneum. The broad greater curvature is attached to the omentum and mesentery of the transverse colon, the transverse mesocolon. The lesser curvature is attached to the liver by connective tissue known as the gastrohepatic ligament.

Internally, the fundus and body are covered by folds or rugae which consist of cores of submucosa covered by mucosa (fig. 8-2). In the antrum, the folds flatten, especially along the lesser curvature. On close inspection, the mucosal surface appears finely granular or nodular as a result of alternating elevations and surrounding depressions. The elevations, about 1 to 3 mm across, are known as the areae gastricae (8).

### Microscopic Anatomy

The normal gastric wall has the same layers as does the rest of the gut: a mucosa composed of epithelium and lamina propria with muscularis mucosae at the base, submucosa, muscularis propria, and subserosa.

**The Epithelium.** The normal stomach has several different types of mucosa, which imperfectly correlate with the gross anatomic divisions: cardiac; body, corpus, or fundic; and antral or pyloric (figs. 8-3–8-6). All mucosae have two components or compartments, the superficial pit or foveolar compartment and the deep glandular

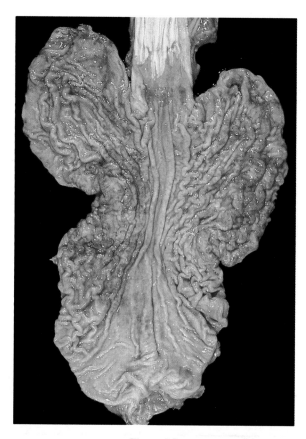

Figure 8-2
MUCOSAL VIEW OF THE STOMACH

Mucosal view of a whole stomach opened along the greater curvature with the esophagus at the top. The parallel folds in the middle of the specimen run along the lesser curvature. The two wings at either side are the fundus. The entire fundus and body are covered by thick, often serpentine, folds or rugae. They flatten distally in the antrum. The bulge at the bottom is the pyloric sphincter.

compartment. The pit compartment contains the surface epithelium that extends into the pits, which are really conduits to the lumen for glandular secretions. The surface and pit epithelia are tall columnar, with apical mucus vacuoles. These appear pale pink when stained with hematoxylin and eosin (H&E), dark red with the periodic acid–Schiff stain, and do not stain with any of the acid mucin stains, such as mucicarmine and Alcian blue (fig. 8-3). These staining characteristics indicate that these cells contain only neutral mucins. While the cells of the superficial compartment are the same throughout the gastric mucosa, the depth of the pits varies, so that in the body mucosa, the pits are short and take up about one fourth of the total mucosal thickness,

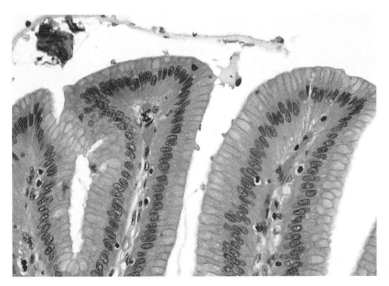

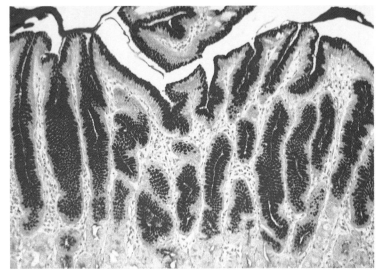

Figure 8-3
NORMAL SUPERFICIAL
AND PIT EPITHELIUM

The normal superficial and pit epithelium is tall columnar. The apical mucin stains pink with H&E, red with the periodic acid–Schiff (PAS) stain and does not stain neutral mucin with Alcian blue. Top: H&E stain; bottom: Alcian blue, periodic acid–Schiff combination stain.

Figure 8-4
NORMAL CARDIAC MUCOSA

The pit and the glandular compartments are approximately equal in height. Scattered glands are dilated.

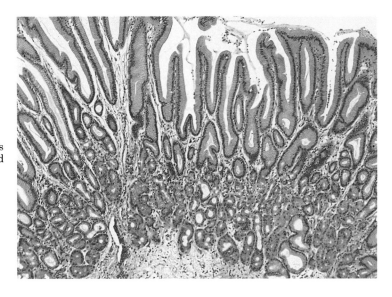

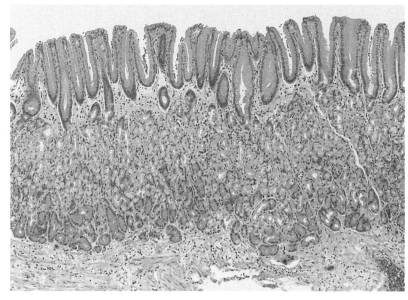

Figure 8-5
NORMAL BODY
(CORPUS, FUNDIC) MUCOSA
The pit compartment is about one fourth of the entire mucosal thickness, resulting in a pit to gland ratio of 1 to 3. The glands are tightly clustered. The superficial lamina propria has few cells.

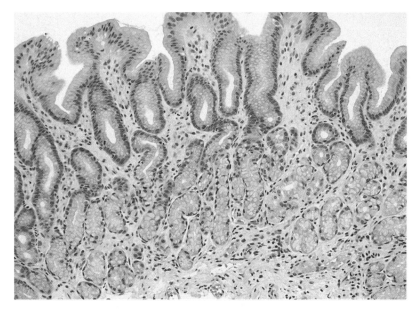

Figure 8-6
NORMAL ANTRAL
(PYLORIC) MUCOSA
The pit and glandular compartments are about the same height. The glands are clustered and less densely packed than are the body glands.

while in the cardia and in the antrum, the pits are about half the total mucosal thickness.

In contrast to the superficial compartment, the deep or glandular compartment differs in different parts of the stomach, not only in thickness, but also in cell type. In the cardia and in the antrum, the glands are arranged in clusters, separated by fine collagenous and smooth muscle septa. The glands contain cells that produce only neutral mucins, much like the cells of the superficial compartment (fig. 8-7). In routine preparations, their cytoplasm appears more granular than the cytoplasm of the superficial cells. In contrast, in the body and fundus, the glands contain highly specialized cells which produce acid (the parietal cells) and enzymes (the chief cells) (fig. 8-8). In H&E stained sections the parietal cells are plump, oval to round, with pale pink and slightly granular cytoplasm, while the columnar cells with darker cytoplasm are the chief or enzyme-producing cells. The parietal cells usually are more prominent in the upper part of the glandular compartment, while the chief cells are concentrated at the base. In the

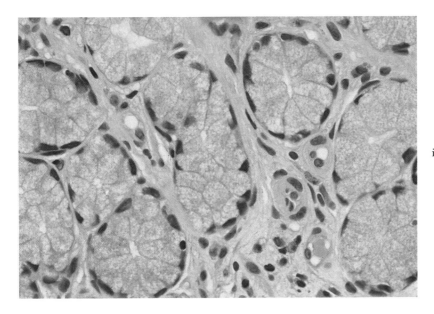

Figure 8-7
MUCOUS GLANDS
Mucous glands of the type that occur
in normal cardiac and antral mucosae.

Figure 8-8
SUPERFICIAL GLANDULAR
COMPARTMENT OF THE
BODY MUCOSA
The glands are tightly packed. The
pale cells with finely granular cyto-
plasm are parietal cells; the cells with
denser, darker cytoplasm are chief cells.

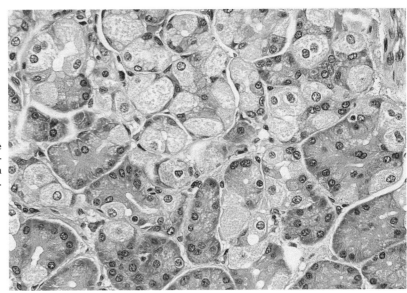

body mucosa, there are alternating areas of concentrated glands and shorter pits, separated by
depressions in which the glandular compartment is thinner and the pits longer, the areae
gastricae which can be seen grossly.

The gastric mucosae contain endocrine cells,
but they differ with the mucosal type (1). In the
antral mucosa, the predominant endocrine cell
is the gastrin-producing cell or G cell. These are
located mostly in the neck and upper gland
areas. In the body mucosa, G cells are rare, while
the histamine-producing enterochromaffin-like

(ECL) cells are more common. These are located
in the lower third of the mucosa, near the chief
cells. All the endocrine cells are seen better with
special staining techniques, especially specific
immunocytochemistry, than with the H&E
stain. However, G cells can often be recognized
as pear-shaped cells with finely granular cytoplasm, situated next to the basement membrane
of the antral necks and glands (fig. 8-9).

At the junction of two different mucosal types,
especially antral and body, there are transitional
zones which share features of both mucosae.

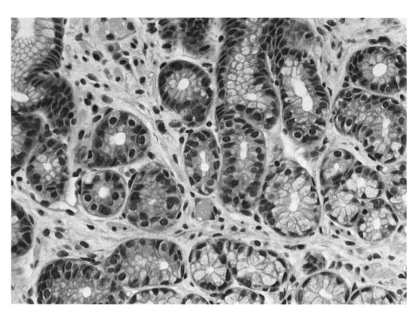

**Figure 8-9**
**NECK REGION**
**OF THE ANTRAL MUCOSA**
The pits are at the top and the glands at the base. In between, the tubules are lined by a mucus-containing epithelium with nuclei that are slightly larger than in either the pits or the glands. This is the neck region, the proliferative zone for all gastric mucosae. The pale, pear-shaped cells with finely granular, gray cytoplasm at the base of the necks and glands are the gastrin-producing or G cells.

This transitional mucosa usually has the structure of antral mucosa, with clustered glands and tall pits; the glands usually contain mucous cells and gastrin-producing cells of antral mucosa mixed with parietal and chief cells of body mucosa. As people age, transitional mucosa seems to gradually creep proximally, especially along the lesser curvature (4). In one study of stomachs of patients with duodenal and gastric ulcers, the size of the transitional mucosa correlated with maximal acid output and the parietal cell density in the body mucosa (9).

Between the pits and the glands in all mucosal types is the neck region, the generative zone for all cells of the gastric glands and pits (fig. 8-9). The cells of this narrow zone are tall, with apical mucus vacuoles, the mucous neck cells. Mitotic figures are sometimes found in this zone, especially in cases of surface epithelial injury.

**The Lamina Propria.** The lamina propria is sparse throughout the normal stomach. In the body mucosa, there is little stroma between the glands, only scant stroma between the pits and necks, and almost no inflammatory cells of any type (fig. 8-5). In the antral and cardiac mucosae, the gland clusters are separated by a few loose collagen fibers and smooth muscle cells and the pits are more widely spaced than in the body mucosa; but even in this more spacious lamina propria, there are few inflammatory cells (figs. 8-4, 8-6). Most of the cells are smooth muscle, a few macrophages, and rare lymphocytes and plasma cells. Arterioles, venules, and capillaries are present at all levels. In contrast, lymphatics are present in the basal lamina propria, but not higher; however, in severe chronic atrophic gastritis, lymphatics may be found much higher in the mucosa (6).

**The Muscularis Mucosae.** The muscularis mucosae is a thin double layer of smooth muscle that defines the base of the mucosa and separates it from the submucosa. Muscle fibers extend from here into the base of the mucosa, especially in the most distal part of the antrum.

**The Submucosa.** This is a loose connective tissue layer containing blood vessels, lymphatics, nerves, and ganglion cells of the submucosal (Meissner) plexus; a few adipocytes; and a variety of scattered spindle cells that are a mix of fibroblasts, smooth muscle cells, and mast cells.

**The Muscularis Propria.** In contrast to other parts of the gut, which have a bilayer of inner circular and outer longitudinal smooth muscle in the muscularis propria, the stomach has three muscle layers: inner oblique, middle circular, and outer longitudinal. The nerves and ganglion cells of the myenteric (Auerbach) plexus are found between the outer two muscle layers.

**The Subserosa and Serosa.** Except where it is attached to omentum, mesocolon, and ligaments, the stomach has a thin covering of subserosal collagen, the subserosa. The subserosa is

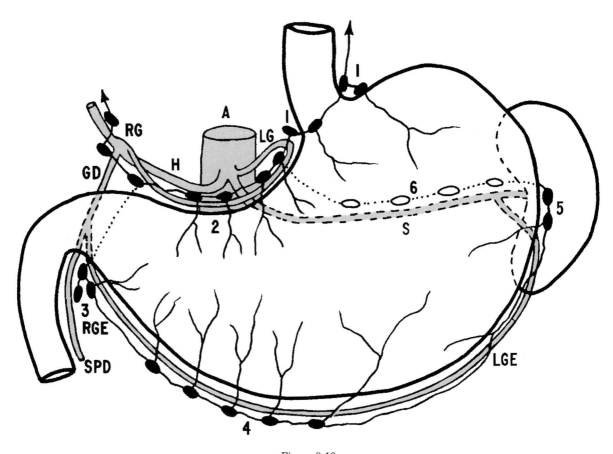

Figure 8-10
ARTERIAL AND LYMPHATIC SUPPLY OF THE STOMACH

A schematic diagram of the arteries of the stomach illustrates: A: aorta; LG: left gastric artery; H: hepatic artery; RG: right gastric artery; GD: gastroduodenal artery; RGE: right gastroepiploic artery; S: splenic artery; LGE: left gastroepiploic artery; and SPD: superior pancreaticoduodenal artery. The lymph nodes are situated along the arteries and consist of six groups: 1) paracardiac nodes; 2) superior gastric nodes; 3) subpyloric nodes; 4) inferior gastric nodes; 5) splenic nodes; and 6) pancreatic nodes. (Fig. 69 from Fascicle 7, Second Series.)

covered by a single layer of flat mesothelium, the serosa proper, a part of the visceral peritoneum.

**Lymphoid Tissue.** There is no agreement as to whether or not the normal stomach contains lymphoid follicles (2,3,8). Lymphoid follicles seem to be easily induced, especially by *Helicobacter pylori,* a bacterium that infects the gastric mucosae, mainly the antral mucosa, so commonly that its associated gastritis may be considered a normal variant in adults in certain populations as they age. Lymphoid follicles are an expected component of that gastritis (2). In our experience, substantial lymphoid aggregates do not occur in normal stomachs in the absence of this organism. Infrequent small aggregates or follicle-like collections of small lymphocytes are occasionally found at the base of otherwise normal-appearing mucosa, but it is never

clear if these lymphocytes are normal or induced by *H. pylori* that may be present in another part of the stomach or another stimulus.

## Blood Supply

The gastric cardia is supplied by the left gastric artery that arises from the celiac axis (fig. 8-10) (7,8). Branches of the hepatic artery, designated as the right gastric artery and the right gastroepiploic artery, supply the lesser and the distal greater curvatures, respectively. The proximal greater curvature is supplied by the left gastroepiploic and short gastric arteries that arise from the splenic artery. These vessels anastomose extensively, resulting in an excellent collateral supply (8). The arteries are accompanied by veins, most of which drain into the portal venous system. The most proximal part of the stomach is drained by veins that communicate with the systemic system by the esophageal veins.

### Lymphatic Supply

The major lymphatics follow the blood vessels, and the nodes are located along the main arteries (fig. 8-10) (7,8). Much of the lesser curvature, from the cardia distally, is drained by lymphatics that extend along the left gastric vessels to the left gastric nodes. From the antral part of the lesser curvature, lymphatics extend to the right gastric and hepatic nodes. Part of the cardia is also drained by the paracardiac nodes. Lymphatics from the proximal greater curvature, including the fundus, drain to nodes in the splenic hilum, while lymphatics from the distal greater curvature drain to the right gastroepiploic nodes in the omentum and to the pyloric or subpyloric nodes near the pancreatic head.

### Nerves

The parasympathetic nerve supply comes from branches of the anterior and posterior vagus nerves that course in the subserosa, mainly along the lesser curvature (8). Sympa-thetic nerves come from the celiac plexus and both phrenic nerves.

## CLASSIFICATION OF GASTRIC TUMORS

In this volume, tumors of the stomach are classified, in general, much as they have been classified by the World Health Organization in its International Histological Classification of Tumours published in 1990 (11). A few modifications have been made in this classification, based upon current reports of mesenchymal tumors, lymphomas, and endocrine neoplasms. The classification of gastric lymphomas has been changed to recognize the special lymphoma types arising in the gut that are different from node-based lymphomas. The classification of stromal tumors has been modified to take into consideration the unique types of stromal proliferations that involve the stomach, but which rarely occur elsewhere. We believe that any classification system involving almost anything in medicine must be looked upon as fluid, since new discoveries, often based upon sophisticated cell biologic techniques, are occurring all the time, and may clarify the status of tumors and tumor-like proliferations that are now either unclear from a nosologic standpoint or placed in a wrong category.

### REFERENCES

1. Dayal Y, Wolfe HJ. Hyperplastic proliferations of the gastrointestinal endocrine cells. In: Dayal Y, ed. Endocrine pathology of the gut and pancreas. Boca Raton: CRC Press, 1991:36–42.
2. Genta RM, Hamner HW, Graham DY. Gastric lymphoid follicles in Helicobacter pylori infection: frequency, distribution, and response to triple therapy. Hum Pathol 1993;24:577–83.
3. Isaacson PG, Spencer J. Is gastric lymphoma an infectious disease? [Editorial] Hum Pathol 1993;24:569–70.
4. Kimura K. Chronological transition of the fundic-pyloric border determined by stepwise biopsy of the lesser and greater curvatures of the stomach. Gastroenterology 1972;63:584–92.
5. Langman J. Medical embryology. Baltimore: Williams & Wilkins, 1975:282–3.
6. Listrom MB, Fenoglio-Preiser CM. Lymphatic distribution of the stomach in normal, inflammatory, hyperplastic, and neoplastic tissue. Gastroenterology 1987;93:506–14.
7. Ming SC. Tumors of the esophagus and stomach. Atlas of Tumor Pathology, 2nd Series, Fascicle 7. Washington, D.C.: Armed Forces Institute of Pathology, 1973:84–5.
8. Owen DA. Normal histology of the stomach. Am J Surg Pathol 1986;10:48–61.
9. Stave R, Brandtzaeg P, Nygaard K, Fausa O. The transitional body-antrum zone in resected human stomachs. Anatomical outline and parietal-cell and gastrin-cell characteristics in peptic ulcer disease. Scand J Gastroenterol 1978;13:685–91.
10. Toner PG, Watt PC, Boyd SM. The gastric mucosa. In: Whitehead R, ed. Gastrointestinal and oesophageal pathology. Edinburgh: Churchill Livingstone, 1989:13–28.
11. Watanabe H, Jass JR, Sobin LH. Histological typing of oesophageal and gastric tumors. 2nd ed. Berlin: Springer-Verlag, 1990:19–39.

# 9

# NON-NEOPLASTIC TUMOR-LIKE LESIONS, PREDOMINANTLY EPITHELIAL

There are three types of non-neoplastic gastric masses that are confused with neoplasms, either endoscopically, by imaging studies, or during gross and microscopic morphologic examinations. They are mainly epithelial, and almost all are mucosal, but a few are intramural. They include a variety of polyps, some of which are thought to be developmental; conditions that are accompanied by expansion of the folds or rugae; and a collection of cysts. Each of these major groups is discussed separately in this chapter.

## GASTRIC MUCOSAL POLYPS

**Definition.** A polyp is a projection that protrudes into the lumen from the mucosal surface, that is, a structure that is elevated above the surrounding mucosa (figs. 9-1, 9-2). Usually, the term polyp is used for grossly visible lesions,

although grossly inapparent but microscopically obvious projections also should be incorporated within the term. Polyps may be produced by mucosal abnormalities, or they may be intramural masses that elevate intact mucosa. From an endoscopic standpoint, mucosal polyps have some surface characteristics that differ from the surrounding mucosa, suggesting an abnormal mucosa (figs. 9-3, 9-4). Intramural lumps, on the other hand, are covered by endoscopically normal-appearing mucosa, unless they are ulcerated. This chapter deals only with benign, non-neoplastic mucosal polyps which are the result of abnormal epithelial structures, including pits and glands, and often accompanied by abnormalities in the lamina propria and muscularis mucosae. Stromal and lymphoid polyp-forming proliferations are discussed in their respective chapters.

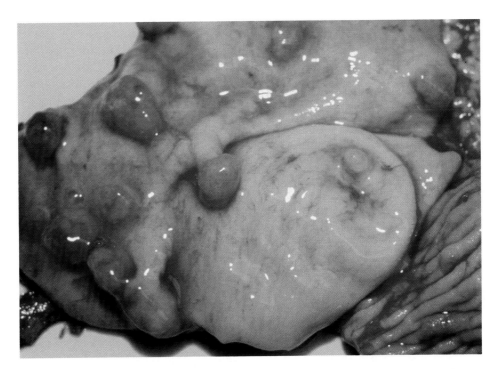

Figure 9-1
MULTIPLE GASTRIC MUCOSAL POLYPS WITH SMOOTH SURFACES
These were all hyperplastic polyps. (Courtesy of Dr. Anne Gideon, Lima, OH.)

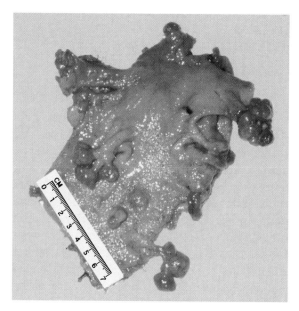

Figure 9-2
MULTIPLE POLYPS

Multiple polyps, some of which have complex surfaces with multiple lobulations. These are a mixture of adenomas and hyperplastic polyps. (Courtesy of Dr. Stefan Tsvetanov, Port Huron, MI.)

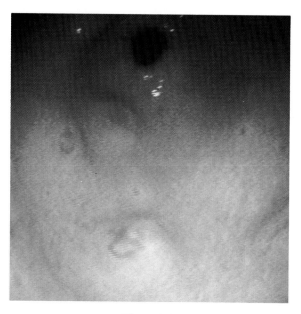

Figure 9-4
MUCOSAL POLYPS

Endoscopic view of multiple small polyps, all of which are hyperplastic, except one of localized lymphocytic gastritis.

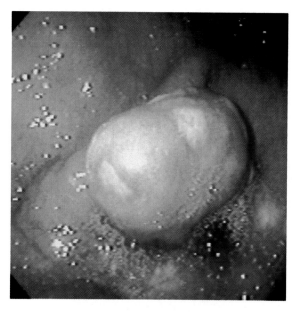

Figure 9-3
MUCOSAL POLYP

Endoscopic view of a solitary mucosal polyp. The surface is altered in several ways. At the top, there are some small lobules projecting slightly above the surface of the polyp. The light depressed areas are erosions. The lower right surface is finely corrugated.

Distinguishing multiple gastric mucosal polyps from polypoid expansions of mucosa in giant fold diseases may be difficult endoscopically, especially when only biopsies of the polypoid mucosa are taken, without samples of the intervening or flat mucosa. For instance, some cases of Menetrier's disease have the endoscopic appearance of multiple polyps. Also, there are no endoscopic features, other than size, location, and multiplicity, that distinguish one type of mucosal polyp from another. A large single polyp is never a focal foveolar hyperplasia and almost never a fundic gland polyp. In contrast, multiple small polyps in the fundus or body are almost always fundic gland polyps.

**Clinical Features.** There are no symptoms that are attributable to gastric polyps (17). On rare occasions, a large antral polyp, especially one that is pedunculated, will prolapse distally and obstruct the pylorus (65). Otherwise, they are incidental findings during endoscopy or in a resection specimen.

**Prevalence.** In contrast to the colon where polyps, especially hyperplastic polyps and polypoid adenomas, are so common that any adult is likely to develop one or more of them, the stomach contains few. They are estimated to occur in

Table 9-1

## INCIDENCE OF GASTRIC POLYPS IN ENDOSCOPIC SERIES

| Author (ref.) | Site | Year | No. Patients/ No. Polyps* | No. Endoscopies | No. Pts. per 1,000 Endos.** |
|---|---|---|---|---|---|
| Santiago (83) | Mexico | 1990 | 54/100 | 15,974 | 3 |
| Niv (75) | Israel | 1985 | 72/99 | 13,500 | 5 |
| Roseau (79) | France | 1990 | 191/? | 13,000 | 15 |
| Laxen (60) | Finland | 1982 | 454/? | 13,200 | 34 |
| Kamiya (48) | Japan | 1981 | 1201/2013[+] | 24,192 | 50 |

*Number of patients who had gastroscopic polyps and total number of gastroscopic polyps found.
**Number of patients with polyps per 1,000 gastroscopic exams.
[+]In this study, the number of patients is the number of patients who had biopsies, and this may not be the same as the number of patients who had gastroscopic exams.

2 to 3 percent of all gastroscopic exams (17). Table 9-1 lists the incidence of gastric polyps in five large endoscopic series: this varies from 3 patients with gastric polyps per 1,000 consecutive gastroscopic examinations in a Mexican series to 34 patients per 1,000 exams in one from Finland (48,60,75,79,83). In a report from Japan in which 711,455 persons were screened by upper gastrointestinal X-ray examinations, gastric polyps were found in 1,616, a frequency of 2.3 polyp-bearing people per 1,000 exams (97). However, since most gastric mucosal polyps are too small to be detected by X ray, endoscopic studies are more reliable for frequency statistics. In the Japanese study, polyps were 1 1/2 times as common in women than men; in both sexes, there was a steady rise in frequency with age, so that people aged 70 years and up had about nine times the frequency of polyps than those in the fourth decade, five times more than those in the fifth decade, and over twice those in the sixth decade. Table 9-1 also summarizes another study from Japan in which approximately 50 patients with gastric polyps were found for every 1,000 patients who had upper endoscopic biopsies, rather than examinations (47). Presumably, there were gastroscopic exams during which no biopsies were taken, so this study has a different data base than the other four summarized in the table. In the biopsied group, males were the predominant polyp formers; there was also an increase in the incidence of polyps with age, up to the seventh decade after which the incidence was stable. The only large series from the United States included 255 patients with mucosal polyps seen in a busy endoscopic service over 8 years, for an average of about 32 new patients with polyps per year, but these numbers were not related to the total number of upper endoscopic procedures performed during the study period (62).

**Classification.** *Historical Perspective.* Gastric mucosal polyps are variable exaggerations of one or both of the two normal compartments of the gastric mucosa, the deep glandular and the superficial pit or foveolar compartments. Most polyps are dominated by expansion of the pit compartment (1).

Some types of polyps are well established and easily recognized, such as adenomas, fully developed hyperplastic polyps, fundic gland polyps, and the polyps that accompany juvenile polyposis, Peutz-Jeghers syndrome, and Cronkhite-Canada syndrome. These form the basis for almost all classification systems. However, there are a substantial number of polyps that do not fit easily into the well-recognized categories. Some of these may be early or incipient stages in the formation of hyperplastic polyps, but some may be different entities altogether. In addition, there are polyps with histologic features of more than one type, indicating that it is not always possible to separate one type from another (60).

The original classification schemes for gastric polyps were based upon information derived from resection specimens and autopsies, and the major concern of most of these early studies was the relationship of all types of polyp to carcinoma (24,67,68,96). In some of these studies all gastric

Table 9-2

## TYPES OF POLYPS IN LARGE SERIES WHEN COMPARABLE TERMINOLOGY IS USED

| Author/Country (ref.) | Year | Number | Aden (%)* | HP/FH (%) | FGP (%) | NL (%) | Other (%) |
|---|---|---|---|---|---|---|---|
| Koch/Germany (53) | 1979 | 802 pts | 6 | 94 | nr** | ns | ns |
| Laxen/Finland (60) | 1982 | 454 pts | 8 | 55 | † | 0 | 36‡ |
| Seifert/Germany (85) | 1983 | 5728 polyps | 6 | 79 | 14 | 0 | 2 |
| Nakamura/Japan (72) | 1985 | 611 polyps | 18 | 82 | ns | ns | ns |
| Niv/Israel (75) | 1985 | 99 polyps | 12 | 49 | ? | 18 | 39§ |
| Deppisch/USA (18) | 1989 | 35 pts | 9 | 74 | 17 | 0 | §§ |
| Roseau/France (79) | 1990 | 191 pts | 3 | 25 | 10 | 18 | 44¶ |
| Santiago/Mexico (83) | 1990 | 54 pts | 22 | 17 | ?13 | 0 | 48 |
| Chua/Singapore (12) | 1990 | 30 pts | 20 | 70 | ?3 | 0 | 6 |
| Lindley/USA (62) | 1993 | 329 polyps | 7 | 48 | 28 | 9 | 9 |

*Aden = adenoma; HP = hyperplastic polyp; FH = focal foveolar hyperplasia; FGP = fundic gland polyp; NL = normal mucosa in an endoscopic polyp.
**nr = not recognized; ns = not included in the study. This study antedated the first identification of the fundic gland polyp.
†Fundic gland polyps either were not recognized or did not exist in this study.
‡All of these were called "inflammatory polyps."
§Mostly "inflammatory polyps."
§§"Inflammatory epithelial polyps" were excluded from the study.
¶All designated as "interstitial gastritis."

mucosal polyps were collectively referred to as "adenomas" (4,68); nonadenomatous mucosal polyps were not recognized. When endoscopic biopsy or polypectomy became the procedure of choice for polyps, there were few modifications of the old classifications. There have been a few endoscopic surveys of polyps from various parts of the world, but surprisingly, there have been none with detailed pathologic analysis from the United States until recently (62).

Table 9-2 lists the classes of polyps removed or biopsied in some large series as diagnosed presumably by the institutional pathologists (12,18, 53,60,62,72,75,79,83,85). It is obvious that the same classification scheme was not used in all series. In some series, fundic gland polyps were either not recognized or did not occur, although the latter possibility is difficult to accept considering how common fundic gland polyps really are. It is also obvious that the types of polyps differ in different populations. Adenomas are uncommon in the European series but much more common in the Asian studies. Not included in the table, because the results are so much at

odds with every study, is a 5-year American study (1973 to 1978) of polyps first detected either by upper gastrointestinal X ray or endoscopy (21). Sixty-four patients had mucosal polyps, of which 63 percent were classified as adenomas, the highest percent of adenomas in any study in almost 25 years, and there was not a single hyperplastic polyp. In nonendoscopic series of gastric polyps, adenomas are larger than hyperplastic polyps (67,96). However, since gastric polyps are virtually always asymptomatic and are detected as incidental findings during upper endoscopic exams for common upper gut symptoms, the size relations are no longer valid. Many published studies refer to generic gastric polyps without classifying them into specific categories (6,82); most of the reported polyps were hyperplastic, however.

*Proposed Classification Scheme.* In this Fascicle, the classification of gastric mucosal polyps is a modified version of the most recently proposed system recommended by the World Health Organization (WHO):

1. Hamartomatous and Other Developmental Polyps and Polyposes
   a. Fundic gland polyps
   b. Peutz-Jeghers polyps
   c. Juvenile polyps
   d. Cowden's disease polyps
   e. Heterotopic (ectopic) pancreas and adenomyomatous hamartomas
   f. Heterotopic gastric gland polyps
2. Focal Foveolar Hyperplasias
3. Hyperplastic Polyps
   a. Usual (sporadic) type
   b. Hyperplastic-like polyps at gastro-enterostomy stomas
   c. Gastroesophageal reflux polyps
4. Polyposis of the Cronkhite-Canada Syndrome
5. Miscellaneous Non-neoplastic Polyps, including those that have not been classified
6. Adenomas

Adenomas are neoplasms. They are included here as they are included in most gastric polyp classification systems. They are discussed in detail in chapter 10.

**The Mucosa in which Gastric Polyps Arise.** According to our experience, the mucosa surrounding or adjacent to gastric polyps is rarely biopsied, so that there is little endoscopically based information about the milieu in which these polyps arise (62). What data we have comes from surgically resected polyps and from biopsy studies from a variety of countries. The data concerning the background mucosa is probably skewed to reflect the types of gastritis which are endemic in different countries, and the information derived from these studies may not be applicable to stomachs from all parts of the world. Nevertheless, some of the available information concerning the background is fascinating.

Both hyperplastic polyps and adenomas commonly occur in stomachs with one of the types of chronic atrophic gastritis. In a combined Japanese and Swedish study, hyperplastic polyps were most likely to occur in stomachs with the immunologic form of atrophic gastritis, the type involving the body and sparing the antrum, which is accompanied by hypergastrinemia (73). In contrast, adenomas, all of which were antral, were much more likely to occur in the presence of multifocal, nonimmunologic atrophic gastritis that involves antral mucosa, and that has much less associated hypergastrinemia. A report from Finland also found that immunologic atrophic gastritis was closely related to hyperplastic polyps and foveolar hyperplasia (59). Peculiarly, however, in only 70 percent of cases did the polyps occur in the atrophic body and fundic areas; the other 30 percent occurred in antral mucosae that were histologically normal.

There is a greater risk of carcinoma in stomachs with hyperplastic polyps and adenomas and for developing carcinomas on follow-up. This is not surprising considering that both types of polyps commonly arise in stomachs with one of the chronic atrophic gastritides, which are associated with an increased cancer frequency. This carcinoma association is much greater for adenomas than for hyperplastic polyps (32). In the case of adenomas, some of the carcinomas are within the adenoma while others are elsewhere in the stomach; with hyperplastic polyps, the associated carcinomas are almost all elsewhere (60). In a study from Japan, both benign gastric polyps and the elevated type of early gastric cancer occurred in stomachs with severe and extensive atrophic changes (82).

**Gastric Mucosal Polyps and Extragastric Diseases.** Gastric mucosal polyps have been associated with several extragastric abnormalities besides the multiple polyposis syndromes. These include multiple hyperplastic polyps in a few patients with functioning parathyroid adenomas and hyperchlorhydria, including one patient with multiple subcutaneous lipomas on his forearms; gastric hyperplastic polyps and adenomas occurring with increasing frequency in patients with increasing numbers of colonic adenomas and colorectal carcinomas who do not have familial adenomatous polyposis; and extragastric gut carcinomas, including primaries in the oral cavity, esophagus, gallbladder, and rectum (6,24,87). In a study from a regional hospital in Finland of families of patients with all types of gastric polyps discovered between 1972 and 1983, the families of men, but not women, with polyps had about 3 1/2 times the frequency of intestinal (probably colorectal) carcinomas as did a control population (33). The families of women, but not men, with polyps had twice the frequency of gastric cancer.

**Treatment.** The only way to determine what type of polyp is present is to examine it histologically. There are no absolute endoscopic criteria that separate neoplastic from non-neoplastic polyps (17). Biopsy may be inconclusive, since many polyps and even some adenomas have pit hyperplasia with inflammation. Therefore, endoscopic polypectomy is the procedure of choice for diagnosis. This is also the treatment for polyps that can be totally removed endoscopically. However, for large polyps, especially those that contain dysplastic epithelium, surgical removal may be required. Because of the association between gastric mucosal polyps and carcinoma, careful evaluation of the nonpolypoid gastric mucosa is essential. This association with cancer is stronger when there are multiple polyps rather than a single polyp (85). Ideally, biopsy of the adjacent mucosa is advisable in order to determine if one of the forms of atrophic gastritis is present, since these, especially the diffuse body or immunologic type, carries a significant risk for carcinomas and carcinoid tumors. (See the discussion on Hyperplastic Polyps for information on follow-up of patients with gastric mucosal polyps.)

## SPECIFIC TYPES OF GASTRIC POLYPS

### Fundic Gland Polyps and Fundic Gland Polyposis

Fundic gland polyps are small sessile lesions that occur in the fundus and upper body of the stomach and which have a characteristic histologic appearance. They do not produce symptoms, and they do not bleed or ulcerate. The first description of fundic gland polyps may have been by Elster in 1977 who designated them by the German name of "drusenkorperzysten" (89). Sipponen et al. (89) called them "cystic hamartomatous polyps." They first appeared in the English language literature in 1978 in a paper from Japan in which they were described as a manifestation of familial adenomatosis coli and were considered to be hamartomatous (100). The name fundic gland polyp seems to have been first used in this paper. For some small lesions in which the glandular cysts dominate the histologic picture, the term fundic gland cyst has also been used. Although fundic gland polyps were considered curiosities at first, it is now clear that they are among the most common of all gastric polyps, possibly the most common in some centers.

Fundic gland polyps occur in three different clinical settings: 1) multiple polyps (fundic gland polyposis) in patients with familial adenomatous polyposis (FAP) (100); 2) multiple polyps (fundic gland polyposis) in patients without FAP (37,41,89,94); and 3) single, or at most two or three polyps also in patients without FAP (29,31). The relative frequency of fundic gland polyposis and gastric adenoma as the gastric expression of FAP are displayed in Table 10-1 in chapter 10. In general, except for a few reports from the Far East, fundic gland polyposis is a far more common manifestation of FAP than are gastric adenomas and occur earlier (45,100). Other than as a gastric manifestation of FAP, fundic gland polyps have no clinical significance. Those not associated with FAP are incidental findings during endoscopic examination performed for other problems. Patients without FAP are about 25 years older than those with FAP, but this may be a manifestation of surveillance of the upper gut in FAP patients. These patients commonly have their first upper endoscopy examination when they are young, for evaluation of adenomas, not fundic gland polyps, especially in the duodenum, because these are potential cancer precursors (37). Non-FAP patients are predominantly female, while the FAP patients are mostly male (37,38,61,89,94). There is evidence that fundic gland polyps, both sporadic and FAP associated, overexpress transforming growth factor alpha and its receptor, the epidermal growth factor receptor (75a). This suggests that these polyps, regardless of their clinical setting, have abnormal cell proliferative characteristics compared to normal gastric mucosa. There is evidence that long-term treatment with omeprazole, a potent inhibitor of gastric acid secretion, may be followed by the development of fundic gland polyps (25a).

**Gross and Endoscopic Findings.** Fundic gland polyps are small, dome-shaped nodules with smooth surfaces (fig. 9-5). Usually, they are multiple, especially those that are FAP associated (37). In one study, there were more than 80 FAP-associated polyps per patient, compared to less than 50 in patients without FAP. Almost all are smaller than 8 mm in diameter; a few not associated with FAP measure 2 cm across or even slightly larger (37,38). As their name suggests, they are located in the fundic or body mucosa exclusively.

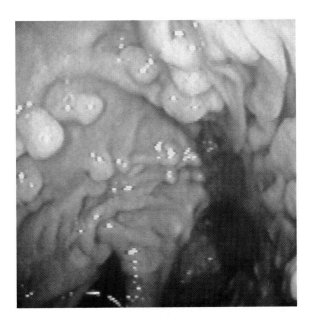

Figure 9-5
FUNDIC GLAND POLYPS
In this characteristic endoscopic view, the polyps appear
as multiple, small, dome-shaped to slightly elongated bumps
on the mucosa.

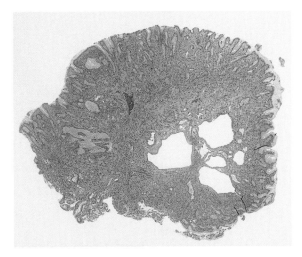

Figure 9-6
FUNDIC GLAND POLYP
This is a larger lesion. The bulk of the polyp is composed
of glands. Several small cystic pits are present to the left,
while on the right there are large glandular cysts.

**Histologic Findings.** Fundic gland polyps, no
matter what the clinical setting, usually have a
normal or shortened pit compartment which leads
into an altered glandular compartment (figs. 9-6,
9-7) (1,61,101). There are two different glandular
abnormalities. In the first, normal or distorted
fundic or body glands with typical chief cells and
parietal cells are close to, or even immediately
below, the surface epithelium, a place where gastric glands are not normally found (fig. 9-7). Some
of these glands seem to bud, resulting in clover leaf
or club-shaped structures (61). Furthermore, these
glands are frequently disorganized and arranged
in clusters separated by a loose stroma which may
be edematous but which is rarely inflamed. The
second alteration in the glandular compartment
is the formation of cystic glands lined by parietal
and chief cells. Cystic pits also may be present
(figs. 9-6–9-8). Some cysts are part pit and part
gland. In one detailed study of the structure of
these cysts based upon serial microscopic sections, it was determined that the cysts often
interconnect (89). In general, the polyps have a
characteristic zonation of changes, with the
short pits and disorganized but cytologically normal glands beneath the surface, the cysts be-

neath these, and additional disorganized glands
deeper. Very tiny polyps may have subtle microscopic changes with very mild and focal gland
distortion and only one or two small cysts (fig.
9-9). These polyps seem to arise not from deep
within the body mucosa, but from the superficial
mucosa, so that they appear to be tacked on to
the surface as mucosal redundancies (100).

When several different polyps are biopsied, it
is common for some to contain normal mucosa.
We do not know why this histologically normal-
appearing mucosa produces an endoscopically
apparant polyp, unless it is the base of one of the
small polyps. In addition, some polyps contain
only a single fundic gland cyst. In the cases of
FAP-associated fundic gland polyposis, adjacent
mucosa has normal histologic features without
metaplasia of any type (34,37,94,100). Because of
the abnormal arrangement of normal mucosal
elements, these polyps have been designated as
hamartomas rather than neoplasms. If this is
truly their niche, then they add a hamartomatous element to the FAP syndrome. This is not
surprising, since this syndrome is not simply a
neoplastic disease, but also includes such disparate aberrations as cysts and fibromatoses.

Rare FAP-associated fundic gland polyps contain foci of dysplastic pit epithelium, mainly low
grade, characterized by cellular crowding, nuclear

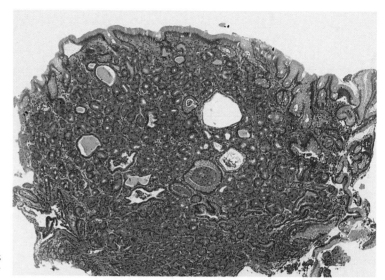

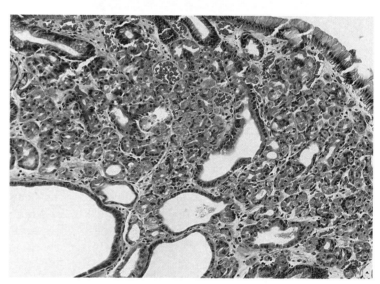

Figure 9-7
FUNDIC GLAND POLYP

Top: This is a typical small polyp with a short pit compartment, disordered glands which extend close to the surface, and deep cysts.

Bottom: At high power, the glands form clusters, some of which virtually touch the surface epithelium on the right. Some glands are dilated and some branch.

enlargement in relation to cytoplasmic volume, nuclear hyperchromasia, little nuclear pleomorphism, increased numbers of mitoses, and decreased cytoplasmic mucin. Such lesions are truly hybrid adenoma-fundic gland polyps.

Although FAP-associated and nonassociated polyps seem to be identical, there may be some subtle differences. In a comparative analysis from Japan of the two types of fundic gland polyps, 10 of 11 cases with FAP had orthoacylated sialic acid in the superficial and pit epithelium, while only 1 of 12 cases without the syndrome had this mucin (74). Orthoacylated sialomucins are identified using the potassium borohydride/potassium hydroxide/periodic acid–

Schiff technique. They are normal in the colon, but are not present in the normal stomach, although they may occur in foci of gastric intestinal metaplasia. These differences in mucin content suggest that syndrome-associated fundic gland polyps may be more than simple hamartomas.

**Natural History.** There are several long-term follow-up studies of patients with both FAP-associated and nonassociated fundic gland polyposes (38–40,89). The results, as displayed in Table 9-3, indicate that the natural history of these polyps is unpredictable, with some regressing, some increasing in number or size, and some staying the same; the course is independent of whether or not the patients have FAP.

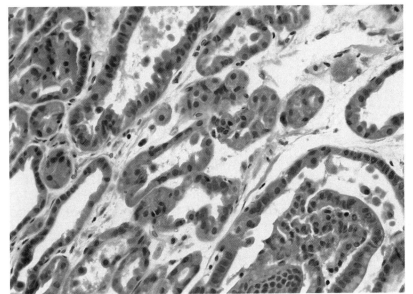

Figure 9-8
GLANDULAR DISTORTION
IN A FUNDIC GLAND POLYP
All of these tubular structures are glands. The large lining cells with pale red cytoplasm are parietal cells, while the darker cells are chief cells. Some glands are cystic, some are branched with small protrusions, and a few are normal.

Figure 9-9
TINY FUNDIC GLAND POLYP
At first glance, this looks like normal mucosa, but closer analysis indicates that the glands are vaguely clustered, some are unusually close to the surface epithelium, and there are a few small cysts in the glandular compartment.

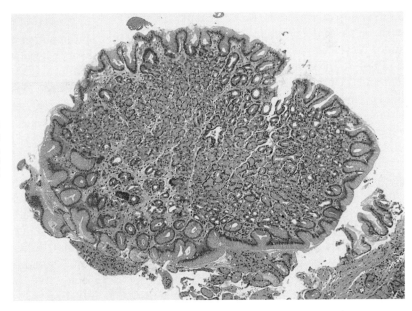

Table 9-3

**FUNDIC GLAND POLYPOSIS: NATURAL HISTORY**

| Author | Year | FAP* | Years Follow-up | Number Patients | Dec.** | Same | Incr. |
|---|---|---|---|---|---|---|---|
| Sipponen (89) | 1983 | no | 1-5 | 7 | 0 | 5 | 2 |
| Iishi (40) | 1989 | no | 1-10 | 14 | 7 | 7 | 0 |
| Iida (38) | 1985 | yes | 1-13 | 9 | 2 | 0 | 7 |

*FAP = The patients in the study had familial adenomatous polyposis.
**Dec. = Number of patients whose polyps decreased in size and/or number; Same = number of patients whose polyps did not change in size and/or number; Incr. = number of patients whose polyps increased in size and/or number.

## Hamartomatous Polyps of the Peutz-Jeghers Type

The Peutz-Jeghers syndrome is a dominantly inherited set of abnormalities characterized by gastrointestinal polyposis and mucocutaneous pigmented spots, involving mainly the perioral skin, gums, and buccal mucosa (1,27). The polyps have been designated as hamartomas because of their disorganized content of normal mucosal elements, including branched muscularis mucosae. In a study of 222 patients, polyps were located within the small intestine in 64 percent of the patients, in the colon in 53 percent, and in the stomach in 49 percent (98). However, in a study from the United States, gastric polyps were found only in about 25 percent of the patients; this study, however, was not based upon endoscopic data (3). The true incidence of gastric polyps awaits long-term endoscopic studies. Most patients present with signs and symptoms resulting from the small bowel polyps, such as intestinal obstruction due to intussusception. Some polyps are silent and the presenting manifestation is the peculiar pigmentation. Gastric polyps are silent, although the authors are aware of a few cases in which a large antral polyp apparently autoamputated and was vomited by the patient.

The WHO defines the gastric Peutz-Jeghers polyp as "a lesion with excessive hyperplasia, elongation and cystic change of foveolar epithelium, reduced lamina propria and prominent cores of branching bands of smooth muscle derived from the muscularis mucosae, the deeper glandular components showing atrophy" (101). Although there is considerable morphologic description of intestinal polyps, there is very little information about the gastric lesions. There may be a variety of gastric polyps, depending upon the type of mucosa in which they arise, so that fundic or body polyps may be different from antral polyps. Most polyps are antral. Like those in the small intestine, gastric polyps are mostly sessile (98). There may be any number of polyps. Most antral polyps are composed of remarkably elongated, branched and sometimes cystic pits which contain inspissated mucin that may secondarily calcify (fig. 9-10) (1,7). The glands usually do not participate in the formation of these polyps, except that they may persist at the base. The epithelium is normal or hyperplastic foveo-lar. There may be only a delicate fibrovascular stroma separating these pits and very little central branched muscularis mucosae is usually present (1,28). Thus gastric polyps differ somewhat from their small intestinal counterparts which have a branched muscularis mucosae as a prominent and possibly the most important component. At one time gastric polyps were even given the name "antral-foveolar" polyps to stress their predominant pit composition, but the name never gained acceptance (24). Peutz-Jeghers–type gastric polyps may occur without other manifestations of the syndrome, and it is not clear if these are formes fruste or not.

Gastric carcinomas have been reported in patients with the syndrome, but there has been little documentation of the carcinomas arising within these hamartomatous polyps, although they are the preferred candidate precursor lesion (13,28,56,98). Inverted growth and epithelial misplacement, in which the abnormal mucosa extends through breaks in the muscularis mucosae into the submucosa, muscularis propria, or even beyond, have been described in small intestinal Peutz-Jeghers polyps but not in the gastric polyps (88).

## Juvenile Polyps

Juvenile polyps are common in the colon, where they tend to occur singly or at most a few. Juvenile polyposis is rare; it is characterized by the formation of multiple juvenile polyps over the entire colon (27). In most cases, the polyposis is familial, inherited as an autosomal dominant trait. Sometimes the juvenile polyposis is generalized, with polyps in the stomach and small intestine as well as the colon. It appears that this generalized form is always familial (81,92). One report even describes familial juvenile polyposis confined to the stomach (99). Juvenile polyposis, whether confined to the colon or disseminated, is associated with carcinomas of the colon and stomach. Some of the polyps have dysplastic epithelium, so that they appear to be mixed juvenile-adenomatous polyps (25,92); therefore, patients with gastric juvenile polyposis should be monitored by regular endoscopy, so as to detect the dysplasias early in their evolution.

Gastric juvenile polyps are structurally characterized by their rounded contour, extensive superficial ulceration, cellular edematous lamina

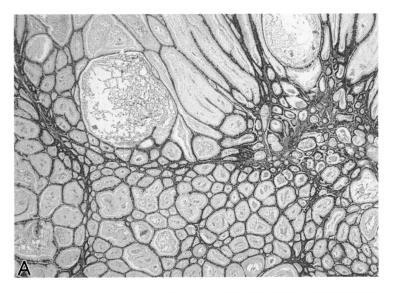

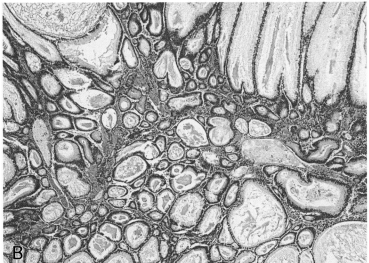

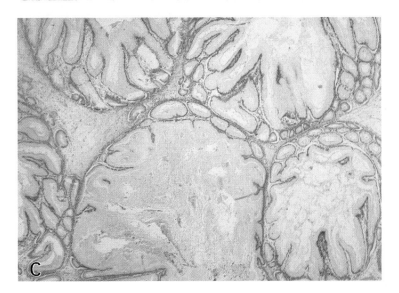

Figure 9-10
HAMARTOMATOUS POLYP
OF THE PEUTZ-JEGHERS TYPE

A: This is the center of the polyp. There is a small amount of branching stroma at the right center which contains a few smooth muscle bundles. Most of the polyp is composed of dilated, mucus-filled pits, some of which branch.

B: At higher power, the core of the polyp has small cysts that are probably residual basal glands and a few smooth muscle bundles.

C: At the periphery there are huge, dilated, branching pits, some of which are filled with inspissated mucus.

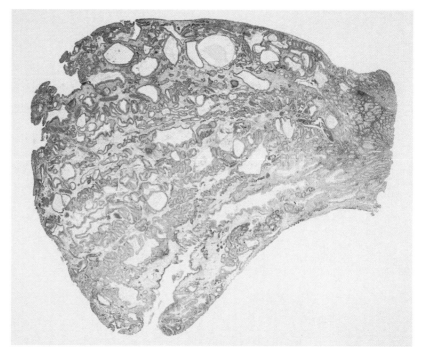

Figure 9-11
JUVENILE POLYP
This roughly mitten-shaped polyp came from the stomach of a patient with juvenile polyposis of the colon. The surface is smooth and eroded, and the center is filled with cystic pits. (Fig. 278 from Fascicle 7 supplement, 2nd Series.)

propria, and distorted tubules lined by normal or hyperplastic foveolar epithelium (fig. 9-11) (1,27). The distorted tubules are commonly cystic, many are branched, and some have serrated lumenal contours. The inflamed lamina propria is often filled with small vessels, and it contains many eosinophils in addition to plasma cells, lymphocytes, and macrophages. Characteristically, there is very little smooth muscle in the expanded lamina propria; the muscularis mucosae does not participate in the formation of juvenile polyps, in contrast to Peutz-Jeghers polyps where it is a predictable, although minor, component. There may be occasional single or grouped smooth muscle cells, most of which may be vascular, but there are no large muscle bundles.

The inflammation and distortion are also the usual features of hyperplastic polyps, which gastric juvenile polyps superficially resemble; however, juvenile polyps have a round contour whereas hyperplastic polyps are often coarsely villiform or lobulated. Solitary mucosal polyps occurring in the colon of children are virtually all of juvenile type. It is possible that single polyps in the stomachs of children are also juvenile, but they may not be reported as such. On the other hand, some hyperplastic polyps in children may be reported as juvenile polyps (65). The confident diagnosis of a gastric juvenile polyp is probably not possible unless the patient is known to have diffuse juvenile polyposis (1).

### Gastric Polyps of Cowden's Disease

Cowden's disease, also known as *multiple hamartoma syndrome,* is a rare genodermatosis with an autosomal dominant inheritance. It is characterized by cutaneous tricholemmomas, oral mucosal papillomas, and gastrointestinal polyps. The cutaneous lesions are the most common. These patients also have an increased risk of breast and thyroid carcinomas (10,27). The incidence of associated gastrointestinal polyps is uncertain, because not all patients have gastrointestinal tract evaluations, either radiologic or endoscopic, but possibly close to three quarters of the patients have polyps (95). The polyps have been referred to as hamartomas, probably because they are usually composed of distorted non-neoplastic mucosa which is often inflamed or fibrotic, or contains excess smooth muscle in the center. A few colonic polyps have been described in detail, but the gastric polyps have not been well characterized, probably because they are so rare. The published photomicrographs suggest that pit hyperplasia, possibly with some pit cysts, may be a component of the gastric polyps (103).

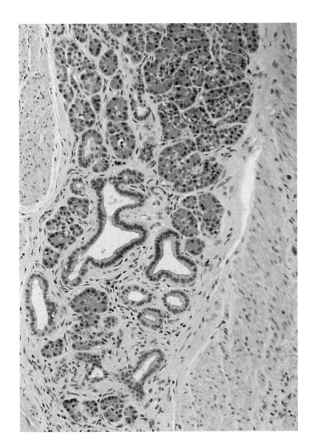 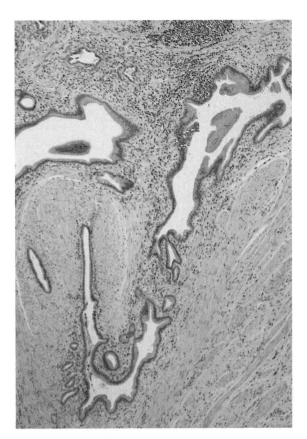

Figure 9-12

HETEROTOPIC PANCREAS–MYOGLANDULAR HAMARTOMA

Left: Pancreatic parenchyma with acini and ducts, surrounded by hypertrophic smooth muscle of the muscularis propria.
Right: Ducts, identical to those of the pancreaticobiliary system, surrounded by similar hypertrophic smooth muscle.

## Heterotopic or Ectopic Pancreas, including Adenomyomatous or Myoglandular Hamartoma

Intramural masses composed of a variety of normal tissues found in the pancreas, biliary tract, and duodenum occur throughout the gastrointestinal tract. The pathogenesis of these lesions is unknown: the theories include transplantation or misplacement of embryonic tissues which develop into mature elements and pancreatic metaplasia of endodermal tissues which for some reason or reasons wound up in the submucosa during embryonic life. The misplacement theory may explain the occurrence of the heterotopia in the upper gut near the pancreas, but it does not explain its occurrence in the colon. Intramural masses are situated primarily within the submucosa, with some extending into the muscularis propria. When pancreatic tissue, including acini,

islets, and ducts, dominates, the masses are called *heterotopic* or *ectopic pancreas* (fig. 9-12, left). When pancreaticobiliary-type ducts dominate, the ducts are surrounded by hypertrophic smooth muscle bundles (fig. 9-12, right); such lesions are commonly designated as *adenomyomatous, myoglandular,* or *myoepithelial hamartomas* or as *adenomyomas* (58). These may have collections of mucous glands resembling Brunner's glands and complex papillae resembling the structures of the ampulla of Vater (16). Grossly, they are firm intramural nodules. Those that contain pancreatic tissue look like a cluster of yellow-white pancreatic lobules (fig. 9-13); those that are mostly ducts and muscle are pale, solid, circumscribed nodules or masses that may have a few small cysts which are dilated ducts. The pancreatic lesions are much more common than the ductal ones. In the largest reported series of 212 cases of heterotopic pancreas, 174 of which were

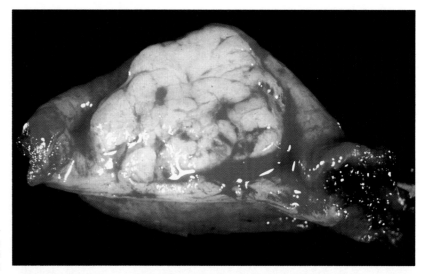

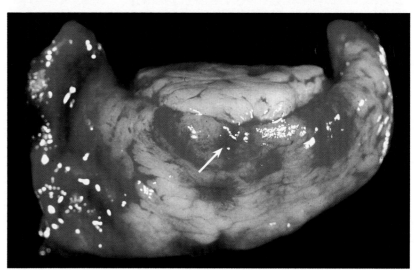

Figure 9-13
HETEROTOPIC PANCREAS:
GROSS VIEWS
Top: Buried deeply within the gastric muscularis propria is this mass that, on cross section, has the same lobulated appearance and yellowish white color as normal pancreas.
Bottom: In the mucosa overlying the mass there is a depression corresponding to the draining duct.

resected or biopsied, 52 percent occurred in the upper small intestine, including the duodenum and proximal jejunum, while 38 percent were found in the stomach, mostly in the prepyloric region on the greater curvature or posterior wall (19,52). In two small series of 37 and 34 cases, 22 and 24 percent, respectively, occurred in the stomach (2,57). They have been reported to occur in as few as 0.5 percent and as much as 13 percent of autopsies. These discrepant figures must reflect the care of the prosectors and the definition of what is acceptable as a pancreatic heterotopia.

Pancreatic heterotopias are most commonly found incidentally, either at the time of laparotomy for another disease, or during radiographic or endoscopic examinations of the upper gut. Very

few produce symptoms although some patients have virtually every upper gastrointestinal symptom imaginable, from epigastric pain to hematemesis to gas, none of which are caused by the lesions (19,52). Usually they are small, with 80 percent or more measuring 3 cm or less in diameter (105). The gastric lesions tend to be larger than those arising elsewhere. Rare distal gastric tumors become big enough or prolapse through the pylorus to produce gastric outlet obstruction. They are discovered at all ages, and there is no sex predilection. The classic roentgenographic and endoscopic appearance is that of a smooth, well-circumscribed, intramural nodule with a central depression or umbilication that may be the site of a duct draining the lesion to

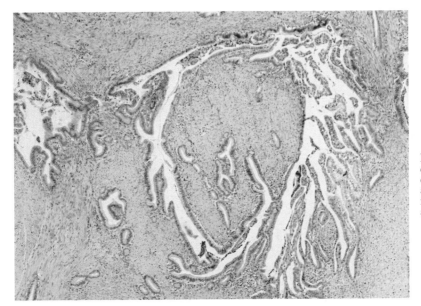

Figure 9-14
INVASIVE ADENOCARCINOMA
ARISING WITHIN AN
ECTOPIC PANCREAS IN
THE DISTAL STOMACH
The dilated, elongated ducts to the left of center are benign remnants of the ectopic pancreas. The ducts to the right of center are carcinomatous. They are architecturally more complex and are identical to carcinomatous ducts that arise in the pancreas.

the mucosal surface (19). However, the umbilication is not a dependable finding, since it occurs in half or less of the lesions (52). In one study, the draining or aberrant duct was cannulated and radiographic contrast material was introduced to produce a ductogram of the lesion (77). If there is no umbilication, then the tumors resemble other intramural masses, especially stromal tumors.

These lesions rarely grow or produce clinical disease (19). However, virtually anything that can happen to the pancreas in its proper site can happen to pancreas that is ectopic, including acute and chronic pancreatitis, abscess, carcinoma, and islet cell–type endocrine tumors, including those that produce insulin and gastrin and the resultant hyperproduction syndromes (fig. 9-14) (36,49).

### Gastric Gland Heterotopia

This is a rare, predominantly submucosal malformation which, by published definition, "consists of gastric glandular elements mixed with thin muscular bundles" from the muscularis mucosae (101). The most common glandular elements are antral-pyloric glands or Brunner-like clusters of mucous glands, but there may be fundic glands as well. Fundic glands may even predominate. Cystic glands or cystic pits may be part of the lesion, and when fundic glands are prominent and when some of them become cystic, parts of the lesion resemble the fundic gland

polyp (fig. 9-15). There is very little literature describing these polyps. One was reported as a "solitary polypoid hamartoma of the oxyntic mucosa" (9). Another probable case was reported as an example of a solitary Peutz-Jeghers polyp (55). A third case was designated as a myoepithelial hamartoma of Brunner's gland (43).

### Focal Foveolar Hyperplasia (Foveolar Hyperplasia)

Foveolar hyperplasia commonly accompanies many gastric diseases. It is a part of several reactive or inflammatory processes, such as chemical gastropathy and the gastritis of *Helicobacter pylori*. It is an integral part of Menetrier's disease, and is an expected finding on the gastric side of a gastrojejunal anastomosis. It often occurs at the margins of neoplasms, and in this setting it can be looked upon as the gastric mucosal equivalent of transitional colonic mucosa, a slightly distorted, elongated mucosa which is full of mucin and which is found next to or over virtually every colonic mass or localized inflammation.

On occasion, foveolar hyperplasia is very focal or localized and produces a polyp characterized by elongated pits; little distortion, except for slight serration or dilatation; a normal deep glandular compartment; and a lamina propria that is normal or no more inflamed than the adjacent mucosa (figs. 9-16–9-18). However, this type of hyperplasia, composed of elongated foveolae or

197

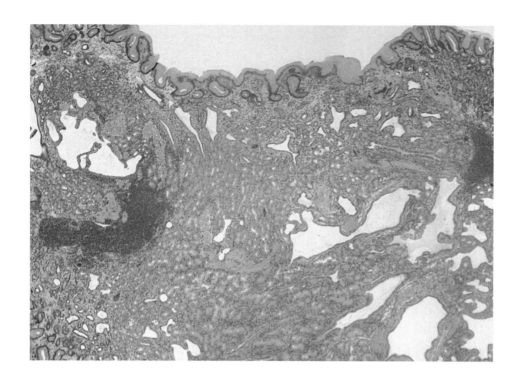

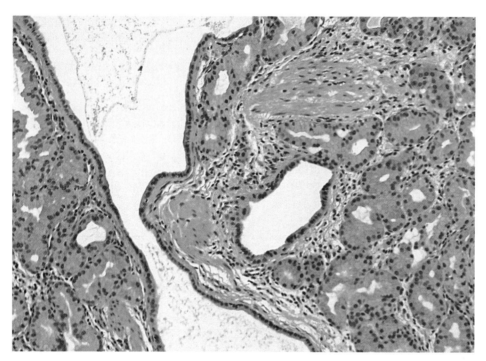

Figure 9-15
GASTRIC GLAND HETEROTOPIA

Top: This lesion, which obliterates the mucosa-submucosa interface, contains cysts and solid glandular clusters. The mucosa wraps around the polyp from the lower left, across the top, to the lower right.

Bottom: Higher power view of the center of the top figure. The cyst is a cystic gland with a cuboidal epithelial lining. Next to it are clusters of mucous glands resembling antral-pyloric glands. In the center is a large bundle of smooth muscle.

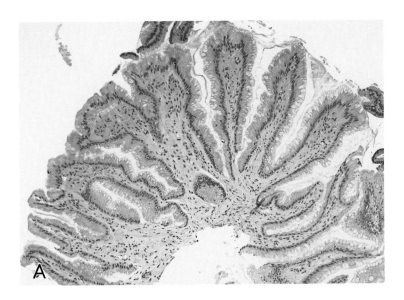

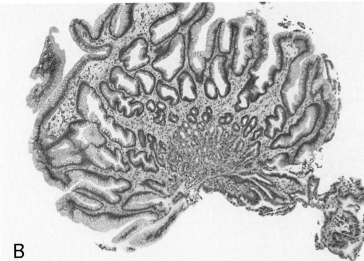

Figure 9-16
### FOCAL FOVEOLAR HYPERPLASIAS

A: A well-oriented section of a tiny antral polyp which contains elongated, slightly tortuous pits separated by normal lamina propria.

B: Also well-oriented, these pits are more tortuous and some have serrated lumens.

C: Bias- or tangential-cut polyp, with prominent dilated pits.

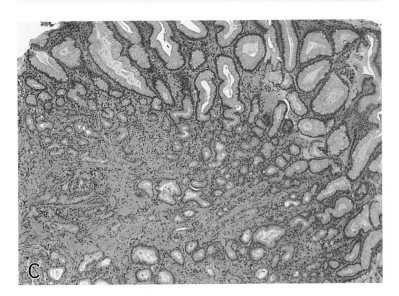

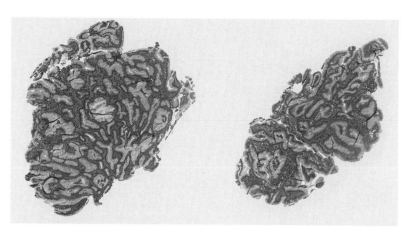

Figure 9-17
FOCAL FOVEOLAR
HYPERPLASIA
These are halves of a small antral polyp which contains excess elongated, branched and occasionally dilated pits.

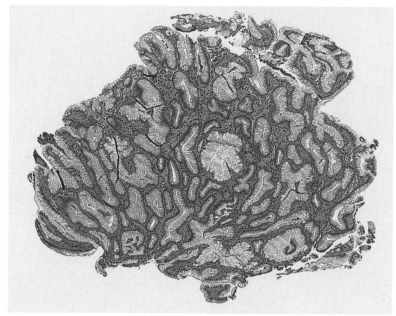

Figure 9-18
FOCAL FOVEOLAR
HYPERPLASIA
This is a medium-power view of a deeper cut of the polyp in figure 9-17. The crowding of the peculiarly shaped pits and the compressed lamina propria resembles the pattern in tubular adenomas as described in chapter 10. However, the epithelium has small uniform basal nuclei, indicating that there is no dysplasia.

pits and nothing more, is not universally accepted as a polyp. It is included as a specific class of polyp by some investigators, particularly in northern Europe (20,53,59,60,70,90); others, however, either do not identify it as a specific type of polyp or include it as a variant of hyperplastic polyp (66). The new WHO histologic classification of gastric polyps does not recognize this entity at all (101). Thus, focal foveolar hyperplasia is caught in the middle of a recognition tug-of-war. Part of the identity crisis results from the fact that foveolar hyperplasia is such a common reaction in the stomach. One author included focal foveolar hyperplasia in his classification of gastric polyps, but said that it is not a "true gastric polyp" but a reactive process (20); some

think focal foveolar hyperplasia is due to a regenerative process in the healing phase of ulcers or erosions (78). Some tiny polyps have crowded pits with little intervening lamina propria, so that they resemble adenomas with foveolar epithelium, but their epithelium has no dysplastic features (fig. 9-18).

Whatever the etiology, there are some small polyps that have no other features than an elongated pit compartment. These tiny lesions may be by far the most common of all gastric polyps, and account for over 90 percent in one series (53). They have a predilection for the antrum as do most other mucosal polyps. The natural history of such tiny bumps is not known, but it is tempting to imagine that some of them serve as precursors of larger polyps, such as hyperplastic polyps, that are also dominated by foveolar hyperplasia but which have other features such as intense inflammation and greater distortion. The potential relationship between focal foveolar hyperplasia and hyperplastic polyps is further discussed below.

### Hyperplastic Polyps

**Definition.** Perhaps the most difficult polyp to define is the hyperplastic polyp. This lesion was given the same name as the innocuous small colonic polyp, yet it has totally different growth characteristics (96). It has several different names, including *hyperplasiogenous, regenerative,* and *type I polyps* in the Nakamura numerical designation system (20,67,72). In several studies up to the early 1970s, hyperplastic polyps were considered to be adenomas (4,68,71) while the fundic gland polyp, now a distinct entity, was considered a hyperplastic polyp.

The definition of hyperplastic polyp varies greatly, but disorganized tubular, branched, or cystic hyperplastic gastric pits is a feature common to all (20,59,66,70,78,96). Additional features of some definitions include extensions of pits deep into the mucosa, hypervascularity, edema, and excess smooth muscle in the lamina propria (14, 20,78). Some definitions insist that the glandular compartment not be a part of the polyp, while others indicate that pyloric glands may participate (14, 20). The WHO classification describes the hyperplastic polyp as "a benign sessile or pedunculated polyp composed of irregular hyperplastic glands, the epithelium being mostly of the foveolar (i.e., superficial gastric) type, but pyloric (antral) glands, chief cells and parietal cells may be present; regenerative atypia in the epithelium (immature regenerating epithelium) and atypical reactive stromal cells may appear frequently after erosion" (101). Unfortunately, this definition uses the word "gland" in more than one way, referring to both pits and glands.

All these definitions recognize the basic abnormality, namely, the hyperplasia or expansion of the pit compartment. Thus any mucosal polyp composed of too many pits or pits that are too long satisfies the definition of a hyperplastic polyp. Also included in the hyperplastic polyp category are small lesions that may be precursors of the more typical large polyps. However, most definitions do not include the profound distortion of the pits and the stromal expansion of the lamina propria that are so much a part of usual hyperplastic polyps. As a result of this seemingly uncompromising series of definitions, the hyperplastic gastric polyp is defined here as a mucosal polyp that contains elongated, distorted pits; very few, if any, glands; and an inflamed, edematous lamina propria which may have smooth muscle fibers. On occasion, residual glands at the base of the polyp appear to add to its bulk, but they probably are not part of the polyp itself. The small polyps composed of non-inflamed mucosa with expanded pits that are only slightly distorted are placed in the focal foveolar hyperplasia category.

**Etiology and Pathogenesis.** In virtually every reported series of gastric mucosal polyps, hyperplastic polyps, especially if combined with focal foveolar hyperplasias, are the most common, by far (see Table 9-2). Yet, the cause or causes of these polyps is unknown. There is a predilection for them to occur in association with atrophic gastritis. One study showed that these polyps arose in patients with atrophic gastritis and very low maximal acid output, low serum pepsinogen I and high serum gastrin levels (34). Peculiarly, in stomachs with severe atrophic gastritis of the gastric body, about 50 percent of both focal foveolar hyperplasias and hyperplastic polyps actually arose in the antrum, where there was no significant atrophy (59). Similar polyps arise on the gastric side of gastrojejunostomy stomas, where they may be manifestations of mucosal prolapse (see Gastritis Cystica and Stomal Changes). Comparable polyps arise at the cardioesophageal junction, supposedly as a result of chronic reflux (see Reflux Polyps). In one study, hyperplastic polyps had a slightly increased tendency to occur in stomachs with erosions surrounded by an elevated border, possibly indicating a progression of the erosion or its elevated border to hyperplastic polyp (50). Finally, there is a recent report of hyperplastic polyps associated with *Helicobacter pylori* infection which were not found on endoscopy 2 years after appropriate antibacterial treatment, but which reappeared 3 months after treatment was discontinued (102). Since part of the gastric mucosal response to chronic *H. pylori* infection is foveolar hyperplasia, this organism may occasionally induce hyperplastic polyp type features.

The evolution of hyperplastic polyps is also unknown. What constitutes the minimal criteria for a diagnostic polyp is likely to determine what may be considered a precursor. Do the tiny focal foveolar hyperplasia polyps with pit hyperplasia alone constitute the small or precursor polyp? In one view, focal foveolar hyperplasias enlarge by continued proliferation of the pits with progressive distortion, possibly accentuated by secondary ulceration and inflammation (1,66). Or perhaps the small focal hyperplasia becomes secondarily inflamed and even ulcerated, with the distortion a secondary phenomenon, much as distortion develops in ulcerative colitis as a result of bouts of mucosal destruction which leads to irregular, distorting repair. These small focal lesions thus enlarge by repeated bouts of ulceration with granulation tissue overgrowth and secondary pit repair and resultant distortion. There are polyps that look like they might be transitional forms, with greater pit expansion, distortion, and inflammation than a focal foveolar hyperplasia but less of all those features than in a full blown hyperplastic polyp (62).

Since fully developed hyperplastic polyps are inflamed, it is logical to suggest they are post-inflammatory phenomena. One author suggests that hyperplastic polyps develop through a process that begins with small inflamed projections with normal pits to later stages with elongated pits (foveolar hyperplasia) to full blown hyperplastic polyps with elongated pits and architectural disorganization (59). This theory is based upon the increase in rapidity of histologic progression of the associated gastritis and in the mean age of the patient beginning with the inflammation, followed by the foveolar hyperplasia, and finally the hyperplastic polyp. One of the older names for the hyperplastic polyp was "regenerative polyp"; inflammation with repair were thought to have something to do with their development (67). The stomach does not produce inflammatory pseudopolyps like the colon does, probably because gastric peptic ulcers are not ulcers of the types found in the ulcerating colitides, that is, serpiginous ulcers, undermining ulcers, and interconnecting ulcers that trap islands of mucosa and submucosa. Gastric ulcers are mostly round and discrete, and do not trap islands of mucosa and submucosa. A polyp arising at the site of a healed gastric ulcer was

reported by Mori et al. (69), but in their illustrations, the polyp looks like an overgrowth of remarkably uniform pits with only a few small cysts, not the significant distortion that characterizes the hyperplastic polyp. Furthermore, this case was reported over 20 years ago, and it is still a curiosity; there have been no comparable cases reported since. As has been emphasized by Elster (20), the gastric hyperplastic polyp "has no counterpart in other parts of the gastrointestinal tract and is thereby organotypical for the stomach."

Since the stimuli for their development and their natural history are not known, the possibility that they are foveolar neoplasms cannot be completely excluded. Some may really be adenomas of surface cell type with very low-grade dysplasia and secondary inflammation. We know that some hyperplastic polyps contain foci of clear-cut high-grade dysplasia and even carcinoma (35). Possibly, hyperplastic polyps such as these are really foveolar adenomas with very low-grade dysplasia, but the morphologic criteria of lowest grade pit cell dysplasia are not yet defined, and as a result, they are not recognized as adenomas.

**Gross and Endoscopic Findings.** The gross appearance of hyperplastic polyps depends upon their size, and whether they are seen in gastrectomy specimens or during endoscopic examination. There is no minimum size; the largest polyps measure several centimeters across. When they are discovered endoscopically, most are 1 cm or less in diameter. The small polyps are dome-shaped sessile lesions with a surface that may be smooth or slightly granular or corrugated; the large ones are frequently lobulated and pedunculated (figs. 9-19–9-21) (14). With age, there is a tendency toward greater numbers of pedunculated, rather than sessile, polyps (47). In one study of gastrectomy specimens, hyperplastic polyps were randomly distributed throughout the stomach, although slightly over half were located in the antrum (96). In a Japanese study of 477 hyperplastic polyps, 46 percent occurred in the distal third of the stomach and 44 percent occurred in the middle third (14). In a third or more of cases, the polyps are multiple (24,67).

**Microscopic Findings.** The basic histologic abnormalities involve the pits, which are elongated and distorted. The elongation is far greater than that encountered in all other polyps, except perhaps in some Peutz-Jeghers and juvenile polyps

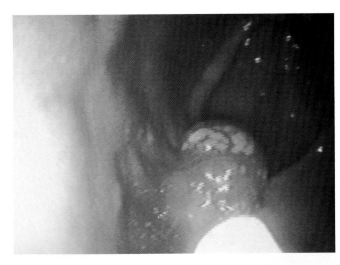

Figure 9-19
HYPERPLASTIC POLYP
Endoscopic view of a small antral hyperplastic polyp which appears as a sessile dome covered by a slightly irregular mucosa with a mix of dark and pale areas. (Courtesy of Dr. Timothy Nostrant, Ann Arbor, MI.)

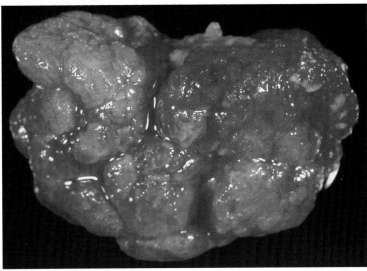

Figure 9-20
HYPERPLASTIC POLYP
Hyperplastic polyp measuring 2.5 cm has a coarsely lobulated surface.

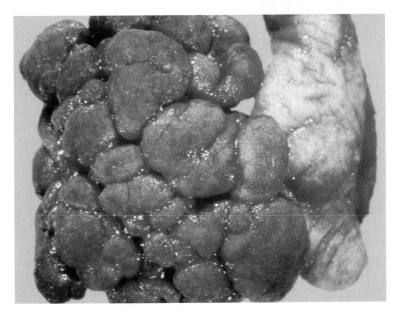

Figure 9-21
HYPERPLASTIC POLYP
Lobulated hyperplastic polyp measuring 4 cm was attached to the mucosa, the pale strip at the right, by a short pedicle.

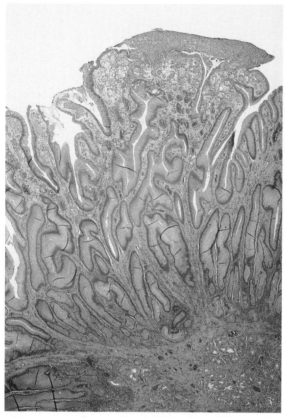

Figure 9-22
HYPERPLASTIC POLYP

In this low-power view the pits are elongated. Many of them are dilated, and some have peculiar shapes with branches or buds. The lamina propria is expanded, especially near the surface. The tip is eroded and covered by exudate. Residual antral glands are at the base on the left.

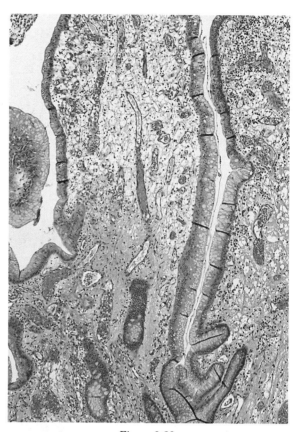

Figure 9-23
HYPERPLASTIC POLYP

These are irregularly shaped surface projections or villi which have edematous, highly vascular cores of lamina propria. The lumen is on the left.

and in the polypoid mucosa of Menetrier's disease (fig. 9-22). This elongation also exaggerates the surface contours, producing coarse or irregular villi (fig. 9-23). The distortion takes several forms. Some of the elongated pits have serrated or cork-screw configurations (fig. 9-24); others are cystic, while still others branch (figs. 9-22, 9-25, 9-26). In one study in which the three-dimensional structure of hyperplastic polyps was analyzed using serial sections, the authors found both horizontal and longitudinal infoldings of the pits, producing the serrated configuration and the two-dimensional appearance of branching, but no true branching was detected (70). The proliferative zone was lengthened and irregular, so that proliferating cells were not confined to the neck area, but were also mixed with mature cells. These distorted

pits are found at all levels, from close to the surface to near the base (figs. 9-25, 9-26).

Superimposed upon the pit changes are inflammatory changes, and it is the inflammation which, in combination with the cystic pits, gives most of the bulk to these polyps (figs. 9-27, 9-28). In most hyperplastic polyps, particularly the large ones, the lamina propria is edematous and contains inflammatory cells, prominent among which are plasma cells, but lymphocytes, eosinophils, mast cells, and macrophages are also present. The peculiar villiform surface may become even coarser and more distorted by ulcers that add granulation tissue to the lamina propria (figs. 9-22, 9-24). It is likely that these peculiar polyps enlarge as repeated ulcers lead to the gradual accumulation of inflammatory tissue. The glands probably do

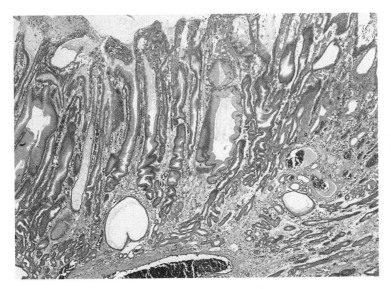

Figure 9-24
HYPERPLASTIC POLYP
Many of the elongated pits have serrated or corkscrew contours. The lamina propria is expanded and inflamed, and the surface, especially on the left, is eroded and covered by exudate.

Figure 9-25
HYPERPLASTIC POLYP
This field includes most of the polyp. The lesion has long, distorted pits, some of which are cystic. The surface is partly villous and the lamina propria is inflamed.

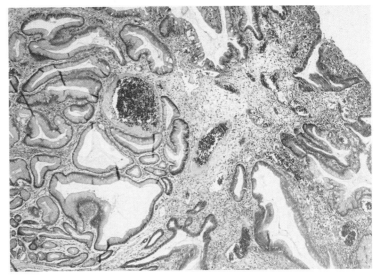

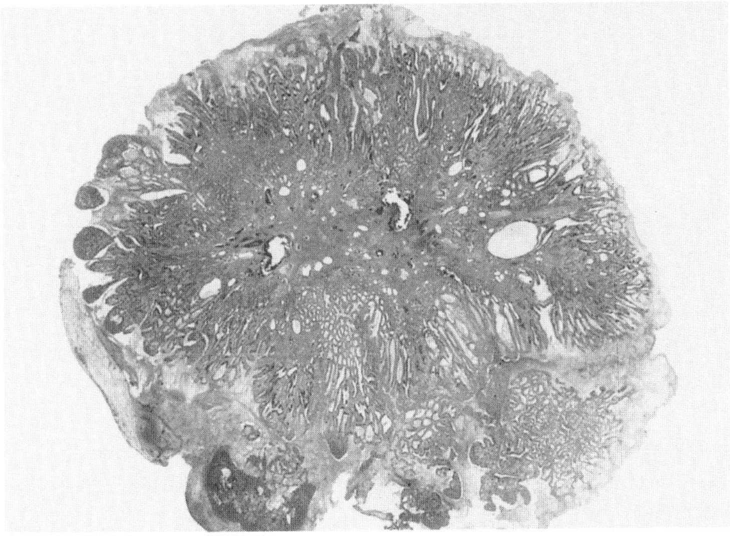

Figure 9-26
HYPERPLASTIC POLYP
This is an entire polyp. The amputation site is at the lower left corner. The bulk of the polyp is composed of long, tortuous pits, some of which are cystic. The surface is focally coarsely villiform.

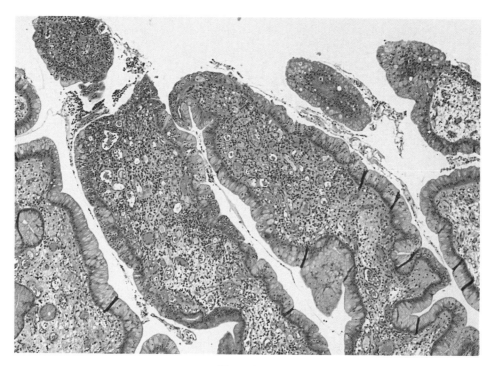

Figure 9-27
SURFACE OF A HYPERPLASTIC POLYP

The lamina propria separating the distorted pits and filling the coarse villi is edematous, hypervascular, and full of inflammatory cells.

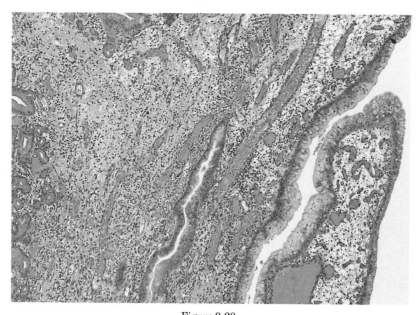

Figure 9-28
HYPERPLASTIC POLYP

This hyperplastic polyp has a lamina propria that is edematous and filled with inflammatory cells and dilated vessels. The small tubules at the base on the left are pits rather than glands.

not participate in the formation of hyperplastic polyps, since the polyps appear to develop from the superficial mucosa. However, glands may persist at the base of a polyp, and they may be captured in a biopsy, especially of a small polyp (fig. 9-22). Nevertheless, there are reports of hyperplastic polyps with hyperplastic glands as an additional component (70). Single smooth muscle fibers or bundles of fibers extending from the muscularis mucosae into the lamina propria between the distorted and elongated pits are often present (fig. 9-23). Whether these are manifestations of prolapse or whether they are intrinsic parts of the polyp is not known.

The epithelium lining the distorted and hyperplastic pits has the features of pit epithelium of all reactive or inflammatory gastric diseases. The epithelium may be normal foveolar epithelium with uniform tall columnar cells containing uniform round basal nuclei and large amounts of apical neutral mucin (fig. 9-29). In very inflamed polyps, particularly at the edges of ulcers, the epithelium may be regenerative with syncytial cells containing undifferentiated eosinophilic cytoplasm and large vesicular nuclei which occasionally bulge the cytoplasm (fig. 9-29). These regenerative nuclei often have prominent nucleoli. Sometimes, especially at the base or in the middle of the polyp, the epithelium may be crowded, more cuboidal than columnar, and the nuclei may be enlarged, hyperchromatic, and vary slightly in size and shape, resembling dysplastic epithelium (fig. 9-29). This is also regenerative and is the type of pit epithelium that is seen in gastric biopsies in which there is significant surface injury, as in chronic bile reflux. The pit cells may be hypertrophied at or near the surface, resulting in large cells with huge apical mucus vacuoles so that the cells resemble goblet cells that contain gastric, rather than intestinal, mucin (fig. 9-29). Small foci of intestinal metaplasia may occur, usually of the incomplete variety, but that is probably not an integral part of these polyps (fig. 9-29) (35); it may reflect the metaplastic status of the gastric mucosa in general.

**Biopsy Diagnosis and Differential Diagnosis.** Many hyperplastic polyps are not removed in total but are biopsied instead. Part of the reason for this is that they may not have a well-defined stalk to serve as an amputation site. The biopsy appearance reflects the surface

changes of pit hyperplasia, pit and mucosal distortion, and inflammation (figs. 9-30, 9-31). The hyperplasia is seen as elongated pits, while the distortion may include coarse surface villi or lobules, cysts, or branching foveolae. The inflammation includes superficial edema, predominately plasma cells and eosinophils, and possibly some granulation tissue from superficial chronic ulcers. This combination of pit hyperplasia, distortion, and inflammation is common to several different lesions, especially the overhanging or prolapsed edges of peptic ulcers; some of the giant fold diseases, especially Menetrier's disease; and less likely, exaggerated cases of chemical gastropathy and *Helicobacter pylori* gastritis. The obvious way to tell all these apart is by correlating the biopsy findings with the endoscopic appearances. A giant fold disease looks quite different from a chronic ulcer, an isolated polyp, and flat gastritis.

**Specific Subtypes of Hyperplastic Polyps.** Hyperplastic polyps may be separated into three epidemiologic types. The most common is the *sporadic type* which tends to occur in stomachs with chronic atrophic gastritis, but also occurs in nonatrophic stomachs. The other two types have similar basic microscopic features, but with certain modifications that relate to their special circumstances.

The second type occurs on the gastric side of gastroenteric anastomoses, especially following a Billroth II procedure combining distal gastrectomy and gastrojejunal anastomosis, but also occurs with gastroduodenal anastomoses. In additional to the simple designation of "hyperplastic polyp," these polyps have been given a bewildering array of names, because of their location at the stoma and because of some morphologic changes within them. An example of such a designation is *gastric stomal polypoid hyperplasia,* and additional names are given in the ensuing discussion (42). Although the exact incidence is not known, they occur in as many as 10 percent of anastomoses (44,84). The development of these polyps is independent of the disease for which the anastomosis is performed (46). Although most reported polyps are found 10 or more years after surgery, many are discovered much earlier, even at 6 months. Therefore, it does not appear that their development is necessarily time-dependent, although, in general,

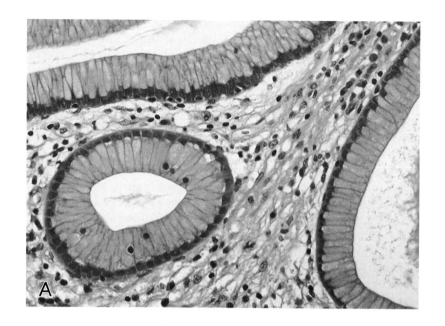

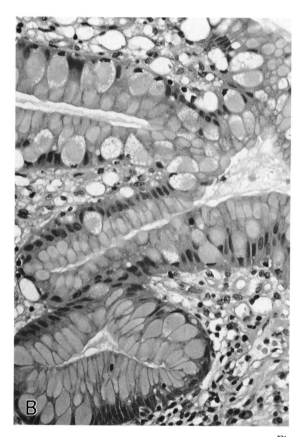

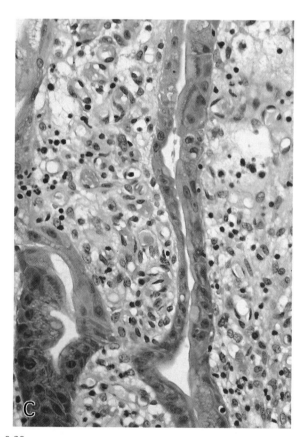

Figure 9-29
EPITHELIA AND STROMA COMMONLY FOUND IN HYPERPLASTIC POLYPS
A: Normal or near-normal foveolar epithelium.
B: Hypertrophic foveolar cells that contain distended mucin vacuoles.
C: Regenerative syncytial epithelium with few mucin-containing cells.

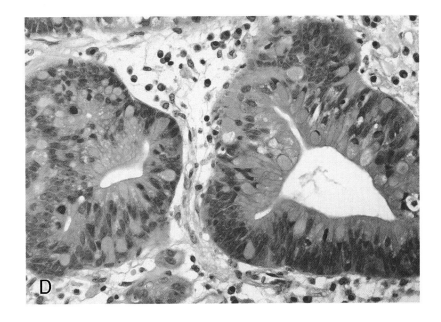

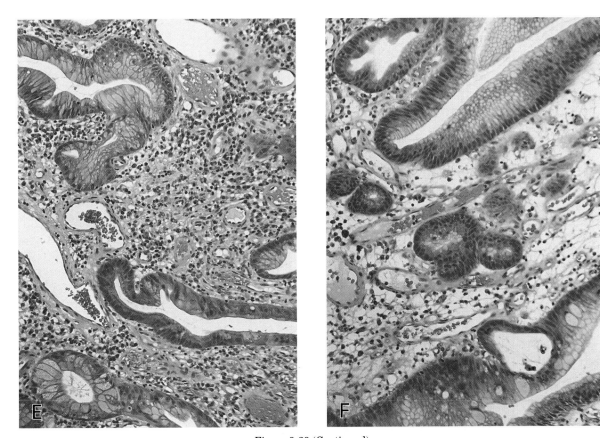

Figure 9-29 (Continued)
D: Hyperplastic epithelium with enlarged, hyperchromatic, stratified nuclei.
E: A mixture of epithelia in a heavily inflamed, vascular stroma.
F: A mixture of epithelia in a less inflamed, but intensely edematous stroma.

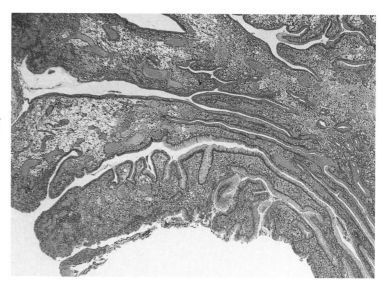

Figure 9-30
HYPERPLASTIC POLYP
Low-power view of a biopsy from the top of
a large hyperplastic polyp. The fragment contains very long pits, some of which branch. The
surface on the left is coarsely villiform and the
stroma is inflamed.

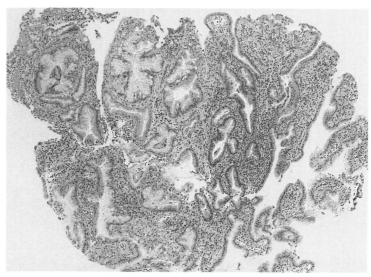

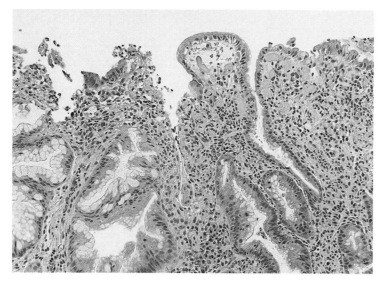

Figure 9-31
BIOPSY OF A
HYPERPLASTIC POLYP
Low-power (top) and high-power (bottom)
views of a hyperplastic polyp. The pits are
distorted, and the pit epithelium varies. Some
pits have normal epithelium; others, such as
those in the center, have cells with crowded
nuclei. The branching pit to the left of center
has epithelium with huge mucus vacuoles.
The lamina propria is expanded and filled
with inflammatory cells.

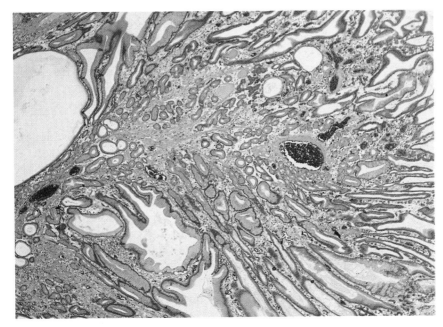

Figure 9-32
STOMAL POLYP
(HYPERPLASTIC POLYP
ARISING ON THE GASTRIC
SIDE OF A GASTROENTERIC
ANASTOMOSIS)
The pits are very long and distorted. Deep cysts are next to a few clusters of residual glands. In the stroma, occasional thin bundles of smooth muscle extend between the strange pits.

their frequency increases with the age of the anastomosis. This type of polyp may be localized or it may appear as a circumferential ring of heaped-up mucosa at the anastomosis site (26, 54). On occasion, there may be multiple polyps, not all of which are right at the stoma. Usually, they are sessile masses with grossly lobulated surfaces, and some can grow to 6 cm or even more in diameter (23). They have all the features mentioned above for sporadic hyperplastic polyps, but the surface is usually more villiform and there is likely to be more smooth muscle emanating from disorganized muscularis mucosae, presumably the result of prolapse of this hyperplastic mucosa distally toward the small bowel. This smooth muscle proliferation appears as excess fibers and bundles of fibers oriented parallel to the pits, often extending from the base to the surface (fig. 9-32) (1). Further extension of these pits through the base of the mucosa into the submucosa results in gastritis cystica, in which the cystic pits are surrounded by hypertrophic bundles of smooth muscle. This phenomenon has led to a variety of cystic descriptors for these polyps, such as *gastritis cystica polyposa, gastric cystic polyposis,* and *polypoid cystic gastritis* (11,26, 63). Illustrations of this phenomenon are found near the end of this chapter in the section covering cysts. The cause of this submucosal extension is not known, but similar changes occur in some

large, left-sided, pedunculated colonic adenomas and at the margins of some solitary rectal ulcers. A study of the gastric mucosa at the gastroenteric anastomosis site of 38 random cases indicated that there were hyperplastic or hypertrophic mucosal changes in two thirds of the cases, comparable to those of the polyps but of less intensity (54). This suggested that the polyps were just exaggerations of a more common alteration, and another name, *stomal polypoid hypertrophic gastritis,* was given. These changes may be partly bile reflux induced, since bile reflux is a predictable consequence of such anastomoses, and foveolar hyperplasia is a common result of chronic bile reflux. In addition, it is on the crests of these polyps that the postanastomosis dysplasias and carcinomas are likely to occur.

The third type of hyperplastic polyp occurs at the cardioesophageal junction. These are thought to be due to chronic gastroesophageal reflux, and have been designated as *reflux gastroesophageal polyps* or *inflammatory esophagogastric polyps* (76,91). Some may be associated with prominent mucosal-submucosal folds (5). Many of the reported cases have been in children and young adults. Histologically, because of their location, they commonly incorporate the squamocolumnar junction, although some polyps are composed entirely of gastric mucosa (93). On the gastric or columnar side, there is pit hyperplasia and distortion with superimposed inflammation. These changes are identical to those found in sporadic hyperplastic polyps. On the esophageal or squamous side, there may be changes of gastroesophageal reflux, including papillomatosis and basal cell hyperplasia; peptic ulcers; or healing or ulcer-edge alterations with long prongs of primitive basal cells extending into granulation tissue.

**Natural History and Relation to Dysplasia and Carcinoma.** Few follow-up studies of hyperplastic polyps are available once they have been viewed endoscopically and biopsied. In the largest published series, 93 polyps in 56 patients were followed from 5 to 12 years by endoscopy and biopsy (48): 63 polyps remained unchanged; 30 changed in size, shape, or number. Three polyps, all less than 1 cm across, disappeared; 25 polyps increased in size; and 2 polyps initially grew larger and then disappeared. In 2 of the polyps that enlarged, dysplastic epithelium, including carcinomatous, developed. The number of polyps increased in 16 patients, usually in the same part of the stomach as the original polyps. Most patients had single polyps at the beginning. As with adenomas, there are two associations between hyperplastic polyps and carcinoma: the presence of dysplastic epithelia of all grades, as well as carcinomatous epithelium, within the polyp and the presence of dysplastic epithelium elsewhere in the stomach.

Of 67 hyperplastic polyps in Japanese patients, Hattori (35) found 11 had dysplastic foci, 9 of the gastric type and 2 of the intestinal type. Three polyps had invasive adenocarcinoma, but it is not clear if these were in the dysplastic polyps. In another Japanese study of 477 hyperplastic polyps, dysplasia was found in 19 and intramucosal carcinoma plus dysplasia in an additional 10 (14). The risk of both dysplasia and carcinoma occurring in hyperplastic polyps increased with the size of the polyps, particularly those over 2 cm in diameter. Patients with carcinoma were about 9 years older, on average, than those without carcinoma. The dysplastic and carcinomatous foci occurred in the superficial parts of the polyps, the same place where adenomas develop. There is a report of a Portuguese family with multiple gastric hyperplastic polyps, gastric carcinoma, and psoriasis (86). The mode of inheritance appears to be autosomal dominant. Photographs of one of the polyps shows it to be centrally cystic, as are many hyperplastic polyps, but the prominent villous surface resembles more the surface of an adenoma. This family may be producing hybrid polyps. There was no mention of whether or not there was atrophic gastritis in the nonpolypoid mucosa.

**Treatment.** The treatment of choice for hyperplastic polyps is excision, and this can be accomplished endoscopically in almost every case. Gastrotomy with open removal is rarely needed. Histologic examination of excised specimens is also the only way to determine the composition of any gastric polyp. Large polyps should be excised to ensure that they are not dysplastic lesions, since dysplasia and even carcinoma can occur in large hyperplastic polyps (14). However, if carcinoma is discovered in such a polyp, there is no data about whether polypectomy alone is adequate therapy, or if some type of gastric resection is necessary. If there are multiple polyps, the larger ones, those 1.5 cm or more, should be excised. If there are only small polyps, then a few should be excised, and the rest may be cauterized or left alone. There is no data about the risk of bleeding from unresected gastric polyps, so potential bleeding may not constitute an indication for resection.

There are follow-up issues. In a study from Finland, 50 percent of patients with polyps developed new or recurrent polyps, usually inflammatory lesions or hyperplastic polyps (89). About 1 percent developed carcinomas on follow-up. Another study of more than 5,700 patients with noncarcinomatous mucosal polyps, most of which were hyperplastic, concluded that over 6 percent of patients developed recurrent polyps at the original site, mostly within the first year after polypectomy (85). Additionally, about one third of the patients developed new polyps in other gastric sites. The recurrent and new polyps were usually of the same type as the original polyp. Gastric carcinomas, usually the early types, developed in 1.3 percent of patients with polyps during 1 to 7 years of follow-up, but for those with adenomas, the rate was 3.4 percent. These studies suggest that patients with gastric mucosal polyps might benefit from endoscopic follow-up (12). However, since the cancer risk is very low, the proper scheduling period for such follow-up has not yet been determined.

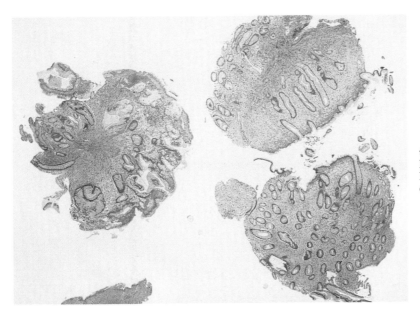

Figure 9-33
CRONKHITE-CANADA POLYPS
Low-power view of three polyps. The two on the right have smooth surfaces like juvenile polyps, while the one on the left resembles a hyperplastic polyp with distorted pits and villiform surface.

## Polyposis of the Cronkhite-Canada Syndrome

The Cronkhite-Canada syndrome is a peculiar complex that includes unrelated endodermal and ectodermal abnormalities (15). The ectodermal features include alopecia, macular hyperpigmentation of the face, and nail dystrophy. The endodermal change is a gastrointestinal polyposis which involves any part of the gut except the esophagus. This polyposis is really part of a diffuse mucosal abnormality, and the clinical manifestations reflect this. These include diarrhea and even steatorrhea with malabsorption as a result of the small intestinal and colonic mucosal disease, and hypoproteinemia secondary to gastrointestinal protein loss. Some patients have profound weight loss and abdominal pain. When the gastric polyposis becomes extensive and exaggerated, the gross appearance can be that of a giant fold disease (22). Thus the clinical, radiographic, and endoscopic features may resemble those of Menetrier's disease (51). Most patients are late middle aged or elderly, and about 60 percent are men. The syndrome is not familial. The clinical course is unpredictable, and many cases are progressive, even fatal; some cases, however, completely or partially resolve (80). A few cases of adenocarcinoma, mostly colonic, have been reported in association with the syndrome (64).

The stomach is involved in almost every case. The typical gastric polyp is sessile with a broad base. Microscopically, it has an expanded, edematous lamina propria and hyperplastic pits, many of which are cystic (figs. 9-33, 9-34) (8). These features are similar to those encountered in both juvenile and hyperplastic polyps. The lamina propria is hypercellular as a result of a mixture of inflammatory cells, including eosinophils and mast cells; fibroblasts; and smooth muscle fibers from the muscularis mucosae. Occasional polyps may be superficially eroded. The glandular compartment is often atrophic. The surrounding flatter mucosa is thickened and is likely to contain many small foci of edema, stromal changes, and cystic pits similar to those found in the polyps. The etiology of this unusual acquired polyposis and diffuse mucosal alteration is unknown. It may be the result of loss of proliferative stimuli or a block in maturation (22,46). No drugs or toxins have been implicated.

## Other Polyps

In any classification scheme, there must be a place to put the lesions that do not conform to the criteria established for known entities. In the case of gastric polyps, there are mucosal lumps that do not fit into established categories. In almost every published series, these are placed into one of the other categories, probably as

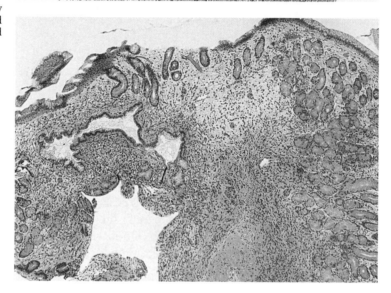

Figure 9-34
CRONKHITE-CANADA POLYPS
Top: In this polyp, the surface is smooth, and the lamina propria is expanded and cellular.
Bottom: This polyp has residual clustered glands; an expanded edematous lamina propria containing spindle cells, presumably smooth muscle cells and fibroblasts, mixed with inflammatory cells; distorted, dilated pits; and a smooth surface.

hyperplastic polyps or foveolar hyperplasia, since no series has ever had an "other" or "none-of-the-above" category. These untitled polyps have a mixture of histologic features that are common to other classifiable polyps, but the features are either not fully enough developed to be diagnostically helpful, or else they are combined in unusual ways. For instance, some antral polyps have prominent pits, disorganized clusters of antral glands, and scattered small cystic pits, so that they seem to be the antral equivalent of the fundic gland polyp. Another polyp has disorganized clusters of body glands, no gland cysts, and plasmacytic and lymphocytic inflammation in a slightly lengthened pit compartment, a mix-

ture of a cystless fundic gland polyp and chronic *Helicobacter*-like gastritis. Another polyp has long pits, an expanded antral gland compartment, and hypertrophy or even hyperplasia of the muscularis mucosae; in essence, too much antral mucosa has produced a polyp, but one without a name (fig. 9-35). Lymphocytic gastritis is one inflammatory condition that produces a polyp from time to time. In fact, its endoscopic or gross appearance has been designated as "varioliform gastritis," a set of features which includes large folds in the fundus and mucosal bulges; the latter may appear as small polyps (30). Lymphocytic gastritis is an inflammation of unknown cause which sometimes accompanies

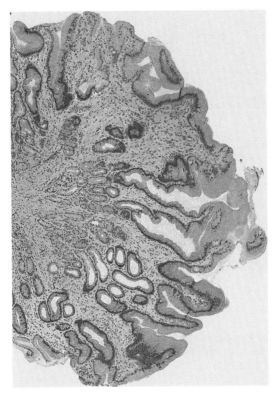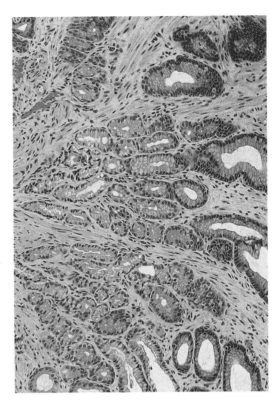

Figure 9-35
A POLYP THAT DOES NOT BELONG TO A WELL-DEFINED CATEGORY
The pits are elongated but widely spaced by a lamina propria that has many smooth muscle fascicles. The glands at the base are normal, except that they too are separated by smooth muscle. (Left: Low-power view of the entire polyp. Right: High-power view of the base.)

one of the sprue conditions and which is characterized by a variably intense infiltrate of T lymphocytes in the surface and pit epithelia, usually with accompanying epithelial damage (fig. 9-36) (104). Thus, the surface looks much like that in sprue. In addition, there is usually some pit expansion or hyperplasia and a superficial plasmacytosis and lymphocytosis.

## GIANT RUGAL HYPERTROPHIES (GIANT FOLDS DISEASES, HYPERPLASTIC GASTROPATHIES)

The normal gastric folds or rugae are composed of cores of submucosa covered by mucosa (fig. 9-37). They are prominent in the fundus and body, but the antrum is generally flat. There is considerable variation in fold size which does not necessarily correlate with age. In addition, the status of the folds depends, to a great extent, upon the degree of gastric distention. Unusually large folds, therefore, are defined as those that persist even in the distended stomach (112). What constitutes giant or unusually large folds has been quantitatively defined: in one definition, radiographic large folds are those greater than 8 mm in width, while endoscopic large folds are greater than 1 cm in height (109); in a second purely radiographic definition, large folds are those that are more than 1 cm wide (120). Some giant folds are accompanied by clinical syndromes; others are not. Enlargement of the rugae is always accounted for, at least in part, by elongation of the submucosal cores. These lengthened cores are covered by various types of mucosa, some of which are so thick that they add to the total thickness of the folds (106). Giant folds may be caused by neoplasms or they may be non-neoplastic conditions that mimic neoplasms. Sometimes giant folds appear endoscopically as diffuse or multiple gastric polyposes.

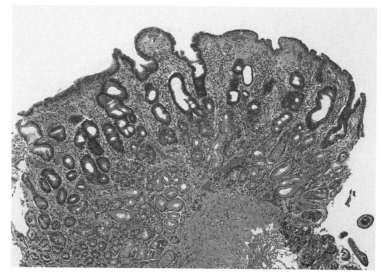

Figure 9-36
LYMPHOCYTIC GASTRITIS

Top: The dilated pits are separated by a cellular lamina propria containing a mixture of plasma cells and lymphocytes. The epithelium covering the surface and the superficial pits is disorganized and contains lymphocytes.

Bottom: High-power view of the surface epithelium, within which is an infiltrate of T lymphocytes. The epithelium is mucus-depleted and the nuclei are stratified, evidence of cell damage.

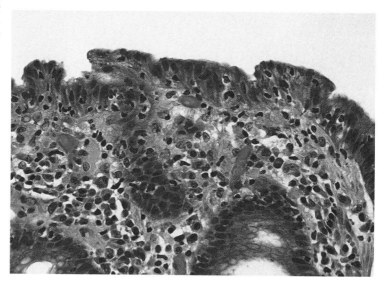

## Classification of Giant Folds, with or without Associated Syndromes

Giant folds are classified by the types of mucosa covering the expanded submucosal folds and the clinical settings in which they occur. The classification is shown in Table 9-4.

Literature on giant folds is confusing because some of the associated conditions or syndromes have not been rigidly defined, incomplete variants of some of the syndromes have been reported, and results of some of the published cases and series do not correlate with histologic changes. As an example, a large series of giant folds cases were defined as Menetrier's disease based only upon the combination of gross giant folds, which the authors referred to as "hypertrophic gastropathy," and hypoproteinemia, with no histologic correlation (123). Furthermore, 43 patients with this combination were compared with 47 patients who also had giant folds but who had normal serum proteins, and this group also had no histologic correlation. In this study, the authors did not include histologic analysis, because all the patients had small gastroscopic biopsies that were considered of "limited value for assessing the extent and depth of inflammation and hypertrophy." Nevertheless, histologic assessment is essential in order to determine what changes are occurring in the big folds.

216

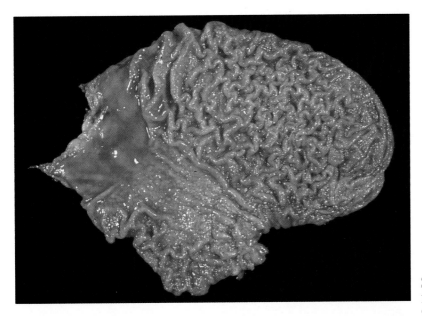

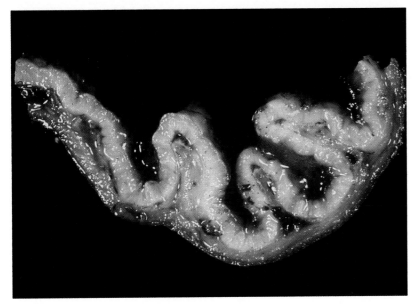

Figure 9-37
PROMINENT RUGAL FOLDS
Top: En face view of the stomach opened along the greater curvature. The antrum is the flattened area to the left. The remainder of the mucosa is covered by long ridges or folds.
Bottom: Cross section shows submucosa in the core of each fold. These cores are covered by thick mucosa, in this case characterized by glandular hyperplasia, part of the Zollinger-Ellison syndrome.

Table 9-4

## CLASSIFICATION OF GIANT FOLDS

1. Normal variant, including common gastritis
2. Menetrier's disease and variants
3. Zollinger-Ellison syndrome
4. Lymphocytic gastritis
5. Extensive or diffuse neoplastic infiltrates
6. Other causes

Recently, large bore biopsy instruments or snare biopsy instruments have been utilized for assessment (119,120). These have the capability to amputate a full thickness chunk of mucosa, including the entire tip of a giant fold. If such instruments are used, the only limitation is histologic analysis of conditions in which irregular or focal, rather than diffuse, changes occur, because a single biopsy, even one taken with a large bore instrument, may not pick up the diagnostic area.

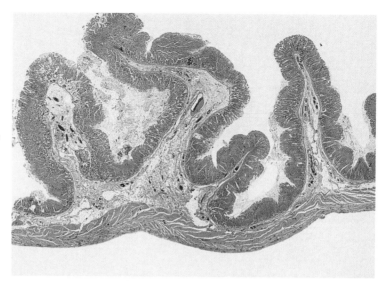

Figure 9-38
GIANT FOLDS
Giant folds covered by normally thick body mucosa.

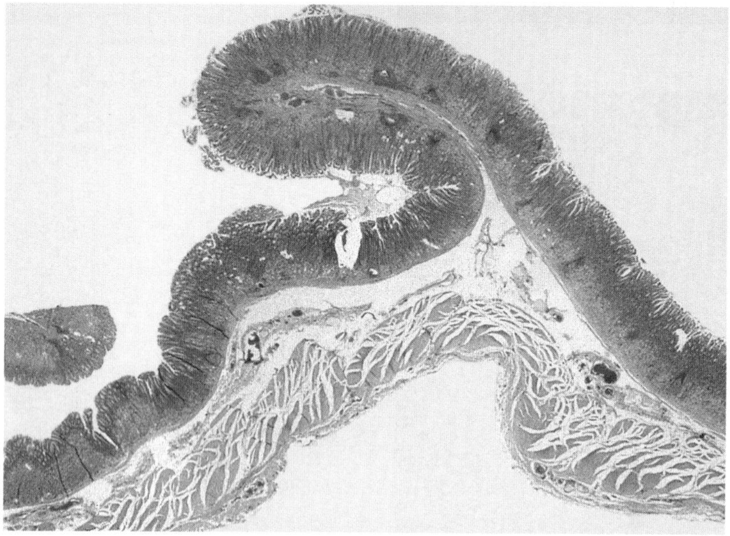

Figure 9-39
GIANT FOLDS
The unusually prominent folds in this stomach were covered by inflamed mucosa. At the base of the mucosa are a series of lymphoid follicles, while the superficial mucosa is hypercellular. This is the characteristic gastritis associated with *Helicobacter pylori*, and *H. pylori* was present on the surface epithelium. It is unlikely that the gastritis caused the giant folds; it probably accidently affected a stomach that had big folds as a normal variant.

## Normal Variant Giant Folds

Endoscopic and radiographic findings of unusually prominent rugae in the body and fundus are not unusual in patients who have no accompanying disease. In one endoscopy text, the author states that large rugal folds occur in about 1 percent of all gastroscopic exams (107). These folds may be covered by normal mucosa or by mucosa with one of the common gastritides, such as *Helicobacter pylori* gastritis (figs. 9-38, 9-39) (119), or rarely, atrophic gastritis. Endoscopic atrophy is usually synonymous with grossly flattened mucosal-submucosal folds. This does not always correlate with histologic atrophy, which is defined as loss of glands at the microscopic level.

## Menetrier's Disease

**Clinical Features.** Menetrier's disease is a giant folds disease syndrome, but all the parts of the syndrome may not be present at the same time, and those that are present may be incompletely developed. The full blown syndrome includes giant folds, gastric protein loss, and decreased gastric acid production, accompanied by a histologic complex that includes foveolar hyperplasia and distortion, glandular atrophy, and edema but little inflammation, in the lamina propria (106, 107). There is no known cause; in fact, there is not even a commonly occurring underlying or associated condition to suggest an etiology. However, it is now being linked to excessive levels of growth

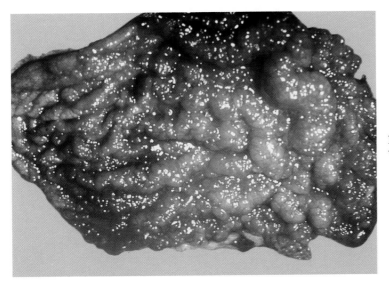

Figure 9-40
MENETRIER'S DISEASE
The body of this stomach is covered by thick
knobby folds with a coarsely granular surface,
the result of irregular pit hyperplasia.

factors. A histologically and clinically identical condition has been produced in transgenic mice that overexpressed transforming growth factor alpha (TGFα) in their stomachs (127). Furthermore, one patient with Menetrier's disease had markedly elevated levels of serum epidermal growth factor, which dropped to near normal levels following therapy with a somatostatin analog thought to inhibit certain growth factors (134). TGFα is normally expressed in surface epithelium and parietal cells of the gastric body mucosa, but it is not found in normal pit epithelium. In Menetrier's disease, it also appears in the hyperplastic pit epithelium (109a). However, this is not a specific reaction in stomachs with Menetrier's disease, since similar pit cell expression has been found in other conditions that have profound pit hyperplasia, such as the diffuse form of lymphocytic gastritis and hyperplastic polyps (109a). Many giant folds cases reported as Menetrier's disease do not have all of the abnormalities listed above. It is not clear if they should or should not be included with other, fully developed cases of the disease; if they are variants; or if they are separate diseases. Some patients have normal serum proteins, while others have normal gastric acid secretion or even hypersecretion (110, 117,122,126). Some cases combine features of both Menetrier's disease and the Zollinger-Ellison syndrome (see the following discussion on Zollinger-Ellison syndrome). In fact, there was a single case report of a patient who had both diseases at the same time (116).

Menetrier's disease usually occurs in adults, with a mean age of 55 to 60 years. There is a self-limited, Menetrier-like, hypoproteinemic giant folds condition in children that is probably postinfectious, particularly following viral illness, and is not the same as the adult disease (111,125). In the adult syndrome, men are affected over twice as often as women. The presenting symptoms include abdominal pain, generally epigastric, and peripheral edema, a consequence of the protein loss and the resulting hypoproteinemia. All cases have enlarged folds in the gastric body and fundus which are detected either radiographically or endoscopically. The antrum is grossly normal, although it may be involved at the microscopic level (132). These folds often have knobby, lobulated, or even cerebriform surfaces, and localized patches may look like polyps (fig. 9-40). Commonly, there is abundant mucus on the surface, sometimes bridging the folds.

**Morphologic Findings.** The expanded folds are covered by mucosa which, in its most advanced state, has florid pit hyperplasia accompanied by loss of (atrophy of) glands, superficial edema, and, at most, mild inflammation. The pits are unusually elongated, and frequently extend from the surface to the base of the mucosa. Occasionally, they penetrate the muscularis mucosae to end as cysts surrounded by smooth muscle bundles in the superficial submucosa, in other words, as patchy gastritis cystica profunda (figs. 9-41–9-43). As more and more pit hyperplasia develops, the glandular compartment is progressively

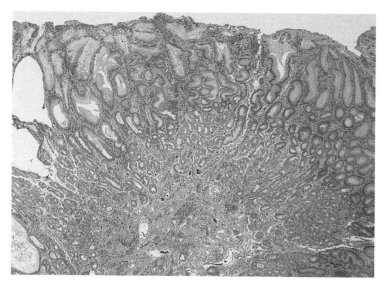

Figure 9-41
MENETRIER'S DISEASE,
BODY MUCOSA

The pits are much longer than normal, and many are dilated. The surrounding lamina propria is edematous. The glands persist at the base, but are fewer than normal for body mucosa, and many are dilated.

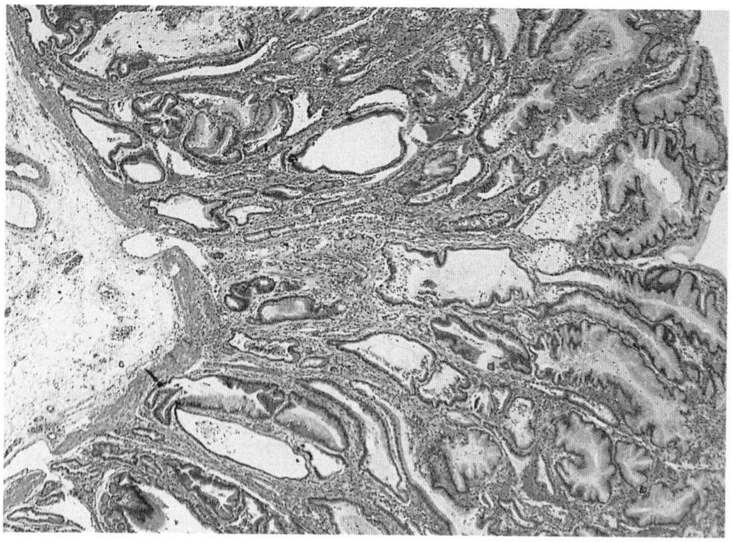

Figure 9-42
MENETRIER'S DISEASE

This is also body mucosa, but compared to figure 9-41, the pits are more prominent, many have a serrated configuration, and many extend to the base of the mucosa, where some of them end as cysts.

Figure 9-43
MENETRIER'S DISEASE

This is the base of the mucosa with the muscularis mucosae at the bottom. The dilated structures are cystic pits. The surrounding lamina propria is edematous and contains very few inflammatory cells.

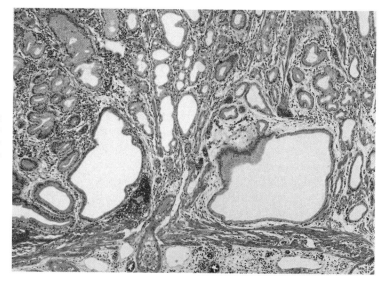

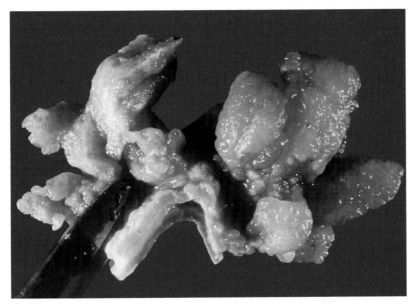

Figure 9-44
MENETRIER'S DISEASE
In this case, there was so much pit hyperplasia that the giant folds appeared to be covered by a myriad of polyps resembling hyperplastic polyps. The muscularis propria is the folded structure at the bottom center.

compromised, resulting in atrophy. The long pits are also distorted, with cystic and branched forms, and pits with serrated lumens. The surface may be villiform. Intestinal metaplasia is not characteristic, although patches of it may be found, as it is found in many adult stomachs. The superficial lamina propria is edematous, and there may be a mild plasmacytosis (132). In some cases, eosinophils or mast cells are conspicuous (132). In general, however, inflammation is not a significant component of this process. The pit hyperplasia and superficial edema seem to be the cause of, or at are least associated with, protein loss, while the replacement of the glandular compartment by the ehpanding pit compartment results in hypochlorhydria or achlorhydria. These changes are not uniform. They tend to be most prominent on the crests of the folds, where the mucosal expansion may be so pronounced that it leads to the polyp-like lesions seen grossly by the endoscopist or radiologist (fig. 9-44). The folds and their polypoid expansions may become so prominent that they prolapse through the pyloric sphincter. There may be stretches of normal or near-normal mucosa interspersed among the areas of pit hyperplasia, so that biopsies from different areas may offer remarkably different views, obscuring the diagnosis in some cases. Some of these foci may have subtle changes, such as a little pit elongation accompanied by a slight decrease in the number of glands.

**Treatment and Prognosis.** The course of Menetrier's disease is unpredictable. In most cases, the signs or symptoms are severe enough to require gastrectomy. The most common indication for resection is the hypoproteinemia that leads to uncontrollable peripheral edema and even anasarca. A few recent reports suggest that treatment with H2 or histamine receptor blockers may be effective in controlling the protein loss and even in reversing the histologic changes (129). Rare adult cases resolve spontaneously, and so resemble childhood cases (130). Sequential biopsies in some cases show end stage atrophic gastritis; at this point, the protein loss stops, suggesting that it is directly related to the pit hyperplasia or the accompanying superficial inflammation (108). A few cases of Menetrier's disease are complicated by adenocarcinoma, but the carcinoma is not necessarily in the same part of the stomach as the giant folds (133); it is uncertain whether this is a precursor lesion for gastric cancer.

### Zollinger-Ellison Syndrome

This syndrome, first described in 1955, is characterized by intractable peptic ulcers, usually duodenal and often multiple, which are the result of profound hypergastrinemia, usually from a gastrin-producing tumor (114). The tumors are often found in the pancreas, but most are in the duodenum. A few patients with the syndrome do not have tumors, but instead, have

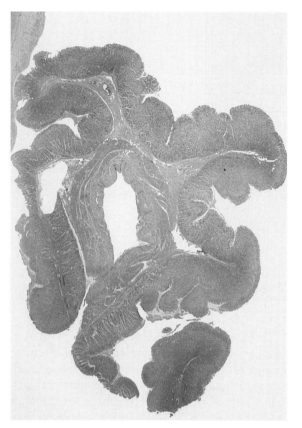 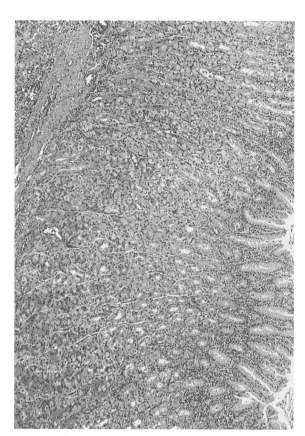

Figure 9-45
ZOLLINGER-ELLISON SYNDROME

Left: This is a cross section of a rolled gastric wall. The C-shaped structure in the center is the muscularis propria. The long submucosal folds are covered by thick body mucosa.

Right: In this typical ZES case, the mucosa has a normally thick pit compartment and an expanded glandular compartment with much of the expansion due to an excess of parietal cells.

hypergastrinemia secondary to antral G cell (gastrin-producing cell) hyperplasia. When gastrin is present in excessive quantities, there is hyperplasia and hypertrophy of the parietal cells in the body mucosa. This is the typical mucosal abnormality in the Zollinger-Ellison syndrome (ZES) (106,119). The glandular compartment of the body mucosa becomes enlarged, so that the pit to gland ratio changes from the usual 1 to 3 to 1 to 4 or even 1 to 5 (fig. 9-45). The parietal cells are often huge and distended; this expanded mucosa covers large submucosal folds, producing the giant folds. The pit compartment is generally normal. In ZES, the folds are not as large as in Menetrier's disease, because the hyperplasia involves the deep glandular compartment diffusely and spares the pit compartment

completely (see fig. 9-37). One other abnormality occurs and that is hyperplasia of the enterochromaffin-like endocrine cells of the gastric body, since they are also responsive to gastrin (124). If ZES is part of the multiple endocrine neoplasia syndrome type 1 (MEN 1), enterochromaffin-like cell micronests and small carcinoid tumors may result, identical to those that occur in the diffuse body form of chronic atrophic gastritis (124).

There is a normogastrinemic form of giant folds disease resembling ZES which has been called *hypertrophic hypersecretory gastropathy* (128). Patients with this syndrome have large folds with a nodular or "cobblestone" appearance, gastric acid hypersecretion, frequent peptic ulcers, and no protein loss.

## Lymphocytic Gastritis

Not only can lymphocytic gastritis produce polyps, but it can produce a giant folds disease that is an exaggerated variant of varioliform gastritis. In several recently reported cases, this combination of lymphocytic gastritis and giant folds was associated with profound protein loss, much as in Menetrier's disease (113,118,131,132). The typical histologic findings are identical to those described for lymphocytic gastritis polyps, but more extensive, involving most of the gastric body and sometimes the antrum as well. They include infiltration of the surface and superficial epithelium by T-lymphocytes (see fig. 9-36). The infiltrated epithelium has changes of injury, including loss of apical mucin, nuclear stratification, and a change from columnar to cuboidal cells. The lamina propria, especially the superficial part, has excessive inflammatory cells, particularly plasma cells. This diffuse giant fold type of lymphocytic gastritis may be complicated by adenocarcinoma, as can Menetrier's disease (121,132).

## Extensive or Diffuse Neoplastic Infiltrates

One of the classic gross and radiographic descriptions of gastric lymphoma is that of fold enlargement. These big folds are usually coarse and irregular. Occasional carcinomas, especially the diffuse or signet ring cell types, infiltrate to produce giant folds. These neoplastic-associated giant folds are not necessarily the result of invasion and expansion of the submucosa. Some tumors may be limited to the mucosa.

## Other Causes of Giant Folds

In some cases of the Cronkhite-Canada syndrome, the diffuse polyposis may appear grossly as giant folds (115). Furthermore, since hypoproteinemia is often a component of this syndrome, and since the mucosa has superficial pit distortion and inflammation, these cases may be confused with Menetrier's disease on biopsy.

# CYSTS OF THE STOMACH

There are three types of gastric cysts: 1) large, usually single, intramural or extramural congenital or developmental cysts that commonly have their own muscularis; 2) small, commonly multiple, intramucosal cysts that have no surrounding smooth muscle; and 3) variably-sized, multiple, submucosal cysts surrounded by smooth muscle, known as gastritis cystica profunda. Each has a different cause, presentation, and clinical significance.

## Developmental Cysts

Most large intramural cysts of the stomach are considered duplication anomalies (fig. 9-46). The literature is full of single case reports of duplications, but the anomaly is so unusual that there are no substantial series reported. Gastric duplications are much less common than those of the esophagus and small intestine, which are also rare. They are composed of a central mucosa-lined lumen surrounded by thick layers of smooth muscle which, in some cases, is in continuity with the smooth muscle of the muscularis propria, or even within it (136). Such cysts only rarely communicate with the gastric lumen. The mucosa may be gastric or any other type of gut mucosa, and there may be superimposed chronic ulcers (fig. 9-47). One reported case contained a focus of ectopic pancreatic parenchyma with ducts and acini in the wall, while a second case had pancreatic islets and ducts but no acini (137, 155). Most have been found on the greater curvature of the stomach where they are likely to produce a palpable mass, or at the pylorus where they may obstruct the gastric outlet (156). They may appear endoscopically as smooth intramural masses resembling stromal tumors. Most are detected in children, but some do not become obvious until adulthood. In children, they are often associated with other anomalies, especially duplication of the esophagus and vertebral abnormalities, including fusions, hemivertabrae, and spina bifida. They are usually over 3 cm in diameter when first discovered, but huge cysts measuring 17 cm or more have been reported. Three cases of gastric duplication cysts in adults containing invasive adenocarcinoma have been reported (135). An intramural gastric cyst lined by respiratory epithelium also had a focus of cartilage in the wall (152). This may not be a duplication, but it seems to be a developmental cyst, perhaps comparable to the bronchogenic cysts that occur in the subcutis of the chest and neck and in the mediastinum (138).

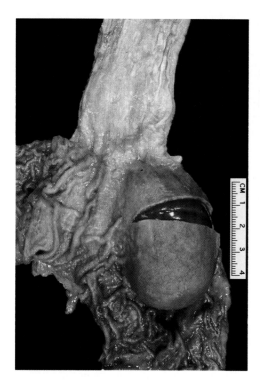
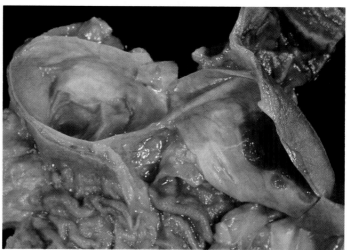

Figure 9-46
INTRAMURAL DEVELOPMENTAL CYST
Left: In the upper stomach, immediately below the esophageal orifice, there is a large cyst that bulges and smooths the overlying mucosa.
Above: This cyst has been opened. Its lining has a few ridges, but is otherwise smooth. The gastric mucosa is at the lower left. The ridge running across the center of the field is an extension of the gastric muscularis propria that envelops the cyst. (Courtesy of Dr. Peter Shireman, Kansas City, MO.)

## Intramucosal Cysts

Epithelial cysts are expected components of virtually every type of gastric mucosal polyp. In fundic gland polyps, the cysts are cystic glands. In hyperplastic polyps, the cysts are cystic pits. Cysts are also common in the deep mucosa of adenomas, possibly because the proliferating dysplastic epithelium may obstruct the foveolar orifices (149). Deep mucosal cysts are also common in Menetrier's disease. Cystic mucosal elements occurring in nonpolypoid or flat mucosa are common incidental findings in gastric mucosal biopsies and resections and their significance is unknown. Virtually any mucosal component may form a cyst, including the pits, body glands with parietal and chief cells, and pure mucous antral or cardiac glands (figs. 9-48, 9-49). Furthermore, intestinalized tubules with goblet cells and parietal cells may become cystic in areas of atrophic gastritis. The relative frequency of the different cyst types may reflect the frequency of atrophic gastritis in the population studied. Rare cysts with ciliated columnar epithelium occur, but have no special significance (144).

Intramucosal cysts have a close association with gastric carcinoma, and there are frequency differences among different populations. Such cysts were found in noncancerous mucosae in 97 percent of 91 stomachs resected for elevated dysplasias or carcinomas in a study from Japan and 70 percent of stomachs resected for carcinoma in a Chinese study (144,158). They were found in 39 percent of 51 stomachs resected for peptic ulcer disease in a Swedish study, in 90 percent of 102 consecutive stomachs resected for peptic ulcers in a Japanese study, and in 43 percent of peptic ulcer stomachs in China (148, 150,158). In the Swedish study, the number of cysts occurring in nontumorous mucosae from stomachs resected for early gastric cancer was far greater than in stomachs resected for peptic ulcer disease (150). In the Chinese study, the cancer-associated cysts were usually intestinal, while those that were ulcer associated were not (158).

## Misplaced Gastric Pits in the Submucosa and Muscularis Mucosae: Gastritis Cystica Profunda and Gastritis Cystica Polyposa

There are several situations in which hyperplastic gastric pits or even mucous glands appear to push through the base of the mucosa into the muscularis mucosae. As they penetrate this

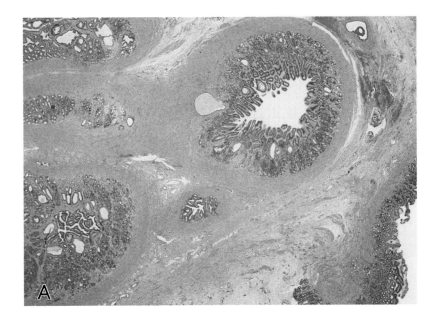

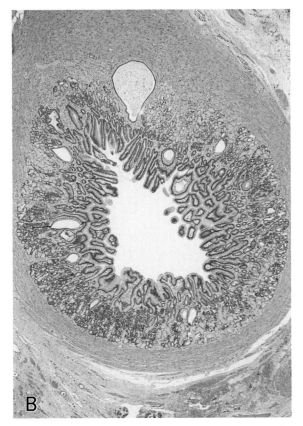

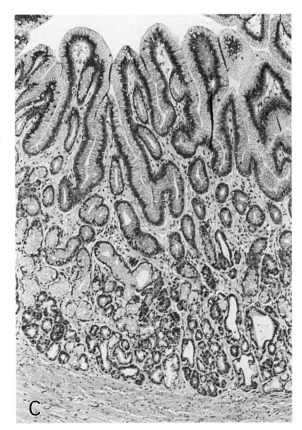

Figure 9-47
INTRAMURAL DEVELOPMENTAL DUPLICATION CYST

A: Within the wall of the gastric antrum are epithelial structures, some of which have lumens and all of which are surrounded by smooth muscle that is continuous with the muscularis propria (out of the field to the left). The mucosa is at the far right.

B: One of the cysts in A. The cyst is lined by gastric type mucosa with superficial pits and deep glands in clusters, and the cyst wall is thick smooth muscle.

C: The cyst mucosa at higher power.

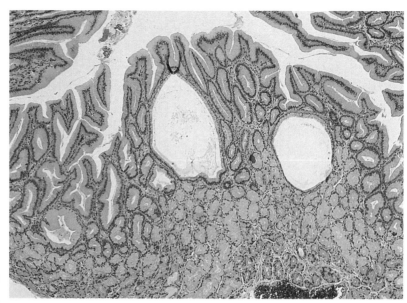

Figure 9-48
MULTIPLE INTRAMURAL
CYSTS OF PIT TYPE

Top: Low-power view of the cysts at all levels of the mucosa.

Bottom: At high power, the cysts are lined by foveolar epithelium with uniform apical mucus vacuoles.

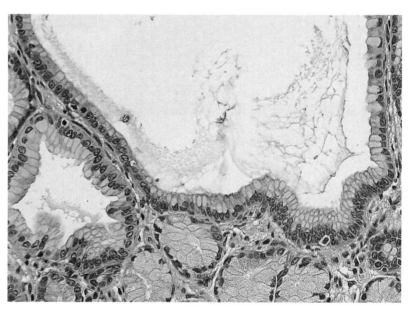

muscle layer and extend into the superficial submucosa, they become enveloped by hypertrophic, disorganized bundles of smooth muscle (fig. 9-50) (147). These muscle bundles are in continuity with the muscularis mucosae. This process has been designated as gastritis cystica profunda to indicate that it is comparable to a somewhat similar colonic alteration, colitis cystica profunda (140). This phenomenon occurs in three settings. First and probably the most common is gastritis cystica profunda at the bases of the hyperplastic-like polyps that develop on the gastric side of a gastroenteric anas-

tomosis. When these polyps contain submucosal cysts, the name changes to *stomal polypoid hypertrophic gastritis, gastritis cystica polyposa,* or *gastric cystic polyposis.* This is discussed in detail in the Hyperplastic Polyp section of this chapter. Second, gastritis cystica profunda occurs deep to the expanded mucosa of Menetrier's disease (see Giant Folds Diseases). In the third setting, which is not disease or syndrome associated, gastritis cystica profunda occurs as plaques of varying sizes, some of which may be so large that they seem to encompass most of the stomach. When the process

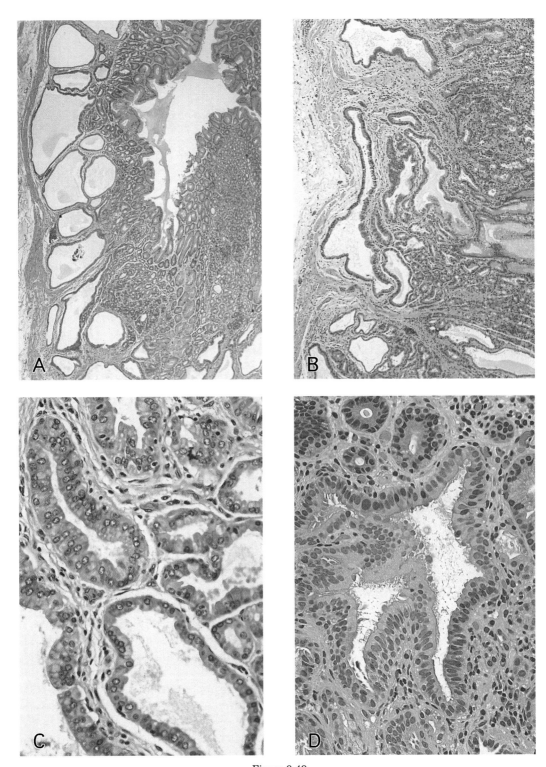

Figure 9-49

MULTIPLE CYSTS, SOME OF WHICH ARE GLAND CYSTS

A: At low power, these cysts are mostly at the mucosal base (at the left) and are round.

B: A low-power view of a different area. Here the cysts are irregularly shaped.

C: At high power, the cells lining some cysts resemble those in antral and body glands, with mucous cells and plump parietal cells.

D: Rare cysts are lined by ciliated epithelium.

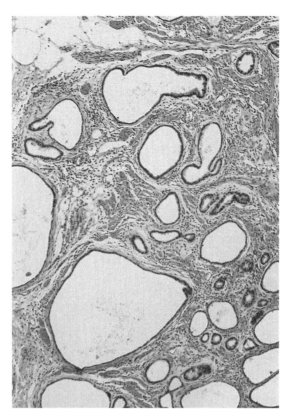 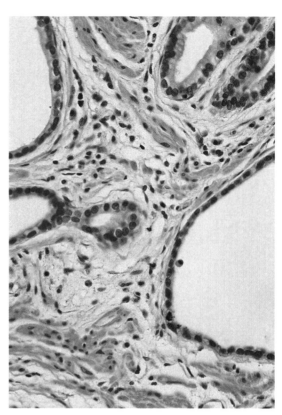

Figure 9-50
SUBMUCOSAL GASTRIC CYSTS (GASTRITIS CYSTICA PROFUNDA)
Left: Superficial submucosa with cysts of different shapes and sizes are separated by a stroma that contains smooth muscle bundles.
Right: In this higher power view, the muscle bundles between the cysts are more easily seen. The cysts are cystic pits with flattened epithelium that have extended from the base of the mucosa into the muscularis mucosae and the superficial submucosa.

is extensive, it can exaggerate the folds pattern to produce a giant folds appearance (142). In some of the earlier descriptions, these foci were looked upon as some type of congenital malformation (145,146,154).

The mechanism that induces this deep pit or gland extension in any of these settings is not known. Experimentally, similar changes have been produced in rats treated with oral aspirin, possibly at the sites of healed ulcers (153). Gastritis cystica-like lesions also occur in monkeys, both spontaneously and secondary to different irritants, such as bezoars, parasites, diesel oil, and other toxins (151). In man, the association with ulcers is not clear, considering that peptic ulcers are common and gastritis cystica at the edges or base of healed ulcers is rare. However, in a Japanese study of 1,500 exhaustively analyzed gastrectomy specimens of all types, the

authors found sporadic deep cysts in 11 percent, but they were found in 15 percent of gastric ulcer cases, indicating that in that population, gastritis cystica profunda and ulcers are frequently associated (157). Its occurrence at gastroenterostomy stomas suggests that mucosal prolapse or ischemia may have some causal relationship to the misplaced mucosal elements, but the dynamics are not understood. Virtually identical changes are seen in the rectum with the solitary rectal ulcer syndrome, also a prolapse disease. One recurring theme in the reported cases and series is the frequent association between gastritis cystica profunda and carcinoma in the overlying mucosa (139,141–143,146). The reasons for this relationship are not known, but chronic ischemia and bile reflux have been suggested, especially since gastritis cystica occurs next to gastroenterostomy stomas where bile reflux is the rule.

## REFERENCES

### Polyps and Polyposis Syndromes

1. Appelman HD. Localized and extensive expansions of the gastric mucosa: mucosal polyps and giant folds. In: Appelman HD, ed. Pathology of the esophagus, stomach, and duodenum. New York: Churchill Livingstone, 1984:79–104.

2. Armstrong CP, King PM, Dixon JM, Macleod IB. The clinical significance of heterotopic pancreas in the gastrointestinal tract. Br J Surg 1981;68:384–7.

3. Bartholomew LG, Dahlin DC, Waugh JM. Intestinal polyposis associated with mucocutaneous melanin pigmentation (Peutz-Jeghers syndrome). Review of the literature and report of six cases with special reference to pathologic findings. Gastroenterology 1957;32:434–51.

4. Berg JW. Histological aspects of the relation between gastric adenomatous polyps and gastric cancer. Cancer 1958;11:1149–55.

5. Bleshman MH, Banner MP, Johnson RC, DeFord JW. The inflammatory esophagogastric polyp and fold. Radiology 1978;128:589–93.

6. Bodily KC, Mowlem A, Hoffman JE. Multiple gastric polyps and parathyroid adenomas. Report of two cases. Am J Surg 1976;132:118–20.

7. Burdick D, Prior JT, Scanlon GT. Peutz-Jeghers syndrome: a clinical-pathological study of a large family with a 10-year follow-up. Cancer 1963;16:854–67.

8. Burke AP, Sobin LH. The pathology of Cronkhite-Canada polyps. A comparison to juvenile polyposis. Am J Surg Pathol 1989;13:940–6.

9. Carfagna G, Pilato FP, Bordi C, Barsotti P, Riva C. Solitary polypoid hamartoma of the oxyntic mucosa of the stomach. Path Res Pract 1987;182:326–30.

10. Carlson GJ, Nivatvongs S, Snover DC. Colorectal polyps in Cowden's disease (multiple hamartoma syndrome). Am J Surg Pathol 1984;8:763–70.

11. Chakravorty RC, Schatzki PF. Gastric cystic polyposis. Am J Dig Dis 1975;20:981–9.

12. Chua CL. Gastric polyps: the case for polypectomy and endoscopic surveillance. J R Coll Surg Edinb 1990;35:163–5.

13. Cochet B, Carrel J, Desbaillets L, Widgren S. Peutz-Jeghers syndrome associated with gastrointestinal carcinoma. Report of two cases in a family. Gut 1979;20:169–75.

14. Daibo M, Itabashi M, Hirota T. Malignant transformation of gastric hyperplastic polyps. Am J Gastroenterol 1987;82:1016–25.

15. Daniel ES, Ludwig SL, Lewin KJ, et al. The Cronkhite-Canada syndrome. An analysis of clinical and pathologic features and therapy in 55 patients. Medicine (Baltimore) 1982;61:293–309.

16. DeBord JR, Majarakis JD, Nyhus LM. An unusual case of heterotopic pancreas of the stomach. Am J Surg 1981;141:269–75.

17. Dekker W. Clinical relevance of gastric and duodenal polyps. Scand J Gastroenterol 1990;25:7–12.

18. Deppisch LM, Rona VT. Gastric epithelial polyps. A 10-year study. J Clin Gastroenterol 1989;11:110–5.

19. Dolan RV, ReMine WH, Dockerty MB. The fate of heterotopic pancreatic tissue. Arch Surg 1974;109:762–5.

20. Elster K. Histologic classification of gastric polyps. In: Morson BC, ed. Pathology of the gastrointestinal tract. Berlin: Springer-Verlag, 1976:77–93.

21. Fabry TL, Frankel A, Waye JD. Gastric polyps. J Clin Gastroenterol 1982;4:23–27.

22. Freeman K, Anthony PP, Miller DS, Warin AP. Cronkhite-Canada syndrome: a new hypothesis. Gut 1985;26:531–6.

23. Glick SN, Teplick SK, Amenta PS. Giant hyperplastic polyps of the gastric remnant simulating carcinoma. Gastrointest Radiol 1990;15:151–5.

24. Goldman DS, Appelman HD. Gastric mucosal polyps. Am J Clin Pathol 1972;58:434–44.

25. Goodman ZD, Yardley JH, Milligan FD. Pathogenesis of colonic polyps in multiple juvenile polyposis: report of a case associated with gastric polyps and carcinoma of the rectum. Cancer 1979;43:1906–13.

25a. Graham JR. Omeprazole and gastric polyposis in humans [Letter]. Gastroenterology 1993;104:1584.

26. Griffel B, Engleberg M, Reiss R, Saba K. Multiple polypoid cystic gastritis in old gastroenteric stoma. Arch Pathol 1974;97:316–8.

27. Haggitt RC, Reid BJ. Hereditary gastrointestinal polyposis syndromes. Am J Surg Pathol 1986;10:871–87.

28. Halbert RE. Peutz-Jeghers syndrome with metastasizing gastric adenocarcinoma. Arch Pathol Lab Med 1982;106:517–20.

29. Hanada M, Takami M, Hirata K, Kishi T, Nakajima T. Hyperplastic fundic gland polyp of the stomach. Acta Pathol Jpn 1983;33:1269–77.

30. Haot J, Berger F, Andre C, Moulinier B, Mainguet P, Lambert R. Lymphocytic gastritis versus varioliform gastritis: a historical series revisited. J Pathol 1989;158:19–22.

31. Hara M, Tsutsumi Y, Watanabe K, Suzuki S, Tani N, Miwa T. Solitary gastric polyps in the fundic gland area. A histochemical study. Acta Pathol Jpn 1985;35:831–40.

32. Harju E. Gastric polyposis and malignancy. Br J Surg 1986;73:532–3.

33. Harju E. Malignancies in the families of patients with gastric polyps. Anticancer Research 1989;9:659–62.

34. Haruma K, Sumii K, Masaharu Y, Watanabe C, Kajiyama G. Gastric mucosa in female patients with fundic gland polyposis. J Clin Gastroenterol 1991;13:565–9.

35. Hattori T. Morphological range of hyperplastic polyps and carcinomas arising in hyperplastic polyps of the stomach. J Clin Pathol 1985;38:622–30.

36. Hickman DM, Frey CF, Carson JW. Adenocarcinoma arising in gastric heterotopic pancreas. West J Med 1981;135:57–62.

37. Iida M, Yao t, Watanabe H, Itoh H, Iwashita A. Fundic gland polyposis in patients without familial adenomatosis coli: its incidence and clinical features. Gastroenterology 1984;86:1437–42.

38. Iida M, Yao T, Itoh H, et al. Natural history of fundic gland polyposis in patients with familial adenomatosis coli/Gardner's syndrome. Gastroenterology 1985;89:1021–5.

39. Iida M, Yao T, Watanabe H, Imamura K, Fuyuno S, Omae T. Spontaneous disappearance of fundic gland polyposis: report of three cases. Gastroenterology 1980;79:725–8.

40. Iishi H, Tatsuta M, Okuda S. Clinicopathological features and natural history of gastric hamartomatous polyps. Dig Dis Sci 1989;34:890–4.

41. Ingram NP, Valentine JC. Unusual gastric polyposis. Br J Clin Pract 1982;36:160–1.

42. Jablokow VR, Aranha GV, Reyes CV. Gastric stomal polypoid hyperplasia: report of four cases. J Surg Oncol 1982;19:106–8.

43. Jacob CO, Batt L, Horovitz A, Scapa E. Myoepithelial hamartoma of Brunner's gland in the stomach [Letter]. Gastrointest Endoscopy 1982;28:48–9.

44. Janunger KG, Domellof L. Gastric polyps and precancerous mucosal changes after partial gastrectomy. Acta Chir Scand 1978;144:293–8.

45. Jarvinen H, Nyberg M, Peltokallio P. Upper gastrointestinal tract polyps in familial adenomatosis coli. Gut 1983;24:333–9.

46. Jenkins D, Stephenson PM, Scott BB. The Cronkhite-Canada syndrome: an ultrastructural study of pathogenesis. J Clin Pathol 1985;38:271–6.

47. Joffe N, Goldman H, Antonioli DA. Recurring hyperplastic gastric polyps following subtotal gastrectomy. AJR Am J Roentgenol 1978;130:301–5.

48. Kamiya T, Morishita T, Asakura H, Miura S, Tsuchiya M. Histoclinical long-standing follow-up study of hyperplastic polyps of the stomach. Am J Gastroenterol 1981;75:275–81.

49. Kaneda M, Yano T, Yamamoto T, et al. Ectopic pancreas in the stomach presenting as an inflammatory abdominal mass. Am J Gastroenterol 1989;84:663–6.

50. Karvonen AL, Sipponen P, Lehtola J, Ruokonen A. Gastric mucosal erosions. An endoscopic, histological, and functional study. Scand J Gastroenterol 1983;18:1051–6.

51. Kilcheski T, Kressel HY, Laufer I, Rogers D. The radiographic appearance of the stomach in Cronkhite-Canada syndrome. Radiology 1981;141:57–60.

52. Kilman WJ, Berk RN. The spectrum of radiographic features of aberrant pancreatic rests involving the stomach. Radiology 1977;123:291–6.

53. Koch HK, Lesch R, Cremer M, Oehlert W. Polyps and polypoid foveolar hyperplasia in gastric biopsy specimens and their precancerous prevalence. Front Gastrointest Res 1979;4:183–91.

54. Koga S, Watanabe H, Enjoji M. Stomal polypoid hypertrophic gastritis: a polypoid gastric lesion at gastroenterostomy site. Cancer 1979;43:647–57.

55. Kuwano H, Takano H, Sugimachi K. Solitary Peutz-Jeghers type polyp of the stomach in the absence of familial polyposis coli in a teenage boy. Endoscopy 1989;21:188–90.

56. Kyle J. Gastric carcinoma in Peutz-Jeghers syndrome. Scott Med J 1984;29:187–91.

57. Lai EC, Tompkins RK. Heterotopic pancreas. Review of a 26 year experience. Am J Surg 1986;151:697–700.

58. Lasser A, Koufman WB. Adenomyoma of the stomach. Am J Dig Dis 1977;22:965–9.

59. Laxen F, Kekki M, Sipponen P, Siurala M. The gastric mucosa in stomachs with polyps: morphologic and dynamic evaluation. Scand J Gastroenterol 1983;18:503–11.

60. Laxen F, Sipponen P, Ihamaki T, Hakkiluoto A, Dortscheva Z. Gastric polyps: their morphological and endoscopical characteristics and relation to gastric carcinoma. Acta Path Microbiol Immunol Scand 1982;90:221–8.

61. Lee RG, Burt RW. The histopathology of fundic gland polyps of the stomach. Am J Clin Pathol 1986;86:498–503.

62. Lindley PR, Appelman HD. Is there a preferred classification scheme for endoscopic gastric polyps? [Abstract] Mod Pathol 1993;6:48A.

63. Littler ER, Gleibermann E. Gastritis cystica polyposa (gastric mucosal prolapse at gastroenterostomy site, with cystic and infiltrative epithelial hyperplasia). Cancer 1972;29:205–9.

64. Malhotra R, Sheffield A. Cronkhite-Canada syndrome associated with colon carcinoma and adenomatous changes in C-C polyps. Am J Gastroenterol 1988;83:772–6.

65. Marcheggiano A, Iannoni C, Agnello M, Paoluzi P, Pallone F. Solitary juvenile polyp of the stomach [Letter]. Hum Pathol 1986;17:1077–8.

66. Ming SC. Epithelial polyps of the stomach. In: Ming SC, Goldman H, eds. Pathology of the gastrointestinal tract. Philadelphia: WB Saunders, 1992:547–69.

67. Ming SC, Goldman H. Gastric polyps. A histogenetic classification and its relation to carcinoma. Cancer 1965;18:721–6.

68. Monaco AP, Roth SI, Castleman B, Welch CE. Adenomatous polyps of the stomach. A clinical and pathological study of 153 cases. Cancer 1962;15:456–67.

69. Mori K, Shinya H, Wolff WI. Polypoid reparative mucosal proliferation at the site of a healed gastric ulcer: sequential gastroscopic, radiological, and histological observations. Gastroenterology 1971;61:523–9.

70. Muller-Lissner SA, Weibecke B. Investigations on hyperplasiogenous gastric polyps by partial reconstruction. Path Res Pract 1982;174:368–78.

71. Muto T, Oota K. Polypogenesis of gastric mucosa. Gann 1970;61:435–42.

72. Nakamura T, Nakano GI. Histopathological classification and malignant change in gastric polyps. J Clin Pathol 1985;38:754–64.

73. Nakano H, Persson B, Slezak P. Study of the gastric mucosal background in patients with gastric polyps. Gastrointest Endosc 1990;36:39–42.

74. Nishiura M, Hirota T, Itabashi M, Ushio K, Yamada T, Oguro Y. A clinical and histopathological study of gastric polyps in familial polyposis coli. Am J Gastroenterol 1984;79:98–103.

75. Niv Y, Bat L. Gastric polyps—a clinical study. Isr J Med Sci 1985;21:841–4.

75a. Odze R, Gallinger S, So K, Antonioli D. Immunohistochemical expression of transforming growth factor alpha (TGF-alpha) and epidermal growth factor receptor (EGF-R) in gastric fundic gland polyps (FGP) [Abstract]. Mod Pathol 1993;6:50A.

76. Rabin MS, Bremner CG, Botha JR. The reflux gastroesophageal polyp. Am J Gastroenterol 1980;73:451–3.

77. Rohrmann CA Jr, Delaney JH Jr, Protell RL. Heterotopic pancreas diagnosed by cannulation and duct study. AJR Am J Roentgenol 1977;128:1044–5.

78. Rosch W. Epidemiology, pathogenesis, diagnosis and treatment of benign gastric tumours. Front Gastrointest Res 1980;6:167–84.

79. Roseau G, Ducreux M, Molas G, et al. Les polypes gastriques epitheliaux. Dans une serie de 13,000 fibroscopies gastriques. Presse Med 1990;19:650–4.

80. Russell DM, Bhathal PS, St John DJ. Complete remission in Cronkhite-Canada syndrome. Gastroenterology 1983;85:180–5.

81. Sachatello CR, Pickren JW, Grace JT Jr. Generalized juvenile gastrointestinal polyposis. A hereditary syndrome. Gastroenterology 1970;58:699–708.

82. Sakurada H, Ishimori A, Arakawa H, et al. Comparative study on gastric secretory function between benign gastric polyp and elevated type of early stomach cancer with special reference to histologic findings of gastric mucosa. Tohoku J Exp Med 1976;11:39–43.

83. Santiago-Gallo R, Rodriguez-Hernandez H, Elizondo-Rivera J. Polypos gastricos. Experiencia en la Departamento de Endoscopia del Instituto Nacional de la Nutricion Salvador Zubiran. Rev Gastroenterol Mex 1990;55:51–4.

84. Savage A, Jones S. Histological appearances of the gastric mucosa 15-27 years after partial gastrectomy. J Clin Pathol 1979;32:179–86.

85. Seifert E, Gail K, Weismuller J. Gastric polypectomy. Long-term results (survey of 23 centres in Germany). Endoscopy 1983;15:8–11.

86. Seruca R, Carneiro F, Castedo S, David L, Lopes C, Sobrinho-Simoes M. Familial gastric polyposis revisited. Autosomal dominant inheritance confirmed. Cancer Genet Cytogenet 1991;53:97–100.

87. Shemesh E, Czerniak A, Pines A, Bat L. Is there an association between gastric polyps and colonic neoplasms? Digestion 1989;42:212–6.

88. Shepherd NA, Bussey HJ, Jass JR. Epithelial misplacement in Peutz-Jeghers polyps. A diagnostic pitfall. Am J Surg Pathol 1987;11:743–9.

89. Sipponen P, Laxen F, Seppala K. Cystic "hamartomatous" gastric polyps: a disorder of oxyntic glands. Histopathology 1983;7:729–37.

90. Snover DC. Benign epithelial polyps of the stomach. Pathol Annu 1985;20:303–29.

91. Stafford EM, Imai WK. Gastroesophageal polyp diagnosed in an adolescent presenting with epigastric pain. J Adolesc Health Care 1987;8:441–4

92. Stemper TJ, Kent TH, Summers RW. Juvenile polyposis and gastrointestinal carcinoma. A study of a kindred. Ann Int Med 1975;83:639–46.

93. Styles RA, Gibb SP, Tarshis A, Silverman ML, Scholz FJ. Esophagogastric polyps: radiographic and endoscopic findings. Radiology 1985;154:307–11.

94. Tatsuta M, Okuda S, Tamura H, Taniguchi H. Gastric hamartomatous polyps in the absence of familial polyposis coli. Cancer 1980;45:818–23.

95. Taylor AJ, Dodds WJ, Stewart ET. Alimentary tract lesions in Cowden's disease. Br J Radiol 1989;62:890–2.

96. Tomasulo J. Gastric polyps. Histologic types and their relationship to gastric carcinoma. Cancer 1971;27:1346–55.

97. Ueno K, Oshiba S, Yamagata S, Mochizuki F, Kitagawa M, Hisamichi S. Histo-clinical classification and follow-up study of gastric polyp. Tohoku J Exp Med 1976;118:23–38.

98. Utsunomiya J, Gocho H, Miyanaga T, Hamaguchi E, Kashimure A. Peutz-Jeghers syndrome: its natural course and management. Johns Hopkins Med J 1975;136:71–82.

99. Watanabe A, Nagashima H, Motoi M, Ogawa K. Familial juvenile polyposis of the stomach. Gastroenterology 1979;77:148–51.

100. Watanabe H, Enjoji M, Yao T, Ohsato K. Gastric lesions in familial adenomatosis coli. Their incidence and histologic analysis. Hum Pathol 1978;9:269–83.

101. Watanabe H, Jass JR, Sobin LH. Histological typing of oesophageal and gastric tumours. Berlin: Springer-Verlag, 1990:34–8.

102. Wauters GV, Ferrell L, Ostroff JW, Heyman MB. Hyperplastic gastric polyps associated with persistent Helicobacter pylori infection and active gastritis. Am J Gastroenterol 1990;85:1395–7.

103. Weinstock JV, Kawanishi H. Gastrointestinal polyposis with orocutaneous hamartomas (Cowden's disease). Gastroenterology 1978;74:890–5.

104. Wolber R, Owen D, DelBuono L, Appelman H, Freeman H. Lymphocytic gastritis in patients with celiac sprue or spruelike intestinal disease. Gastroenterology 1990;98:310–5.

105. Yamagiwa H, Ishihara A, Sekoguchi T, Matsuzaki O. Heterotopic pancreas in surgically resected stomach. Gastroenterol Jpn 1977;12:380–6.

## Giant Folds

106. Appelman HD. Localized and extensive expansions of the gastric mucosa: mucosal polyps and giant folds. In: Appelman HD, ed. Pathology of the esophagus, stomach, and duodenum. New York: Churchill Livingstone, 1984:104–19.

107. Appelman HD. Menetrier's disease. In: Haggitt RC, Appelman HD, Riddell RH, eds. Diseases of the gastrointestinal tract. Chicago: ASCP Press, 1989:25–30.

108. Berenson MM, Sannella J, Freston JW. Menetrier's disease. Serial morphological, secretory, and serological observations. Gastroenterology 1976;70:257–63.

109. Blackstone MO. Endoscopic interpretation. Normal and pathologic appearances of the gastrointestinal tract. New York: Raven Press, 1984:100–14.

109a. Bluth RF, Carpenter HA, Pittelkow MR, et al. Immunolocalization of transforming growth factor-α in normal and diseased human gastric mucosa. Hum Pathol 1995;26:1333–40.

110. Brown WG, Van Pelt MW. Hypertrophic hyposecretory gastropathy. A case report. Cancer 1969;23:1163–70.

111. Chouraqui JP, Roy CC, Brochu RP, Gregoire H, Morin CL, Weber AM. Menetrier's disease in children: report of a patient and review of sixteen other cases. Gastroenterology 1981;80:1042–7.

112. Cotton PB, Williams CB. Practical gastrointestinal endoscopy. Oxford: Blackwell Scientific, 1990:45.

113. Crampton JR, Hunter JO, Neale G, Wight DG. Chronic lymphocytic gastritis and protein losing gastropathy. Gut 1989;30:71–4.

114. Creutzfeldt W, Arnold R, Creutzfeldt C, Track NS. Pathomorphologic, biochemical, and diagnostic aspects of gastrinomas (Zollinger-Ellison syndrome). Hum Pathol 1975;6:47–76.

115. Daniel ES, Ludwig SL, Lewin KJ, Ruprecht RM, Rajacich GM, Schwabe AD. The Cronkhite-Canada syndrome. An analysis of clinical and pathological features and therapy in 55 patients. Medicine (Baltimore) 1982;61:293–309.

116. Fegan C, Sunter JP, Miller IA. Menetrier's disease complicated by the development of the Zollinger-Ellison syndrome. Br J Surg 1985;72:929–30.

117. Fieber SS, Rickert RR. Hyperplastic gastropathy. Analysis of 50 selected cases from 1955-1980. Am J Gastroenterol 1981;76:321–9.

118. Haot J, Bogomoletz WV, Jouret A, Mainguet P. Menetrier's disease with lymphocytic gastritis: an unusual association with possible pathogenic implications. Hum Pathol 1991;22:379–86.

119. Komorowski RA, Caya JG. Hyperplastic gastropathy. Clinicopathologic correlation. Am J Surg Pathol 1991;15:577–85.

120. Komorowski RA, Caya JG, Geenen JE. The morphologic spectrum of large gastric folds: utility of the snare biopsy. Gastrointest Endosc 1986;32:190–2.

121. Mosnier JF, Flejou JF, Amouyal G, Molas G, Henin D, Potet F. Hypertrophic gastropathy with gastric adenocarcinoma: Menetrier's disease and lymphocytic gastritis? Gut 1991;32:1565–7.

122. Overholt BF, Jeffries GH. Hypertrophic, hypersecretory protein-losing gastropathy. Gastroenterology 1970;56:80–7.

123. Searcy RM, Malagelada JR. Menetrier's disease and idiopathic hypertrophic gastropathy. Ann Int Med 1984;100:565–70.

124. Solcia E, Capella C, Fiocca R, Rindi G, Rosai J. Gastric argyrophil carcinoidosis in patients with Zollinger-Ellison syndrome due to type I multiple endocrine neoplasia. A newly recognized association. Am J Surg Pathol 1990;14:503–13.

125. Stillman FE, Sieber O, Manthel U, Pinnas J. Transient protein-losing enteropathy and enlarged gastric rugae in childhood. Am J Dis Child 1981;135:29–33.

126. Sundt TM III, Compton CC, Malt RA. Menetrier's disease. A trivalent gastropathy. Ann Surg 1988;208:694–701.

127. Takagi H, Jhappan C, Sharp R, Merlino G. Hypertrophic gastropathy resembling Menetrier's disease in transgenic mice overexpressing transforming growth factor alpha in the stomach. J Clin Invest 1992;90:1161–7.

128. Tan DT, Stempien SJ, Dagradi AE. The clinical spectrum of hypertrophic hypersecretory gastropathy. Report of 50 patients. Gastrointest Endosc 1971;18:69–73.

129. Vendelboe M, Jaspersen J. Hypertrophic protein-losing gastritis (Menetrier's disease) treated with cimetidine. Acta Med Scand 1981;209:125–7.

130. Walker FB IV. Spontaneous remission in hypertrophic gastropathy (Menetrier's disease). South Med J 1981;74:1273–6.

131. Wolber RA, Owen DA, Anderson FH, Freeman HJ. Lymphocytic gastritis and giant gastric folds associated with gastrointestinal protein loss. Mod Pathol 1991;4:13–5.

132. Wolfsen HC, Carpenter HA, Talley NJ. Menetrier's disease: a form of hypertrophic gastropathy or gastritis? Gastroenterology 1993;104:1310–19.

133. Wood GM, Bates C, Brown RC, Losowsky MS. Intramucosal carcinoma of the gastric antrum complicating Menetrier's disease. J Clin Pathol 1983;36:1071–5.

134. Yeaton P, Frierson HF Jr. Octreotide reduces enteral protein losses in Menetrier's disease. Am J Gastroenterol 1993;88:95–8.

### Cysts

135. Coit DG, Mies C. Adenocarcinoma arising within a gastric duplication cyst. J Surg Oncol 1992;50:274–7.

136. Dehner LP. Pediatric surgical pathology. Baltimore: Williams & Wilkins, 1987:339.

137. Floros D, Dosios T, Gourtsoyiannis N, Vyssoulis C. Gastric duplication associated with adenomyoma. J Surg Oncol 1982;19:98–100.

138. Fraga S, Helwig EB, Rosen SH. Bronchogenic cysts in the skin and subcutaneous tissue. Am J Clin Pathol 1971;56:230–8.

139. Franzin G, Musola R, Zamboni G, Manfrini C. Gastritis cystica polyposa: a possible precancerous lesion. Tumori 1985;71:13–18.

140. Franzin G, Novelli P. Gastritis cystica profunda. Histopathology 1981; 5:535–47.

141. Honore LH, Lewis AS, O'Hara KE. Gastritis glandularis et cystica profunda. A report of three cases with discussion of etiology and pathogenesis. Dig Dis Sci 1979;24:48–52.

142. Ignatius JA, Armstrong CD, Eversole SL. Case reports. Multiple diffuse cystic disease of the stomach in association with carcinoma. Gastroenterology 1970;59:610–4.

143. Iwanaga T. Koyoma H, Takahashi Y, Taniguchi H, Wada A. Diffuse submucosal cysts and carcinoma of the stomach. Cancer 1975;36:606–14.

144. Kato Y, Sugano H, Rubio CA. Classification of intramucosal cysts of the stomach. Histopathology 1983;7:931–8.

145. Oberman HA, Lodmell JG, Sower ND. Diffuse heterotopic cystic malformation of the stomach. N Engl J Med 1963;269:909–11.

146. Pillay I, Petrelli M. Diffuse cystic glandular malformation of the stomach associated with adenocarcinoma. Case report and review of the literature. Cancer 1976;38:915–20.

147. Rubio CA. Intramucosal gastric cysts simulating submucosal cysts. Path Res Pract 1989;184:418–21.

148. Rubio CA, Hirota T, Itabashi M. The intramucosal cysts of the stomach. III. In Japanese subjects with gastric or duodenal ulcers. Scand J Gastroenterol 1983;18:125–8.

149. Rubio CA, Kato Y, Kitagawa T, Sugano H, Grimelius L. Intramucosal cysts of the stomach. VIII: Histochemical studies. APMIS 1988;96:627–34.

150. Rubio CA, Ohman U. The intramucosal cysts of the stomach. I. In Swedish subjects with gastric or duodenal ulcers. Acta Pathol Microbiol Immunol Scand 1982;90:363–6.

151. Scott TM. Simian gastropathy with submucosal glands and cysts. Arch Pathol 1973;96:403–8.

152. Shireman PK. Intramural cyst of the stomach. Hum Pathol 1987;18:857–8.

153. St John DJ, Yoemans ND, Bourne CA, de Boer WG. Aspirin-induced glandular dysplasia of the stomach. Arch Pathol Lab Med 1977;101:44–8.

154. Tchertkoff V, Wagner BM. Diffuse cystic malformation of stomach. NY State J Med 1966;66:2049–52.

155. Ueda D, Taketazu M, Itoh S, Azuma H, Oshima H. A case of gastric duplication cyst with aberrant pancreas. Pediatr Radiol 1991;21:379–80.

156. Wieczorek RL, Seidman I, Ransom JH, Ruoff M. Congenital duplication of the stomach: case report and review of the English literature. Am J Gastroenterol 1984;79:597–602.

157. Yamagiwa H, Matsuzaki O, Ishihara A, Yoshimura H. Heterotopic gastric glands in the submucosa of the stomach. Acta Path Jpn 1979;29:347–50.

158. Zhu FG, Deng XJ, Cheng NJ. Intramucosal cysts in gastric mucosa adjacent to carcinoma and peptic ulcer: a histochemical study. Histopathology 1987;631–8.

# 10

# ADENOMAS

**Definition.** An adenoma is defined by the World Health Organization (WHO) as "a circumscribed benign neoplasm composed of tubular and/or villous structures lined by dysplastic epithelium" (28). This definition has both cytologic (dysplasia) and architectural (tubular and villous) components. In this chapter, the designation adenoma is limited to dysplasias of all grades of severity and of all architectural patterns that are circumscribed or localized and polypoid, meaning that they are elevated above the surrounding flat mucosa. The "depressed adenoma" recently described in several Japanese studies is not discussed here, since it is not polypoid but is actually a focus that is thinner than the surrounding flat mucosa (11,19,29). However, it is clearly a form of dysplasia.

The cytologic features of all gastric dysplasias are the same, whether they are elevated, flat, or depressed. As a result, the concept of adenoma/dysplasia as a single entity has emerged. This is discussed in greater detail in chapter 11 on Carcinomas of the Stomach.

Adenomas are uncommon neoplasms in the stomach, in contrast to the colon where they are frequent. However, there is considerable variation in frequency of gastric adenomas, depending upon the population analyzed: they are much more common in Japanese series than in series reported from Western countries (4).

Adenomas often arise in the stomachs of patients with familial adenomatous polyposis (FAP), but more commonly, they arise sporadically, especially in one of the forms of chronic atrophic gastritis, usually the nonimmunologic, multifocal type that is so common in populations at high risk for gastric cancer. No matter the background, adenomas are almost always antral; they rarely arise in the body mucosa, even when it is atrophic.

**Clinical Features.** Adenomas, much like other gastric polyps, produce no symptoms, so that they are accidental findings encountered during endoscopic procedures performed for other symptomatic problems. The frequency of sporadic adenomas probably increases with age,

and may be a function of the age of the population that has endoscopic examinations. In contrast, the FAP-associated adenomas are likely to be detected when the patients are younger because of widespread use of upper endoscopy early in the course of FAP to detect duodenal as well as gastric adenomas.

**Gross Findings.** Gastric adenomas have the same gross features as do their colonic counterparts, but in different proportions. Nodules connected to the mucosa by stalks, that is, pedunculated adenomas, are rare. Some are nodules without stalks that seem to adhere to the mucosal surface. Others are plaque-like mucosal thickenings or sessile adenomas. In one report from Japan, the authors were able to recognize macroscopic or gross types of gastric adenoma which corresponded to types of early gastric carcinoma, including sessile, pedunculated, flat, elevated, and depressed forms (8). In fact, it may be very difficult on gross examination alone to distinguish an adenoma from one of the protruding types of early gastric cancer (26). In the past, adenomas were thought to be the largest gastric polyps, but this conclusion was based upon resection and autopsy specimens (17,24). Since neither adenomas nor any other kind of polyps produce symptoms and since all are found incidentally, endoscopically there is really no size difference between them, particularly hyperplastic polyps. In fact, adenomas that occur in patients with FAP are usually smaller than those that occur sporadically in older adults, since patients with newly diagnosed FAP, who often are teenagers, have upper endoscopy to detect gastric and duodenal adenomas when they are small. In perhaps two thirds of patients, especially those with sporadic adenomas, the lesions are solitary.

**Microscopic Findings.** Many gastric adenomas, regardless of whether they are FAP-associated or sporadic, seem to arise within the surface and superficial pit epithelia, much like their counterparts in the colon (fig. 10-1). It is possible that some arise deeper in the mucosa, perhaps from the generative zone in the gastric neck

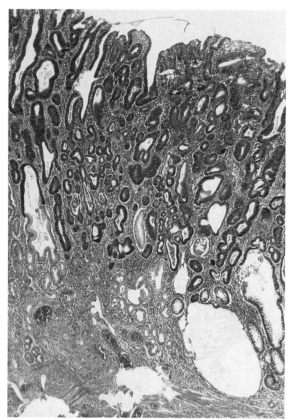

Figure 10-1
SMALL SESSILE TUBULAR ADENOMA
The superficial half of the mucosa is the adenoma, with its darkly staining dysplastic epithelium. The basal half is residual antral mucosa with a few cystic tubules. This adenoma was only slightly elevated above the surrounding nondysplastic mucosa.

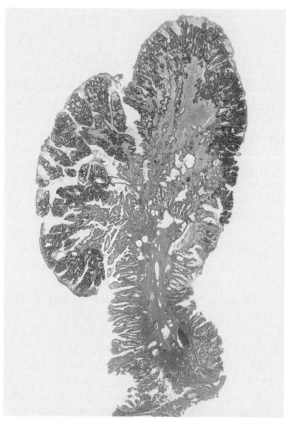

Figure 10-2
PEDUNCULATED TUBULOVILLOUS ADENOMA
The stalk is at the bottom. The darkly staining superficial adenomatous tubules are in sharp contrast to the residual, nondysplastic mucosa at the base, in which there are scattered cysts.

region. However, we are not aware of any published studies that have analyzed the mucosal dynamics of gastric adenomas, comparable to such studies of colonic adenomas. Nevertheless, in small adenomas, the abnormal neoplastic epithelium is usually confined to the superficial mucosa (17). Often, beneath the adenomatous epithelium, the mid-mucosa contains cysts which are cystic pits, perhaps trapped and obstructed by the dysplastic tubules above (figs. 10-1, 10-2).

Nakamura (20) divided all gastric polyps into four types, two of which were non-neoplastic and included hyperplastic polyps and two of which were adenomas. One type of adenoma had tubules clustered near the surface, and cystic pits were situated below them. The other type included the larger, sessile or pedunculated, often

lobulated adenomas. However, this classification, based upon low-power microscopic characteristics, is rarely used except in some studies from Japan. As in the colon, the most commonly used architectural classification and the one proposed by the WHO includes tubular, tubulovillous, and villous patterns (28). The tubular pattern has clusters of adenomatous tubules or pits which appear as rounded or oval structures in two-dimensional study (figs. 10-3, 10-4). These may vary in size and shape, and bud or branch. The villous pattern has elongated cores of attenuated lamina propria covered by dysplastic epithelium (fig. 10-5). In gastric villous adenomas, in contrast to those in the colon, the villi often have a papillary modification in which multiple branches arise from the surface villi (fig. 10-6).

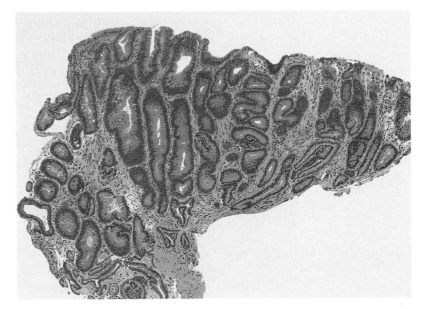

Figure 10-3
SMALL SESSILE
TUBULAR ADENOMA
Small sessile tubular adenoma in which many of the tubules extend from surface to base and appear elongated.

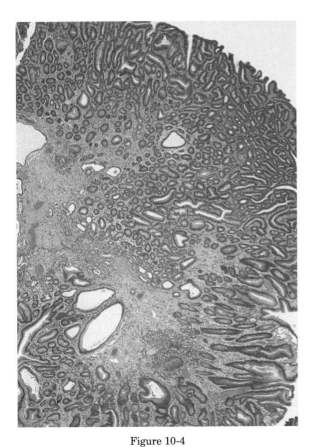

Figure 10-4
LARGE TUBULAR ADENOMA
In contrast to figure 10-3, the tubules here appear mainly as cross sectional profiles.

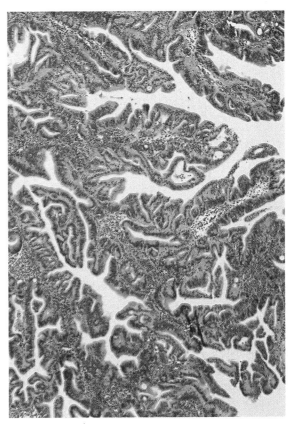

Figure 10-5
VILLOUS ADENOMA
The mucosa has been converted into a series of parallel elongated structures or villi that are covered by dysplastic epithelium.

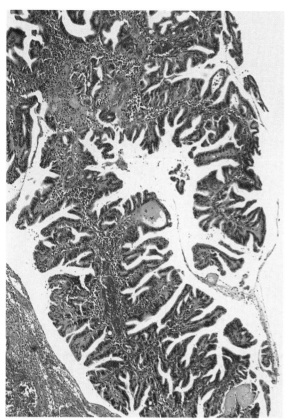

Figure 10-6
VILLOUS ADENOMA
This villous adenoma has a papillary surface with multiple branches extending from each villus.

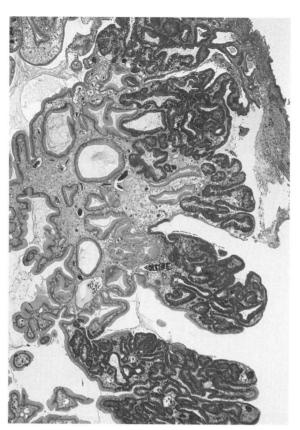

Figure 10-7
TUBULOVILLOUS ADENOMA
Part of the adenoma is composed of cross sections of tubular structures, while part of the surface, especially on the right, is covered by villi.

As a result, the villous pattern has been referred to as the papillary pattern in some published series. The tubulovillous adenoma has a mixture of patterns, with each pattern contributing at least 20 percent of the total (fig. 10-7) (28). There is an imperfect correlation between microscopic and gross features. Pure tubular adenomas tend to be broad sessile lesions, while villous and tubulovillous adenomas are more likely to be dome shaped or pedunculated (12). This is different from the colon where pure tubular adenomas are the most common pedunculated adenomas, while predominantly villous adenomas are usually sessile.

Also in contrast to the colon, in which all adenomatous epithelium caricatures colonic epithelium, in the stomach, there are probably at least two separate types of dysplastic epithelium which appear in adenomas and in the flat mucosa (6,8,18,20). The most common, the intesti-

nal type, is composed of dysplastic-metaplastic intestinal epithelial cells, including the dominant undifferentiated or primitive cell, along with a group of differentiated cells such as goblet cells, Paneth cells, possibly absorptive cells, and endocrine cells (figs. 10-8, 10-9). This dysplastic epithelium is indistinguishable from that which occurs in colonic adenomas. The second type, the gastric type, is composed of dysplastic cells resembling gastric foveolar and surface cells with apical neutral mucin vacuoles (figs. 10-10, 10-11). Some adenomas have both types of dysplasia. Actually, there is a third type with a mix of dysplastic intestinal type goblet cells and dysplastic gastric type surface cells. Perhaps this latter epithelium is the dysplastic equivalent of incomplete intestinal metaplasia. The intestinal type has the colonic-style tubular, villous, and tubulovillous growth patterns, while the gastric

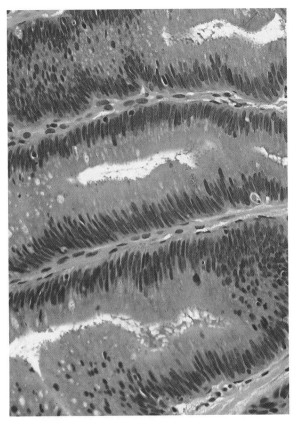

Figure 10-8
INTESTINAL TYPE DYSPLASIA, LOW GRADE

This epithelium is identical to that in many colorectal adenomas. The cells are elongated, as are their nuclei. The nuclei are stratified, but the stratification is mostly confined to the basal half of the cells. There is no nuclear pleomorphism. Small mucus vacuoles within dysplastic goblet cells are present in the luminal cytoplasm of many cells.

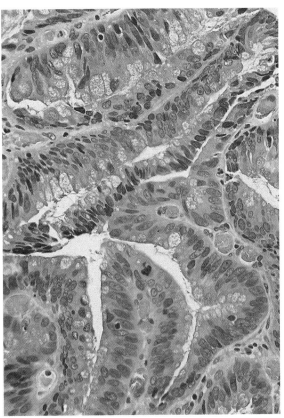

Figure 10-9
INTESTINAL TYPE DYSPLASIA, HIGH GRADE

The cells resemble those in figure 10-8, but the nuclei are larger and take up more of the cell volume, nuclear stratification is often full thickness, and there are scattered mitoses.

type has tubular and villous patterns, the latter with the papillary modification. Probably, there are no significant differences between these different types of dysplastic epithelia in terms of cancer association and the background mucosa from which they originate. In FAP patients, the adenomas may all be of the intestinal type.

The dysplasias, regardless of type, are of all grades of severity, ranging from the lowest grade which closely caricatures normal or metaplastic epithelium to the highest grade which is so disorganized and anaplastic that it is essentially carcinomatous (fig. 10-12). There are subtle morphologic differences, depending upon which type of dysplasia is present in the adenoma. In the lower grades of intestinal dysplasia, the cells

and their nuclei are elongated but uniform; the nuclei are larger than normal and take up more of the cytoplasmic volume; the nuclei are stratified, but the stratification is generally not higher than the basal half of the cells; mitoses are increased, but usually not abnormal; and the nuclei are hyperchromatic, but not pleomorphic, and their nucleoli are small (figs. 10-8, 10-9). Goblet cells are usually randomly dispersed, and there may be scattered Paneth cells and endocrine cells. Architecturally, low-grade dysplasias have tubules of relatively uniform shape and size. With progressively higher grades, the nuclei become more pleomorphic, the nucleoli larger, stratification closer to full-thickness, mitoses more irregular and more numerous, and there is more variation in cell size and shape. Goblet cells are progressively lost as are Paneth cells and endocrine cells,

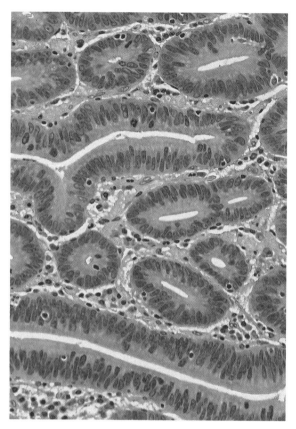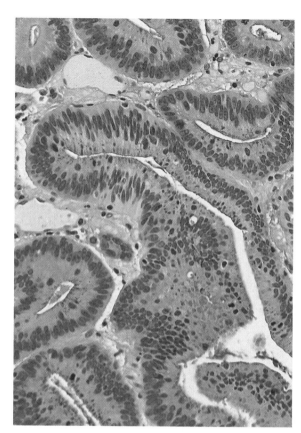

Figure 10-10
GASTRIC OR FOVEOLAR CELL TYPE DYSPLASIA, LOW GRADE

Left: The cells are columnar, but less so than in the intestinal type in figure 10-8. Many cells contain apical mucin vacuoles. The nuclei are oval to round, and many have small nuclei. Nuclear stratification is limited to the basal half of the epithelium. (Hematoxylin and eosin stain)

Right: Many of the cells have small apical neutral mucin vacuoles that stain red with periodic acid–Schiff, but there is no staining with Alcian blue. (Alcian blue/PAS stain)

so that the whole cell population may be undifferentiated columnar cells with basophilic cytoplasm (12). In addition, there is progressive architectural disorganization with the formation of peculiarly shaped tubular structures, great variation in tubule size, compromise of the lamina propria so that the tubules are adjacent to one another, budding of tubules, and proliferation of dysplastic epithelial bridges across the tubular lumens resulting in cribriform foci.

The gastric type dysplasia has nuclei that are commonly round and basal, rather than elongated. In low-grade gastric dysplasia, the cells often have apical neutral mucin droplets (figs. 10-10, 10-11). With higher grades, these droplets are gradually lost, resulting in a population of columnar to cuboidal cells with dark eosinophilic cytoplasm. The

nuclei enlarge, become more hyperchromatic and more pleomorphic, and nucleoli appear.

As in the colon, in general, the more villous the adenoma and the larger its diameter, the higher the grade of dysplasia and the more likely there will be the highest dysplastic grade or carcinomatous epithelium (5,8,12). This applies no matter the type of dysplasia.

A few morphologic peculiarities occur in rare adenomas. An adenoma in which 95 percent of the cells were dysplastic Paneth cells has been reported (10) as has another adenoma in which a tiny carcinoid tumor arose (22).

**Differential Diagnosis.** Gastric adenomas, like other gastric polyps, are detected during endoscopic examinations. Smaller lesions are removed in total, while larger ones are biopsied. Only

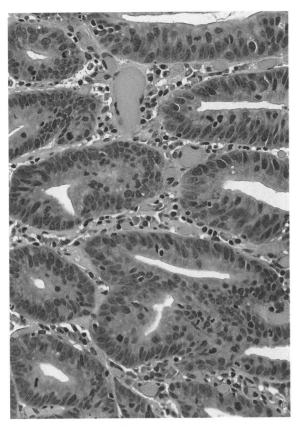

Figure 10-11
GASTRIC OR FOVEOLAR CELL TYPE
DYSPLASIA, HIGH GRADE

The cells resemble those in figure 10-9, but the nuclei are larger in relation to the cytoplasmic volume, stratification is often full thickness, and mitoses are common.

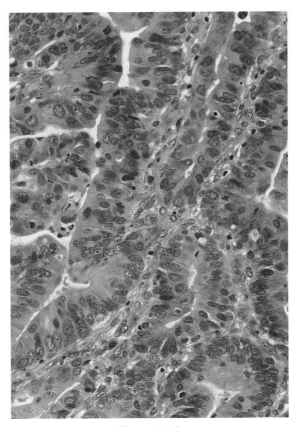

Figure 10-12
HIGH-GRADE DYSPLASIA

The nuclei are stratified through the full thickness, they vary in size and shape, and there are irregular thickenings of the epithelium. When the epithelium looks like this, it is impossible to determine the type of dysplasia.

the endoscopist knows the size for certain. The diagnosis depends upon the finding of dysplastic epithelium in the polyp. As with colonic adenomas, the architectural subtype and the presence of high-grade dysplasia should be identified as part of the pathologic diagnosis, because of the associations among architecture, grade of dysplasia, and invasive carcinoma. Occasional adenomas, particularly large ones, contain invasive carcinoma, and this may be sampled by the biopsy procedure. As a corollary, a biopsy of a polypoid invasive carcinoma can contain some dysplastic mucosa from the margin with a tubular, villous, or mixed pattern: this may be an adenoma within which the carcinoma arose. In our experience, the surrounding mucosa is rarely biopsied. The differential diagnosis mostly consists of the various forms of pit hyper-

plasia and regeneration that can resemble low-grade dysplasia (fig. 10-13), such as chemical gastropathy which has pit hyperplasia as one of its components. The resultant features of elongated pits lined by cuboidal epithelium with large, hyperchromatic nuclei and occasional mitoses, which sometimes extends onto the surface, mimics low-grade dysplasia. Since this usually occurs in flat mucosa, and adenomas are polyps of some form or other, this differential diagnosis is an issue only in the case of flat dysplasias. However, another polyp that can be confused with an adenoma on histologic grounds is the hyperplastic polyp that contains a large component of proliferating foveolar epithelium. Some of these are impossible to differentiate from adenomas with pit or foveolar cell dysplasia. Since both polyps can have deep cystic tubules, telling them

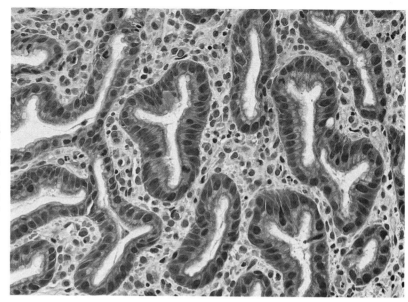

Figure 10-13
REGENERATIVE FOVEOLAR
EPITHELIUM RESEMBLING
LOW-GRADE
FOVEOLAR CELL DYSPLASIA
Much of the epithelium along these tubules have enlarged nuclei, many of which are vesicular and some of which are stratified. Apical mucus vacuoles are present throughout, but they are much smaller than normal. This is a reactive pit epithelium in a patient with chemical gastropathy, such as occurs with bile reflux.

apart based upon architecture is not always possible. Furthermore, rare hyperplastic polyps have foci of true dysplasia. In such situations, diagnostic honesty is the best policy, and the patient should be treated as if he had an adenoma.

**Natural History and the Importance of Adenomas as Cancer Precursors.** Carcinomatous foci occasionally develop in adenomas (fig. 10-14). In contrast to the colon, where adenomas are considered to be the major precursor of ordinary adenocarcinoma, adenomas, as specific elevated or polypoid dysplastic lesions, have never been implicated as common precursors of invasive gastric carcinoma, although flat dysplasias have. It is conceivable that this situation has resulted, at least in part, because most gastric carcinomas in Western populations are advanced tumors when they are first detected, and in such cases, any precursor adenoma might have been obliterated or overgrown by the carcinoma. If this assumption is valid, then adenomas should comprise a significant precursor population for early gastric carcinomas, that group of small tumors which have invaded no deeper than the submucosa. In a review of 1,900 early gastric cancers at the National Cancer Center Hospital in Tokyo, only 47 or 2.5 percent were thought to arise from adenomas (7). It is now accepted that the polypoid gastric dysplasias which we refer to as adenomas are not common precursors of clinically important invasive or even early gastric

carcinomas. As in the colon, the larger the gastric adenoma, the more likely it will contain carcinomatous epithelium (8). In one study from Japan, none of 29 adenomas 1 cm or less in diameter had carcinoma, while 5 of 38 (13 percent) adenomas between 1.1 and 4.0 cm and 5 of 6 (83 percent) adenomas larger then 4 cm did (26). Another study, also from Japan, in which adenomas were followed with endoscopic and biopsy examinations for over 3 years, found that high-grade dysplasia evolved only in those adenomas in which a carcinoma developed (16a). Furthermore, compared to those adenomas in which carcinoma did not develop, adenomas with carcinoma were more likely to have a prominent villous component, were more likely to enlarge, and were more likely to have sulfomucins in the adenomatous epithelium.

There is little information on the natural history of adenomas. In one study, 85 adenomas in 74 patients were biopsied and followed for from 6 months to 12 years: 4 became smaller, 4 enlarged, and 77 stayed the same (15). The little data on the microscopic natural history of adenomas indicate that most are stable lesions, although there is a risk of carcinoma and higher dysplasia grades developing in about 20 percent, especially those that are large and start with at least a level of dysplasia somewhere between low and high grades. In a 1- to 7-year follow-up biopsy study of 85 adenomas, 9 developed foci of carcinoma which

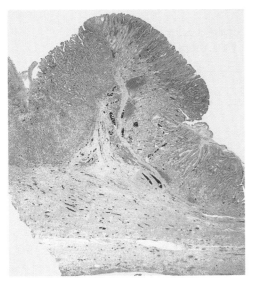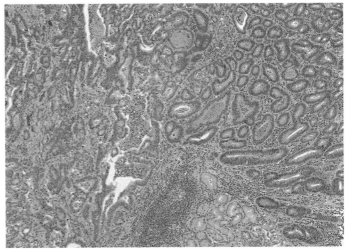

Figure 10-14
CARCINOMA INVADING THE LAMINA PROPRIA WITHIN AN ADENOMA
Left: Low magnification view of an adenoma (right) with the dysplastic tubules appearing relatively uniform, evenly spaced by lamina propria, and lined by a single layer of cells with basal nuclei. To the center and lower left is the invasive carcinoma. Here, the tubular shapes are uneven, the cells lining the tubules are less uniform, there is stratification of epithelium and nuclei, and the stroma separating the tubules is irregular and even lost as the tubules appear to be immediately adjacent to one another.
Right: Higher magnification view.

invaded the lamina propria but no deeper (15). Seven of these 9 adenomas were larger than 2 cm in diameter. Six other adenomas developed higher grades of dysplasia between 6 months and 2 years, and 3 actually had decreases in dysplasia grade between 6 months and 3 years after diagnosis. Several other adenomas had transient changes in dysplasia grade, but this may have been due to sampling. However, in this study, there was no change in microscopic appearance of 75 percent of the adenomas over an average follow-up period of 49 months. In another report from Japan, of 42 adenomas followed for over 3 years, 9 or 21 percent developed invasive carinomas after an average of 6 1/2 years of follow-up (16a).

There are probably some genetic alterations which occur in the gastric adenoma-carcinoma sequence. In one study, point mutations of c-Ki-*ras* oncogenes were detected using the polymerase chain reaction in 3 of 3 tubular adenomas and in 3 of 14 tubular carcinomas, but not in 18 poorly differentiated or signet ring cell carcinomas, suggesting that activation of this oncogene may be a relatively early step in at least some adenoma-carcinoma sequences (16).

The issue of adenomas as part of gastric dysplasias in general is covered in greater detail in chapter 11 in the discussion of the precursors of carcinomas of the stomach. Adenomas seem to be markers of overall gastric carcinoma predisposition. In one endoscopic study, coexistent gastric carcinomas occurred in 14 of 178 patients (8 percent) with adenomas (15).

**Gastric Adenomas in Familial Adenomatous Polyposis (FAP).** Table 10-1 compares the prevalence of both gastric and duodenal adenomas with the prevalence of fundic gland polyps in patients with FAP in eight studies from different parts of the world. There is striking variation from one report to another, suggesting that factors other than the FAP itself must be active. There may be population differences, possibly environmental, to explain the much higher frequency of FAP-associated gastric adenomas in Japan and Italy than in Finland, England, and the United States (1). There may be specific familial characteristics: duodenal adenomas are more likely to occur in patients with the Gardner's syndrome variant of FAP than in those without the syndrome, while fundic gland polyps

Table 10-1
## UPPER GASTROINTESTINAL MANIFESTATIONS
## OF FAMILIAL ADENOMATOUS POLYPOSIS

| Author | Year | Country | FAP* | FGP | St Ad | Duod Ad | Misc. |
|---|---|---|---|---|---|---|---|
| Jarvinen (14) | 1983 | Finland | 34 | 18 (53%) | 4 (12%) | 16 (47%) | 1 duodenal carcinoma |
| Burt (2) | 1984 | USA | 11 | 5 (45%) | 1 ( 9%) | 7 (64%) | Gardner's syndrome |
| Ranzi (21) | 1981 | Italy | 9 | 4 (44%) | 4 (44%) | 6 (67%) | |
| Domizio (5) | 1990 | England | 102 | 44 (43%) | 6 ( 6%) | 94 (92%) | |
| Watanabe (27) | 1978 | Japan | 22 | 6 (27%) | 9 (41%) | NS** | 1 stomach carcinoma |
| Sarre (23) | 1987 | USA | 100 | 26 (26%) | 2 (2%) | 33 (33%) | |
| Bulow (1) | 1985 | Denmark | 26 | 6 (23%) | 1 ( 4%) | 12 (43%) | |
| Tonelli (25) | 1985 | Italy | 24 | 3 (13%) | 3 (13%) | 14 (58%) | |

*FAP = Number of patients with FAP; FGP = number of patients with fundic gland polyposis; St Ad = number of patients with adenomas in the stomach; Duod Ad = number of patients with adenomas in the duodenum. **NS = not stated.

are less common with Gardner's syndrome (23). There are few long-term follow-up studies of patients with FAP to determine if there is a change in frequency of adenomas or fundic gland polyps with time. The limited data suggest that the prevalence and size of adenomas increase with age (9,21,23,25). In the most detailed follow-up study of 26 Japanese patients, 11 had adenomas initially, all in the antrum; on follow-up, 4 of these developed new adenomas, while there was no change in adenoma number, size and histologic features in the other 7 (9). One patient developed new adenomas and a high-grade dysplasia equivalent to in situ carcinoma in one of the original adenoma sites. Only 2 of the 15 patients who did not have gastric adenomas at the beginning of the study developed adenomas during the median follow-up of 7 years 3 months. Almost all FAP-associated adenomas occur in the antrum and about two thirds are multiple. Most gastric adenomas occur in patients who also have duodenal adenomas (14,21). Nonpolypoid microadenomas in the flat antral mucosa, comparable to the single and double crypt adenomas that are found in the FAP colons, also have been reported (5,21). A few examples of dysplastic foci in fundic gland polyps, essentially mixed fundic gland and adenomatous polyps, have been seen (2,5). Finally, there are a few reported cases of gastric adenocarcinoma in FAP patients, some of which are multiple, suggesting that the adenoma-carcinoma sequence is working in the stomach, much as it is working in the colon and duodenum (3,13,27). However, considering that gastric adenomas are much more common in stomachs with FAP, there are very few gastric cancers in these patients, suggesting that the FAP gastric adenomas are not highly predisposed to progress through the adenoma-carcinoma sequence.

**Treatment:** Remarkably little information has been published about the proper treatment for gastric adenomas. It seems reasonable that they should be removed completely and that the rest of the gastric mucosa be examined thoroughly to ensure that there are no other adenomas. Endoscopic removal is adequate treatment for small tumors; large ones may require surgical resection (26). In all cases, the patient needs follow-up because of the association between adenoma and carcinoma elsewhere in the stomach. However, there are no widely accepted standards for the follow-up interval.

# REFERENCES

1. Bülow S, Lauritsen KB, Johansen A, Svendsen LB, Sondergaard JO. Gastroduodenal polyps in familial polyposis coli. Dis Colon Rectum 1985;28:90–3.

2. Burt RW, Berenson MM, Lee RG, Tolman KG, Preston JW, Gardner EJ. Upper gastrointestinal polyps in Gardner's syndrome. Gastroenterol 1984;86:295–301.

3. Coffey RJ Jr, Knight CD Jr, van Heerden JA, Weiland LH. Gastric adenocarcinoma complicating Gardner's syndrome in a North American woman. Gastroenterol 1985;88:1263–6.

4. den Orth JO, Dekker W. Gastric adenomas. Radiology 1981;141:289–93.

5. Domizio P, Talbot IC, Spigelman AD, Williams CB, Phillips RK. Upper gastrointestinal pathology in familial adenomatous polyposis: results from a prospective study of 102 patients. J Clin Pathol 1990;43:738–43.

6. Hattori T. Morphological range of hyperplastic polyps and carcinomas arising in hyperplastic polyps of the stomach. J Clin Pathol 1985;38:622–30.

7. Hirota T, Ming SC. Early gastric carcinoma. In: Ming SC, Goldman H, eds. Pathology of the gastrointestinal tract. Philadelphia: WB Saunders, 1992:570–82.

8. Hirota T, Okada M, Itabashi M, Kitaoka. Histogenesis of human gastric cancer—with special reference to the significance of adenoma as a precancerous lesion. In: Ming SC, ed. Precursors of gastric cancer. New York: Praeger, 1984:233–52.

9. Iida M, Yao T, Itoh H. Natural history of gastric adenomas in patients with familial adenomatosis coli/Gardner's syndrome. Cancer 1988;61:605–11.

10. Ito H, Ito M, Tahara E. Minute carcinoid arising in gastric tubular adenoma. Histopathology 1989;15:96–9.

11. Ito H, Yasui W, Yoshida K, Nakayama H, Tahara E. Depressed tubular adenoma of the stomach: pathological and immunohistochemical features. Histopathology 1990;17:419–26.

12. Ito H, Yokozaki H, Ito M, Tahara E. Papillary adenoma of the stomach. Pathologic and immunohistochemical study. Arch Pathol Lab Med 1989;113:1030–4.

13. Jagelman DG, DeCosse JJ, Bussey HJ. Upper gastrointestinal cancer in familial adenomatous polyposis. Lancet 1988;1:1149–51.

14. Jarvinen H, Nyberg M, Peltokallio P. Upper gastrointestinal tract polyps in familial adenomatosis coli. Gut 1983;24:333–9.

15. Kamiya T, Morishita T, Asakura H, Miura S, Munakata Y, Tsuchiya M. Long-term follow-up study on gastric adenoma and its relation to gastric protruded carcinoma. Cancer 1982;50:2496–503.

16. Kihana T, Tsuda H, Hirota T, et al. Point mutation of c-Ki-ras oncogene in gastric adenoma and adenocarcinoma with tubular differentiation. Jpn J Cancer Res 1991;82:308–14.

16a. Kolodziejczyk P, Yao T, Oya M, et al. Long-term follow-up study of patients with gastric adenomas with malignant transformation. An immunohistochemical and histochemical analysis. Cancer 1994;74:2896–907.

17. Ming SC, Goldman H. Gastric polyps. A histogenetic classification and its relation to carcinoma. Cancer 1965;18:721–6.

18. Muratani M, Nakamura T, Nakano GI, Mukawa. Ultrastructural study of two subtypes of gastric adenoma. J Clin Pathol 1989;42:352–9.

19. Nakamura K, Sakaguchi H, Enjoji M. Depressed adenoma of the stomach. Cancer 1988;62:2197–202.

20. Nakamura T, Nakano GI. Histopathological classification and malignant change in gastric polyps. J Clin Pathol 1985;38:754–64.

21. Ranzi T, Castagnone D, Velio P, Bianchi P, Polli EE. Gastric and duodenal polyps in familial polyposis coli. Gut 1981;22:363–7.

22. Rubio CA. Paneth cell adenoma of the stomach. Am J Surg Pathol 1989;13:325–8.

23. Sarre RG, Frost AG, Jagelman DG, Petras RE, Sivak MV. Gastric and duodenal polyps in familial adenomatous polyposis: a prospective study of the nature and prevalence of upper gastrointestinal polyps. Gut 1987;28:306–14.

24. Tomasulo J. Gastric polyps. Histologic types and their relationship to gastric carcinoma. Cancer 1971;27:1346–55.

25. Tonelli F, Nardi F, Bechi P, Taddei G, Gozzo P, Romagnoli P. Extracolonic polyps in familial polyposis coli and Gardner's syndrome. Dis Colon Rectum 1985;28:664–8.

26. Tsujitani S, Furusawa M, Hayashi I. Morphological factors aid in therapeutic decisions concerning gastric adenomas. Hepato-Gastroenterol 1992;39:56–8.

27. Watanabe H, Enjoji M, Yao T, Ohsato K. Gastric lesions in familial adenomatosis coli. Their incidence and histologic analysis. Hum Pathol 1978;9:269–83.

28. Watanabe H, Jass JR, Sobin LH. Histological typing of oesophageal and gastric tumours. Berlin: Springer-Verlag, 1990:34–8.

29. Xuan ZX, Ambe K, Enjoji E. Depressed adenoma of the stomach, revisited. Histologic, histochemical, and immunohistochemical profiles. Cancer 1991;67:2382–9.

# 11

# CARCINOMA OF THE STOMACH

There are a number of histologically distinct types of gastric carcinoma, although the majority are adenocarcinomas. Many of the other types of carcinoma appear to be variants of, or derived from, adenocarcinomas. This chapter discusses the usual types of adenocarcinoma and the rarer forms.

## ADENOCARCINOMA OF THE STOMACH

Carcinoma of the stomach is one of the most common neoplasms in the world, and most are adenocarcinomas. They are not, however, a homogeneous group of tumors but rather several distinct clinicopathologic entities with different predisposing conditions and probable etiologies. For example, it is now clear that *Helicobacter pylori* plays an important role in the pathogenesis of carcinomas of the gastric antrum and fundus whereas carcinomas of the gastric cardia, which now account for a third or more of gastric carcinomas in the United States, are pathogenetically more similar to esophageal adenocarcinoma than gastric carcinoma (6).

Another interesting group of lesions are the early gastric cancers, which have been described primarily in the Japanese literature and now increasingly in that from the United States and Europe. These tumors appear to represent the earliest stages of common gastric carcinomas. They are important because they are essentially curable. However, since most patients with these early tumors are asymptomatic, detection is possible only with massive screening programs. Currently this is economically feasible only in high incidence areas such as Japan.

The prognosis of advanced gastric carcinoma remains poor but in some countries such as Japan it has greatly improved as a result of more accurate staging procedures and consequently more precise and radical surgery.

Gastric adenocarcinoma is the most common cancer in Japan and much of the excellent detailed data regarding etiology, pathogenesis, pathology, and management originates there. However, not all the data applicable to Japan are necessarily relevant to gastric carcinoma found in the United States and Europe; these lesions may be different from their Japanese counterparts.

## Prevalence and Incidence

The incidence of gastric adenocarcinoma varies greatly from country to country: it is particularly high in Japan (with an incidence of about 80 cases per 100,000 people), Costa Rica, Columbia, Chile, and Finland, and very low in Thailand and many parts of Africa (75,172,226). In the United States there has been a steady decline in incidence over the last 50 years (172) and is presently 10 cases per 100,000. Nevertheless, there are still approximately 23,000 to 25,000 new cases per year and approximately 14,000 deaths (6,226).

There has been a steady decline in the mortality rate in most countries, including Japan. In 1990, the age-adjusted incidence of deaths per 100,000 population reported in the United States was 7.4 for males and 3.4 for females; in 1993, it was 5.3 and 2.3, respectively. A similar trend was noted in Japan where the death rates for males and females were 54.6 and 25.1 in 1990 and 37.9 and 17.2 in 1993 (7,14,22,172,226). The precise cause for this decline in mortality is not clear but is probably due to early diagnosis and treatment and to a fall in the incidence of the intestinal type of carcinoma (128), which is commonly associated with atrophic gastritis, a condition that is decreasing in incidence.

## Pathogenesis

Much of the data on the pathogenic mechanisms of gastric carcinoma have come from high incidence areas, such as Japan, Columbia, and Scandinavia. In these countries the populations are more racially homogeneous and thus some data may not apply to relatively low incidence areas such as the United States where populations are genetically more heterogeneous.

**Risk Factors.** These are attributes that confer a higher than expected incidence of cancer on a population (75). For gastric carcinoma there are marked geographic variations in incidence, due possibly to dietary factors and genetic predisposition. Epidemiologic studies have shown that migration from a high risk (e.g., Japan) to a low risk region (e.g., Hawaii) is associated with a decline in incidence of gastric carcinoma, most notably in the second generation (34,35,73,75). Similar findings have been reported from Columbia (35,38). These studies have also shown that environmental factors, principally diet, are important in the genesis of carcinoma.

**Dietary Factors.** High salt consumption, associated with salted fish and meat; starchy (rice), pickled, and smoked foods; and low caloric intake have been implicated in gastric cancer. Conversely, the intake of fresh fruit, vegetables, and vitamins C, E, and A and trace metals appears to be beneficial. Smoking and alcohol consumption may also contribute. Nitrosamines, resulting from the conversion of dietary nitrates in the acid milieu of the stomach, have been proposed but unconfirmed as important carcinogenic agents in gastric carcinoma (73,217,238). This suggests the possibility that antioxidants (which can prevent the conversion of nitrates to nitrosamine), such as carotenoids, vitamins C and E, and trace elements such as selenium, zinc, copper, iron, and manganese, which are essential components of antioxidant enzymes, may lower the risk of carcinoma (51,260).

**Genetic Factors.** Patients with blood group A have a higher incidence of gastric cancer than those with other blood groups (2). There is also a difference in the incidence of gastric cancers between whites and blacks in the United States. In the Surveillance, Epidemiology, and End Results (SEER) data, between 1983 and 1987 the age-adjusted incidence of gastric adenocarcinoma for black males was 16.8 per 100,000 compared to 9.5 for white males; the figures for black and white females were 6.9 and 4.0, respectively. In contrast, the age-adjusted incidence for gastric cardia adenocarcinomas was 1.7 per 100,000 for whites and 0.9 for blacks (Dr. L. Sobin, Armed Forces Institute of Pathology, 1994). Family clusters of carcinoma of the stomach have been described, and relatives of cancer patients appear to have a threefold risk of developing cancer. However, these individuals also may be influenced by the same environmental factors as the patient. It is probable that environmental factors are of greater importance, and enhanced, in patients with a genetic predisposition (2,34,186).

**The Role of Oncogenes, Tumor Suppressor Genes, and Other Chromosome Abnormalities.** It appears that the activation of cellular oncogenes is important in the development of gastric adenocarcinomas. Oncogenes are present in all normal cells and are often associated with cell growth and regulation. When activated, they act in a dominant fashion to cause a cell to express the malignant phenotype. Another important mechanism in tumor formation is the loss of suppresser genes. Probably both mechanisms are important in tumor formation, and the activation of one or more oncogenes and the loss of one or more suppresser genes is required for a tumor to progress from initiation through promotion to a metastasizing malignancy (76).

Gastric carcinomas display some of the same genetic alterations observed in other carcinomas. These changes include aberrant expression of *bcl*-2 protein; reduction or dysfunction of cadherim-e and K-sam amplification; point mutation of the *ras* oncogene and the p53 tumor suppresser gene, gene amplification of epidermal growth factor (EGF), transforming growth factor-alpha (TGF-alpha), platelet derived growth factor (PDGF), insulin growth factor (IGF), and p185 (*ERB*B2) gene; and chromosomal loss of heterozygosity in chromosomes 7p, 17p, 1q, and 5q (85,94,95,110, 116,151,177,178,210,243,245,264,266). Some of these genetic and oncogene changes may have prognostic implications. For example, loss of heterozygosity on chromosomes 5q and 17p is associated most commonly with well-differentiated carcinoma, whereas allele loss on chromosomes 1q and 7p may be involved in the progression to less well-differentiated adenocarcinoma (210). Amplification of *ERB*B2 seems to be an indicator of metastatic ability and overexpression of the EGF receptor system is a biologic marker for high malignancy. The synchronous expression of EGF, TGF-alpha and *ras* p21 is associated with tumor invasion and metastasis, and overexpression of TGF-beta, IGF, and PDGF is associated with collagen synthesis in poorly differentiated gastric carcinomas resulting in linitis plastica (243). However, further work is needed before the aforementioned findings can be applied to clinical practice.

**Predisposing Conditions.** These are pathologic processes associated with an increased risk of carcinoma. They include severe *H. pylori* infection, atrophic gastritis, subtotal gastrectomy with gastrojejunal anastomosis, immunodeficiency syndromes, chronic gastric ulcers, and Menetrier's disease. The association of some disorders to cancer, such as atrophic gastritis and the postgastrectomy state, appear to be more important in high-risk countries (Table 11-1).

*Chronic Gastric Ulceration.* The association of chronic gastric ulcers with carcinoma is controversial and often difficult to prove. In order to convincingly demonstrate this association it is necessary to document a longstanding ulcer with carcinoma developing at the edge late in the course of the disease. This may be difficult in advanced cases of carcinoma in which the tumor may have overrun much of the ulcer.

Early studies from Japan reported carcinomas around ulcers in up to 70 percent of cases and a recent study from the United States reported that 25 percent of patients with gastric carcinoma had a history of gastric ulcer (210). However, studies now rarely report a relationship to ulcer (Table 11-1) (172,210,257). In one follow-up study on 481 patients with gastric ulcer over a period of 16 years, seven gastric carcinomas developed (25). However, these were located at sites distant from the ulcers. The same is true for studies from other countries, which show that the incidence of gastric carcinoma in patients with gastric ulcer is no higher than in the general population (92,203). Furthermore, histologic examination of minute gastric carcinomas (less than 5 mm) almost never reveals evidence of an underlying chronic ulcer (173).

Recent work on the association of *H. pylori* may explain the association of chronic gastric ulcer with gastric cancer. We now know that most cases of gastric ulcer are due to *H. pylori* infection, and also that *H. pylori* plays some part in the development of gastric cancer and lymphoma. Thus the relationship of chronic gastric ulceration to cancer may be due to the underlying *H. pylori* infection rather than the ulcer per se. Also, early gastric carcinoma may closely resemble a benign peptic ulcer (149). Up to 65 percent of early gastric carcinomas have superficial ulcers or features of ulcer scars characterized by mucosal folds radiating towards the carcinoma. The latter are the result of secondary chronic ulcers extending into the submucosa with ulceration and fibrosis.

*Severe Atrophic Gastritis and Intestinal Metaplasia.* These are by far the most important precursor lesions of gastric carcinoma (172,236a). In one study in Japan chronic atrophic gastritis was

Table 11-1

**RELATIVE FREQUENCY OF EARLY GASTRIC CARCINOMA ARISING IN VARIOUS PRECANCEROUS LESIONS***

| Precursor Lesion | Percent of Malignancies with Precursor Lesions |
|---|---|
| Hyperplastic polyp | 0.5 |
| Adenoma | 2.5 |
| Chronic ulcer | 0.7 |
| Atrophic gastritis | 95.0 |
| Chronic erosive gastritis | 1.4 |
| Stomach remnant | 0.1 |

*Diagnosed at the National Cancer Center Hospital, Tokyo, Japan. Data obtained from reference 10.

found in the stomach of 80 to 95 percent of cancer patients (90,170). The incidence of gastritis increases with age and is the highest in the elderly population; however, in high-risk areas chronic gastritis is commonly present in the young (38). Long-term follow-up studies in Finland on patients with atrophic gastritis, with or without pernicious anemia, have shown an incidence of 10 percent of associated gastric carcinoma (231).

Correa (31) stressed that only some forms of gastritis appear to be associated with an increased risk of gastric cancer, namely those associated with atrophic gastritis. He divided chronic gastritis into four morphologic patterns, two of which are associated with gastric atrophy, intestinal metaplasia, and an increased risk of gastric carcinoma. The first is diffuse corporal atrophic gastritis which is confined to the body and fundus and mainly associated with pernicious anemia, an autoimmune disorder. The second is multifocal atrophic gastritis, which is haphazardly distributed throughout the stomach but concentrated mainly around the antrofundic junction. It is common in developing countries and is often associated with *H. pylori* infection. The other two morphologic patterns of gastritis are not associated with gastric atrophy, intestinal metaplasia, and cancer. They are chronic superficial gastritis and diffuse antral gastritis. The latter may be confused with multifocal atrophic gastritis because there is a dense, full-thickness mucosal lymphoplasmacytic infiltrate. However, there is no glandular atrophy or intestinal metaplasia and the lesion is confined to the antrum. Currently there is no unanimity of opinion as to whether diffuse antral gastritis predisposes to cancer. Diffuse antral gastritis is commonly associated with duodenal and pyloric channel ulcers and *H. pylori* infection appears to be the chief cause (30). Since *H. pylori* is now known to predispose to gastric cancer it would seem logical that diffuse antral gastritis may also be a cancer precursor (30,36).

Intestinal metaplasia is commonly found in atrophic gactritis and appears to be an important precursor of gastric carcinoma, primarily of the intestinal type (236a). In the stomach, intestinal metaplasia first develops in the mid-crypt or neck region, the site of the glandular stem cell. From here the metaplastic mucosa migrates first upwards to the mucosal surface and eventually downwards to reach the gland base, resulting in the formation of a metaplastic crypt. This replacement of gastric glands by intestinalized epithelium is accompanied by expansion of the proliferative zone which may occupy most of the metaplastic crypt (fig. 11-1) (49).

There are several types of intestinal metaplasia: one resembles normal small intestinal mucosa and is called mature or complete intestinal metaplasia (fig. 11-1); another lacks cells normally found in the small intestine, such as Paneth cells and goblet cells, or has immature cells, and is designated colonic, incomplete or immature intestinal metaplasia. The majority of gastric carcinomas arise in areas of incomplete intestinal metaplasia (fig. 11-2) (144,260). Jass and Felipe (104,105) have subdivided intestinal metaplasia into three types on the basis of the mucin content of the columnar cells: type I consists of mature intestinal metaplasia, type II contains sialylated acidic glycoprotein, and type III sulfated acidic glycoprotein (60,104,144,260). Recent studies by Filipe et al. (58,59) have shown that intestinal metaplasia of a subgroup of type III carries a greater risk of gastric cancer than types I and II. These studies remain to be corroborated.

The different types of metaplasia can also be distinguished on the basis of their morphology and mucin stains (Table 11-2) (68,103,172,204,249). The mature type of intestinal metaplasia, type I, resembles normal small intestine (fig. 11-1). The intestinal crypts are straight and lined by ab-

sorptive cells with well-formed microvilli, goblet cells, and sometimes Paneth cells (fig 11-1F). The absorptive cells have well-developed microvilli which contain alkaline phosphatase and digestive enzymes such as disaccharidases and peptidases. The goblet cells secrete sialomucins. This subtype has not been shown to be precancerous.

In incomplete or immature intestinal metaplasia, there are goblet cells but no Paneth cells and the mucous cells between the goblet cells are immature, with short blunted microvilli and no digestive enzymes (fig. 11-2). These are called intermediate cells and contain primarily acidic glycoproteins (mucins) or sulfomucins as in the colon (170).

Histologically, incomplete metaplasia of type II shows mild architectural distortion, with irregular crypts lined by goblet cells and columnar cells showing variable stages of differentiation. The columnar cells contain a mixture of neutral mucins and sialomucins and the goblet cells contain sialomucins.

Type III intestinal metaplasia shows more extensive architectural distortion: the crypts are tortuous and branched and the columnar cells are more undifferentiated with larger, irregular, and more hyperchromatic nuclei. These histologic features may be confused with low-grade dysplasia, especially at low power. The columnar cells secrete sulfomucins and the goblet cells contain sialomucins or sulfomucins (fig. 11-2).

*Helicobacter Pylori.* The significance of *H. pylori* in the pathogenesis of gastritis and gastric carcinoma has received much attention in the recent literature: it has been clearly established that *H. pylori* infection is associated with noncardiac gastric carcinoma. Studies have shown that compared to a noncancerous control population, patients with gastric carcinoma have a higher incidence of infection with *H. pylori,* not only at the time of diagnosis of the gastric carcinoma (as demonstrated by Giemsa staining and by antibody studies) but also many years prior to the onset of carcinoma (shown by antibody studies). A number of strains of *H. pylori* which include variation in lipopolysaccharide structure, expression of cagA-encoded protein, production of vacuolating cytotoxin, and enhanced activation of neutrophils appear more likely to predispose the patients to cancer (11a). Furthermore, it has

Table 11-2
## INTESTINAL METAPLASIA IN ATROPHIC GASTRITIS

| A. MUCIN CONTENT | | |
|---|---|---|
| Type of Metaplasia | Goblet Cells | Columnar Cells |
| Type I Complete (mature) | Sialomucins* Sulfomucins** | Negative |
| Type II Incomplete (immature) | Sialomucins Sulfomucins | Sialomucins Neutral mucins |
| Type III Incomplete (immature) | Sialomucins Sulfomucins | Sulfomucins |

| B. HISTOCHEMICAL DEMONSTRATION OF VARIOUS MUCINS | | |
|---|---|---|
| Stain | Histologic Color | Type of Mucin |
| Periodic acid–Schiff (PAS) | Magenta | Neutral glycoproteins (mucin) Sialomucins |
| Alcian blue pH 2.5 | Blue | Acid mucins Sialomucins Sulfated mucins |
| pH 1.0 | Blue | Sulfated mucins only |
| High iron diamine Alcian blue | Brown Blue | Sulfomucins Sialomucins |

*Sialyated acidic glycoproteins.
**Sulfated acidic gylycoproteins.

been shown that both the diffuse and intestinal types of gastric carcinoma are associated with previous *H. pylori* exposure (32,33,61,182,193, 230,248), although it is more common in the intestinal type (52a). *H. pylori*–associated chronic gastritis is the common general background factor for gastric carcinoma (229,230). However, an epidemiologic association between *H. pylori* and gastric carcinoma does not necessarily prove that there is a causal relationship. There are a number of contradictory findings which complicate the role of *H. pylori* in the etiology of gastric carcinoma. For one, gastric carcinoma develops in only a small proportion of patients infected with *H. pylori,* and occasionally gastric carcinoma occurs in patients who are uninfected. Secondly, patients with diffuse antral gastritis, which is known to be associated with duodenal ulceration and *H. pylori* infection, have a lower risk of gastric carcinoma (193). Thirdly, there are some population groups with a high prevalence of *H. pylori* gastritis, notably in China and Africa, in whom the

risk of gastric carcinoma appears to be low (61). Thus, *H. pylori* by itself is insufficient to give rise to gastric carcinoma and other cofactors must play a role in the etiology and pathogenesis of this tumor. Some of these cofactors are the age of onset of *H. pylori* infection; dietary factors such as deficiencies of some vitamins, minerals, and antioxidants (due to dietary deficiencies in fresh fruit and vegetables), and excessive salt intake; and altered immune status (32,61,193).

The age of onset of *H. pylori* infection seems to be one of the important factors predisposing to gastric carcinoma (228). In developing countries, where the incidence of gastric carcinoma is high, more than half of the children may be infected as compared to developed countries where half of the older population have gastritis (228). Studies of Japanese immigrants to Hawaii have shown that the risk of gastric carcinoma is determined to a large extent in childhood, that is those immigrants born in Japan had a higher incidence of gastric carcinoma than their descendants who

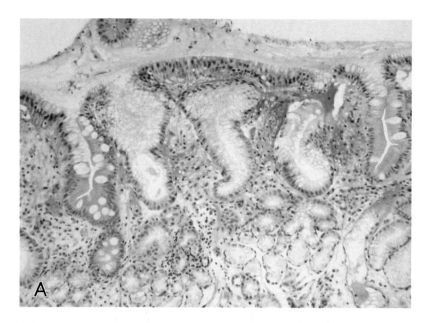

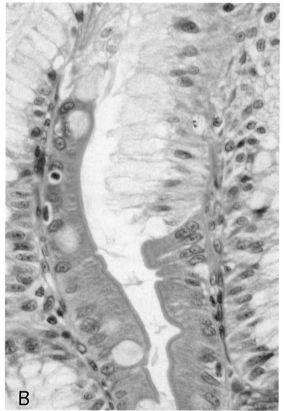

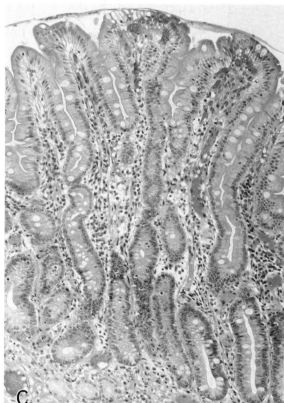

Figure 11-1
GASTRIC MUCOSA SHOWING MATURE INTESTINAL METAPLASIA

A: Severe atrophic gastritis. Note the presence of two foci of intestinal metaplasia in the foveolar region.

B: Higher magnification of A showing typical small intestinal columnar cells and interspersed goblet cells.

C: Atrophic gastritis of the antral mucosa showing intestinal metaplasia occupying the full thickness of the mucosa. Note the presence of intestinal villi lined by goblet cells, absorptive columnar cells containing the characteristic brush border, and a few remaining gastric columnar cells with clear cytoplasm at the top of the central villus. Three residual antral gland profiles are visible at the bottom of the field.

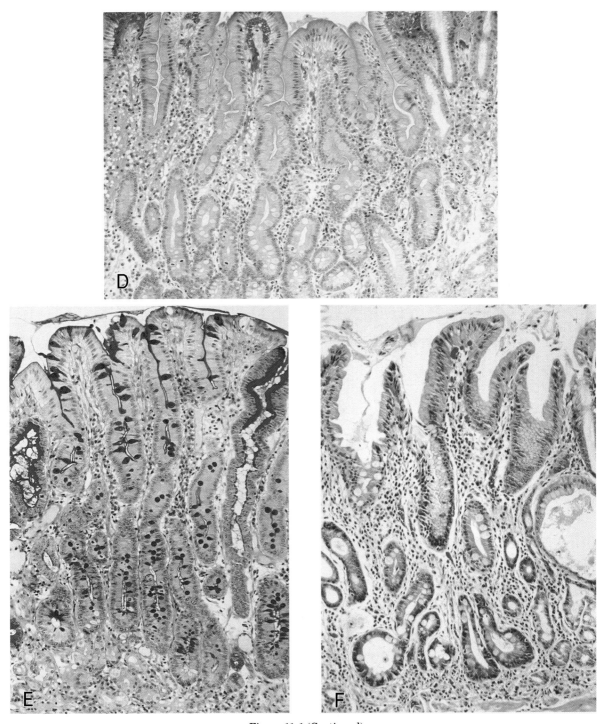

Figure 11-1 (Continued)

D: Acid mucins are seen in atrophic fundic gland gastritis with intestinal metaplasia stained with Alcian blue at pH 2.5. Most of the mucosa has been replaced by intestinalized epithelium with only a few residual antral mucous glands at the bottom of the figure. The goblet cells stain blue with Alcian blue stain in contrast to the surface of clear-staining normal gastric columnar cells, pit cells, and the pyloric glands.

E: Atrophic antral gland gastritis with intestinal metaplasia stained with periodic acid–Schiff (PAS) which stains sialylated acid and neutral mucins. There is intense purple staining of foveolar cells of the residual antrum (top right). The metaplastic mucosa shows intensely purple staining of the goblet cells and negative staining of the intervening columnar cells. A weak PAS-positive outline of the striated border of the columnar cells is seen.

F: Full-thickness intestinal metaplasia with Paneth cells at the base of the crypts.

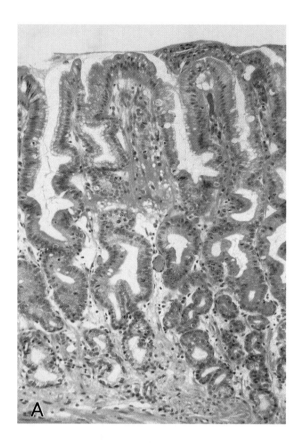

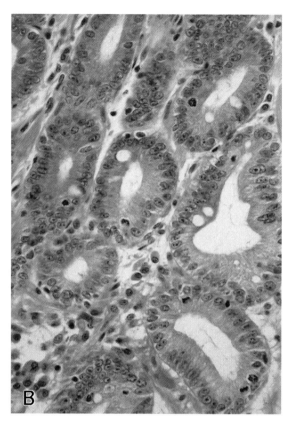

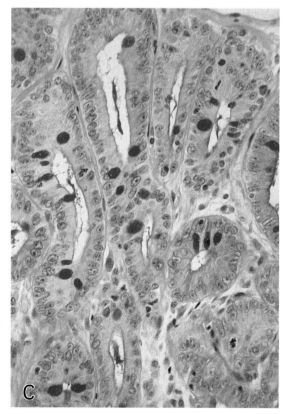

### Figure 11-2
### GASTRIC MUCOSA SHOWING
### INCOMPLETE METAPLASIA

Gastric biopsy from a patient with severe atrophic gastritis showing replacement of the normal body mucosa by incomplete intestinal metaplasia.

A: Low-power view showing intestinalized change primarily in the mid-portion of the mucosa.

B: Higher magnification showing glands containing goblet cells and columnar cells. The latter differ from mature small intestinal columnar cells in that they lack the distinctive brush border.

C: PAS stain shows the numerous goblet cells. The columnar cells lack the distinctive PAS-positive brush border seen in the normal intestine as well as the PAS-positive apical cytoplasm normally seen in the gastric columnar cells.

were born in Hawaii. This suggests that the risk of gastric carcinoma is determined by an environmental factor present in Japan and this might well be *H. pylori* infection (74,228, 248). The persistence of inflammatory products over decades probably exposes dividing stem cells to mutations and malignant transformation. This may be further aggravated by dietary factors such as nitrates, carbohydrates, and excessive salt which could amplify the risk of mutation beyond that due to inflammation. Protective factors such as antioxidants, which are present in fresh fruits and vegetables, may limit the inflammation-related oxidative damage. Thus, dietary deficiency of these foods may further aggravate the cancerous predisposition of the stomach (32,193).

The clinical implications of *H. pylori* infection in gastric carcinoma are unclear. The elimination of the organism, even if it were shown to be effective on a long-term basis, is not cost effective or even practical since such a large percentage of the population is infected. However, populations considered to be at particular high risk might benefit from screening for *H. pylori* infection since other preventative measures might be indicated such as prophylactic treatment with antioxidants (193).

*Other Infections.* Epstein-Barr virus (EBV) has been shown to be associated with some gastric adenocarcinomas, including gastric carcinoma with lymphoid stroma (discussed later) (71a,224). In one study, EBV sequences were detected by polymerase chain reaction in tumor cells of 16 percent of typical gastric adenocarcinomas as well as in the adjacent dysplastic epithelium (224).

*Postgastrectomy* (fig. 11-3). The risk of carcinoma developing in the gastric remnant following gastrectomy, usually for peptic ulcer disease, has been estimated at between 5 and 10 percent but is probably much lower. It occurs most frequently in gastric resections with Billroth II anastomoses (172), and has been blamed on reflux of duodenal contents (including activated pancreatic enzymes). It is a late complication of gastrectomy, occurring 15 to 25 years after gastric resection and thereafter the risk keeps increasing although it is not high enough to justify surveillance (5,172,205,235,254). These findings have been disputed by Schafer (215) and others, who in their long-term follow-up studies in the United States, found that the incidence of gastric carcinoma is no more common among patients with prior gastric surgery for ulcer disease than among the general population.

Carcinomas in the gastric remnant may occur anywhere in the residual stump or at the stoma and are adenocarcinomas of either diffuse or intestinal type (fig. 11-3). They may be associated with bile reflux gastropathy, polypoid prolapsing mucosa, and superimposed dysplasia (219). It may well be that the increased risk of carcinoma in these patients is related to the preexisting atrophic gastritis and not the postgastrectomy state.

Because of the apparent rarity of carcinoma in postgastrectomy patients, surveillance for gastric dysplasia and carcinoma is not currently advocated in most centers in the United States unless there is some indication for it such as the chance finding of dysplasia. This is especially important in those patients who develop high-grade dysplasia since a high percentage (up to 40 percent in one study) are prone to the development of carcinoma (235).

*Immunodeficiency Disorders.* The risk of cancer in some of the primary immunodeficiency disorders, such as common variable immunodeficiency, X-linked immunodeficiency, and infantile X-linked agammaglobulinemia, ranges from 2 to 10 percent (41,73,82,134,194). Most of the tumors are lymphomas but gastric carcinoma has also been reported.

*Menetrier's Disease.* The association of Menetrier's disease with gastric carcinoma has been reported (24,126,216,263), and we have seen several such cases (fig. 11-4). Unfortunately, Menetrier's disease is poorly defined in the literature; some gastroenterologists equate it merely with any disease associated with giant gastric folds. More accurate information is needed before it can be labeled a premalignant condition.

**Premalignant (Preinvasive) Lesions of the Stomach.** These consist primarily of adenomas that have the potential to become carcinoma. They usually arise in individuals who have one or more predisposing conditions, such as atrophic gastritis or less commonly familial polyposis, and probably represent the final common pathway through which these conditions give rise to carcinoma.

Occasionally other gastric polyps, such as hyperplastic polyps and those of familial juvenile polyposis, also show malignant transformation, but this is the exception rather than the rule (45,129).

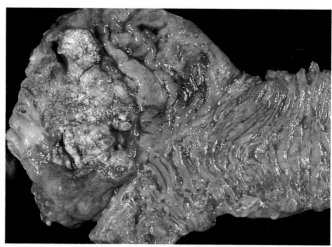

Figure 11-3
GASTRIC CARCINOMA IN
POSTGASTRECTOMY REMNANT
(GASTRIC STUMP CANCER)

Top: Resection specimen from a gastric stump anastomosed to jejunum. The tumor in the gastric remnant consists of an elevated nodular mass with surface erosions.

Bottom: Low-power view of the gastric stump. The carcinoma is on the left, within the gastric mucosa and infiltrating the submucosa.

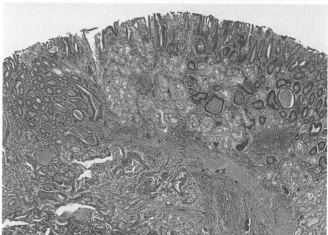

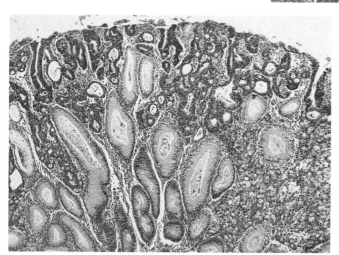

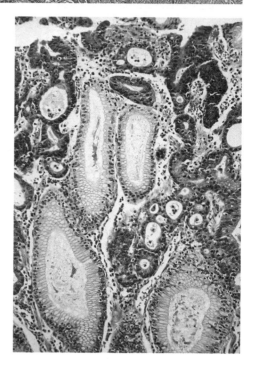

Figure 11-4
GASTRIC ADENOCARCINOMA WITH MENETRIER'S DISEASE

Above: Low-power view of gastric mucosa showing great thickening due to foveolar hyperplasia and marked elongation of the gastric pits. The carcinoma can be seen infiltrating between the upper ends of the gastric pits.

Right: Higher magnification shows the carcinoma infiltrating between the foveolar epithelium.

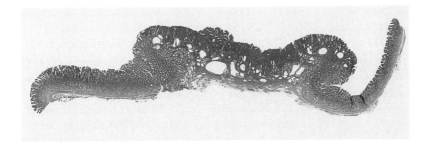

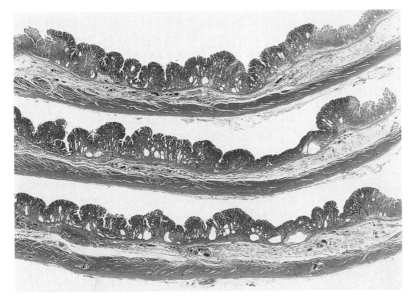

Figure 11-5
GASTRIC ADENOMA
AND DYSPLASIA:
MORPHOLOGIC PATTERNS
Top: Sessile adenoma.
Bottom: Dysplasia characterized by a
flat lesion.

## GASTRIC DYSPLASIA

Dysplasia is defined as an unequivocal neoplastic epithelial alteration. It is characterized by a set of morphologic features that include cytoplasmic changes such as mucin loss, cellular crowding, nuclear stratification, increased nuclear size in relation to cytoplasmic volume, nuclear hyperchromatism, nuclear and cellular pleomorphism, and increased mitoses. The grade of dysplasia is based on the intensity of each of these changes (figs. 11-5–11-11).

Two types of dysplastic lesions are recognized: dysplasia and adenoma. Both adenomas and nonadenomatous dysplasias have identical epithelia. Because of this, it is tempting to lump all adenomas and all dysplasias not specifically referred to as adenomas together into a single category. Unfortunately, gastric adenomas, comparable to colonic adenomas, have a long literary history behind them. They are defined by the World Health Organization (WHO) as "a circumscribed benign neoplasm composed of tubular and/or villous structures lined by dysplastic epithelium." It is not clear whether this definition includes within the adenoma category all dysplastic foci in the stomach, as long as each focus is circumscribed. If so, many, if not all gastric dysplasias automatically become adenomas, since most of such foci are circumscribed. We suspect that this was not the intention of the WHO since they defined a separate category of gastric epithelial abnormalities as "dysplasia," which is defined as "atypical changes in the epithelium considered to be precancerous." Therefore, tempting as it is to group all dysplastic lesions together, we have elected to follow tradition and separate adenomas from dysplasias by adding the additional requirement that they be polypoid or elevated, in contrast to dysplasias that involve flat mucosa (fig. 11-5). Adenomas are discussed in detail in chapter 10. The separation of adenomas from other dysplasias is sometimes arbitrary, and published studies of adenomas or nonadenoma dysplasias do not use the terms the same way. Furthermore, recent additions to the list of terms, such as flat adenomas and depressed adenomas add further nosologic confusion by using the adenoma designation for nonelevated or even depressed lesions, although they do fit the WHO definition of adenoma because they are circumscribed. We define these as dysplasias.

The diagnosis of carcinoma in situ of the stomach and its differentiation from high-grade dysplasia is often difficult, if not impossible, and therefore we have combined the two categories under high-grade dysplasia. The behavior and management of both lesions is similar. Another designation used by some for these high-grade dysplasias and carcinomas in situ is "possible cancer." In Japan, possible cancer, as the name implies, is not a definitive diagnosis and is understood by the clinician to be a temporary designation until the issue can be resolved by urgent rebiopsy.

High-grade dysplasia is a noninvasive neoplastic lesion. In contrast, early gastric cancer is an invasive lesion traversing the lamina propria or submucosa, and often eliciting a desmoplastic response as a result.

**Grading.** Dysplasia is graded according to the degree of histologic abnormality as low grade or high grade, or mild, moderate, or severe dysplasia (48,66,102,125,153,156,163,164,171, 206,270). As is true for other sites, low-grade dysplasia may be difficult to differentiate from epithelial atypia associated with inflammation and regeneration. This difficulty in interpretation may account for reports on the reversibility of low-grade dysplasia (3,27,154,184,211). The Pathology Panel of the International Study Group on Gastric Cancer has recommended that regenerative and mild dysplastic changes be grouped under hyperplasia, whereas moderate and severe dysplasia be grouped into one category of dysplasia because they cannot be sharply separated and often coexist (156). In addition, the degree of interobserver agreement for high-grade dysplasia is much higher than for the other categories (125,153).

In keeping with the current nomenclature of dysplasia for ulcerative colitis (200) and Barrett's esophagus (198), we prefer to use low and high grades for dysplasia. For those cases in which there is difficulty in differentiating between reactive change and dysplasia the term "indefinite for dysplasia" is recommended.

**Clinical Significance of Dysplasia.** Data on the prevalence of gastric dysplasia and the progression of low-grade dysplasia to high-grade dysplasia and carcinoma are scant and not always consistent. Furthermore, the definitions of carcinoma vary as well: in some studies carcinoma denotes invasive lesions (206) whereas in others it is not always clear and may include in situ lesions, which we regard as high-grade dysplasia. In addition, all studies on dysplasia are based on symptomatic patients and its true incidence in the general population is unclear (206,227). Despite these limitations, a number of important factors regarding gastric dysplasia are becoming apparent.

Gastric dysplasia appears to be an important marker for carcinoma risk and is almost certainly a precursor lesion for gastric carcinoma, primarily for the intestinal type. In retrospective studies of gastric resection specimens, dysplasia adjacent to early gastric cancers occurred in 50 to 100 percent of cases and in up to 80 percent of advanced cancers (90,146,185,270). In another study (206) in which 134 cases of gastric dysplasia were followed prospectively, it was found that there was progression of the degree of dysplasia and the development of gastric carcinoma in many: mild dysplasia appeared to regress in 66 percent, persist in 15 percent, and progress in 19 percent (3 cases to moderate dysplasia, 1 to severe dysplasia, and 5 to invasive carcinoma); moderate dysplasia persisted in 30 percent of cases and progressed in 40 percent (1 case to severe dysplasia and 7 to invasive carcinoma); severe dysplasia appeared to regress in 12.5 percent of cases, persist in 12.5 percent, and progress to invasive carcinoma in 75 percent. These findings support the notion that a significant proportion of high-grade dysplasias progress to carcinoma.

The time frame for the transformation of dysplastic lesions into carcinoma is not clear because detailed information is lacking, particular for diminutive flat lesions (less than 5 mm in diameter). It probably varies from case to case depending on the severity of the dysplasia. However, high-grade dysplasia is highly predictive for gastric carcinoma. In fact, a high proportion of cases already have coexisting carcinoma or it develops within months of diagnosis (206,227).

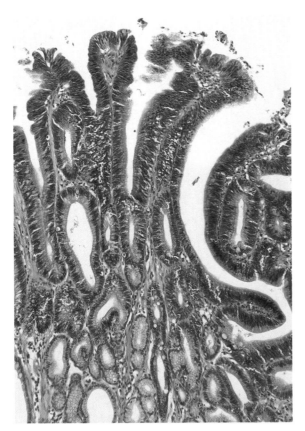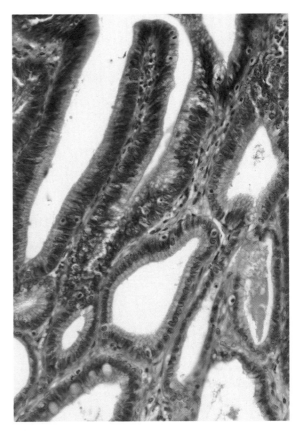

Figure 11-6
HIGH-GRADE DYSPLASIA
High-grade dysplasia showing a villous pattern (left) and a tubulovillous pattern (right).

It is unclear whether all grades of gastric dysplasia can transform directly into carcinoma or whether there is a stepwise progression from low-grade through high-grade dysplasia before carcinoma can develop. However, in general it has been found that low-grade dysplastic lesions remain stable for many years, in contrast to those of high grade, which are frequently associated with carcinoma (from 30 to 80 percent of cases) either at the time of diagnosis of dysplasia or within 1 or 2 years (27,43,55,57,206,211).

The size of the adenoma appears to be an important indicator of the likelihood of malignant change. The incidence of malignant change is low in small lesions but rises with increasing size. The reported incidence of malignant change for small adenomas is 6 to 18 percent, compared to around 35 percent for the larger lesions (174,240). However, the incidence figures re-ported in the literature vary greatly, from a low of 6 percent to a high of 76 percent (155).

Independent coexisting carcinomas are common in patients with gastric dysplasia. In one study of 121 cases of gastric adenoma, there were 55 concomitant early gastric carcinomas and 29 advanced carcinomas (90).

**Microscopic Findings.** The dysplastic epithelium has either a tubular, villous, or mixed tubular villous configuration (figs. 11-6, 11-7). In tubular lesions, there are two types of dysplastic cells which have been designated by some as adenomatous dysplasia and hyperplastic dysplasia. Because the latter term may cast doubt about the neoplastic nature of dysplasia, we prefer not to use these qualifiers and just refer to dysplasia generically, while recognizing that there may be several patterns and that these may occur together (39,102).

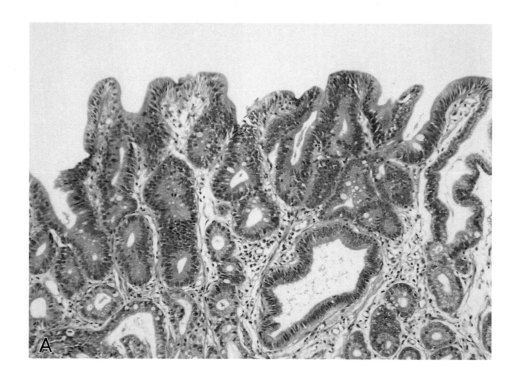

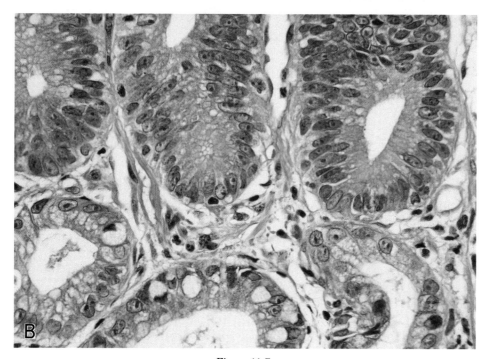

Figure 11-7
LOW-GRADE DYSPLASIA OF THE STOMACH: HISTOLOGIC SPECTRUM

A: This lesion is characterized by dysplastic tubules which occupy the superficial half of the mucosa. At low power the dysplastic epithelium is distinctive because of the enlarged basal nuclei and prominent basophilic cytoplasm, resulting from failure of the epithelium to differentiate into mucin-producing cells.

B: Higher magnification of A showing dysplastic tubules lined by cells with basophilic cytoplasm and basally oriented, enlarged nuclei containing tiny nucleoli. The histologic changes are at the low end of dysplasia and may be interpreted by some as indefinite or reactive atypia.

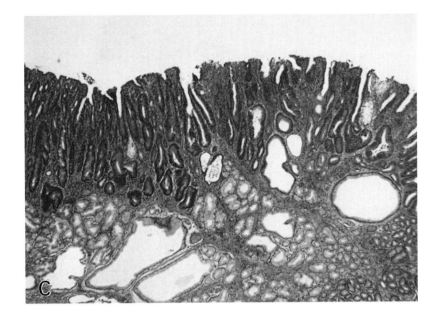

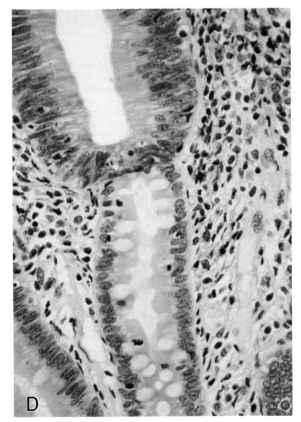

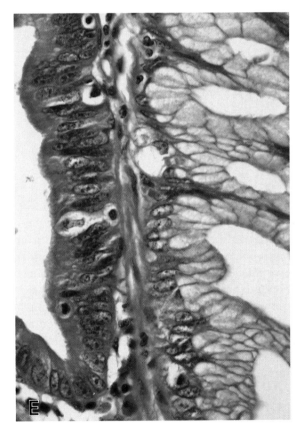

Figure 11-7 (Continued)

C: Low-power view of another dysplastic lesion of the antrum. The superficial half of the mucosa is dysplastic. The lower half consists of normal antral glands, some of which are cystically dilated.

D: Low-grade dysplasia occupying the superficial half of the gland, lower half of which appears normal.

E: Higher magnification showing the dysplastic epithelium on the left compared to normal epithelium on the right. In contrast to C the severity of the dysplasia is greater but still low grade. Note that the nuclei are larger and pseudostratified and occupy more than half the length of the cell.

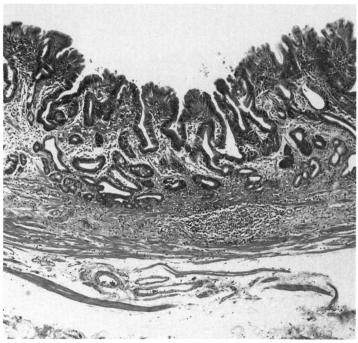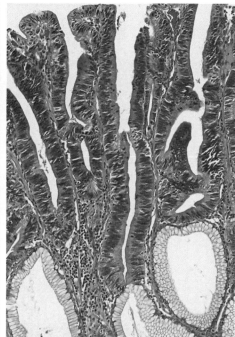

Figure 11-8
HIGH-GRADE DYSPLASIA

Left: There is extensive glandular proliferation and budding involving most of the mucosa with the exception of the lowermost portion. The latter contains atrophic antral glands and a focus of intestinal metaplasia at the base in the center.

Right: Higher magnification of the dysplastic glands showing marked pseudostratification with enlarged spindle-shaped nuclei occupying most of the cell. Note the normal crypts at the bottom characterized by small, basally oriented nuclei and clear-staining cytoplasm. The degree of dysplasia is clearly at the low end of high grade and would be graded moderate if a three-grade system was used.

One type of dysplasia, which is commonly associated with intestinal metaplasia, is characterized by cells that are crowded together and peudostratified with cigar-shaped nuclei, inconspicuous nucleoli, and abundant amphophilic cytoplasm (figs. 11-7D, 11-8, right). The nuclei occupy the basal half of each cell and mitoses may be prominent. As the severity of dysplasia increases the nuclei become less hyperchromatic and more vesicular, and the number of mitoses increases. The cell cytoplasm frequently contains mucin which may be neutral (periodic acid–Schiff [PAS] positive) or acidic (Alcian blue positive at pH 2.5). Enterochromaffin and Paneth cells are common.

The second histologic pattern is often found in the setting of chronic atrophic gastritis and immature or incomplete intestinal metaplasia. This type of dysplasia sometimes resembles, and is confused with, regenerative change. There are architectural derangements of the mucosa consisting of abnormal glands with budding, irregular branching, and crowding. Both goblet cells and columnar cells may be present. There is variation in size and shape of the cells and an increased nuclear/cytoplasmic ratio. The cytoplasm of the dysplastic cells is pale and sparse; the nuclei show loss of polarity, and are enlarged, rounded, and vesicular with enlarged single nucleoli. In high-grade dysplasia the cells are round and have large vesicular nuclei, a prominent nucleolus, and many mitoses (fig. 11-9). A number of Japanese pathologists consider the latter cytologic features to be diagnostic of gastric carcinoma irrespective of whether there is invasion into the lamina propria.

The histologic features of the different grades of dysplasia depend upon the architectural complexity and the degree of cytologic atypia. The two components however do not always go hand in hand.

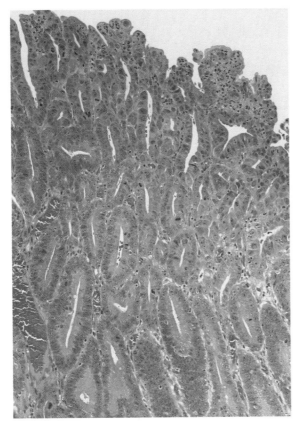
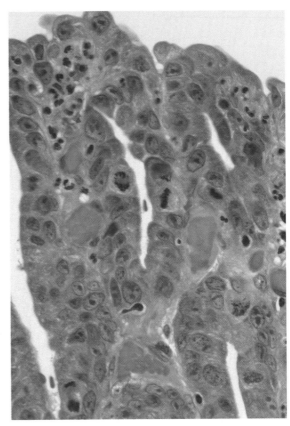

Figure 11-9
HIGH-GRADE DYSPLASIA

High-grade dysplasia with mild architectural changes but marked cytologic atypia.

Left: The tubules are crowded and almost touching one another, barely separated by the fibrovascular stroma of the lamina propria.

Right: High-power magnification of the dysplastic tubules. The dysplastic cells have enlarged vesicular nuclei each containing one or more prominent nucleoli (in contrast to the pseudostratified dysplasias which contain small indistinct nucleoli). They occupy much of the cell and scant cytoplasm. Also note the many mitotic figures.

*Low-Grade Dysplasia.* This lesion usually occupies the superficial portion of the mucosa, and is characterized by simple dysplastic tubules with little branching, connecting to the underlying normal foveolar epithelium (fig. 11-6). Some dysplasias involve the full thickness of the mucosa. The dysplastic cells may be of the different types described above but they tend to retain their basal nuclear polarity and have small indistinct nucleoli. Mitoses are present but usually sparse, increasing in number with progressive dysplasia.

*High-Grade Dysplasia.* The dysplastic tubules often show pronounced architectural changes, with elongation and complex budding producing a cribriform pattern in the most extreme cases. The dysplastic cells show marked variation in size and shape and loss of basal nuclear polarity. The nuclei are large, often vesicular, with irregularly clumped chromatin and large nucleoli (fig. 11-9). Mitoses are common and often atypical (fig. 11-9, right). The extreme form of high-grade dysplasia, which is considered carcinoma in situ by some, is characterized by marked cytologic atypia, with or without architectural complexity of the glands. The glands proliferate and bud, resulting in an abnormal network of loop-shaped glands with anastomoses producing a cribriform pattern. The cytologic atypia is characterized by round cells with large, spherical, vesicular nuclei; irregularly clumped chromatin; and numerous large distinct and irregular nucleoli, considered by some as the hallmark of carcinoma (fig. 11-11). Mitoses, which often are atypical, are frequently prominent.

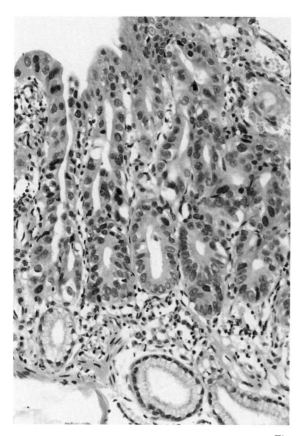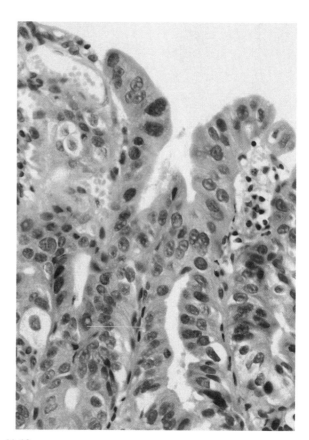

Figure 11-10
HIGH-GRADE DYSPLASIA

Left: Low-power magnification showing marked crowding of the dysplastic tubules, which are relatively simple without much architectural distortion. The lower third of the mucosa contains nondysplastic, cystically dilated antral glands.

Right: Higher magnification shows variation in size and shape of the dysplastic cells. The nuclei are greatly enlarged, some are hyperchromatic, others vesicular with prominent nucleoli.

*Lesions Indefinite for Dysplasia.* Reactive and regenerative epithelium in gastric mucosa may sometimes be difficult to differentiate from adenoma (fig. 11-12). The nuclei may be larger and denser than those normally seen in regenerative epithelium and may have bigger and more prominent nucleoli. In addition, there is often increased cytoplasmic basophilia (fig. 11-12E). Those lesions in which the distinction between regenerative and dysplastic epithelium is not clear have been called indefinite for dysplasia.

*Dysplasia Involving Nonmetaplastic Mucosa.* The precursor lesion of the diffuse type of gastric carcinoma is much more subtle than that occurring in intestinal mucosa. This is because tumor cells, such as those from signet ring carcinoma, frequently appear to extrude from gastric pits that look virtually normal morphologically. Careful examination of many of these pits reveals that the nuclei vary slightly in size and shape. In one study the dysplasia was characterized by cytologic atypia in the absence of architectural glandular derangement and replacement of the differentiated cells lining the glands by cells with varying degrees of cytologic abnormalities (crowding, loss of nuclear polarity, and nuclear pleomorphism) (66). The nuclei are enlarged, vesicular or hyperchromatic, with numerous nucleoli and the cytoplasm is frequently scant (fig. 11-13). The severity of the changes can be graded by the degree of involvement of the gland as measured from the proliferative zone (situated in the lower third of the gastric pit and the isthmus) and by the degree of cytologic abnormality. By analogy with dysplasia in inflammatory bowel disease, the authors of this study found that in a number of cases the histologic changes were equivocal and were categorized as indefinite for dysplasia (66).

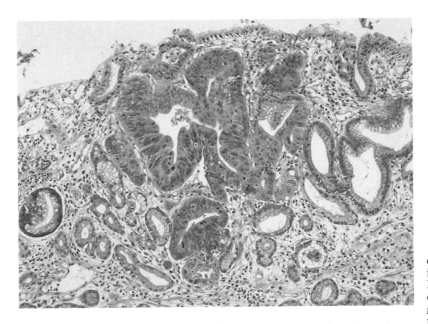

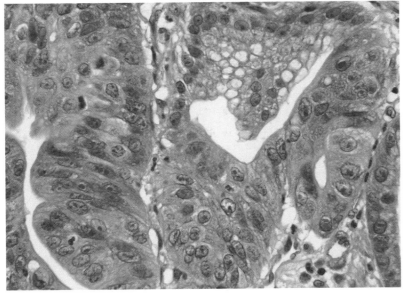

Figure 11-11
HIGH-GRADE DYSPLASIA

Top: Low-power view of gastric mucosa showing a small focus of highly irregular branched dysplastic tubules. In this sort of biopsy it is sometimes difficult to differentiate dysplastic glands from an early invasive intramucosal carcinoma. Unless there is definite invasion into the lamina propria, this is not diagnosed as intramucosal carcinoma.

Bottom: High-power view showing a highly irregular, branched tubule with a multilayered epithelium.

A second change that is frequently observed at the edge of the carcinoma is markedly thickened, distorted, hyperplastic foveolar epithelium which may be the gastric equivalent of the transitional mucosa seen in the large bowel rather than a genuine precancerous lesion. It occurs with both intestinal and diffuse carcinomas.

**Differential Diagnosis.** The major histologic differences between dysplastic, and reactive and regenerative gastric epithelia are listed in Table 11-3. The regenerative changes are characterized by a gradual transition of the normal surrounding epithelium to reactive epithelium; regular arrangement of tubules; uniform enlargement of nuclei, with homogeneous basophilia; and small, frequently multiple nucleoli (fig. 11-12A–D). Other changes are syncytial epithelial cells with red cytoplasm and inflamed vascular stroma. However, occasionally, the epithelial nuclear changes are almost identical to those seen in gastric dysplasia and cannot be relied upon to separate the two.

**Treatment.** There is no agreement on the management of gastric dysplasia. Some clinicians believe that this is a neoplastic lesion and

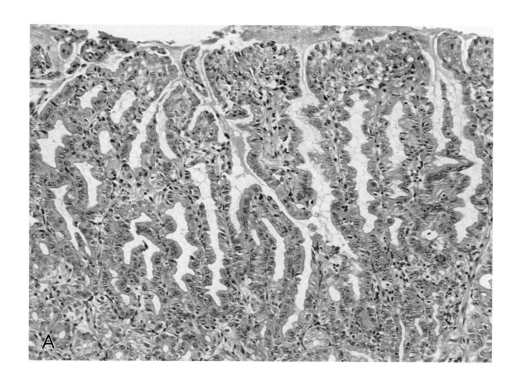

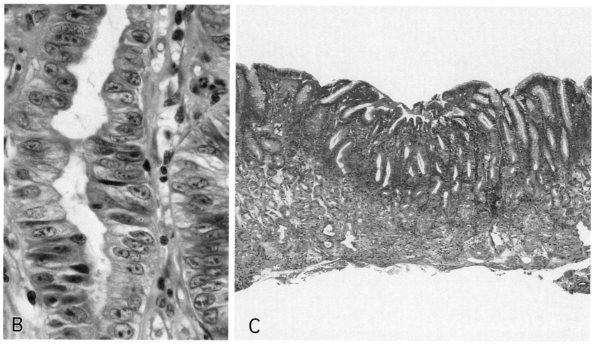

Figure 11-12
GASTRIC REGENERATIVE HYPERPLASIA (REACTIVE GASTROPATHY)
AND EPITHELIAL ATYPIA INDEFINITE FOR DYSPLASIA

A: Low-power view of gastric mucosa of a patient who previously underwent a partial gastrectomy (postoperative stomach). The regenerative features are characterized by elongation of the foveolae, producing a corkscrew-like appearance. There is relatively little inflammation.

B: High-power magnification of one of the gastric pits. The nuclei of the epithelial cells have maintained their basal location but are enlarged and contain small but sometimes multiple nucleoli. In the older literature these changes were misdiagnosed as dysplasia.

C: Low-power view of an NSAID-induced healed erosion. In the center of the field the foveolae are crowded together.

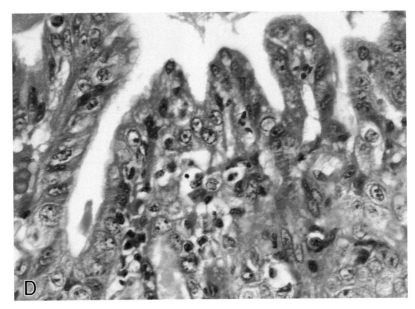

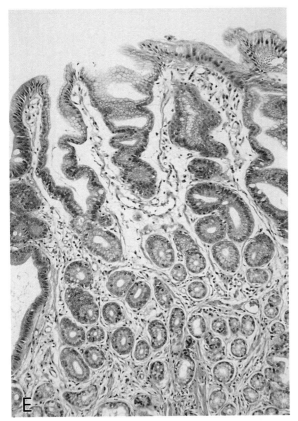

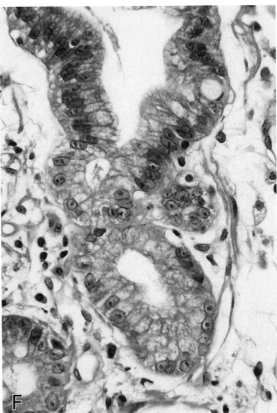

Figure 11-12 (Continued)

D: Higher magnification of C showing regenerative epithelial changes which superficially may be confused with dysplastic cells because of their enlarged nuclei and mucin depletion. However, the overall appearance of the lesion at low power should help distinguish the two.

E: Low-power view of gastric mucosa showing epithelial atypia indefinite for dysplasia. The increased basophilia of the gastric pits draws attention to this lesion.

F: High-power view of E showing a tubule lined by epithelium containing enlarged basophilic nuclei. This is an example of a biopsy that might be called by some reactive epithelial atypia with resemblance to incomplete intestinal metaplasia and by others low-grade dysplasia. It is our philosophy to call these lesions indefinite for dysplasia whenever there is any doubt as to the diagnosis.

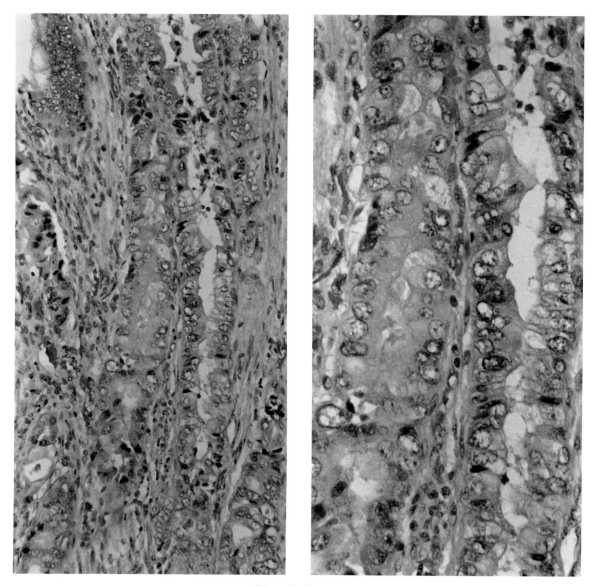

Figure 11-13
HIGH-GRADE DYSPLASIA INVOLVING NONMETAPLASTIC MUCOSA
Left: The tubules are lined by dysplastic cells showing loss of nuclear polarity.
Right: Higher power magnification of the tubular epithelium showing large irregular vesicular nuclei and scant cytoplasm.
A few tumor cells have foamy cytoplasm. (Courtesy of Dr. L. Ghandur Mnaymneh, Miami, FL.)

should be managed by surgical resection, especially high-grade lesions (19,50,105,146,153, 163,171,211,221). Others argue that since dysplastic lesions of the stomach are frequently multifocal, unpredictable in location, and sometimes regress, low-grade dysplasias are best handled conservatively with regular follow-up endoscopy (3). In Japan, where most cases are seen, the consensus is for the conservative approach. However, as already noted, since coincident gastric carcinoma may already be present at the time of diagnosis of gastric dysplasia, it is imperative to examine the stomach meticulously by biopsies if the conservative approach to management is undertaken. In contrast to gastric dysplasia, most authorities recommend excision of pedunculated and sessile adenomas because of their well-circumscribed nature.

Table 11-3

## MAJOR HISTOLOGIC FEATURES DISTINGUISHING ADENOMA FROM REGENERATIVE HYPERPLASIA

| Architectural Changes | |
|---|---|
| **Regenerative Hyperplasia (excluding postinjury phase)** | **Dysplasia** |
| Foveolar hyperplasia<br>Surface maturation | Foveolar proliferation and crowding with loss of surface maturation; tubular budding and branching producing "back to back configuration" and cribriform pattern; cystic dilation |
| | Glandular atrophy |

| Cytologic Abnormalities | |
|---|---|
| **Regenerative Hyperplasia** | **Dysplasia*** |
| Regenerating immature cells in hyperplastic zones | Cytologic changes seen throughout epithelium |
| Reduced mucin; low columnar cells; vesicular nuclei; prominent but small regular nucleoli | Cellular pleomorphism with loss of nuclear polarity, pseudostratification, mucin depletion, hyperchromatic enlarged nuclei; large irregular and multiple nucleoli; prominent mitoses |

*The intensity of these changes is related to the degree of the dysplasia: less in low grade and more in high grade.

## GASTRIC CARCINOMA

On the basis of clinical presentation and prognosis, gastric cancers can be subdivided into two major subtypes: early gastric cancer and advanced gastric cancer.

**Definition and Clinical Features.** Early gastric carcinoma is defined as an invasive gastric carcinoma which is confined to the mucosa and submucosa, irrespective of whether lymph node metastases are present. This corresponds to T1 of the TNM classification. They occur about twice as frequently in males than females and the majority occur in patients over 50 years of age (Table 11-4); the exception is the excavated and large eroded subtype, which is found predominantly in young and middle-aged patients (53,172).

Most early gastric carcinomas are asymptomatic; they are detected by massive screening programs, usually by X ray but increasingly by endoscopy. Those that are symptomatic present with peptic ulcer symptoms (239). They have been described primarily in the Japanese literature, where these tumors now account for 55 percent of all gastric carcinomas. Reports of early carcinoma in the United States indicate that they closely resemble those reported in Japan and Europe (71). With increasing endoscopic biopsy and recognition, these lesions are being diagnosed more often in the United States and Europe (5,7,71).

Is early gastric carcinoma and the so-called advanced gastric carcinoma of the Western hemisphere a similar tumor at different stages of development? Tsukama et al. (251) followed 43 cases of early gastric carcinoma for 6 to 88 months. They found that while 16 remained unchanged, 27 developed into advanced carcinoma. These results and similar studies by others (172) suggest that most early gastric carcinomas progress with time to typical advanced gastric carcinomas.

In its earliest form, carcinoma of the stomach develops from dysplastic epithelium from the generative cell zone of the atrophic gastric glands and intestinal metaplastic glands. It then buds or branches from the glands and infiltrates into the lamina propria (fig. 11-14) (207). Growth is usually very slow (91,181): it has been estimated that the doubling time is from 555 to 3076 days (63). However, once the tumor increases in size and invades the submucosa doubling time accelerates to 17 to 90 days. Still, it may take up to 6 years for a tumor of several millimeters to develop (62,135, 181). The time interval for early gastric carcinoma to transform into advanced carcinoma is also long but variable, ranging from 6 months to 21 years (63,109,135,176,251). The time period for transformation depends in part on the stage of the early cancer: 10 years for the mucosal carcinomas and several months to a year for carcinomas extending into the submucosa (109,111,176,181). Some

Table 11-4

## AGE DISTRIBUTION OF EARLY GASTRIC CANCER IN JAPAN*

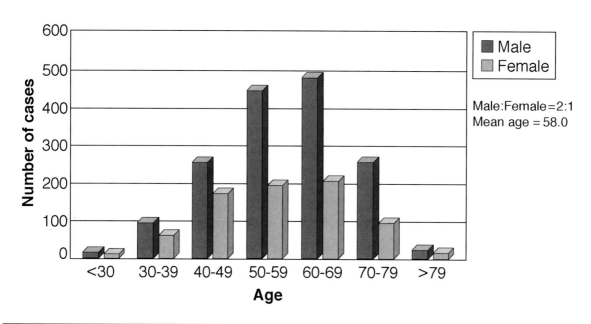

*The data in this table are from the National Cancer Center Hospital, Tokyo. Represented are 2,300 cases and 2,562 lesions. (Courtesy of Dr. T. Hirota, National Cancer Center, Tokyo, Japan.)

early gastric carcinomas have transformed to advanced carcinomas and metastasized soon after diagnosis (63); these lesions may already have had a focus of carcinoma in an unbiopsied area or they may have been intrinsically highly aggressive.

In Japan where the incidence of gastric carcinoma is high, approximately 50 percent of gastric carcinomas are early carcinomas (87). Early diagnosis is achieved by mass X-ray screening and lately by endoscopy, which is becoming increasingly more common. However, these procedures are not practical in the United States where the incidence is considerably lower. Nevertheless, because of a greater awareness of these tumors and the widespread use of endoscopy, more early gastric cancers (as high as 15 percent in one recent report) are being diagnosed in the United States and Europe (239).

Advanced gastric cancers are defined as cancers that have invaded the stomach into or beyond the muscularis propria, irrespective of whether lymph node metastases are present. This corresponds to T2 to T4 of the TNM classification.

These tumors mainly involve the middle-aged and elderly, with a male to female ratio of 2 to 1 (152,257). There is a secondary group of patients who usually have a very aggressive (probably related to the advanced stage of the disease at presentation), diffuse type of adenocarcinoma, frequently of signet-ring cell type (69). These patients are usually under 40 years, the male to female ratio is about 1 to 1, and women sometimes present with ovarian (Krukenberg) tumors. While the incidence of the usual type of gastric carcinoma is falling worldwide, the relative frequency of tumors in younger patients is increasing (172) as is the incidence of tumors of the gastric cardia (12,257).

In most countries except Japan, gastric carcinomas are advanced at the time of presentation. Symptoms are commonly vague, consisting of weight loss and anemia. Other types of presentation consist of ulcer-type pain, occult or overt gastrointestinal bleeding, or gastric outlet obstruction in tumors near the pylorus. Some patients present with wide metastatic disease.

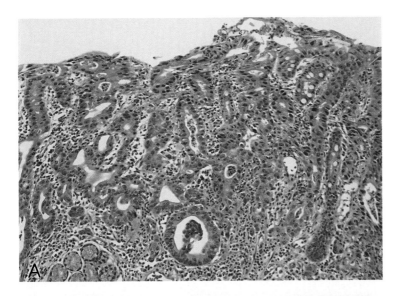

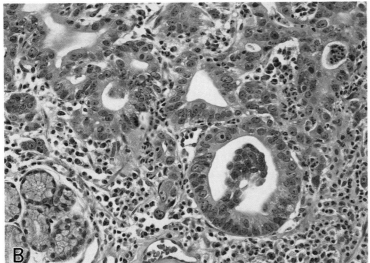

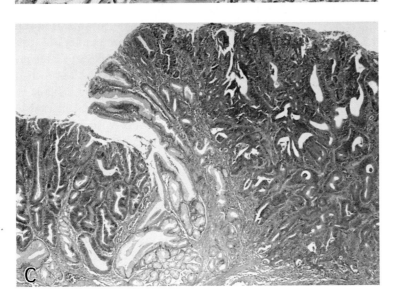

Figure 11-14
### HIGH-GRADE DYSPLASIA AND EARLY GASTRIC CARCINOMA

A: Much of this biopsy specimen shows high-grade dysplasia with crowding and branching of dysplastic tubules. However, at the bottom center of the illustration there is a focus of carcinoma characterized by distorted irregular tubules infiltrating the lamina propria and an accompanying inflammatory infiltrate.

B: High-power magnification of the malignant glandular profiles demonstrate the marked atypia of the malignant cells, some of which infiltrate the lamina propria as single cells or in small clumps. The malignant cells have greatly enlarged vesicular nuclei with prominent nucleoli and often scant cytoplasm. There is an accompanying lymphocytic infiltrate.

C: Low-power view of gastric mucosa showing high-grade dysplasia (on the left) adjacent to intramucosal carcinoma. Note the diffuse infiltration of the lamina propria by atypical glandular profiles.

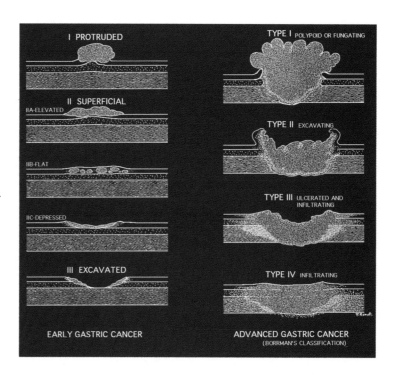

Figure 11-15
EARLY GASTRIC CARCINOMA
Diagrammatic representation of tumor types.

Once carcinoma is diagnosed or suspected further evaluation by ultrasound and computerized tomography (CT) is performed to determine the clinical stage of disease. Endoscopic ultrasonography is another technique that is increasingly used to determine depth of invasion and lymph node metastasis (80).

**Gross and Endoscopic Findings.** The standard classification of early gastric carcinomas was established in 1962 by the Japanese Research Society for Gastric Carcinoma (158,166). Early gastric carcinomas are divided on the basis of macroscopic appearance into three main groups: protruded or polypoid (type I), superficial (type II), and excavated (type III) (figs. 11-15–11-22). The superficial type is further divided into three subtypes: IIa, IIb, and IIc. Combinations of the three major types and subtypes are common (87).

The endoscopic and gross appearances of these lesions are summarized and illustrated in figures 11-15–11-22. Type I lesions are distinctly polypoid, in contrast to the type II lesions which have an irregular and frequently nodular surface. Type IIb lesions are essentially flat and may be difficult to detect. They may have shallow ulcers whose margins show focal discoloration and depression. The elevated type IIa has a mucosa approximately twice as thick as that of the surrounding mucosa. Type IIc is slightly depressed due to surface erosion and there is commonly a convergence of mucosal folds towards the erosion. Sometimes a small ulcer scar occurs within the depressed lesion. Type III early gastric carcinoma is characterized by a deep ulcer rimmed by a narrow margin of tumor, and may resemble a chronic gastric ulcer.

Early gastric carcinomas may resemble healing peptic ulcers grossly. Endoscopically there are two features which help to differentiate between the benign and malignant lesions. First is the difference in the appearance of the mucosal folds at the margin of the ulcer: in early carcinomas they appear to be "cut off" in contrast to the gentle termination of benign ulcers. Second is the difference in the erythema associated with the two lesions: in carcinoma it is intense and diffuse in contrast to the stippled, raised red dots with intervening white lines representing regenerative epithelium (11). In up to 20 percent of cases, however, it is still difficult to separate benign from malignant lesions and in these cases multiple biopsies and careful follow-up are necessary (119).

The above subclassifications obviate unnecessary verbal description and, more importantly, the different gross appearances are associated with disparate growth patterns.

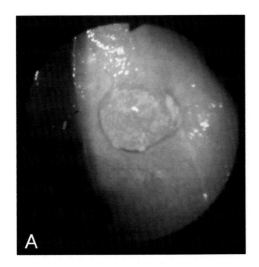

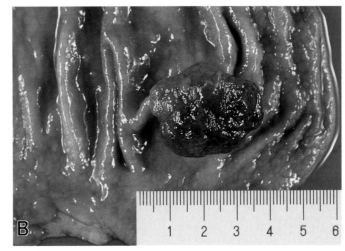

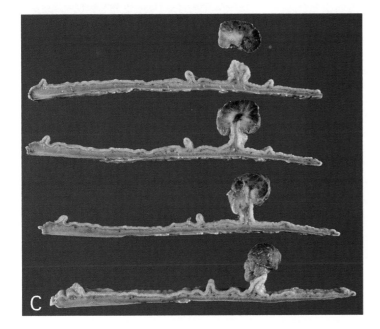

Figure 11-16
EARLY GASTRIC CARCINOMA:
TYPE I (POLYPOID TYPE)

A: Endoscopic appearance.

B: Gross appearance of specimen from gastric resection.

C: Cross-sectional cuts of gross specimen.

D: Scanning power view of histologic section.

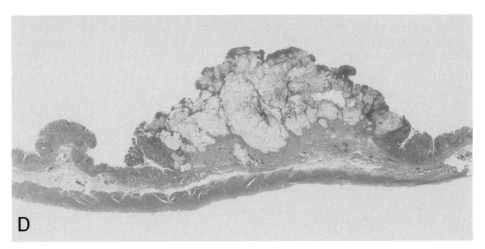

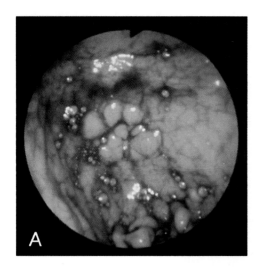

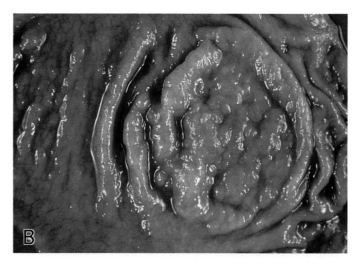

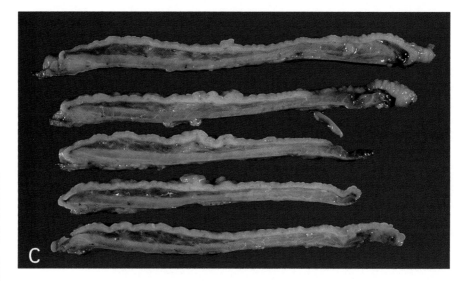

Figure 11-17
EARLY GASTRIC
CARCINOMA:
TYPE IIA
(SUPERFICIAL
[ELEVATED] TYPE)

A: Endoscopic appearance of slightly elevated mucosal nodules. The blue dye (indigo carmine) in the background has been sprayed onto the mucosa to produce a contrast between the lesion and the surrounding mucosa.

B: Gross appearance of a resection specimen showing nodular mucosa in the center surrounded by a number of thickened, elevated, concentric mucosal folds.

C: Cross-sectional cuts of gross specimen. (A, B, and C courtesy of Drs. Itabashi and Saito, Tokyo, Japan.)

D: Scanning power view of histologic section illustrating the thickened elevated mucosa.

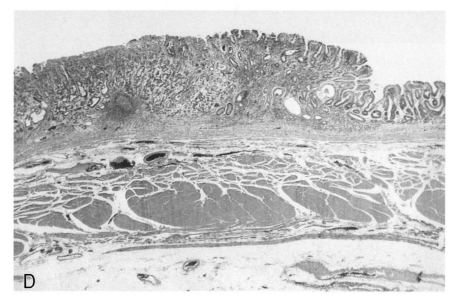

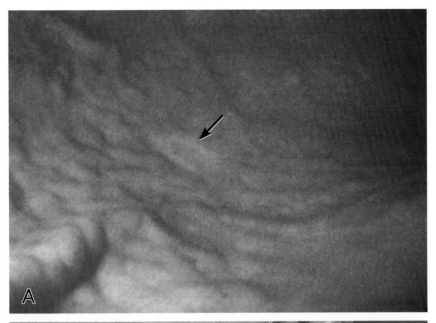

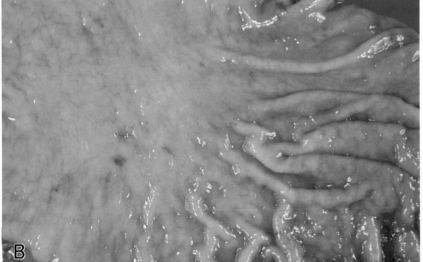

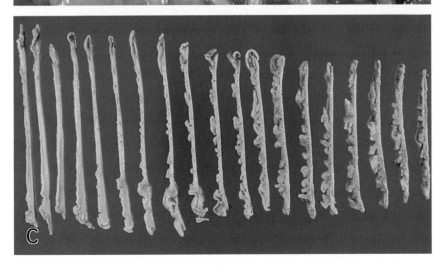

Figure 11-18
EARLY GASTRIC
CARCINOMA:
TYPE IIB
(FLAT TYPE)

These lesions can be difficult to visualize as they merge with the surrounding mucosa.

A: Endoscopic appearance of a barely perceptible mucosal depression (arrow).

B: Resection specimen showing flat mucosa devoid of the normal folds which are present to the right of the lesion.

C: Cross-sectional cuts showing irregular thickening of the mucosa. (A and B courtesy of Drs. Itabashi and Saito, Tokyo, Japan.)

Figure 11-19
EARLY GASTRIC CARCINOMA:
TYPE IIC (DEPRESSED TYPE)

A: Endoscopic view of a small depressed ulcer with a blue base due to the indigo carmine dye.

B: Resection specimen showing shallow ulcer.

C: Scanning power view of the ulcer in histologic section. (Courtesy of Drs. Itabashi and Saito, Tokyo, Japan.)

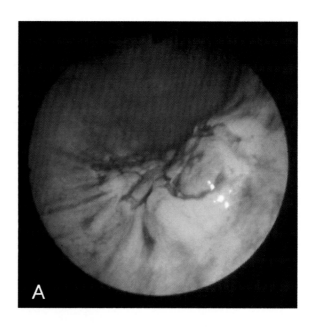

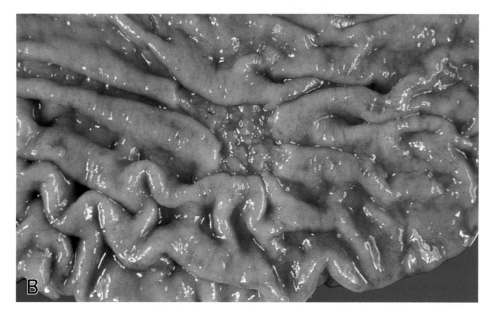

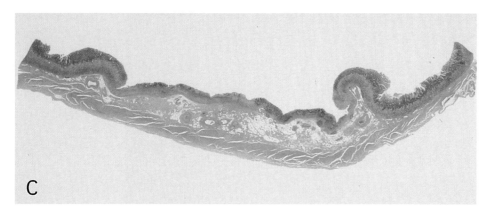

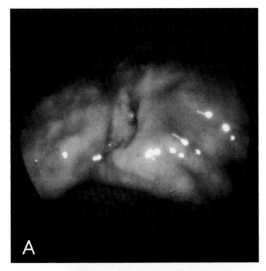

Figure 11-20
EARLY GASTRIC CARCINOMA:
TYPE III (EXCAVATED TYPE WITH WELL-
CIRCUMSCRIBED DEEP ULCER)

A: Endoscopic view.
B: Resection specimen.
C: Scanning view of histologic section of ulcer which
is lined by tumor both at the base and the sides. (Courtesy
of Drs. Itabashi and Saito, Tokyo, Japan.)

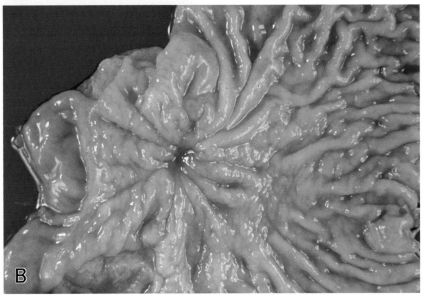

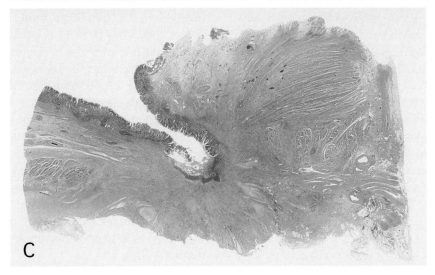

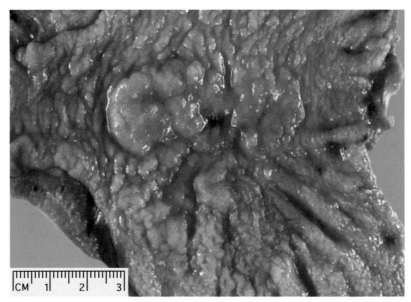

**Figure 11-21**
**EARLY GASTRIC CARCINOMA:**
**TYPES IIA TO IIC**
Resection specimen showing an elevated, centrally ulcerated lesion. (Courtesy of Dr. T. Hirota, Tokyo, Japan.)

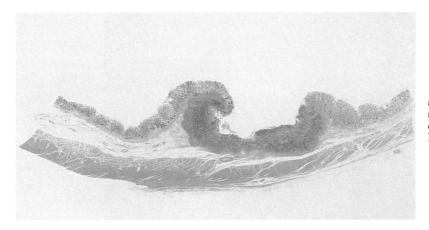

**Figure 11-22**
**EARLY GASTRIC CARCINOMA**
Scanning view of histologic section of an early gastric cancer type IIa to IIc showing elevated margins and central depression of the tumor. (Courtesy of Drs. Itabashi and Saito, Tokyo, Japan.)

*Location and Frequency of Early Gastric Carcinoma.* Early gastric carcinomas can occur anywhere in the stomach but the majority of tumors occur on the lesser curvature and around the angulus, most frequently in fundic mucosa showing transitional mucosa (Table 11-5). About 10 percent are multifocal (16,87), and there is evidence that some of the larger early gastric carcinomas (those over 3 cm) may result from "collision" of smaller ones. Multiplicity of early gastric carcinomas is twice as common in patients over age 65 (87).

*Prevalence of Macroscopic Types of Early Gastric Carcinoma.* The superficial type II tumors are by far the most common, accounting for just under 80 percent of early gastric carcinomas; the other two types account for less than 10 percent each (172,209). The depressed type IIb is almost always smaller than 5 mm, indicating that as the tumor grows larger, the originally flat lesions become either depressed or protruded. It has also been noted that the incidence of some of the macroscopic types of early carcinoma has changed in the last 25 years: the elevated type is decreasing in frequency whereas the superficial type IIc is increasing, probably indicating earlier diagnosis of these tumors. This is further supported by the study by Hirota (86) in which it was found that prior to 1964, 40 percent of early gastric carcinomas were larger than 5 cm in diameter whereas by 1983 only 10 percent were that large and 40 percent were less than 2 cm in diameter (86).

276

Table 11-5
## LOCATION OF EARLY GASTRIC CANCER*

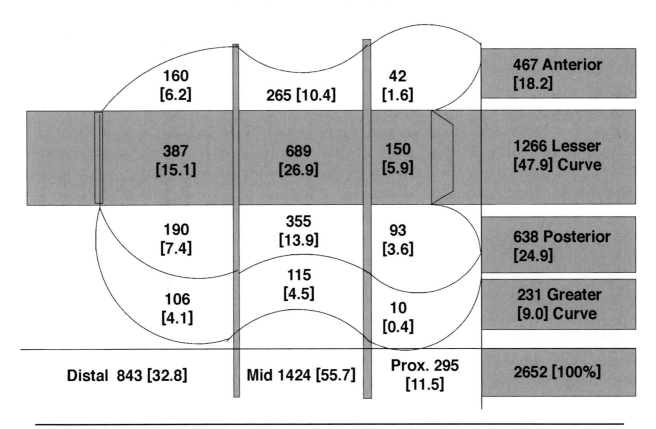

| | | | |
|---|---|---|---|
| 160 [6.2] | 265 [10.4] | 42 [1.6] | **467 Anterior** [18.2] |
| 387 [15.1] | 689 [26.9] | 150 [5.9] | **1266 Lesser** [47.9] **Curve** |
| 190 [7.4] | 355 [13.9] | 93 [3.6] | **638 Posterior** [24.9] |
| 106 [4.1] | 115 [4.5] | 10 [0.4] | **231 Greater** [9.0] **Curve** |
| **Distal 843 [32.8]** | **Mid 1424 [55.7]** | **Prox. 295** [11.5] | **2652 [100%]** |

*The data in this table is compiled from 2,300 cases and 2,562 lesions observed from 1962 to 1991 at the National Cancer Hospital in Tokyo. (Courtesy of Dr. T. Hirota, National Cancer Center, Tokyo.)

*Advanced Gastric Carcinoma.* Advanced gastric carcinomas can occur anywhere in the stomach. They are often very large and involve several sites when discovered. The majority occur in the antrum (50 percent) and lesser curvature of the body (15 percent). About 6 percent occupy the whole stomach and a few are distributed randomly throughout the stomach (15). The frequency of carcinomas of the gastric cardia, which is discussed separately, is rising at the expense of tumors from the antrum and lesser curvature and in some series now accounts for over 30 percent of gastric tumors (12).

Advanced gastric carcinoma is characterized by exophytic intraluminal or infiltrative growth modified by surface erosion and ulceration (figs. 11-23–11-26) (172). At the time of diagnosis, these tumors can vary from less than 2 cm to more than 15 cm in diameter and can involve the entire stomach (linitis plastica). The majority are in the 2- to 6-cm (44 percent) and 6- to 10-cm (30 percent) range (159). Exophytic tumors are typically solitary, well-circumscribed, broad-based polypoid lesions, which may be superficially ulcerated or severely excavated at the dome of the mass. The base of these tumors is commonly situated above the level of the stomach wall and rugal folds appear to terminate around the edge. Endoscopically, these tumors have a nodular, irregular, gray-pink appearance and are commonly superficially eroded in contrast to the smooth textured, orange-pink surrounding mucosa (fig. 11-23) (11). Another common variety of gastric carcinoma consists of an ulcerated tumor with slightly raised, irregular peripheral margins that infiltrate into the adjacent gastric wall (fig. 11-25). These tumors may sometimes mimic chronic gastric ulcer (fig. 11-25B), but careful examination

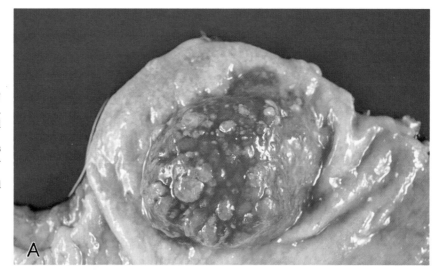

Figure 11-23
ADVANCED GASTRIC
CANCER: POLYPOID
(BORRMANN TYPE 1) LESION
A: Resection specimen show-
ing polypoid tumor with inflamed
nodular surface.
B: Cross-sectional cuts of gross
specimen. (Courtesy of Drs. Oc-
hiai and Saito, Tokyo, Japan.)
C: Endoscopic view of polypoid
lesion with surface erosions.

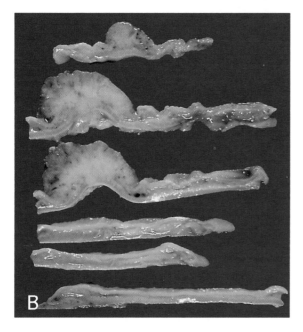

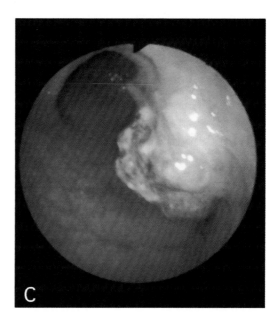

usually allows differentiation of the two lesions. Gastric ulcers are usually small, well-circum-scribed, punched-out lesions with a clean base and smooth, edematous ulcer margins. In con-trast, ulcerated carcinomas have fuzzy borders which are firm, fixed, and often raised and an ulcer that is of variable depth, necrotic, and often hemorrhagic. A minority of gastric carcinomas diffusely infiltrate the greater part of the stom-ach. These tumors are characteristically associ-ated with a marked desmoplastic reaction result-ing in a grossly thickened stomach which has been likened to a leather bottle (linitis plastica:

leather bottle stomach) (fig. 11-26). Frequently there is concomitant giant hypertrophy of the mu-cosal folds. These tumors have also been referred to as *scirrhous carcinomas* because of the intense fibrosis. About two thirds of these tumors show ulceration, thus facilitating the diagnosis of carci-noma, although the intense fibrosis and the often sparsely distributed, undifferentiated nature of the tumor cells sometimes leads to histologic misinter-pretation as chronic peptic ulcer. Diagnosing non-ulcerated tumors can also be difficult. Endoscopi-cally, there are two helpful signs. One is the "shelf effect" which consists of a sharply demarcated area

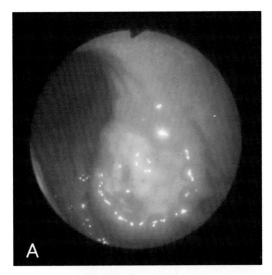

Figure 11-24
ADVANCED GASTRIC CANCER:
EXCAVATING (BORRMANN TYPE II) LESION
A: Endoscopic view of an elevated tumor mass, with central ulceration, crater formation, and raised rolled margins.
B: Resection specimen showing features similar to those in A.
C: Resection specimen of stomach showing central ulceration and a raised rolled margin.

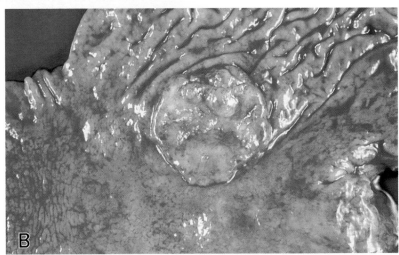

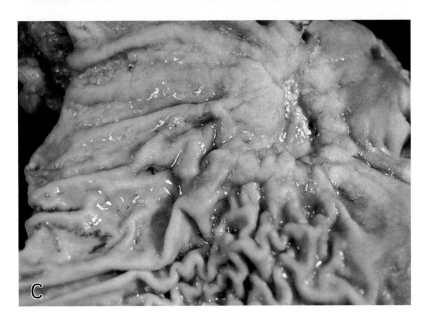

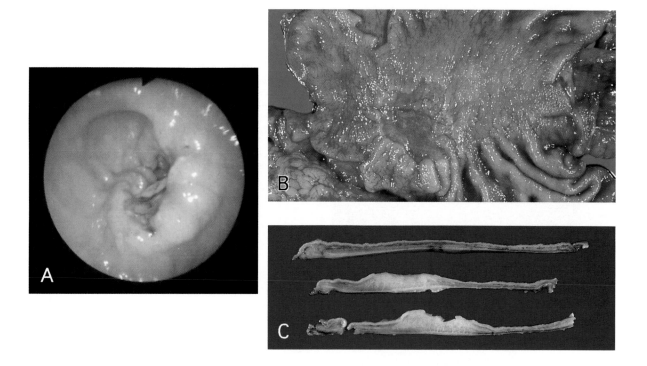

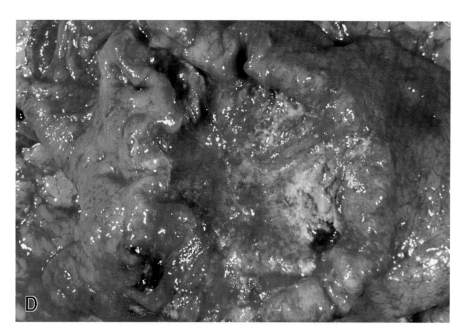

Figure 11-25

ADVANCED GASTRIC CANCER: ULCERATED AND INFILTRATING (BORRMANN TYPE III) LESION

A: Endoscopic view of an ulcerated tumor with slightly raised peripheral margins.

B: Resection specimen showing a centrally ulcerated lesion with a serpiginous raised margin. The mucosa above and to the right appears to be atrophic and devoid of folds.

C: Cross-sectional view of gross specimen showing features similar to B. In addition, a well-circumscribed lateral tumor margin is seen.

D: Gross appearance of a resection specimen of another Borrman type III adenocarcinoma showing a large central crater surrounded by a raised rolled margin.

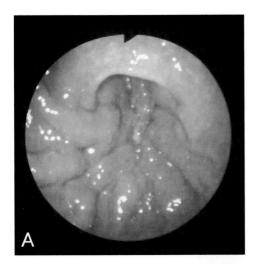

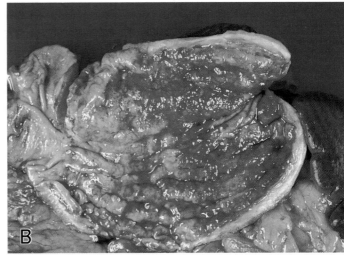

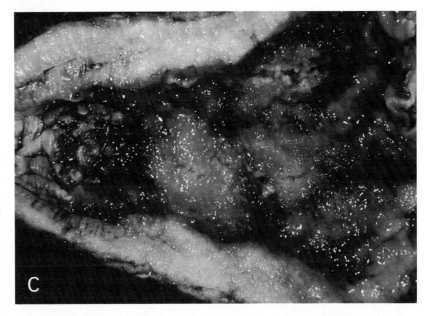

Figure 11-26
ADVANCED GASTRIC CANCER:
DIFFUSELY INFILTRATING
(BORRMANN TYPE IV,
LINITIS PLASTICA) LESION

A: Endoscopic view shows marked thickening and irregularity of the mucosal folds producing a cobblestone appearance.

B: Resection specimen showing involvement of the major portion of the stomach. There is marked thickening of the wall producing the so-called leather-bottle stomach. There is swelling of the mucosa which is covered with blood but otherwise intact. (Fig. 17-10 from Lewin KJ, Riddell RH, Weinstein WM. Gastrointestinal pathology and its clinical implications. New York: Igaku Shoin, 1992:639.)

C: Resected specimen of stomach shows diffuse thickening of the gastric wall.

D: Cross-sectional view of gross specimen shows the diffusely infiltrating tumor, which is white.

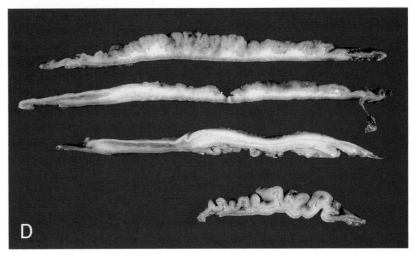

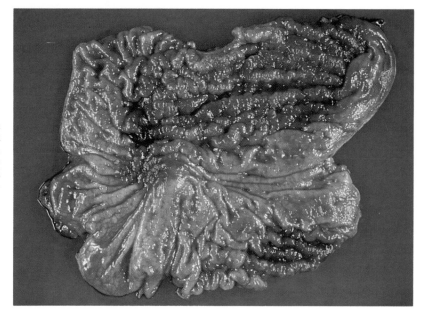

**Figure 11-27**
**SUPERFICIAL**
**SPREADING CARCINOMA**
In this gastric resection specimen a large superficial gastric carcinoma occupies about half the specimen. Histologically, the tumor was confined to the mucosa and superficial submucosa. (Courtesy of Dr. A. Ochiai, Tokyo, Japan.)

between the tumor and the adjacent normal mucosa, the result of tumor infiltration raising the level of the mucosa. The second consists of loss of mucosal tenting. Normally the gastric mucosa can be pulled out (tented) in the lumen but in diffusely infiltrative carcinoma it is firmly attached to the submucosa because of tumor infiltration (11).

There are a number of classifications for the gross appearance of gastric carcinoma; the most widely adopted is that of Borrmann (15). Gastric carcinomas are subdivided into four types: type I for the well-circumscribed polypoid lesions, type II for polypoid tumors with marked central ulceration, type III for the ulcerated tumors with infiltrative margins, and type IV for the linitis plastica variety. The main value of Borrmann's classification is that it eliminates the need of excessive verbal description of the gross appearance of the tumor.

As with early gastric carcinoma, advanced gastric carcinoma shows some correlation between gross characteristics, histologic appearance, and patient age. The exophytic and expanding lesions tend to be well or moderately well-differentiated, associated with intestinal metaplasia, and occur in elderly patients, whereas the diffusely thickened and infiltrative lesions are frequently poorly differentiated and are prominent in younger patients.

**Unusual Variants.** *Minute Gastric Carcinoma.* These are tiny early gastric carcinomas less than 5 mm in diameter. They are mostly unifocal, but may coexist with a larger cancerous lesion. Only a minority of these lesions have associated dysplasia. Fifty percent of these carcinomas invade the submucosa but do not metastasize to a lymph node. They are often overlooked endoscopically and are difficult to differentiate from benign erosions (97,172).

*Superficial Spreading Carcinoma.* These are early gastric carcinomas that frequently have a long history of gastric symptoms. By definition they should measure at least 25 cm$^2$ in area, although they frequently measure up to 10 cm in diameter, but remain confined to the mucosa and submucosa (fig. 11-27) (189).

**Handling of Resection Specimens and Intraoperative Evaluation.** The importance of the stage of gastric carcinoma in determining prognosis cannot be overstressed. Thus, it is critically important for the pathologist to determine in the gross examination the precise distance of the tumor from the resection margins, the extent of penetration into or through the gastric wall, the degree of serosal involvement, and whether adjacent structures are involved. Just as important as examining the primary tumor is the determination of lymph node metastases. In many centers the precise sites of origin of lymph node biopsies are not properly identified to the pathologist, thus creating problems in accurate tumor staging. Evaluation of lymph node involvement for staging entails: 1) the location of the nodes in relation to the tumor, i.e., whether less than or greater than 3 cm from the tumor edge which is indicative of whether the tumor has skipped beyond the local lymph nodes; and 2) whether the nodes are regional or distant.

Table 11-6 summarizes our method of handling stomachs removed because of gastric carcinoma. Because the prognosis of diffuse type gastric carcinoma is adversely affected by tumor within 5 cm of the resection margin (as discussed under prognosis) (4,93), we believe it is most important to measure the distance between the proximal resection margin and the neoplasm intraoperatively. We recommend a frozen section of the proximal margin because of microscopic lymphatic dissemination, which is not grossly visible or palpable. The number of sections taken for frozen section depends on the specimen. If the proximal margin is at the esophagogastric junction, then frozen section of the entire circumference of the resection margin is recommended. For partial gastrectomies, we recommend one or two sections parallel to the resection margin at the point where it comes closest to the tumor.

The resected specimen should be carefully opened, pinned out, and fixed in buffered formalin. The size and extent of tumor penetration should be carefully assessed, particularly whether there has been invasion of the muscularis propria and beyond. Also, it is important to sample all perigastric lymph nodes to determine the number containing metastases. In Japan all lymph nodes dissected from the gastrectomy specimen as well as all biopsied nodes removed are labeled according to their exact location and this accounts for the excellent statistical data on staging and prognosis produced by that country. It remains to be determined whether such detailed examination of lymph nodes in routine gastrectomies is necessary or whether a simplified staging technique related to the major drainage sites, such as around the stomach in the lesser omentum, peripancreatic and hilar regions, and para-aortic region, is adequate for prognostic purposes. Since gastric car-

Table 11-6

## EXAMINATION OF GASTRIC RESECTION SPECIMENS

### Intraoperative
1. Measure distance of tumor from proximal resection margin in the fresh unstretched specimen
2. Do frozen section of proximal resection margin to exclude tumor at any level (i.e., mucosa to serosa)
3. Photograph

### Fixed Specimen
Extent of surgery
  1. Stomach
  2. Other tissues and organs
Location
Gross pathology
  Borrmann's growth patterns
    Type 1. Polypoid
    Type 2. Excavated
    Type 3. Ulcerated
    Type 4. Diffuse thickening
  Depth of penetration and involvement of other structures
  Lymph node involvement: number and distance from tumor
Histology
  1. Tumor
    Type (e.g., WHO classification) and differentiation
    Lauren's classification (intestinal or diffuse)
  2. Lymphatic and/or venous infiltration, especially extramural
  3. Depth of invasion
  4. Resection margins
  5. Lymph node involvement and number
Associated lesions
  Gastritis, intestinal metaplasia, dysplasia, and polyps
Summary statement
  TNM staging
  Likely behavior of tumor and prognosis

cinomas may be multifocal, the remainder of the stomach should be carefully examined.

A modification of the above procedure has been reported from Britain (56,220). The lymph node groups related to the major arteries are identified on the gross fresh specimen. The fat/omentum representing each specific lymph node group is then dissected off the specimen prior to fixation and placed in a separate labeled specimen pot with 1 percent formalin. After fixation each piece of fat/omentum is finely sliced.

Table 11-7

## HISTOLOGIC TYPES OF EARLY GASTRIC CARCINOMA

**Differentiated Carcinomas**
Tubular adenocarcinoma
Papillary adenocarcinoma
Mucinous carcinoma
Squamous cell carcinoma
Adenosquamous cell carcinoma

**Less-Differentiated Carcinomas**
Poorly differentiated carcinomas of the above types
Signet-ring cell carcinoma
Small cell carcinoma
Undifferentiated carcinoma

Table 11-8

## FREQUENCY OF HISTOLOGIC TYPES OF EARLY GASTRIC CANCER*

| Histologic Type | Lesions | Incidence(%) |
|---|---|---|
| Papillary adenocarcinoma | 168 | 6.6 ⌉ |
| | | ⊢ 60.5 |
| Tubular adenocarcinoma | 1381 | 53.9 ⌋ |
| Poorly differentiated adenocarcinoma | 343 | 13.4 ⌉ |
| Signet-ring cell carcinoma | 651 | 25.4 ⊢ 39.5 |
| Mucinous adenocarcinoma | 19 | 0.7 |
| Total | 2562 | 100.0 ⌋ |

*Data from 2,300 cases and 2,562 lesions observed at the National Cancer Center Hospital, Tokyo from May 1962 until May 1991. (Courtesy of Dr. T. Hirota, Tokyo, Japan.)

All lymph nodes found are then sampled. The authors have found that this method results in high yields of lymph node metastases and identifies the location of these nodes accurately.

The handling of gastric resections for palliation only (for example, in cases with liver metastases or extensive intra-abdominal spread) obviously need not be as detailed. Sections should be taken to confirm the diagnosis, assess the depth of invasion, and determine whether there is tumor involvement of the resection margins. In addition, it is important to confirm the presence of metastases by biopsy, because on rare occasions lesions that are thought to be metastatic prove to be something else, for example fibrosis or granulomata.

The evaluation of resection specimens for early gastric carcinoma requires the same meticulous handling as advanced gastric carcinoma. The carcinoma should be examined in its entirety histologically, and special attention should be taken to sample all the regional lymph nodes.

**Histologic Classification and Microscopic Findings.** *Early Gastric Carcinoma.* Early gastric cancers are subdivided into two categories: intramucosal and submucosal. The intramucosal type invades through the epithelial basement membrane into the lamina propria (123,207). The histologic distinction between intramucosal carcinoma and high-grade dysplasia is sometimes difficult and it is our distinct impression that a number of studies on early gastric

carcinomas have included cases of high-grade dysplasia, thus skewing the survival statistics.

Early gastric carcinoma shows the same histologic spectrum as advanced carcinoma (Table 11-7). The better differentiated tumors include the well-differentiated and the moderately differentiated tubular, papillary, and mucinous carcinomas. The less differentiated tumors include signet-ring cell carcinoma and poorly differentiated and undifferentiated carcinomas. The relative frequency of these early gastric cancers is shown in Table 11-8. Signet-ring cell carcinomas are often found in association with poorly differentiated carcinomas, frequently at the periphery of the tumor. Signet-ring cell carcinoma confined to the mucosa may have a three-layered pattern similar to that seen in the normal mucosa: the uppermost layer contains signet-ring cells with neutral mucin of gastric surface epithelial type; the middle layer cells have no mucin; and the lowest layer cells resemble pyloric glandular epithelium. Once these signet-ring carcinomas invade the deeper mucosa and submucosa they lose this pattern (259). The mucinous adenocarcinomas are included with the less-differentiated adenocarcinomas when associated with signet-ring cell carcinomas (see Advanced Gastric Carcinoma for detailed histology). Rarely, other histologic types of gastric carcinoma may be found, such as adenosquamous and squamous carcinomas.

Frequency of Histologic Types. Differentiated early gastric carcinomas are more common than poorly differentiated and undifferentiated types. In one study, 52 percent of early gastric carcinomas were tubular adenocarcinoma, 7 percent were papillary adenocarcinoma, 26 percent signet-ring cell carcinoma, and 14 percent poorly differentiated adenocarcinoma (87). Pure mucinous adenocarcinomas accounted for less than 1 percent of cases.

Correlation Between Macroscopic and Microscopic Types of Tumor. There is a good correlation between the gross appearance, morphologic type, and depth of invasion (172). Polypoid or elevated lesions are usually well-differentiated, whereas excavated and large depressed lesions are poorly differentiated. Small lesions (less than 3 cm) with well-defined margins are usually well differentiated and show only microscopic invasion, whereas larger lesions with serrated margins are often poorly differentiated with signet-ring cells, and invade deep into the submucosa (106,172).

Each subtype of early gastric cancer is most likely to give rise to a specific type of advanced cancer. For example, polypoid lesions tend to produce subtypes of early gastric polypoid carcinoma and type II lesions give rise to ulcerative infiltrating carcinomas. The large eroded type and the excavated types may result in a wider variety of advanced carcinomas ranging from ulcerative infiltrating carcinomas to diffusely infiltrative carcinomas (172). Surface erosion by tumor can sometimes be an indicator of submucosal invasion. There is a far greater likelihood of submucosal invasion in ulcerated small (less than 3 cm) type IIc lesions than in nonulcerated ones (87).

Patterns of Invasion and Relationship to Histologic Type. The pattern of invasion in early gastric carcinoma varies from a few cells into the lamina propria to large and well-demarcated cancerous masses that occupy a large portion of the submucosa and press the muscularis propria downwards. The 10-year survival rate is lowest (being about 85 percent) in the latter (89). Additionally, vascular invasion occurs primarily in the differentiated types of carcinoma while predominantly lymphatic invasion occurs in the undifferentiated diffuse type. (See Advanced Carcinoma for a detailed description of dissemination of gastric carcinoma.)

*Advanced Gastric Carcinoma.* Gastric adenocarcinomas show a great diversity of epithelial cell types that may or may not be indigenous to the stomach, such as goblet cells, Paneth cells, and endocrine cells (167); of growth patterns; of host reactions such as desmoplasia and calcification (168,175); and of degrees of differentiation. Sometimes, there are associated benign submucosal cysts which may cause difficulty in determining the depth of invasion of the carcinoma. Occasionally a specific cell type dominates and is seen as a unique clinicopathologic entity such as carcinoma with lymphoid stroma, parietal cell carcinoma, hepatoid tumor, Paneth cell carcinoma, and mixed signet-ring/endocrine cell carcinoma. These tumors are described separately.

In addition to the cell types, a variety of factors, such as stage, growth pattern, infiltrating or pushing margins, and degree of differentiation, need to be considered in the classification of these tumors. Tumor differentiation is determined by both the cellular and architectural components of the tumor and although the two often go hand in hand, this is not invariable.

In general, well-differentiated adenocarcinoma is associated with intestinal metaplasia, usually occurs in the elderly, and generally corresponds to the intestinal type of carcinoma. Poorly differentiated and signet-ring cell carcinomas often occur together, are not associated with intestinal metaplasia, typically occur in young or middle aged patients, and generally correspond to the diffuse type of carcinoma (172).

**Histologic Types of Gastric Adenocarcinoma.** There are a variety of histologic classifications in use, the most frequent being the WHO, Lauren, and Ming classifications (figs. 11-28, 11-29). No one is ideal, in part because many tumors are not uniform and show considerable overlap of histologic patterns. For pathologists everywhere to be able to clearly understand and compare the precise nature of gastric tumors, it is important for there to be uniformity of nomenclature. The WHO histologic classification is the simplest and most reproducible and also the most widely used; therefore, it was chosen for this chapter (259).

The WHO classification divides gastric adenocarcinomas into four main histologic types: tubular, papillary, mucinous, and signet-ring cell carcinomas (Table 11-7) (259). It is still unproven whether stage for stage the different histologic

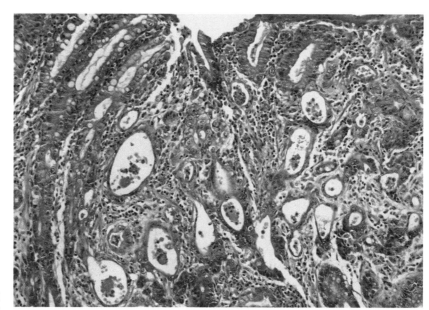

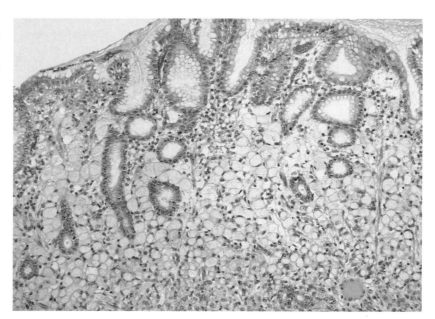

Figure 11-28
GASTRIC ADENOCARCINOMA
OF THE INTESTINAL
AND DIFFUSE TYPES
(LAUREN'S CLASSIFICATION)

Top: Carcinoma of intestinal type. Normal mucosa is replaced by infiltrating tubular profiles.

Bottom: Signet-ring cell carcinoma of the diffuse type. There is diffuse infiltration of the mucosa by signet-ring cells. The gastric pits appear normal and there is no evidence of gastritis or intestinal metaplasia.

types affect prognosis. In part this may be due to the variation in histologic pattern from one area to another (26). For example, an adenocarcinoma may have a papillary pattern superficially and be mucinous in the deeper portions. When metastases are present the tumor is classified by the predominant pattern. It is still uncertain whether histologic subtypes are independent prognostic factors irrespective of tumor stage.

*Tubular Adenocarcinoma.* This is made up mainly of simple or branching tubules resem-

bling colonic carcinoma and less commonly small, acinar structures sometimes resembling antral glands (fig. 11-30A–E). The glands may be cystically dilated and contain mucus or inflammatory debris (fig. 11-30E). Adenocarcinomas containing both glandular and solid structures are included under tubular carcinomas (fig. 11-30F–H). The tumor cells are columnar, cuboidal, or flattened and contain variable amounts of intracytoplasmic mucin. Occasional psammoma bodies may be found (fig. 11-30I,J) (168).

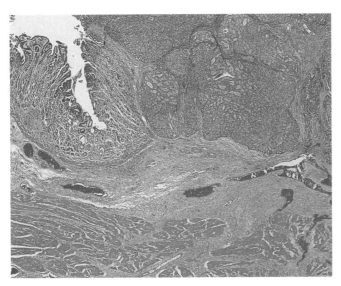

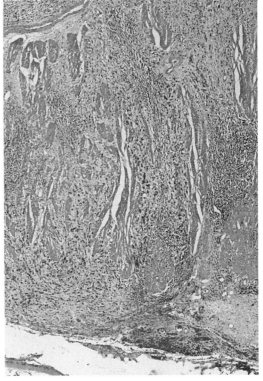

Figure 11-29
GASTRIC ADENOCARCINOMA OF THE
EXPANDING AND INFILTRATIVE TYPES

Above: Low-power view of an early gastric cancer. There is normal mucosa on the left and carcinoma on the right. The carcinoma is expanding in a pushing manner into the submucosa.

Right: A poorly differentiated gastric carcinoma showing diffuse infiltration through the muscularis propria into the serosa.

*Papillary Adenocarcinoma.* This tumor type is composed of finger-like epithelial processes with fibrovascular cores. The finger-like processes can be fine and lined by a single layer of cells (fig. 11-31), or they may consist of more solid processes lined by several layers of cells. The tumor cells are cylindrical or cuboidal, have basally oriented nuclei and well-formed striated borders, and often secrete mucus as small droplets. Goblet cells may also be present. A number of tumors show tubular differentiation but are classified by the predominant histologic pattern (tubulovillous). These carcinomas typically grow as polypoid masses protruding into the gastric lumen, deeply in an expansile manner with "pushing" margins.

*Mucinous Adenocarcinoma.* These are tumors producing abundant intracellular and extracellular mucus (more than 50 percent of the tumor) which may be visible grossly (fig. 11-32). There is often cystic dilatation of glands which may rupture into the interstitial tissues and produce mucus lakes in which scant fragments of disrupted glands appear to float. Sometimes these tumors undergo calcification (168,175). Synonyms include *mucoid, mucus, colloid,* and *muconodular adenocarcinoma.* The WHO classification subdivides these tumors into well differentiated, characterized by glands lined by a columnar, mucus-secreting epithelium together with interstitial mucus and poorly differentiated, composed of chains or irregular clusters of cells surrounded by mucus. Some tumors show an admixture of both growth patterns. Signet-ring cells may be found in some of these tumors (fig. 11-32C); if they comprise more than 50 percent of the tumor they are designated as *signet-ring cell carcinoma.*

The term *mucin-producing carcinoma* has been used as a synonym for mucinous carcinoma and as a descriptive term for adenocarcinomas producing any amount of mucin. Because there is no standard definition for mucin-producing carcinoma, the term should not be used for diagnosis.

*Poorly Differentiated Carcinoma of Diffuse and Signet-Ring Cell Types.* Signet-ring cell carcinomas are adenocarcinomas with a predominant component (more than 50 percent of the tumor cells) of signet-ring cells containing intracytoplasmic mucin (fig. 11-33). This tumor appears to arise from nonmetaplastic foveolar or

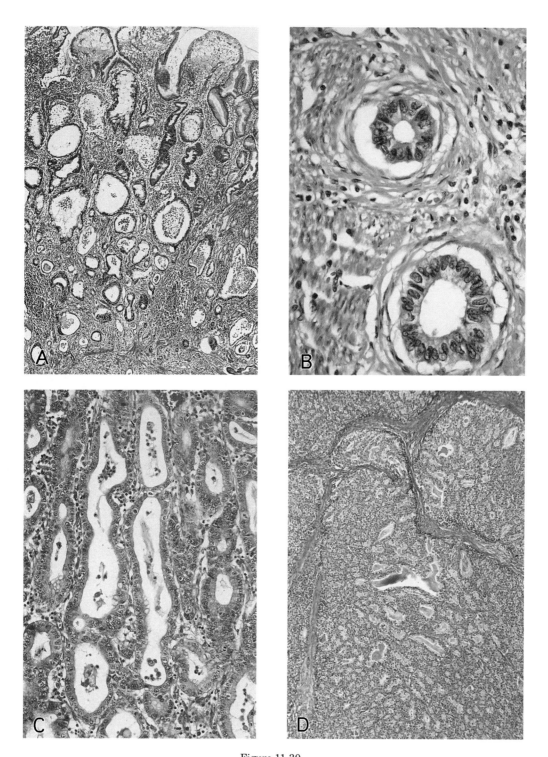

Figure 11-30
HISTOLOGIC SPECTRUM OF TUBULAR ADENOCARCINOMA OF THE STOMACH

A: Well-differentiated tubular adenocarcinoma. There are well-developed tubular profiles, many of which are cystically dilated. As the tumor infiltrates into the submucosa, seen in the lower portion of the picture, it elicits a desmoplastic reaction. There is a moderately severe accompanying inflammatory reaction.

B: High-power magnification of the desmoplastic reaction of A showing two well-developed tubules surrounded by dense collagen.

C: Well-differentiated tubular adenocarcinoma showing well-defined, closely packed tubules with minimal intervening stroma.

D: Moderately differentiated tubular adenocarcinoma composed primarily of closely packed acinar structures.

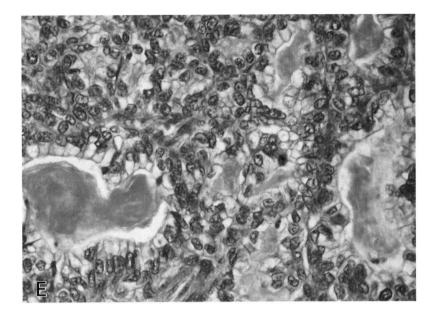

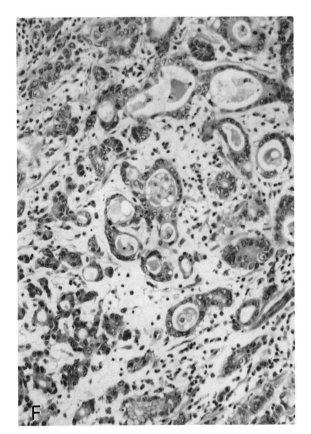

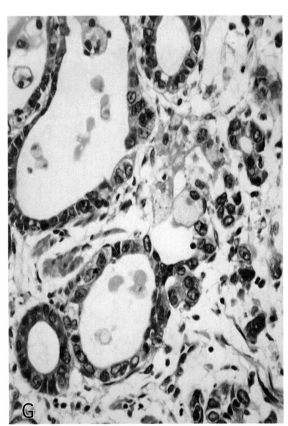

Figure 11-30 (Continued)

E: Higher power magnification of D. The acini contain colloid-like material producing a superficial resemblance to a follicular thyroid tumor.

F: Poorly differentiated tubular adenocarcinoma composed of numerous irregular tubular structures, irregular clumps, and single cells with edematous intervening stroma infiltrated by inflammatory cells.

G: Higher magnification of F. The glandular structures are dilated and lined by cuboidal cells with scant cytoplasm and hyperchromatic nuclei.

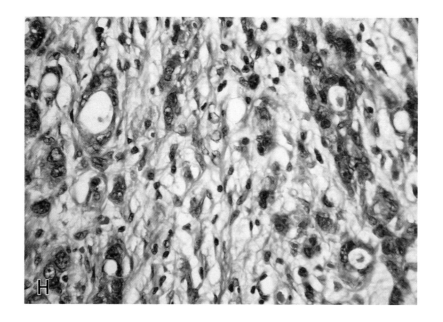

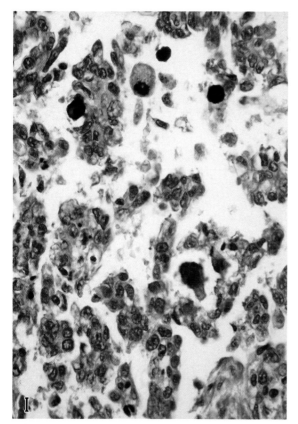

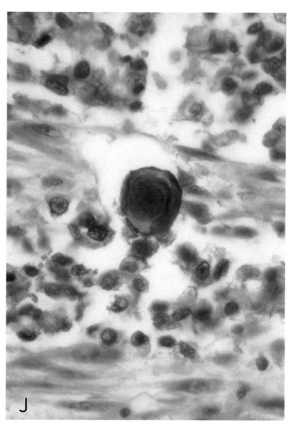

Figure 11-30 (Continued)

HISTOLOGIC SPECTRUM OF TUBULAR ADENOCARCINOMA OF THE STOMACH

H: Poorly differentiated tubular adenocarcinoma. High-power magnification showing poorly formed glandular profiles set in a desmoplastic stroma. There are also many scattered single tumor cells with hyperchromatic nuclei and scant indistinct cytoplasm. Poorly differentiated adenocarcinomas are frequently part of the spectrum of signet-ring cell carcinoma.

I: Poorly differentiated adenocarcinoma with psammoma bodies.

J: Higher magnification to show laminated psammoma body in the center of the field.

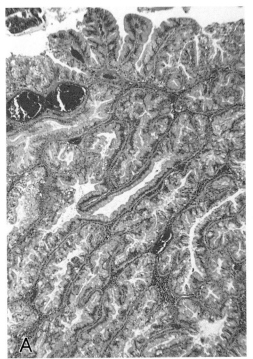

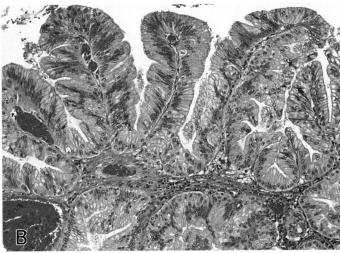

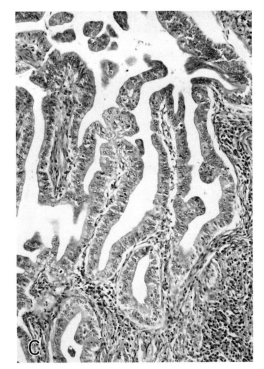

Figure 11-31
HISTOLOGIC SPECTRUM OF
PAPILLARY CARCINOMA OF THE STOMACH

A: Well-differentiated papillary adenocarcinoma. On the surface, finger-like epithelial proliferations can be seen. Deeper down, the papillary processes are compressed together often giving the appearance of tubules, depending on the plane of sectioning. Papillary structures can be seen in the center and the upper field.

B: Higher magnification shows the finger-like surface proliferations. These are composed of villi with a fibrovascular core lined by rounded or elongated basally oriented nuclei showing pseudostratification and clear staining cytoplasm.

C: Moderately differentiated papillary adenocarcinoma. The papillae are less regular than the foregoing examples of papillary carcinoma and are lined by cuboidal cells showing marked atypia with greatly enlarged nuclei. The stroma shows a heavy chronic inflammatory infiltrate.

mucous neck cells that proliferate as single cells or in small clumps. However, there is often an admixture of glandular elements, frequently in the deeper portions of the tumor. Typically the intracytoplasmic mucin compresses the nucleus against the periphery of the cell giving it its characteristic signet-ring appearance. The type and amount of intracytoplasmic mucus vary and four types of tumor cells are seen: 1) a signet-ring cell filled with acid mucin; 2) a cell filled with secretory granules containing acid or neutral mucin; 3) a signet-ring cell with eosinophilic granules containing neutral mucin; and 4) cells without mucin. The last are most common in the deepest layers of the gastric wall.

The detection of signet-ring cells within the mucosa is sometimes subtle and easily missed as they may occur in rather normal looking mucosa.

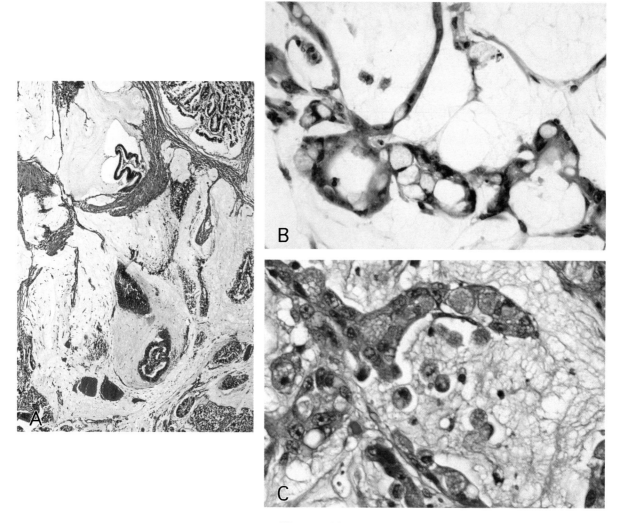

Figure 11-32
MUCINOUS ADENOCARCINOMA OF THE STOMACH
A: There is a large amount of extracellular mucin and much of the malignant epithelium appears to float within it.
B: Higher magnification of mucinous carcinoma showing irregular glandular profiles, lined by attenuated epithelium and occasional goblet cells. These appear to float within the pools of mucin.
C: Strands of tumor cells are interspersed between the extracellular mucin. Intracellular mucin is also abundant in some tumor cells and appears as signet-ring cells. The presence of the latter makes this a poorly differentiated mucinous adenocarcinoma.

(fig. 11-33E,F). The PAS with diastase stain (the most sensitive) and mucin stains, such as mucicarmine or Alcian blue, are often useful for highlighting them (fig. 11-33D). In poorly differentiated carcinomas there is often little nuclear atypia and more tumor cells are demonstrated by mucin stains than by hematoxylin and eosin–stained sections (fig. 11-34). When signet-ring cells infiltrate the submucosa and deeper tissues, they often provoke a dense fibrous reaction which frequently results in a markedly thickened leather bottle–like stomach, namely linitis plastica (figs. 11-26B, 11-34F). However, this lesion is not unique to signet-ring cell carcinoma, and can be seen with other adenocarcinomas (see fig. 11-30A,B) and sometimes with metastatic tumors, especially from the breast (29). Furthermore, diffusely infiltrating, poorly differentiated carcinomas do not always evoke a desmoplastic reaction (259).

A number of conditions may occasionally be confused with signet-ring cell carcinoma. Rare instances of signet-ring cell lymphoma, characterized by lymphoid cells distended with immunoglobulin, may mimic carcinoma. Detailed histologic study of the entire tumor usually resolves the problem but if doubt remains immunohistochemical studies for cytokeratin and common leukocyte antigen are diagnostic. The distinction between macrophage infiltration and signet-ring cell carcinoma is discussed under differential diagnosis of early gastric adenocarcinomas.

In addition to the foregoing histologic types of adenocarcinoma, there are a number of other descriptors of growth patterns or stromal reactions, some of which have already been alluded to, that are not necessarily associated with one specific histologic type of carcinoma. *Scirrhous tumors* are carcinomas with a marked desmoplastic reaction, often associated with relatively few tumor cells. *Solid tumors* are closely packed neoplasms with well-defined boundaries that may be well or poorly differentiated. *Carcinoma with lymphoid stroma* contains a dominant lymphoid infiltrate and is discussed separately.

**Vascular and Lymphatic Invasion.** Gastric carcinomas frequently show venous and lymphatic invasion (fig. 11-36). Tubular carcinomas are predisposed to venous invasion in contrast to signet-ring cell carcinomas which tend to spread by the lymphatics. For further details see section on spread of gastric carcinoma.

**Degree of Tumor Differentiation.** Gastric adenocarcinoma has been subdivided into three types based on the degree of glandular formation and cytologic abnormality. These degrees of differentiation apply primarily to tubular, papillary, and mucinous carcinomas. Signet-ring cell carcinoma is by nature almost always poorly differentiated.

*Well-Differentiated Adenocarcinoma.* These tumors have well-developed glands lined by mature-type tumor cells, are rich in capillaries, and sparse in stroma (see fig. 11-30A–C). The tumor cells consist predominantly of mucus-secreting goblet cells; tall columnar intestinal absorptive cells with striated brush borders; and less commonly, other specialized cells such as endocrine cells, Paneth cells, and parietal cells. The tumor cells typically have large oval to round vesicular nuclei, irregular clumped chromatin, and numerous large distinct irregular nucleoli. Mitoses

are frequently prominent. Ultrastructurally, these well-differentiated carcinomas tend to have well-defined cell junctions (214).

*Moderately Well-Differentiated Adenocarcinoma.* These are clearly defined carcinomas of glandular origin, but their architecture is less well defined than the well-differentiated tumors. The glands frequently have a cribriform or acinar pattern with a variable amount of intervening stroma (see fig. 11-30D,E).

*Poorly Differentiated Adenocarcinoma.* These tumors show poor glandular formation and loss of cell cohesion, and they tend to proliferate diffusely in small clumps or as isolated cells, often eliciting a dense fibroblastic reaction (figs. 11-34–11-36). Cytologically, the tumor cells are small and immature, and this is reflected ultrastructurally by scant microvilli, small mucin granules, and few tight intercellular junctions. As tumor dedifferentiation occurs the nuclei show loss of basal polarity and nucleoli become increasingly more irregular, atypical, and bizarre. Mitoses are frequently prominent and atypical.

*Undifferentiated Carcinoma.* This category is for tumors lacking all evidence of structural and functional differentiation beyond being epithelial, i.e., solid sheets of cells and cohesive growth pattern (fig. 11-37). A tumor that is largely undifferentiated but has foci of tubules, papillae, or mucin is best considered a poorly differentiated adenocarcinoma; the term undifferentiated adenocarcinoma is not recommended as it is contradictory. These tumors resemble poorly differentiated adenocarcinomas, small cell carcinomas, lymphomas (167), leukemia, and poorly differentiated sarcomas. The most important tumor to differentiate is lymphoma which may be treatable and has a better prognosis. The most useful markers for differentiation are immunohistochemical antibody stains demonstrating cytokeratin, and antigens for common leukocyte, S-100 protein, and Ki-1.

**Lauren and Ming Classifications.** Lauren (127) proposed classifying gastric carcinomas into two types: intestinal and diffuse (see fig. 11-28). The intestinal type (presumed to be derived from intestinalized gastric mucosa) is more common in males, usually has a polypoid or fungating gross appearance, and has an expansile growth pattern. Histologically, it is characterized by well-defined glandular structures and is almost invariably

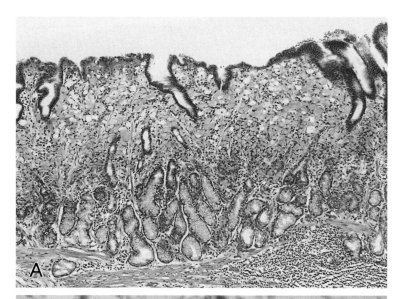

### Figure 11-33
#### HISTOLOGIC SPECTRUM OF SIGNET-RING CELL CARCINOMA

A: Early gastric cancer of signet-ring cell type. There is diffuse infiltration of the superficial lamina propria by sheets of signet-ring cells with preservation of the normal gastric foveolae. The signet-ring cells result from distention of the cells by intracellular mucin which pushes and compresses the nucleus towards the periphery of the cell. The pyloric glands in the lower half of the mucosa appear normal.

B: Higher magnification of signet-ring cells.

C: Neutral mucin stain (PAS) shows the numerous densely staining signet-ring cells (purple) in the upper half of the mucosa and the tubular profiles of the normal antral glands in the lower half.

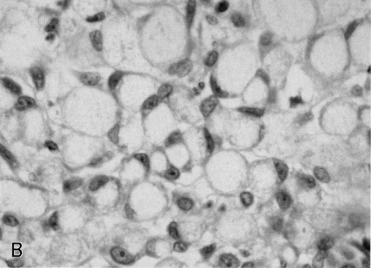

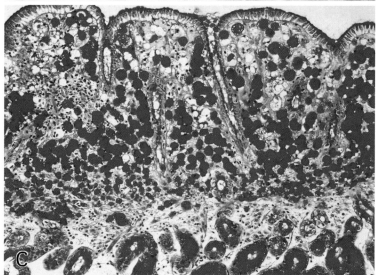

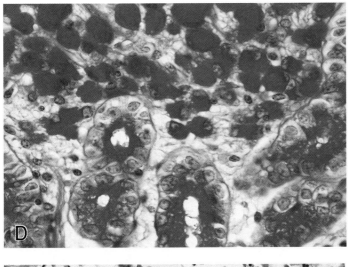

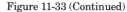

Figure 11-33 (Continued)

D: Higher magnification of C shows the signet-ring cells and the antral glands.

E: Biopsy specimen of signet-ring cell carcinoma of the stomach. In this section, ill-defined glandular profiles are intermixed with signet-ring cells.

F: High-power magnification of the deep mucosa and the superficial submucosa of a signet-ring cell carcinoma showing extensive lymphatic permeation of the tumor.

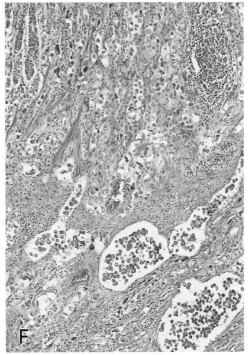

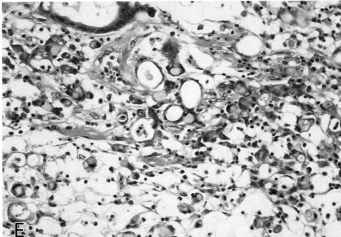

associated with severe atrophic gastritis and intestinal metaplasia. In contrast, the diffuse type (thought to arise from gastric mucous cells) has a similar male to female incidence, an ulcerative or infiltrative gross appearance, and a diffuse infiltrative growth pattern. Histologically it is usually a poorly differentiated adenocarcinoma, often with signet-ring cells and features of linitis plastica. About 15 percent of gastric carcinomas have a mixed diffuse and intestinal pattern.

Ming's classification, based on the nature of the advancing margins of the tumors, is subdivided into expanding or infiltrative carcinomas (see fig. 11-29) (152). In general, Ming's expansile and infiltrative tumors correspond to Lauren's intestinal and diffuse tumor types, with a similar number of cases with overlapping patterns.

Tumors have been further subdivided by some according to their stromal content. Cellular tumors with minimal intervening stroma have been called medullary, whereas those which elicite a dense desmoplastic reaction, scirrhous carcinomas. Scirrhous carcinomas that involve the entire stomach are known as linitis plastica.

Subdividing gastric tumors according to the Lauren or Ming classification system has proven useful in a number of ways, even though 15 percent of cases have overlapping patterns and are impossible to classify (127,152). The intestinal and diffuse types of gastric tumor tend to grow within and disseminate beyond the stomach in different ways. This has important surgical management and prognostic implications. For example, a subtotal gastrectomy might be

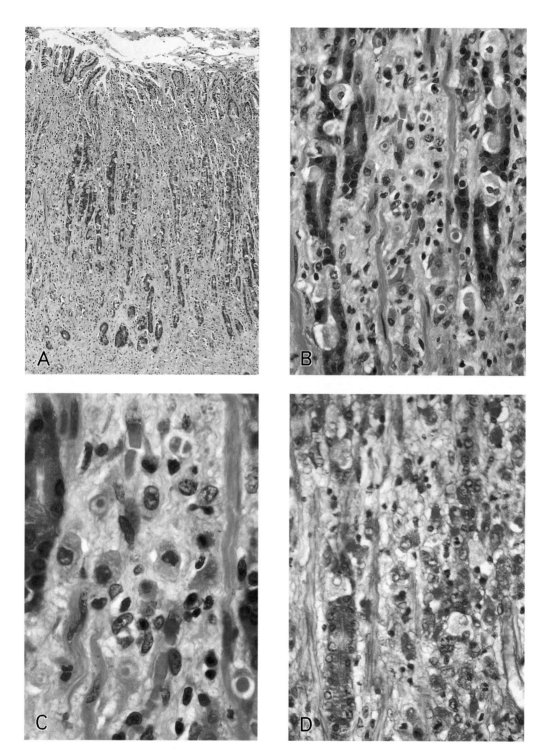

Figure 11-34
POORLY DIFFERENTIATED DIFFUSE ADENOCARCINOMA

A: Low-power magnification of the mucosa of the gastric body showing the normal gastric pits and glands surrounded and separated from one another by a rather indistinct neoplastic and fibroinflammatory infiltrate.

B, C: Higher magnification of A showing normal glands of the gastric body, containing parietal and chief cells, separated by indistinct tumor cells with small hyperchromatic nuclei and scant eosinophilic cytoplasm, resembling macrophages.

D: Diffuse carcinoma stained for neutral mucin with PAS shows the poorly differentiated infiltrating tumor cells between the gastric glands which contain purplish cytoplasm.

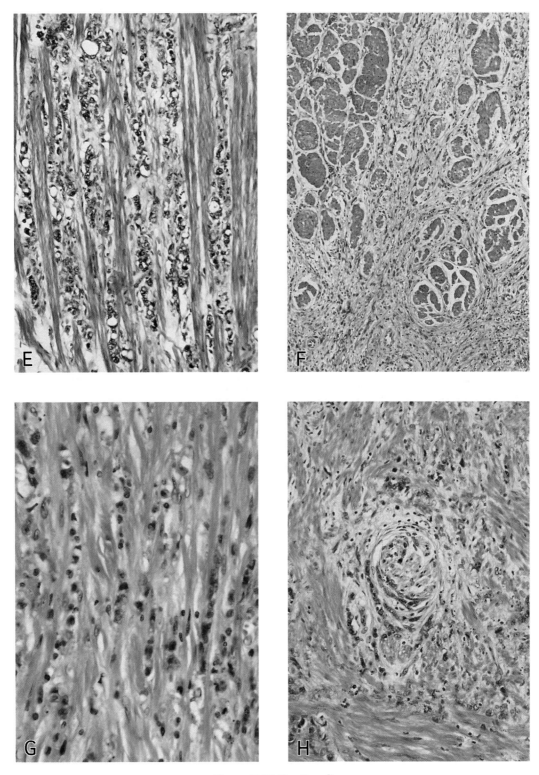

Figure 11-34 (Continued)

E: Separation of the muscle bundles by the diffuse infiltrating tumor is seen in the muscularis propria.

F: Marked desmoplastic reaction of muscularis propria.

G: High-power magnification of F illustrating a single file pattern of tumor infiltration between the fibrous tissue.

H: High-power magnification of a nerve bundle in the intermyenteric region showing perineural tumor invasion.

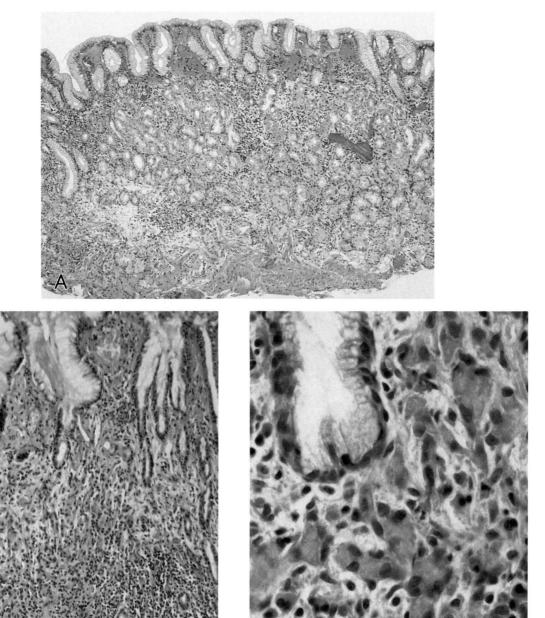

Figure 11-35
ENDOSCOPIC BIOPSY SPECIMENS WITH SUBTLE CHANGES
OF DIFFUSE AND SIGNET-RING CELL CARCINOMA

These are among the most common gastric biopsy specimens sent for a second opinion. The following examples illustrate some subtle changes sometimes aggravated by small specimen size and artefactual distortion.

A: Low-power view of gastric mucosa showing a severe gastritis.

B: Higher magnification of the antral portion of A showing pink-staining cords of cells in the center of the field.

C: High-power magnification shows poorly differentiated epithelial profiles infiltrating the lamina propria.

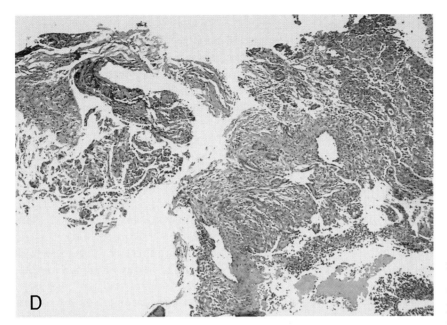

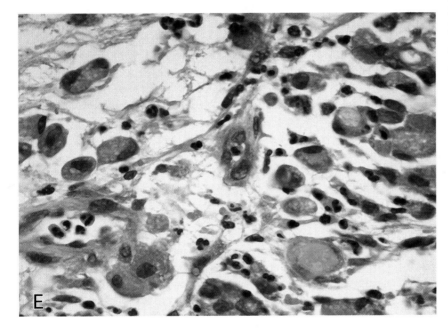

Figure 11-35 (Continued)

D: Low-power view of a very fragmented gastric biopsy specimen.

E: Higher magnification shows scattered signet-ring cells. A frequent question is whether these signet-ring cells could be muciphages. The latter are almost never present in the stomach, thus, as a general rule, when these types of cells are found in gastric biopsy specimens they should be considered carcinoma until proven otherwise.

sufficient for the Lauren intestinal type of carcinoma (well- and moderately differentiated adenocarcinomas), whereas a total gastrectomy is recommended for diffuse type tumors (signet-ring cell carcinomas). Lauren's classification has also been valuable for comparative epidemiologic studies: intestinal type carcinoma is found most frequently in the antrum, is usually associated with intestinal metaplasia, and appears to be environmentally related; the diffuse type is relatively common in younger patients, occurs more commonly in the body of the stomach, is not associated with intestinal metaplasia, and may be determined by genetic predisposition (69,127). Differentiating between expanding and infiltrative growth patterns has prognostic implications independent of other factors, such as histology: patients with well-circumscribed tumors have survival periods almost twice as long as those with infiltrating tumors (192,199,222).

**Special (Histochemical and Immunohistochemical) Stains and Tumor Markers.** The most useful special stains for the demonstration of gastric carcinoma are PAS with diastase or Alcian blue/PAS and cytokeratin (fig. 11-36). As previously discussed, a variety of other mucins may be found in gastric cancer (see Intestinal Metaplasia); however, since these are not always present staining for them is not as helpful as using PAS which stains almost all mucins. Mucicarmine is another commonly used stain for the demonstration of mucin in gastric cancers; in our experience, this stain is generally unreliable since there is much variability in staining results from one laboratory to another.

Some tumors contain intestinal enzymes such as alkaline phosphatase, aminopeptidase, and β-glucuronidase (132,195,236). Carcinoembryonic antigen, an oncofetal antigen, is commonly found in metaplastic, dysplastic, and tumor tissue but may be absent in undifferentiated tumors. It is normally found at the luminal margin of tumor cells and diffusely within the cytoplasm of signet-ring cells (160). Other antigens, such as keratin and milk fat globulin, may also be demonstrated within tumor cells. Of all the above, immunolocalization of cytokeratin is the most reliable method of identifying a poorly or undifferentiated carcinoma. None of these stains or tumor markers are sufficiently distinctive to provide accurate classification or prognosis of gastric tumors, nor do they allow definitive identification of metastatic gastric tumors or adenocarcinomas metastatic to the stomach, as from a lung or breast primary. However, in one study, the demonstration of carcinoembryonic antigen within the stroma of the tumor and the presence of S-100 protein–positive dendritic mononuclear cells infiltrating the tumor was associated statistically with only short-term survival (160).

**Chromosome Abnormalities, DNA Ploidy Patterns, Nucleolar Organizer Regions, and Oncogene Studies.** Abnormalities of DNA ploidy have been demonstrated in many early and advanced gastric adenocarcinomas. Up to 70 percent of adenocarcinomas are aneuploid (46, 47,212,264,268) although superficial carcinomas are mostly diploid. The same is true for signet-ring cell carcinomas confined to the mucosa, whereas invasive signet-ring cell tumors show scattered aneuploidy (44,46,183,190,241). Interestingly, the incidence of aneuploidy is higher in differentiated tubular and papillary carcinomas than in signet-ring cell carcinomas. In general, tumors showing deeper invasion, lymph node metastasis, and vascular invasion are polyploid or aneuploid (77,122, 212,268,269), although this was not confirmed by Sasaki (212). There is no correlation between the ploidy pattern and the histologic type (234).

A number of oncogene studies of gastric tumors have shown gene amplification, particularly of the c-*myc* and *ras* genes (151). The frequency of gene amplification appears to be related to the depth of tumor invasion (177,245, 266). In one study, 11 percent of early gastric carcinoma showed amplification of the *ras* gene compared to 44 percent in advanced carcinoma.

Many chromosome abnormalities have been demonstrated in gastric carcinoma but no consistent karyotype patterns have emerged (151,264). In addition, although nucleolar organizer counts correlate with the degree of dysplasia, the technique appears to be of little practical use (18).

The value of DNA chromosome analysis, ploidy studies, and oncogene determination in diagnostic pathology is uncertain and remains to be defined, but they tend to correlate with certain growth characteristics. For further details see Chromosome Abnormalities, Role of Oncogenes, and Tumor Suppressor Genes.

**Differential Diagnosis.** Benign gastric erosions and ulcers must be differentiated from ulcerating carcinomas while signet-ring cell carcinoma must be differentiated from histiocytes, muciphages, and gastric lipid islands.

Early gastric carcinomas may be difficult to differentiate by endoscopic appearance from benign erosions and ulcers. Furthermore, some early carcinomas may mimic gastric ulcers in their behavior by undergoing cycles of healing and reulceration (208). Malignancy should be suspected whenever a gastric erosion or ulcer looks atypical (e.g., heaped margins) and multiple biopsies taken from the margins of the lesion (an arbitrary four samples is suggested). It should also be noted that ulcerated carcinomas can occasionally be confused with a chronic gastric ulcer.

Morphologically, there are two major issues associated with biopsies. First, the tissue may be tiny, poorly oriented, and distorted so that adequate evaluation is impossible. In these cases serial sections may help but usually it is necessary to

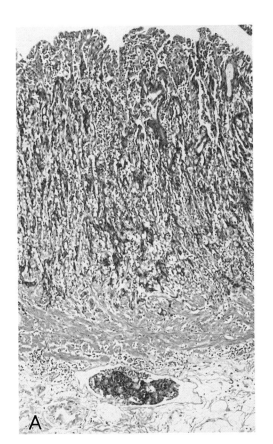

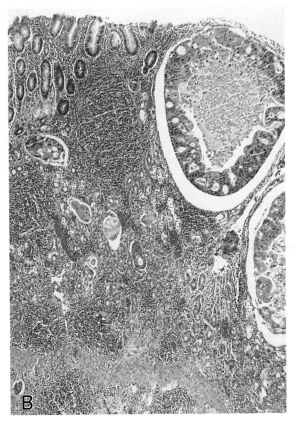

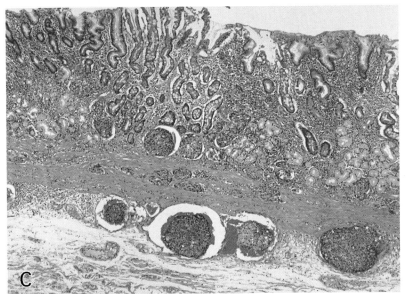

Figure 11-36

ADENOCARCINOMA OF THE STOMACH WITH EXTENSIVE VASCULAR INVASION

A: Low-power view of the mucosa and submucosa of a poorly differentiated diffuse adenocarcinoma of the gastric fundus. The tumor is not well visualized in this section but is interspersed between normal oxyntic glands. Just below the muscularis mucosae, tumor is present in a vascular space.

B: Low-power view of inflamed gastric antrum with extensive vascular tumor invasion.

C: A severely inflamed antrum showing extensive vascular tumor infiltration primarily in vessels just below the muscularis mucosae. The presence of blood within the vascular spaces indicates that they are venous.

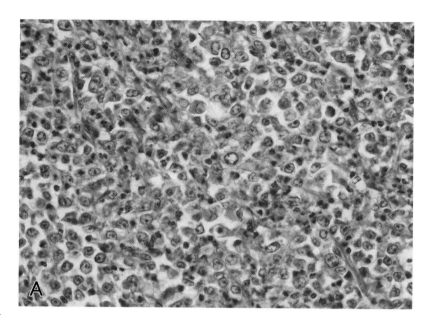

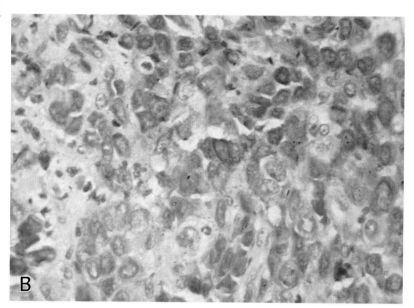

Figure 11-37
UNDIFFERENTIATED
GASTRIC CARCINOMA:
VALUE OF
IMMUNOHISTOCHEMISTRY

A: This tumor is composed of sheets of spheroidal tumor cells with scant indistinct cytoplasm and large round nuclei containing large irregular nucleoli. Keratin stains would be positive in this tumor allowing differentiation from other undifferentiated tumors.

B: Immunoperoxidase reaction for keratin stains the majority of cells.

request more tissue. The second problem is an interpretative one. Occasionally, reactive and regenerative epithelia in gastric mucosa may be difficult to differentiate from dysplasia or mucosal carcinoma. The major histologic differences between reactive and regenerative gastric epithelia are listed in Table 11-3 and discussed under differential diagnosis of adenoma.

Sometimes bland-appearing tumor cells, including signet-ring cells, lying singly or in clusters in the lamina propria may be overlooked or confused with histiocytes or muciphages and, less frequently, with gastric lipid islands. We have seen a gastric mucosal biopsy from a patient who had received polyvinyl pyrrolidone (PVP) as a plasma expander infiltrated with macrophages containing PVP, which resembled signet-ring cell carcinoma (fig. 11-38) (83). Of interest is a recent report describing reactive signet ring cell proliferations arising from foveolar epithelium, in a fair number of gastric MALTomas (269b). Muciphages in the stomach are very rare, and therefore, from a practical point of view, atypical goblet cells and signet-ring cells indicate carcinoma until proven

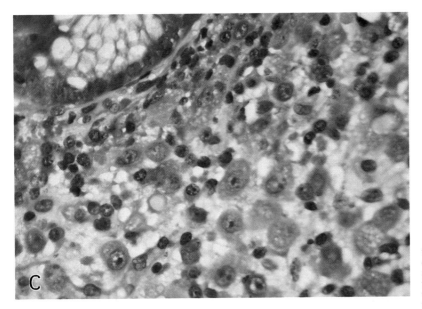

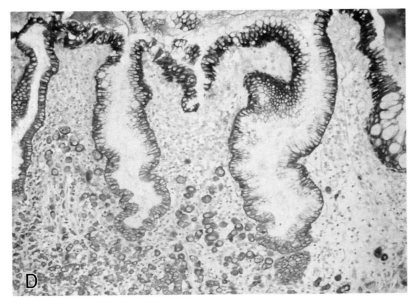

Figure 11-37 (Continued)

C: High-power magnification of gastric mucosa showing scattered tumor cells infiltrating the lamina propria and admixed chronic inflammatory infiltrate. The tumor cells are rounded with vacuolated cytoplasm in some and vesicular nuclei containing a prominent nucleolus. Mucin stains were negative.

D: Immunoperoxidase reaction for cytokeratin. The diffuse staining of the tumor cells confirms their epithelial nature. Also note the positivity in the epithelium which is a good internal control.

otherwise. We have seen consultation cases of signet-ring carcinoma which have been confused with "metabolic disorders." In our experience there are no metabolic disorders in which an infiltration of macrophages mimics carcinoma cells. There is a report of benign histiocytosis X of the stomach in the literature (179). This case was characterized by a dense monotonous histiocytoid infiltration of the lamina propria. It should not cause confusion with carcinoma because the cells lack mucin and they have the typical bean-shaped nuclei described in histiocytosis X.

Gastric lipid islands (xanthelasmas) may occasionally on superficial examination resemble signet-ring cell carcinoma. However, closer examination shows clusters of foamy cells with small, regular, centrally located nuclei within the lamina propria (fig. 11-38). These cells are PAS and keratin negative. If the cells are devoid of mucin and if fresh tissue is available, cytoplasmic lipid can be demonstrated by frozen section. However, in most cases special stains are unnecessary. (Also see discussion of lipid islands under Stromal Tumors.)

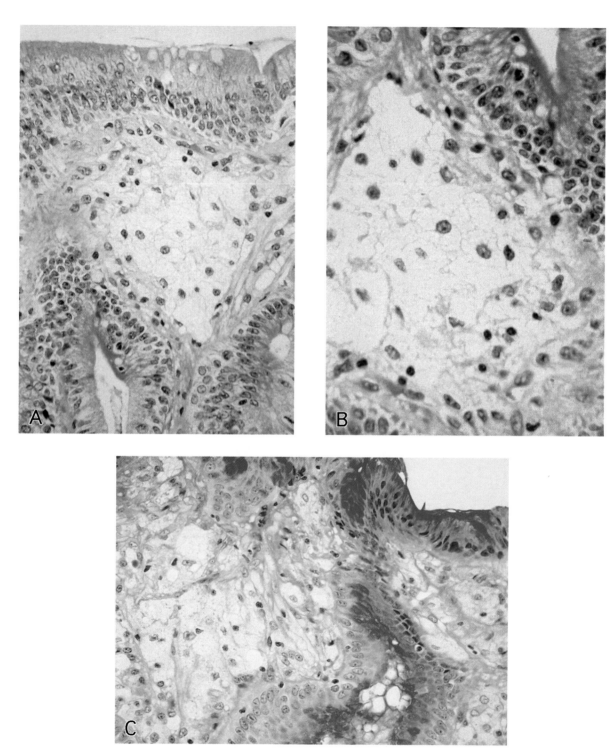

Figure 11-38
COMPARISON OF SIGNET-RING CELL CARCINOMA WITH LIPID ISLANDS
(GASTRIC XANTHELASMA) AND MACROPHAGES IN GASTRIC MUCOSA

A: A small lipid island is seen in the gastric mucosa.

B: Higher magnification shows lipid-laden histiocytes with clear cytoplasm and a small centrally located nucleus.

C: The lipid islands are stained with PAS to show lack of cytoplasmic mucin. There are clusters of bland-appearing clear cells with small, regular, centrally located nuclei. However, the surface and foveolar epithelium stain for mucin.

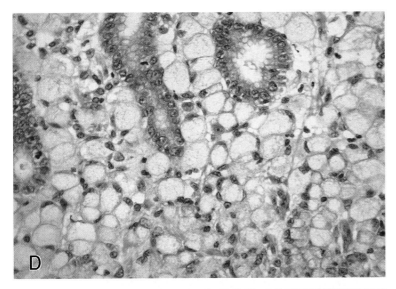

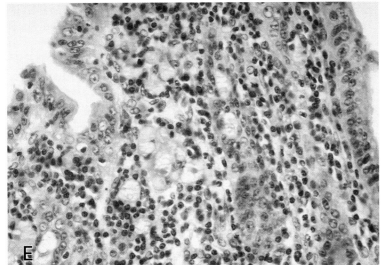

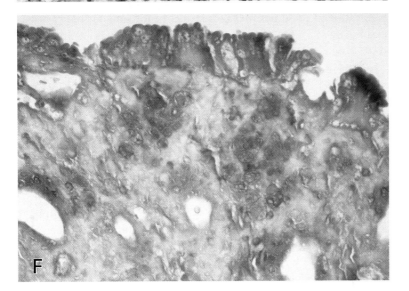

Figure 11-38 (Continued)

D: High-power magnification of a signet-ring cell carcinoma (compare with A).

E: Polyvinyl pyrrolidone (PVP) infiltration of the stomach mimicking signet-ring cell carcinoma. The PVP was given to the patient as a plasma expander. Groups of macrophages containing PVP infiltrate the lamina propria beneath the surface epithelium and look like signet-ring cells. There is also a dense lymphocytic infiltrate. (Courtesy of Dr. L. Sobin, Washington, D.C.)

F: The signet-ring–like cells in E stained intensely red with the Congo red stain. These cells are PAS and keratin negative. If the cells are devoid of mucin and if fresh tissue is available, cytoplasmic lipid can be demonstrated by frozen section. However, in most cases special stains are unnecessary. (See discussion of lipid islands under Stromal Tumors.)

*Lymphoma.* Differentiating poorly differentiated or undifferentiated carcinoma from diffuse large cell lymphoma may sometimes be difficult. Evidence of mucin production may confirm the diagnosis; however, this is often unsuccessful. Demonstrating the presence of desmosomes within the tumor by electron microscopy is another way of confirming the tumor, but is time consuming and expensive. The best way to differentiate lymphoma is by immunohistochemistry. Good markers are now available for epithelial cells (cytokeratin or carcinoembryonic antigen) and lymphoid cells (leukocyte common antigen), making the distinction between them easy most of the time (see chapter 13).

*Metastatic Carcinoma.* Tumor metastatic to the stomach occurs in approximately 2 percent of patients with extraintestinal primaries (147). The most common metastatic tumors are carcinomas of the breast and lung, and melanoma. These may mimic primary gastric carcinoma if they involve the mucosa. Features of metastatic lesions are multicentricity and an absence of metaplastic or dysplastic change in the gastric mucosa. Occasionally, the main part of the tumor seems to lie deep within the stomach wall and it is easily recognized that the mucosa is secondarily involved from below. Some metastatic tumors, particularly those from the breast, may evoke a marked desmoplastic reaction and resemble linitis plastica (29). Immunohistochemistry is usually not helpful in separating the different carcinomas except for S-100 protein and HMB 45 positivity in the case of metastatic melanoma.

*Carcinoid Tumors.* Distinguishing well-differentiated carcinoid tumors from carcinoma is usually easy. However, poorly differentiated carcinoid tumors may be difficult or impossible to distinguish from undifferentiated carcinomas, since the usual markers for gastrointestinal endocrine cells, such as the silver stains, chromogranin, or synaptophysin, are not present and the tumors rarely contain demonstrable peptide hormones. Neuron-specific enolase is generally of limited value here because of its lack of specificity. The most definitive way to make the diagnosis is to demonstrate dense core granules by electron microscopy. However, in order to reliably distinguish between poorly differentiated carcinoids and carcinomas, the granules should be demonstrable in the majority of the tumor cells since standard adenocarcinomas also

normally contain interspersed endocrine cells. Differentiating between poorly differentiated carcinoids and carcinomas is more an academic exercise since the treatment of both tumors is the same and the prognosis is equally poor.

*Granular Cell Tumors.* These occasionally mimic poorly differentiated carcinomas. They differ from carcinoma in that they are usually found in the submucosa without connection to the overlying mucosa. They are PAS positive, may be multiple, and may show a mild desmoplastic response. Histologically, they show small bland nuclei, lack of mitoses, granular eosinophilic cytoplasm, absence of mucin, and S-100 protein positivity.

*Reactive Epithelial Changes and Bizarre Undifferentiated Stromal Cells.* Gastric erosions and ulcers may sometimes contain bizarre undifferentiated stromal cells which may be confused with undifferentiated carcinoma. Distinguishing features of the reactive lesions are the admixed granulation tissue, the presence of ulcers, the gradual merging of the lesions with the adjacent normal tissue, the paucity of mitoses, and the absence of cytokeratin (4,98). Granulation tissue containing prominent arterioles lined by plump endothelial cells may occasionally mimic glands of well-differentiated adenocarcinoma on frozen section, but the associated inflammatory cells and absence of cytokeratin help differentiate it from carcinoma. Reactive atypical epithelium overlying eroded hyperplastic polyps can also sometimes simulate carcinoma.

*Radiation and Chemotherapy.* These may sometimes induce ulceration and epithelial atypia with architectural distortion, pleomorphism, and hyperchromasia. Other histologic changes that differentiate these changes from carcinoma are a history of prior irradiation or chemotherapy, and smudged nuclei with a lack of mitoses. Features of radiation injury, such as bizarre fibroblasts and arterial vascular changes that are predominantly submucosal, and rarely present in biopsies.

**Biopsy Diagnosis.** Approximately 50 percent of biopsy specimens from any given gastric carcinoma contain carcinoma cells (197,236). Obviously, the more specimens taken, the greater the diagnostic yield. More important than some magic number of biopsies is their quality. The endoscopist or endoscopy assistant should examine the specimens before they are placed in the fixative container to ensure that adequate tissue samples are submitted. Fragments of mucus or blood clot should not be considered an adequate biopsy specimen. When only a tiny or shallow fragment has been obtained, the endoscopist should rebiopsy the same site (70,78,133). We recommend at least four to six biopsy samples be taken from suspected gastric carcinomas. For gastric ulcers that are suspected to be malignant, most of the biopsies should be taken from the edges, right at the interface between ulcer and normal mucosal edge, and one or two from the base (78). For sessile polypoid lesions, several biopsies should be obtained from the base, in addition to those taken from the top of the lesion. Tumors in areas of the stomach that are difficult to biopsy because of site (e.g., high lesser curvature of the cardia) or firmness of tissue, require more biopsies. Routine brush cytology may offer additional diagnostic help, especially if a gastrointestinal laboratory with experienced personnel is available (43). The same is true for fine-needle aspiration, which is useful for predominantly invasive tumors such as linitis plastica.

Prior to partial gastrectomy for gastric carcinoma for cure, biopsies should be taken stepwise proximal to the planned resection zone. The rationale for this practice is to minimize the risk of leaving behind tumor that has spread intramucosally or leaving behind high-grade dysplasia. For example, with a carcinoma located in the proximal antrum, biopsies should be taken along the same and opposite walls beginning in the distal body and extending to the cardia. In this case, four equidistantly spaced biopsies could be taken along the same wall and four taken from the opposite wall. If there is difficulty in biopsy interpretation, rebiopsy should be recommended and some material frozen for immunohistochemistry if lymphoma is suspected.

Although biopsying areas around the tumor is valuable to determine whether there is mucosal spread beyond the visible lesion, it is important not to be lulled into a false sense of security by negative results. Some gastric adenocarcinomas, notably the poorly differentiated variants, commonly show diffuse submucosal and lymphatic spread. It is important to examine carefully the margins of gastric resections intraoperatively by frozen section analysis.

Table 11-9

**CAUSES OF DIAGNOSTIC ERRORS IN GASTRIC ADENOCARCINOMA BIOPSIES**

**False Negatives**
1. Inadequate tumor sampling
   a. Tumor site difficult to biopsy, e.g., cardia
   b. Failure to recognize tumor cells because of necrosis or diffuse infiltration (linitis plastica)
   c. Insufficient and inadequately targeted biopsies

**False Positives**
1. Atypical regenerative epithelium aggravated by necrosis, granulation tissue, and crush artifact
2. Bizarre stromal cells beneath ulcers
3. Radiation and chemotherapy effects

The common reasons for false-negative biopsy results are listed in Table 11-9. The major reason is inadequate sampling of the tumor. If the lesion is in a location difficult to biopsy, brush cytology may be helpful. Sometimes biopsy specimens are small, crushed, or necrotic and thus technically inadequate. A less common but important cause of a false-negative result is failure to recognize the tumor. In some cases of poorly differentiated carcinoma, diffuse infiltrating single tumor cells between apparently normal-looking gastric glands may be confused with histiocytes. Mucin stains and especially PAS can identify infiltrating tumor cells.

In addition to false-negative results, regenerating mucosa, particularly at the margins of ulcers, may be misinterpreted as carcinoma. The regenerative epithelium is characterized by nuclear enlargement, often with prominent and sometimes multiple nucleoli, but in contrast to carcinoma, the nuclei are not usually hyperchromatic and the chromatin tends to be regular and diffusely dispersed. However, in the presence of severe inflammation and granulation tissue diagnosis may be difficult and repeat biopsy may be necessary. Florid foveolar hyperplasia, as in the postgastrectomy gastric stump secondary to bile reflux, may be mistaken for high-grade dysplasia.

**Cytology.** Brush cytology is particularly helpful in diagnosis, especially for lesions that are difficult to biopsy. However, about 20 percent of specimens are diagnostically inadequate because of scanty material (4,197,233). Smith et al. (233) greatly improved results by forcefully rinsing the gastric brush in saline after making direct smears and processing the washing by the millipore technique, leaving only 2 percent of esophagogastric biopsies unsatisfactory. Endoscopic fine-needle aspirates can be helpful in cases of diffusely infiltrative carcinoma characterized by thick gastric folds, providing that they are seen by a cytopathologist experienced in gastric cytology.

**Spread of Gastric Adenocarcinoma.** *Local Spread.* Early gastric carcinomas usually arise in the middle and upper mucosa and remain localized for a long time. This is in part because there are virtually no lymphatics in the upper mucosa; mucosal lymphatics appear mostly in the lower mucosa and drain into large sinusoidal channels in the submucosa (130).

Once gastric tumors start to grow more actively, they characteristically progress by local extension from the mucosa to submucosa, through muscularis propria to subserosal tissues, sometimes into surrounding organs and throughout the peritoneal cavity. They may invade lymphatics and veins with resultant widespread metastasis. The manner of tumor dissemination is not usually random but appears to be related to tumor type (172). Signet-ring cell carcinoma or Lauren's diffuse type of carcinoma usually invades the lymphatics. Once within the lymphatics, the tumor grows rapidly into the submucosa; lateral growth may be much greater than is apparent from inspection of the mucosal surface (54). Metastasis to lymph nodes occurs in up to 30 percent of tumors, when they are still early carcinomas (64). Diffuse-type carcinoma continues to spread through the wall by direct extension and also via lymphatic channels and typically disseminates widely by celomic spread to involve adjacent viscera, omentum, peritoneum, and ovary.

In contrast, the differentiated types of adenocarcinoma (Lauren's intestinal type or well- to moderately differentiated tubular or papillary adenocarcinomas) (127), are usually bulky tumors and have an expansile growth pattern with a pushing margin. They frequently show vascular invasion and widespread vascular dissemination with metasta-sis to the liver, lung, and bone. Lymph node metastasis may occur but dissemination through the peritoneal cavity is uncommon (79). Mucinous tumors behave in a manner similar to signet-ring cell tumors (172). All three types of tumor spread to additional sites in 10 percent of cases.

Gastric carcinomas also grow proximally or distally intramurally, sometimes involving the entire stomach. Tumors of the cardia frequently extend into the lower esophagus and it is sometimes difficult to be certain whether they originated in the stomach or esophagus. Tumors in the distal antrum usually appear to stop abruptly at the pyloric sphincter on gross examination. However, microscopically there is often evidence of subserosal invasion, especially within lymphatics (136).

Gastric carcinomas frequently recur in the gastric remnant following gastrectomy (20 to 50 percent of cases), usually because tumor is left behind at the time of the original surgery. Occasionally, a new primary carcinoma develops in the gastric remnant (265).

Spread beyond the stomach is by peritoneal seeding and by lymphatic and vascular dissemination. Peritoneal dissemination occurs in about 40 percent of cases and involves the omentum, peritoneum, and serosa of the intestines (201).

*Metastases.* Lymph node metastasis occurs in 75 to 90 percent of advanced gastric carcinomas (141,201), depending in part on the size of the tumor and the depth of invasion, degree of histologic differentiation, and lymphatic invasion (266a). In one study, the likelihood of metastasis to lymph node in tumors extending to the submucosa, muscularis propria, and subserosa was 18 percent, 48 percent, and 62 percent, respectively (89). Usually there is a predictable spread of tumor to lymph nodes in the immediate lymphatic drainage site, which is related to tumor site. Further dissemination occurs to more distal drainage groups along identifiable lymphatic chains situated along the arteries. These then converge to the area around the upper abdominal aorta. Occasionally, however, metastases skip to more distal sites, sparing the perigastric nodes (141). The superior gastric nodes are the most commonly involved primary metastatic lymph nodes; occasionally, the left gastric artery nodes and splenic hilar lymph nodes are the primary nodal sites of involvement especially in tumors of the mid-portion of the stomach. In 15 percent of cases, metastases to Virchow's nodes (left supraclavicular nodes) are found (201).

Blood-borne metastases are fairly common, usually to liver or lung (35 percent of cases) (201), although any organ can be involved. Ovarian metastases are found in about 10 percent of gastric tumors, usually those of signet-ring cell type. Grossly, the ovaries show bilateral smooth enlargement and microscopically there is diffuse tumor infiltration usually by signet-ring cells (Krukenberg tumors). These ovarian metastases often present before the primary is diagnosed and may be associated with ovarian dysfunction, such as virilization.

The cause of death in cases of gastric carcinoma is usually the result of local recurrence, peritoneal dissemination, and hepatic metastases.

**Prognosis.** The overall prognosis of gastric cancer varies greatly from country to country. The best results are from Japan, with survival rates around 70 percent; survival rates in Germany are around 35 percent, and in the United States only about 20 percent. The major reason for these differences is the more frequent diagnosis of early gastric cancers and the more aggressive surgical approaches in Japan (81a).

*Early Gastric Carcinoma.* The prognosis of early gastric carcinoma after surgery is excellent, with a reported overall 5-year patient survival of about 95 percent: 97 percent for mucosal and 85 to 91 percent for submucosal carcinomas in Japan (89,115). Because these early carcinomas are infrequently diagnosed in Europe and the United States there are not many studies similar to those from Japan detailing early treatment and prognosis. However, in one survey of 319 patients from Great Britain prognosis of early gastric carcinoma was similar to that of Japan (48). Not all the survival figures are quite as high as those quoted above, for reasons that are not always clear. For example, in one study from Germany, the 5-year survival rates were 84 percent for mucosal lesions and 75 percent for submucosal tumors (81), and in two studies from the United States, the 5-year survival rate for early gastric carcinomas not further specified was 70 percent and 50 percent (71,257). The latter study is of interest because none of the patients died of gastric carcinoma although 7 percent (2 of 28) did have recurrent tumor, while 18 percent (5 of 28 patients) died of a second, nonintestinal malignancy.

A number of studies have analyzed the factors responsible for deaths in early gastric carcinoma; primary factors are local recurrences and liver metastasis (89,120,145).

*Factors Influencing Lymph Node Metastasis.* Tumor size and depth of invasion are significant predictors of spread. As the tumors enlarge in their horizontal mucosal diameter, they progressively invade deeper so that there is nearly a direct correlation between the size of the tumor and the degree of invasion and lymph node metastasis. In one study (106), approximately 30 percent of early gastric carcinomas less than 2 cm in mucosal diameter showed submucosal invasion, whereas 65 and 90 percent of lesions measuring 3 cm and 4 cm, respectively, showed submucosal extension. Also tumors less than 1 cm in diameter only had a 4 percent likelihood of lymph node metastasis versus 18 percent for tumors larger than 4 cm (64,87,106). In turn, depth of invasion relates to the probability of regional lymph node metastasis and a reduced 5-year survival. Thus, for intramucosal carcinomas the likelihood of lymph node metastasis is 0-4 percent; the 5-year survival rate is approximately 94 percent without lymph node metastasis and 92 percent with metastasis. The likelihood of lymph node metastasis in early gastric carcinoma with submucosal invasion is about 15 percent and the 5-year survival rate of these patients, with and without lymph node metastasis, is 89 and 80 percent, respectively. It has also been found that the frequency of lymph node metastasis increases in tumors that are ulcerated (87,88).

The distribution of lymph node metastases varies with the depth of invasion. For mucosal carcinomas, metastases are usually limited to the primary regional nodes, whereas for submucosal carcinomas they may spread to secondary or tertiary lymph nodes (165).

*Causes of Tumor Recurrence.* Residual or recurrent carcinoma in the gastric remnant following resection is most likely in superficial depressed lesions (type IIc). Because these tumors frequently have poorly defined lateral margins, the primary resection may not remove the entire neoplasm.

Another early carcinoma with a tendency towards recurrence is elevated, well-differentiated adenocarcinoma with an expansile growth pattern. These tumors cause destruction of the muscularis mucosae and replacement of the submucosa (120).

Twenty-five percent of these lesions have venous invasion, 40 percent invade the submucosal lymphatics, and 25 percent metastasize to perigastric nodes. The overall 10-year survival rate of patients with these tumors is 65 percent.

*Correlation of Histologic Type of Gastric Tumor to Prognosis.* All histologic types of gastric tumor confined to the superficial mucosa do well and rarely metastasize to lymph node. However, when the deeper mucosa and submucosa are invaded, where the lymphatics are more abundant, papillary adenocarcinoma and poorly differentiated carcinomas have a greater propensity than other carcinomas to metastasize (89,135). Diffuse and poorly differentiated carcinomas tend to metastasize to the regional lymph nodes, whereas glandular tumors with vascular invasion metastasize to the liver, lungs, and bones (247). Paradoxically for early gastric carcinoma the differentiated tumors have a worse prognosis because of their tendency towards widespread vascular dissemination.

It is important to be aware that extensive invasion may occur with very small carcinomas (less than 5 mm in diameter) and these therefore require the same definitive surgery as more advanced carcinomas (86).

*Advanced Gastric Carcinoma.* The prognosis of advanced gastric carcinoma worldwide is poor, with an overall 5-year patient survival rate of 10 percent (10,52,257). The results in the United States are not much better. In a recent large multicenter trial the overall survival rate was 14 percent among 10,891 patients (257). The survival rate after resection was 19 percent and 21 percent for cancers in the lower and mid-third of the stomach, respectively; 10 percent for those in the upper third; and 4 percent when the entire stomach was involved. Survival figures related to stage were 50 percent for patients with stage I tumors, 29 percent for stage II, 13 percent for stage III, and 3 percent for stage IV. Patients with tumor-free margins did much better than those with microscopic margin involvement (35 versus 13 percent). However, recent improvements in carcinoma diagnosis and treatment, such as extended lymph node resections, have achieved 5-year survival rates of around 60 percent for all tumors in certain countries, notably Japan (89), and 50 percent for stage III disease (140). This is quite an advance considering that less than 50 percent of gastric carcino-

mas worldwide are resectable for cure. The resectability figure is considerably higher in Japan because of the large number of early gastric carcinomas detected, and approaches 95 percent in some centers (140). The survival rate for patients with resectable advanced carcinoma is about 73 percent (4,10,37,148,180,267). It has been suggested that there may be biologic differences between Japanese and Western gastric carcinomas that account for the marked differences in survival and operability of these tumors. These factors are difficult to evaluate but it is of interest that in several German and British studies the prognostic factors, stage for stage, were similar to those in Japan (13,48,65,134a).

Several tumor characteristics, primarily tumor stage and type, and others, namely tumor differentiation, size, and growth pattern, have prognostic significance. Thus, accurate staging and grading are important in the management of these patients (9,72,114,140,218). In some cases, an enhanced host defense may influence prognosis.

*Prognostic Factors Related to Growth.* Much of the detailed data comes from studies done in Japan; however, recent studies from Europe have indicated similar findings (13,113). The most important prognostic factors relate to tumor stage, specifically depth of invasion; involvement of resection margins; and regional node involvement, including number of lymph nodes involved. Of the various staging systems, the TNM classification of the American Joint Committee on Cancer (AJCC) and its international counterpart the Union Internationale Contre De Cancer (UICC) is currently the most widely used method of staging. Survival figures have been shown to be accurately related to stage. The staging system also allows accurate comparisons between different studies (96,114,118,140,157,188,225,257). The best survival occurs with superficial gastric tumors without lymph node involvement (for details of TNM staging see chapter 1).

Patients with early gastric cancer confined to the mucosa and submucosa (T1) have a 5-year survival rate of about 95 percent. With invasion into the muscularis propria (T2) this falls to between 85 and 60 percent and to 50 percent if there is spread into the subserosa (77a,269a). With involvement of the contiguous structures (T4) there is a further drop to about 30 percent (42,81, 89,114,180,188). The proximity of the tumor to the proximal resection margin affects survival for patients with the diffuse type of gastric carcinoma: survival is greatly reduced if proximity is 5 to 6 cm as measured on a fresh, unstretched specimen (93) and zero if at the margin of resection (4,93). Survival also drops steeply once lymph nodes are involved: the comparable 5-year survival figures cited above fall to 10 and 20 percent (4,6,180). Furthermore, there is evidence that the number of lymph nodes involved both in early and advanced carcinomas influences prognosis: 5-year survival rate for patients with three or less involved lymph nodes is about twice as good as for those with more involved nodes (45 percent versus 25 percent) (96,117, 192). Unfortunately, most advanced gastric carcinomas already have lymph node involvement by the time of diagnosis.

The size of tumor affects prognosis, probably because it is related to stage. Patients with tumors larger than 4 cm in diameter have a 43 percent chance of having lymph node metastases (28,106). The site of the tumor is only important in relation to tumors of the cardia. These do poorly because of their late presentation (42,232). In one report, the 5-year survival rate for patients with tumors in the upper third of the stomach was 33 percent compared to 57 percent for those with tumors in the rest of the stomach, including many cases of early gastric carcinoma (140).

The growth pattern of the tumor also affects prognosis. Patients with carcinomas with an expanding margin do about twice as well as those with infiltrative carcinomas; those with Lauren's intestinal type of carcinoma do better than those with the diffuse type (127,152,192, 199,222,237). The latter is due in part to lymphatic spread and the extensive serosal and peritoneal involvement by the diffuse type.

*Histologic Type and Grade of Tumor.* It is still unclear whether the variations in behavior of gastric tumors are due to stage and grade independently or are interrelated; that is, are the more undifferentiated tumors more likely to be associated with more advanced stages. In one study, which was not biased with early carcinoma cases, there was a significant association between tumor grade and survival. The overall 5-year survival rates for patients with highly differentiated carcinomas was 50 percent; for those with moderately and poorly differentiated carcinomas, 18 percent;

and only 3 percent for those with linitis plastica (188). Similarly, those with adenocarcinomas with massive lymphoid stroma do about twice as well, stage for stage, as those with other advanced gastric carcinomas (258). This is attributed to an enhanced host defense mechanism. When duration of symptoms was analyzed, better differentiated tumors were slower to spread and increase in size than poorly differentiated tumors; however, when stage was taken into consideration, there were no statistically significant differences in survival between the histologic groups (188). Hermanek and others (86,93), on the other hand, have demonstrated differences in survival according to type of tumor in advanced gastric carcinoma (but not in early gastric carcinoma). For surgically resectable cases of advanced gastric carcinoma, stage for stage, the 5-year survival rate for patients with the intestinal type of carcinoma was significantly better than for those with the diffuse type: T2, 64 versus 45 percent; T3, 42 versus 17 percent. Patients with papillary tumors generally did worse than those with other types of carcinomas, probably because of early vascular invasion; those with signet-ring cell carcinomas confined to the stomach did better than those with other types of adenocarcinoma. Once the tumor had extended to the serosa and beyond, there was no significant difference in prognosis between the histologic types (86). Recently, a grading system based on tubular differentiation and mucus production was shown to correlate with tumor spread (138).

The prognostic figures quoted above are changing in certain geographic areas but not in others. The survival statistics for all grades and stages of gastric carcinoma, except for widely disseminated tumors, are improving with the more radical surgical procedures practiced in Japan and elsewhere (140).

*General Prognostic Factors.* Sex and race of the patient do not affect prognosis but there is some evidence that age does, since prognosis is worse in young patients. However, this appears to be related to delay in diagnosis and because many of these tumors are high grade rather than to an intrinsic tumor difference (17,67,69). Whether length of symptoms affects prognosis is unclear, although it has been stated that patients with a long history of symptoms are likely to be those with tumors of low growth rates (67).

A number of tumor markers have been proposed as indicators of unfavorable prognosis. These include carcinoembryonic antigen (CEA), epidermal growth factor, human chorionic gonadotropin, heterogeneous DNA ploidy, and oncogene *ras* and c-*myc* amplification (67,101, 121,244,266). The precise role of these markers in the routine work-up of these tumors remains to be determined.

*Prognosis Related to Early Diagnosis and Treatment.* In Japan, there has been a remarkable improvement in the overall survival rate of patients with gastric carcinoma, which is now about 50 percent for 5 years and longer (37,139). This is attributable in great part to the extensive screening programs, so that approximately 55 percent of patients are now diagnosed at the stage of early gastric carcinoma. However, another factor that has contributed to the increased survival rate in Japan, in marked contrast to the United States, is the aggressive surgical approach to advanced carcinoma by means of extended lymphadenectomy; 5-year survival rates approaching 40 percent are now being reported for advanced gastric carcinomas (139,143). In addition to removing R1 nodes (those immediately adjacent and within 3 cm of the neoplasm) as performed for cure in the United States, Japanese surgeons also remove the R2 nodes (those located more than 3 cm from the tumor including nodes adjacent to the left gastric artery, the common hepatic artery, and the celiac axis); in some cases R3 nodes (those along the aorta, porta hepatis, and retroperitoneum) are removed as well.

So far, adjuvant chemotherapy and radiotherapy have not contributed to survival, although they may produce prolonged remission (40,124, 196,250,262).

**Treatment.** In Japan, some centers are now treating early gastric carcinoma by endoscopic resection by means of snare biopsies (mucosectomy or strip biopsy). The obvious advantages of this limited resection is decreased morbidity, improved quality of life, and low cost. It is the treatment of choice for borderline lesions in which there is uncertainty whether they are high-grade dysplasias or early gastric carcinomas. The selection criteria for this form of treatment are that the lesions be of type I or IIa, nonulcerated, and less than 1.5 cm in diameter. These criteria are based on the fact that tumors

of this type have not been found to metastasize. Careful histologic examination of the resection specimen is necessary in order to verify that the tumor is well or moderately differentiated with no vascular or lymphatic invasion and that the tumor is confined to the mucosa and not present at the resection margins. If any of these factors are positive, then the tumors are handled the same way as advanced carcinomas, namely surgically, because of the increased risk of nodal metastasis (84,187,213,242,246).

Treatment of advanced gastric carcinoma is surgical if the tumor is resectable. In Japan the extent of the gastric resection depends on the distance between the upper border of the tumor and the gastroesophageal junction. For those tumors that are at least 6 cm from the gastroesophageal junction, a distal or partial gastrectomy may be sufficient. For all the others, including all diffuse carcinomas, a total gastrectomy, splenectomy, and sometimes partial pancreatectomy is necessary (107,140).

There is an ongoing debate concerning the extent of lymph node resection. While it is generally accepted that incomplete removal of tumor at the time of resection increases the likelihood of local recurrence, the effect of local recurrence on overall survival remains debatable. In Japan the accepted surgical procedure is to remove all suspected lymph nodes, and it is felt that this accounts for their enhanced survival rate compared to that reported in the West (37,139,142,161,180). However, other factors such as better staging procedures, patient and tumor related factors, and perioperative circumstances may also contribute to the enhanced survival rates (107).

In order to minimize postoperative morbidity, it is important to limit the extent of surgery. Presently in Japan abdominal lymph nodes are numbered according to their location; these are then allocated to lymph node groups according to the site of the tumor. N1 and N2 are considered the regional nodes (see chapter 1, fig. 1-18). Initially it was thought that gastric tumors metastasized from one group to the next. Unfortunately, as already indicated, the site of lymph node metastasis is not always predictable according to the site of origin of the tumor, since tumor sometimes skips beyond the proximal lymph nodes to more distant ones. Maruyama (107,108) has partially overcome this problem of unpredictability of lymph node spread by developing a computer program, based on the clinicopathologic data of 3,843 cases, to predict the likely sites and extent of lymph node invasion and the prognosis for gastric tumor in any given site. This has become a valuable guide for surgeons in determining the extent of lymph node dissection necessary for any given individual with gastric carcinoma. The value of these findings has been independently confirmed in a study from Germany (13,107,108).

## MORPHOLOGIC VARIANTS OF GASTRIC ADENOCARCINOMA

### Undifferentiated Carcinoma with Lymphoid Stroma (Medullary Carcinoma, Gastric Lymphoepithelioma-like Carcinoma)

These are uncommon, undifferentiated gastric carcinomas characterized by a dense lymphocytic infiltrate and resembling lymphoepitheliomas at other sites such as the salivary glands and the nasopharynx (100,131,258). They behave differently from the usual gastric carcinomas, being considerably less aggressive and are morphologically distinctive. Their importance to the pathologist is that they may be confused with lymphoma.

**Clinical Features and Pathogenesis.** The age of presentation and presenting symptoms are similar to those of usual gastric carcinomas. However, there is a higher male to female ratio (approximately 3 to 1 compared to the usual 2 to 1) (258).

The pathogenesis of this tumor is unclear but it is felt that the dense lymphoid infiltrate indicates an intense host reaction, which may explain the favorable prognosis of most of these tumors. It has been shown that many tumor cells contain interleukin-1 (IL-1) and it has been postulated that release of IL-1–related substances might induce migration of T cells with IL-1 receptors to the tumor (131). A number of recent studies have demonstrated the Epstein-Barr virus (EBV) by polymerase chain reaction and in situ hybridization. The role of EBV in the pathogenesis of this tumor and lymphoepitheliomas in general remains to be clarified (20,150,223,261).

**Gross Findings.** These tumors are usually found at the junction of the antrum and body but can occur anywhere in the stomach. Grossly, they are usually centrally ulcerated, circumscribed lesions with eversion of the mucosa at the ulcer margin. On cut section the tumor has an expansive growth pattern with a homogeneous gray or gray-white moist surface, resembling lymphoma. Early medullary carcinomas have the same gross features of any of the types of early gastric carcinoma previously described.

**Histologic Findings.** Microscopically, medullary carcinoma is characterized by nests of tumor cells widely separated by a dense lymphoplasmacytic infiltrate. This infiltrate consists of mature lymphocytes, plasma cells, and occasional neutrophils, eosinophils, and lymphoid follicles (fig. 11-39). The tumor consists of small polygonal cells with clear or slightly eosinophilic cytoplasm arranged as single cells or in trabeculae, small alveoli, primitive tubuloglandular patterns, or syncytial aggregates. Nuclei are usually regular and vesicular, with small nucleoli and scant mitoses, although poorly differentiated forms have also been described (1). The metastatic lesions show similar morphologic changes as the primary tumor.

**Differential Diagnosis.** This tumor may be confused histologically with malignant lymphoma. The diagnosis is usually made by demonstration of cytoplasmic mucin. If the PAS stain is negative or equivocal, immunohistochemical demonstration of cytokeratin and carcinoembryonic antigen confirms the epithelial nature of the tumor cells.

**Prognosis.** The behavior of early gastric carcinoma with lymphoid stroma is similar to that of other early gastric carcinomas. However, the 5-year patient survival rate of advanced tumors is considerably better than that for ordinary carcinomas, averaging about 77 percent. There are no available figures for metastatic lesions (258).

### Diffuse Gastric Carcinoma with Gastric Endocrine Cells

These are poorly differentiated, frequently signet-ring cell gastric carcinomas that contain a large number of admixed endocrine cells. They are considered by some to be ECLomas because of the ultrastructural similarities of the endocrine cells with the normal gastric enterochromaffin-like (ECL) cells (256).

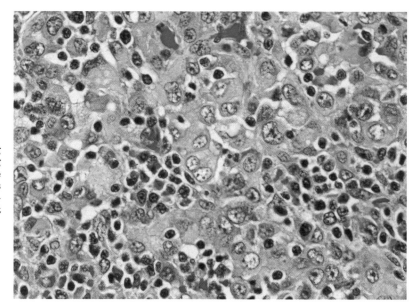

Figure 11-39
UNDIFFERENTIATED
GASTRIC CARCINOMA
WITH LYMPHOID STROMA
(MEDULLARY CARCINOMA)
High-power magnification showing undifferentiated tumor cells bearing some resemblance to lymphoma. The tumor consists of small polygonal cells arranged in syncytial masses, with vesicular nuclei containing prominent nucleoli and interspersed lymphocytes.

## Parietal Cell Carcinoma

This is a rare gastric tumor with histologic features of parietal cells and occurrence in elderly patients (21,23,202). The few tumors that have been described have been huge and transmural, and have involved the gastric body and antrum (23). Histologically, tumors are characterized by solid sheets of polygonal cells with abundant eosinophilic cytoplasm (fig. 11-40). Like parietal cells they stain with phosphotungstic acid hematoxylin. Ultrastructurally, they show features typical of parietal cells: abundant mitochondria, tubulovesicles, and intracellular canaliculi (fig. 11-40) (23). In one case report the tumor cells were poorly cohesive and resembled lymphoma (202).

These tumors appear to behave less aggressively than the usual gastric carcinomas (21,23). Of three patients reported by Capella et al. (23), two are alive and well at 1 and 2 years after tumor resection. However, more information is needed before the prognosis of these lesions can be accurately determined.

## Hepatoid Adenocarcinoma

This is a distinctive but rare tumor consisting of adenocarcinoma admixed with foci of tumor resembling mature and neoplastic hepatocytes (99,169,255).

Patients present with the usual features of advanced gastric carcinoma, and have a very poor prognosis with widespread tumor dissemination due to pronounced vascular infiltration. The patients have a very high serum alpha-fetoprotein level (in the thousands).

The tumor usually has two components, hepatoid-like foci and adenocarcinoma. The hepatoid areas may be well or poorly differentiated (fig. 11-41) and show the full spectrum of hepatocellular carcinoma features, including bile production and vascular invasion. Alpha-fetoprotein, alpha-1-antitrypsin, and albumin can also be demonstrated. Histologically, the adenocarcinomatous component may be well or poorly differentiated, often with clear cells and a papillary pattern.

Hepatoid adenocarcinoma is easy to diagnose if hepatoid areas are clearly distinguishable within the gastric tumor. However, in anaplastic variants or cases with massive liver metastases, it may be difficult. In these cases the gross findings in the stomach coupled with the very high serum alpha-fetoprotein levels are distinctive.

## Composite Gastric Carcinoma

These tumors have discrete areas of two types of neoplastic differentiation. They are thought to represent multidirectional differentiation of a single neoplasm. Only one such tumor has been reported in the stomach (253); this was in a 60-year-old man with a large ulcerating mass in the antrum and metastases to the perigastric

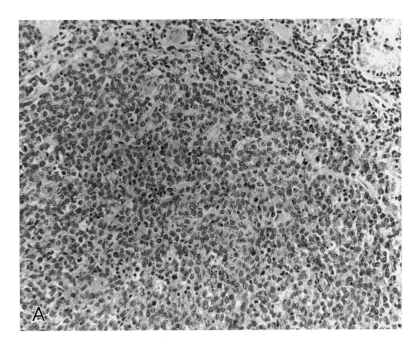

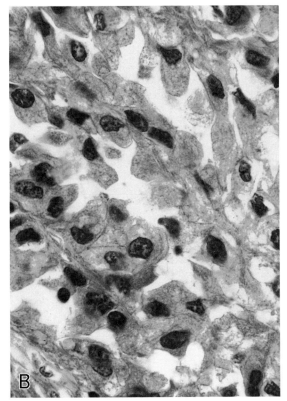

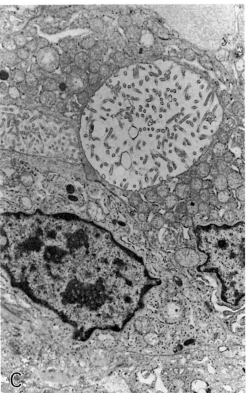

Figure 11-40
GASTRIC PARIETAL CELL CARCINOMA

A: Low-power view showing a solid sheet of fairly cohesive tumor cells. Residual pyloric glands can be seen in the upper right field.

B: High-power magnification showing tubular differentiation.

C: Electron microscopy of two tumor cells showing the well-differentiated parietal cells with abundant mitochondria. One cell contains a distended intracellular canaliculus covered with microvilli. (Courtesy of Dr. C. Capella, Pavia, Italy.)

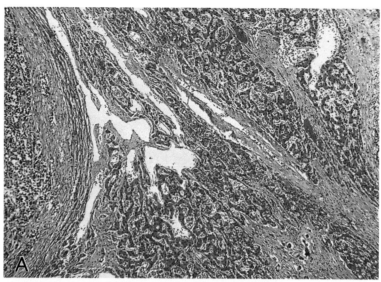

Figure 11-41
HEPATOID CARCINOMA
OF THE STOMACH

A: Low-power magnification showing well-differentiated hepatoid carcinoma occupying much of the center of the field and poorly differentiated tumor resembling hepatoblastoma at the side.

B: High-power magnification of the well-differentiated hepatoid tumor showing cords of liver-like cells separated by sinusoids.

C: High-power magnification of the undifferentiated component consisting predominantly of small cells, with rare tumor cells containing greatly enlarged hyperchromatic nuclei. (Courtesy of Dr. P.A. Allevato, USA.)

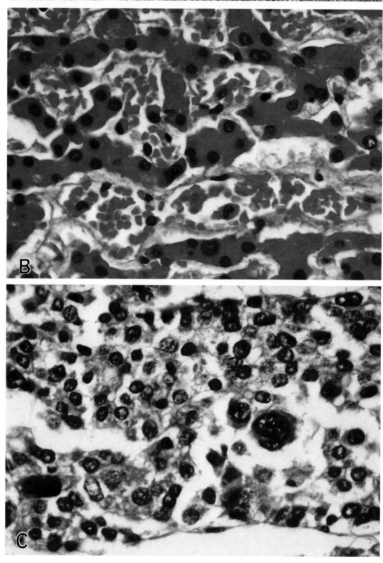

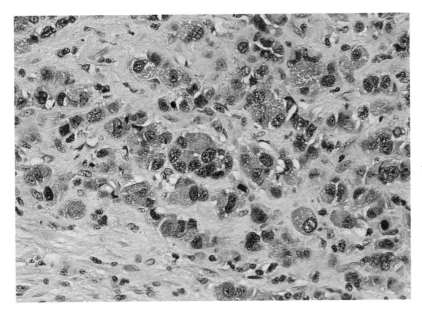

Figure 11-42
PANETH CELL CARCINOMA
The tumor cells contain the characteristic granular eosinophilic cytoplasm.

lymph nodes and liver. Histologically, the tumor showed adenocarcinoma and poorly differentiated carcinoid, which was confirmed by argyrophilia, chromogranin, and serotonin, demonstrated immunohistochemically. It may be difficult to distinguish these tumors from metastatic lesions and collision tumors. Collision tumors are composed of two distinct tumors growing in close proximity to one another (137,253).

### Paneth Cell Carcinoma

This is essentially an adenocarcinoma with a predominance of Paneth cells. These tumors are exceedingly rare and have no distinctive clinicopathologic features (112,191). Histologically, the Paneth cells are identified by their distinctive large, eosinophilic cytoplasmic granules and by the demonstration of lysozyme within the granules (fig. 11-42). The granules are also distinctive ultrastructurally.

### Gastric Carcinoma with Rhabdoid Features

This is a recently described rare variant of gastric carcinoma with a poor prognosis. The tumor has a diffuse or alveolar arrangement and is composed of round to polygonal tumor cells with eosinophilic or clear cytoplasm and large eccentric vesicular nuclei similar to those seen in malignant rhabdoid tumors of the kidney. In all cases, there was coexpression of vimentin and cytokeratin in the cytoplasm (252).

### Collision Tumors

These are rare in the stomach and essentially consist of two distinct neoplasms of any variety arising next to one another and sometimes growing into one another. When the latter occurs it may be impossible to differentiate these tumors from composite tumors (162).

## ADENOCARCINOMA OF THE GASTRIC CARDIA AND PROXIMAL STOMACH

**Definition.** These are tumors of the proximal stomach that are normally located within 1 cm proximal and 2 cm distal to the esophagogastric junction, provided there is no Barrett's mucosa above it (278). It should be noted that the gastric cardia is a very short, frequently variable and indistinct segment of stomach at the esophagogastric junction and it is uncertain whether all proximal gastric tumors originate from this site or from both the cardia and the adjacent fundic mucosa. The differentiation of some cardia tumors from adenocarcinoma of the esophagus arising from short-segment Barrett's esophagus can be difficult since intestinalized epithelium may occur at both sites and therefore does not help differentiate the two. The finding of specialized columnar-lined epithelium adjacent to the proximal margin of the tumor and extending up into the lower esophagus suggests that the tumor arose in a Barrett's esophagus. Similarly, dysplasia of

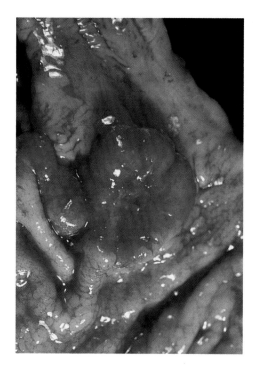
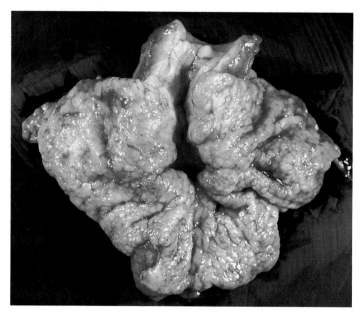

Figure 11-43
GROSS APPEARANCES OF ADENOCARCINOMA OF THE GASTRIC CARDIA
Left: Nodular tumor at the esophagogastric junction.
Right: Marked thickening and nodularity of the cardia encircling the esophagogastric junction.

gastric cardia mucosa is a strong indicator of a primary gastric origin. However, compared to carcinoma in Barrett's esophagus, dysplasia in the gastric cardia is usually sparse (272). Nevertheless, there remains a significant number of tumors which straddle the gastroesophageal junction, where it may be impossible to be certain whether the tumor arose in the gastric cardia or the lower esophagus. If the epicenter of the tumor is clearly above the esophagogastric junction (about 3 cm), this is presumptive evidence that it originated in the columnar-lined esophagus. From a practical point, the differentiation of these tumors is more of academic interest than of practical value since their behavior is similar and because they appear to share similar etiopathogenic characteristics.

**Pathogenesis and Clinical Features.** The incidence of carcinoma of the gastric cardia and proximal stomach is increasing worldwide for reasons that are unclear; this tumor now accounts for approximately a third of all gastric carcinomas (7,12,282). It is a distinctive tumor, differing clinicopathologically from carcinoma of the rest of the stomach and showing many similarities to eso-

phageal adenocarcinoma (272,275, 283). Compared to other gastric carcinomas, cardia carcinomas are associated with a lower mean age (65 years), predominance among white males, a male to female ratio of 6 to 1, greater frequency of hiatal hernia (40 percent), esophageal reflux and duodenal ulcer, and rarity of atrophic gastritis and signet-ring cell carcinomas (276,284). Dietary factors have not been associated with tumors of the cardia but as in the esophagus there seems to be a strong association with alcohol and tobacco (7,275,276).

Clinically, the tumors spread into the esophagus and present with dysphagia. They commonly present at a more advanced stage than other gastric tumors and consequently appear to have a worse prognosis (273,277,281,283). Postoperatively, patients are especially prone to gastroesophageal leakage (283).

**Gross and Microscopic Findings.** Grossly, these tumors are generally larger than gastric tumors at other sites and are predominantly ulcerating and infiltrative in type (Borrmann types 3 and 4) (figs. 11-43, 11-44) (281). The tumors often invade the esophagus (fig. 11-44) (274), and lymph node

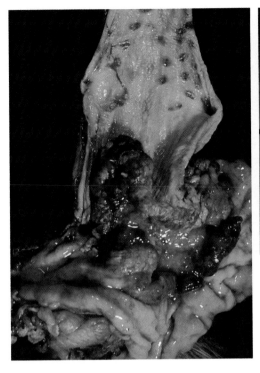

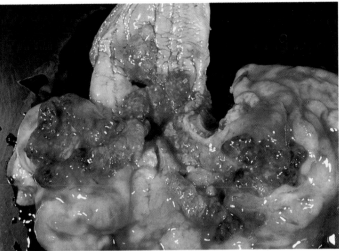

Figure 11-44
GROSS APPEARANCES OF ADENOCARCINOMA
OF THE GASTRIC CARDIA
Left: Exophytic mass protruding into the esophageal lumen.
Above: Exophytic fungating tumor growing into the esophagus.

metastases are common, primarily to the upper gastric, paraceliac, and para-aortic nodes and infrequently to mediastinal nodes (1). With the exception of signet-ring cell carcinomas, which are exceedingly rare, the histology and mode of metastasis of carcinoma of the gastric cardia is most similar to adenocarcinoma of the esophagus associated with Barrett's mucosa (272) and less to other gastric carcinomas. As in other parts of the stomach, cases of early gastric carcinoma have been detected. However, grossly elevated forms and histologically well-differentiated early carcinomas are more common in the gastric cardia (279,280).

## ADENOCARCINOMA IN HETEROTOPIC PANCREAS

These are exceedingly rare with only a handful described, one of which arose in a hiatal hernia (293,293a). Due to the site of origin of heterotopic gastric pancreas, frequently within the gastric wall, the tumors form an intramural mass with relatively late involvement of the mucosa, making early biopsy diagnosis difficult (293a). Histologically, the lesions are ductal adenocarcinomas. To confirm the heterotopic origin, pancreatic tis-

sue must be demonstrated within, or adjacent to, the tumor. The prognosis of these tumors is poor because of their late diagnosis.

## CARCINOMAS WITH INTERSPERSED ENDOCRINE DIFFERENTIATION (ADENOENDOCRINE CELL CARCINOMA, SCIRRHOUS ARGYROPHIL CELL CARCINOMA)

Many gastric adenocarcinomas contain scattered endocrine cells. In addition, occasional signet-ring cell carcinomas contain numerous interspersed argyrophil cells. Their clinical behavior is similar to that of signet-ring cell carcinoma (see Gastric Carcinoids).

### SMALL CELL (OAT CELL) CARCINOMA

These tumors are similar to oat cell cancers of the lung; only a few cases have been reported in the stomach. The prognosis is poor, and most patients die within 1 year of diagnosis (287,289, 291,294,296).

Grossly, early lesions appear to be polypoid and advanced lesions develop deep ulcerations (296). Microscopically, the tumors tend to grow in

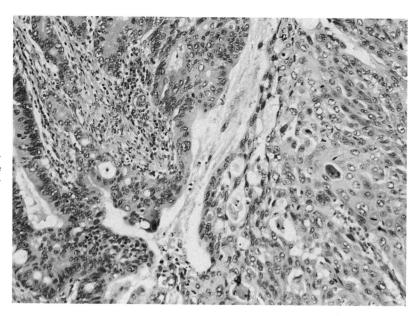

Figure 11-45
ADENOSQUAMOUS CARCINOMA
OF THE STOMACH
There is a well-defined focus of keratinizing squamous cell carcinoma in the
right half of the field and adenocarcinoma on the left.

sheets, cords, and trabecular or alveolar-like patterns, separated by thin bands of vascularized connective tissue, similar to oat cell carcinoma of the lung. The tumor cells may be small lymphocyte–like or of intermediate cell type, characterized by small polygonal or fusiform cells with scant cytoplasm. The nuclei are hyperchromatic, with a "salt and pepper" chromatin pattern, frequently exhibiting nuclear molding. A number of these tumors show foci of adenocarcinomatous or squamous differentiation (291,296).

Small cell carcinomas of the stomach are commonly, but not invariably, argyrophilic; often stain for chromogranin and neuron-specific enolase; and do not usually contain carcinoembryonic antigen. The hallmark of these tumors is the presence of dense core granules, albeit sometimes in sparse numbers, as demonstrated by electron microscopy. As is true for oat cell tumors of the lung, not all the reported small cell tumors of the stomach have features of endocrine cells, namely argyrophilia, immunoreactivity to chromogranin, ob the presence of dense core granules (296). This may be because some tumors are so poorly differentiated that the endocrine cell markers are not sufficiently sensitive. However, it is probable that some poorly differentiated tumors are indistinguishable from small cell carcinomas. From a practical point of view the behavior and treatment of these tumors is the same, irrespective of their cell of origin. Lymphatic and vascular invasion is common.

## ADENOSQUAMOUS AND SQUAMOUS CELL CARCINOMA OF THE STOMACH

These tumors account for less than 1 percent of all gastric carcinomas (285,286,299,306). Clinically and on gross examination they are indistinguishable from usual adenocarcinomas (285, 299). Sixty percent are found in the distal half of the stomach. Tumors that initially are considered to be pure squamous cell carcinomas, on meticulous histologic study almost always reveal at least small foci of adenocarcinoma (299). Squamous cell carcinomas are believed to arise from foci of squamous metaplasia, although they might also arise from primitive cells with the ability to differentiate towards both glandular and squamous epithelium (288,290,298).

Histologically, poorly differentiated adenocarcinomas that do not make lumens may sometimes resemble equally poorly differentiated squamous carcinomas and thus it is imperative to demonstrate unequivocal features of squamous differentiation, namely squamous pearls or definite intercellular bridges by light microscopy (fig. 11-45) and high molecular weight cytokeratin. The degree of squamous and glandular components is variable and may range from almost pure squamous cell carcinoma to only microscopic foci. Occasionally, individual cells containing both tonofibrils and mucus vacuoles are observed (300). Other morphologic patterns, such

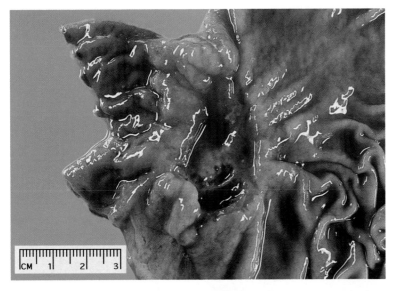

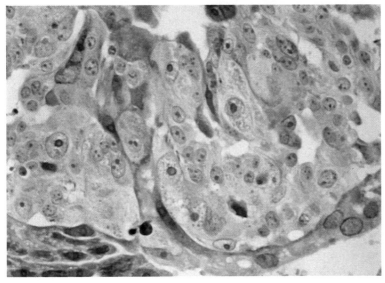

Figure 11-46
CHORIOCARCINOMA
OF THE STOMACH

Top: Resected specimen showing ulcerated lesion in the antrum.

Bottom: High-power magnification of the tumor showing cytotrophoblastic cells bordered by multinucleated syncytiotrophoblasts. (Courtesy of Dr. T. Hirota, Tokyo, Japan.)

as a mucoepidermoid carcinoma (300) and a collision tumor at the esophagogastric junction consisting of squamous cell carcinoma and adenocarcinoma, have also been described (137,300).

Adenosquamous carcinomas behave more aggressively than pure adenocarcinomas because of their greater invasiveness and lymphatic and vascular modes of dissemination (298).

## ADENOCARCINOMA AND CHORIOCARCINOMA

These are exceedingly rare gastric tumors that occur in the absence of gonadal tumors or other primary sites of choriocarcinoma. Histologically,

they show the typical features of choriocarcinoma with both cytotrophoblastic and syncitiotrophoblastic cells (fig. 11-46). They are almost invariably associated with foci of adenocarcinoma, supporting the hypothesis that these tumors are derived by retrodifferentiation of neoplastic mucosal epithelial cells (292,295, 301–303,305).

The patients range in age from 30 to 80 years, but tend to be elderly and are more commonly male (2 to 1) (292,295,297,302,304). They present with symptoms similar to those of carcinoma and their prognosis is poor. For a detailed description of this tumor see chapter 15.

## REFERENCES

### Adenocarcinoma of the Stomach

1. Adachi Y, Mori M, Maehara Y, Sugimachi K. Poorly differentiated medullary carcinoma of the stomach. Cancer 1992;70:1462–6.

2. Aird I, Bentall HH, Roberts JA. A relationship between cancer of the stomach and the ABO blood groups. BMJ 1953;1:799–801.

3. Andersson AP, Lauritsen KB, West F, Johansen A. Dysplasia in the gastric mucosa: prognostic significance. Acta Chir Scand 1987;157:29–31.

4. Antonioli DA. Current concepts in carcinoma of the stomach. In: Appleman HD, ed. Pathology of the esophagus, stomach and duodenum. New York: Churchill Livingstone, 1984:121–44.

5. Antonioli DA. Precursors of gastric carcinoma: a critical review with a brief description of early (curable) gastric cancer. Human Pathology 1994;25:994–1005.

6. Antonioli DA, Goldman H. Changes in the location and type of gastric adenocarcinoma. Cancer 1982;50:775–81.

7. Aoki K, Tominaga S, Kuroishi T. Age-adjusted death rates for cancer by site in 50 countries in 1975. Jpn J Cancer Res 1981;26:251–74.

8. Appelman HD. Localized and extensive expansions of the gastric mucosa: mucosal polyps and giant folds. In: Appelman HD, ed. Pathology of the esophagus, stomach and duodenum. New York: Churchill Livingstone, 1984:79–119.

9. Beahrs OH, Henson DE, Hutter RV, Kennedy BJ. American Joint Committee on Cancer. Manual for staging of cancer. 4th ed. Philadelphia: JB Lippincott, 1992.

10. Bizer LS. Adenocarcinoma of the stomach: current results of treatment. Cancer 1983;51:743–5.

11. Blackstone MO. Endoscopic interpretation. Normal and pathologic appearances of the gastrointestinal tract. New York: Raven Press, 1984.

11a. Blaser MJ. Helicobacter pylori phenotypes associated with peptic ulceration. Scand J Gastroenterol 1994;29(Suppl):205:1–5.

11b. Blaser MJ, Perez-Perez GI, Kleanthous H, et al. Infection with Helicobacter pylori strains possessing cagA is associated with an increased risk of developing adenocarcinoma of the stomach. Cancer Research 1995;55:2111–5.

12. Blot WJ, Devesa SS, Kneller RW, Fraumeni JF. Rising incidence of adenocarcinoma of the esophagus and gastric cardia. JAMA 1991;265:1287–9.

13. Bollschweiler E, Boettcher K, Hoelscher AH, et al. Preoperative assessment of lymph node metastases in patients with gastric cancer: evaluation of the Maruyama computer program. Br J Surg 1992;79:156–60.

14. Boring CC, Squires BA, Tong T. Cancer statistics 1993. CA Cancer J Clin 1993;43:7–26.

15. Borrmann R. Geschwulste des magens und duodenums. In: Henke F, Lubarsch O, eds. Handbuch der speziellen pathologischen anatomie und histologie. Berlin: Springer, 1926:865.

16. Brandt D, Muramatsu Y, Ushio K, et al. Synchronous early gastric cancer. Radiology 1989;173:649–52.

17. Brookes VS, Waterhouse JA, Dowell DJ. Carcinoma of the stomach: a 10 year survey of results and factors affecting prognosis. BMJ 1965;1:1577–83.

18. Burke AP, Sobin LH, Shekitka KM, Avallone FA. Correlation of nucleolar organizer regions and glandular dysplasia of the stomach and esophagus. Mod Pathol 1990;3:357–60.

19. Burke AP, Sobin LH, Shekitka KM, Helvig EB. Dysplasia of the stomach and Barrett esophagus: a follow-up study. Mod Pathol 1991;4:336–41.

20. Burke AP, Yen TS, Shekitka KM, Sobin LH. Lymphoepithelial carcinoma of the stomach with Epstein-Barr virus demonstrated by polymerase chain reaction. Mod Pathol 1990;3:377–80.

21. Byrne D, Holley MP, Cushieri A. Parietal cell carcinoma of the stomach: asssociation with long-term survival after curative resection. Br J Cancer 1988;58:85–7.

22. Campbell H. Cancer mortality in Europe. Site-specific patterns and trends 1955 to 1974. World Health Stat Q 1980;33:251–74.

23. Capella C, Frigerio B, Cornaggia M, Solcia E, Pinzon-Trujillo Y, Chejfec G. Gastric parietal cell carcinoma—a newly recognized entity: light microscopic and ultrastructural features. Histopathology 1984;8:813–24.

24. Case records of the Massachusetts General Hospital. N Engl J Med 1988;318:100–9.

25. Chang FM, Saito T, Ashizawa S. Follow-up endoscopic study of gastric mucosal changes secondary to gastric ulcer. Endoscopy 1978;10:33–40.

26. Collins WT, Gall EA. Gastric carcinoma: a multicentric lesion. Cancer 1952;5:62–72.

27. Coma del Corral MJ, Pardo-Mindan FJ, Razquin S, Ojeda C. Risk of cancer in patients with gastric dysplasia. Follow-up study of 67 patients. Cancer 1990;65:2078–85.

28. Comfort MW, Gray HK, Dockerty MB, et al. Small gastric cancer. Arch Intern Med 1954;94:513–24.

29. Cormier WJ, Gaffey TA, Welch JM, Welch JS, Edmondson JH. Linitis plastica caused by metastatic lobular carcinoma of the breast. Mayo Clin Proc 1980;55:747–53.

30. Correa P. Chronic gastritis: a clinico-pathological classification. Am J Gastroenterol 1988;83:504–9.

31. Correa P. Chronic gastritis as a cancer precursor. Scand J Gastroenterol 1985;104(Suppl):131–6.

32. Correa P. Is gastric carcinoma an infectious disease? N Engl J Med 1991;25:1170–1.

33. Correa P, Fox J, Fontham E, et al. Helicobacter pylori and gastric carcinoma. Serum antibody prevalence in populations with contrasting cancer risks. Cancer 1990;66:2569–74.

34. Correa P, Haenszel W, Tannenbaum S. Epidemiology of gastric carcinoma: review and future prospects. Natl Cancer Inst Monogr 1982;62:129–34.

35. Correa P, Sasano N, Stemmermann GN, Haenszel W. Pathology of gastric carcinoma in Japanese populations: comparisons between Miyagi prefecture, Japan and Hawaii. JNCI 1973;51:1449–59.

36. Correa P, Yardley JH. Grading and classification of chronic gastritis: one American response to the Sydney system. Gastroenterology 1992;102:355–9.

37. Craven JL. Radical surgery for gastric cancer. In: Preece PE, Cuschieri A, Wellwood JM, eds. Cancer of the stomach. London: Grune and Stratton, 1986:165–87.

38. Cuello C, Correa P, Haenszel W, et al. Gastric cancer in Colombia. 1.Cancer risk and suspect environmental agents. JNCI 1976;7:1015–20.

39. Cuello C, Correa P, Zarama G, Lopez J, Murray J, Gordillo G. Histopathology of gastric dysplasias: correlations with gastric juice chemistry. Am J Surg Pathol 1979;3:491–500.

40. Cunningham D, Coombes RC. Current approaches to the chemotherapy of gastric cancer. In: Preece PE, Cuschieri A, Wellwood JM, eds. Cancer of the stomach. London: Grune and Stratton, 1986:243–8.

41. Cunningham-Rundles C. Clinical and immunologic analyses of 103 patients with common variable immunodeficiency. J Clin Immunol 1989;9:22–33.

42. Curtis RE, Kennedy BJ, Myers MH, Hankey BF. Evaluation of AJC stomach cancer staging using the SEER population. Semin Oncol 1985;12:21–31.

43. Cusso X, Mones J, Ocana J, Mendez C, Vilardell F. Is endoscopic gastric cytology worthwhile? An evaluation of 903 cases of carcinoma. J Clin Gastroenterol 1993;16:336–9.

44. Czerniak B, Herz F, Koss LG. DNA distribution patterns in early gastric carcinomas: a Feulgen cytometric study of gastric brush smears. Cancer 1987;59:113–7.

45. Daibo M, Itabashi M, Hirota T. Malignant transformation of gastric hyperplastic polyps. Am J Gastroenterol 1987;82:1016–25.

46. Danova M, Mazzini G, Wilson G, et al. Ploidy and proliferative activity of human gastric carcinoma: a cytofluorometric study on fresh and on paraffin embedded material. Basic Appl Histochem 1987;31:73–82.

47. Danova M, Riccardi A, Mazzini G, et al. Flow cytometric analysis of paraffin-embedded material in human gastric cancer. Anal Quant Cytol Histol 1988;10:200–6.

48. de Dombal FT, Price AB, Thompson H, et al. The British Society of Gastroenterology early gastric cancer/dysplasia survey: an interim report. Gut 1990;31:115–20.

49. Deschner EE, Lipkin N. Proliferation and differentiation of gastrointestinal cells in health and disease. In: Lipkin N, Good R, eds. Gastrointestinal tract cancer. New York: Plenum, 1978:3–27.

50. DiGregorio C, Morandi P, Fante R, De Gaetani C. Gastric dysplasia. A follow-up study. Am J Gastroenterol 1993;88:1714–9.

51. Dorgan JF, Schatzkin A. Antioxidant micronutrients in cancer prevention. Hematol Oncol Clin North Am 1991;5:43–68.

52. Dupont BJ Jr, Cohn I Jr. Gastric adenocarcinoma. Curr Probl Cancer 1980;4:1–46.

52a.Endo S, Ohkusa T, Saito Y, Fujiki K, Okayasu I, Sato C. Detection of Helicobacter pylori infection in early stage gastric cancer. A comparison between intestinal- and diffuse-type adenocarcinomas. Cancer 1995;75:2203–8.

53. Esaki Y, Hirokawa K, Yamashiro M. Multiple gastric cancers in the aged with special reference to intramucosal cancers. Cancer 1987;59:560–5.

54. Evans DD, Craven JL, Murphy F, Cleary BK. Comparison of early gastric cancer in Britain and Japan. J Clin Pathol 1978;19:1–9.

55. Farinati F, Rugge M, Di Mario F, Valiante F, Baffa R. Early and advanced gastric cancer in the follow-up of moderate and severe gastric dysplasia patients. A prospective study. IGGED- Interdisciplinary Group on Gastric Epithelial Dysplasia. Endoscopy 1993;25:261–4.

56. Farrell DJ, Scott DJ. Method for improving lymph node retrievel from gastrectomy specimens. J Clin Pathol 1993;46:580.

57. Fertitta AM, Comin U, Terruzzi V, et al. Clinical significance of gastric dysplasia: a multicenter follow-up study. Gastrointestinal Endoscopic Pathology Study Group. Endoscopy 1993;25:265–8.

58. Filipe MI. Borderline lesions of the gastric epithelium: new indicators of cancer risk and clinical implications. In: Fenoglio-Preiser CM, Wolff M, Rilke F, eds. Progress in surgical pathology. Vol. 12. Philadelphia: Field & Wood, 1992:269–90.

59. Filipe MI, Munoz N, Matko I, et al. Intestinal metaplasia types and the risk of gastric cancer: a cohort study in Slovenia. Int J Cancer 1994;57:324–9.

60. Filipe MI, Potet F, Bogomoletz WV, et al. Incomplete sulphomucin-secreting intestinal metaplasia for gastric cancer. Preliminary data from a prospective study from three centres. Gut 1985;26:1319–26.

61. Forman D. Helicobacter pylori infection: a novel risk factor in the etiology of gastric cancer. JNCI 1991;83:1702–3.

62. Fujita S. Kinetics of cancer cell proliferations and cancer growth. Cancer 1976;15:248–61.

63. Fujita S. Biology of early gastric carcinoma. Pathol Res Pract 1978;163:297–309.

64. Fukutomi H, Sakita T. Analysis of early gastric cancer collected from major hospitals and institutes in Japan. Jpn J Clin Oncol 1984;14:169–79.

65. Gall FP, Hermanek P. New aspects in the surgical treatment of gastric carcinoma-—a comparative study of 1636 patients operated on between 1969 and 1982. Eur J Surg Oncol 1985;11:219–25.

66. Ghandur-Mnaymneh L, Paz J, Roldan E, Cassady J. Dysplasia of nonmetaplastic gastric mucosa. A proposal for its classification and its possible relationship to diffuse-type gastric carcinoma. Am J Surg Pathol 1988;12:96–114.

67. Giles GR. Staging and prognostic determinations of gastric cancer. In: Preece PE, Cuschieri A, Wellwood JM, eds. Cancer of the stomach. London: Grune and Stratton, 1986:89–105.

68. Goldman H, Ming SC. Mucins in normal and neoplastic gastrointestinal epithelium. Histochemical distribution. Arch Pathol 1968;85:580–6.

69. Grabiec J, Owen DA. Carcinoma of the stomach in young persons. Cancer 1985;56:388–96.

70. Graham DY, Schwartz JT, Cain GD, Gyorkey F. Prospective efaluation of biopsy number in the diagnosis of esophageal and gastric carcinoma. Gastroenterology 1982;82:228–31.

71. Green PH, O'Toole KM, Weinberg LM, Goldfarb JP. Early gastric cancer. Gastroenterology 1981;81:247–56.

71a.Gulley ML, Pulitzer DR, Eagan PA, Schneider BG. Epstein-Barr virus infection is an early event in gastric carcinogenesis and is independent of bcl-2 expression and p53 accumulation. Hum Pathol 1996;27:20–7.

72. Gunven P, Maruyama K, Okabayashi K, Sasako M, Kinoshita T. Non-ominous micrometastases of gastric cancer. Br J Surg 1991;78:352–4.

73. Haas JF, Schottenfeld D. Epidemiology of gastric cancer. In: Lipkin M, Good RA, eds. Gastrointestinal tract cancer. New York: Plenum Medical Book Co, 1978:173–206.

74. Haenszel W, Kurihara M, Segi M, Lee RK. Stomach cancer among Japanese in Hawaii. JNCI 1972;49:969–88.

75. Haggitt RC. Premalignant lesions of the gastrointestinal tract. View Dig Dis 1985;17:1–4.

76. Hall EJ. From Chimney sweeps to oncogenes: the quest for the causes of cancer. Radiology 1991; 179:297–306.

77. Haraguchi M, Okamura T, Korenaga D, Tsujitani J, Marin P, Sugimachi K. Heterogeneity of DNA ploidy in patients with undifferentiated carcinomas of the stomach. Cancer 1987;59:922–4.

77a. Harrison JC, Dean PJ, Vander Zwaag R, El-Zeky K, Wruble LD. Adenocarcinoma of the stomach with invasion limited to the muscularis propria. Hum Pathol 1991;22:111–7.

78. Hatfield AR, Slavin G, Segal AW, Levi AJ. Importance of the site of endoscopic gastric biopsy in ulcerating lesions of the stomach. Gut 1975;16:884–6.

79. Hayashida T. End results of early gastric cancer collected from twenty-two institutions. Stom Intest 1969;4:1077–85.

80. Heintz A, Junginger T. Endosonographic staging of cancers of the esophagus and stomach. Comparison with surgical and histopathologic staging. Bildgebung 1991;48:4–8.

81. Hermanek P. Prognostic factors in stomach cancer surgery. Eur J Surg Oncol 1986;12:241–6.

81a. Hermanek P, Maruyama K, Sobin LH. Stomach carcinoma. In: Hermanek P, Gospodarowicz MK, Henson DE, Hutter RV, Sobin LH, eds. Prognostic factors in cancer. UICC, International Union Against Cancer. Berlin: Springer-Verlag, 1995:47–63.

82. Hermans PE, Diaz-Buxo JA, Stobo JD. Idiopathic late-onset immunoglobulin deficiency. Clinical observations in 50 patients. Am J Med 1976;61:221–37.

83. Hewan-Lowe K, Hammers Y, Lyons JM, Wilcox CM. Polyvinylpyrrolidone storage disease: a source of error in the diagnosis of signet ring cell gastric adenocarcinoma. Ultrastruct Pathol 1994;18:271–5.

84. Hirao M, Asanuma T, Masuda K, Miyazaki A. Endoscopic resection of early gastric cancer following locally injecting hypertonic saline-epinephrine. Stom Intest 1988;23:399–409.

85. Hirohashi S, Sugimura T. Genetic alterations in human gastric cancer. Cancer Cells 1991;3:49–52.

86. Hirota T, Itabashi M, Suzuki K, Yoshida S. Clinicopathologic study of minute and small early gastric cancer. Histogenesis of gastric cancer. Pathol Annu 1980;15:1–19.

87. Hirota T, Ming SC. Early gastric carcinoma. In: Ming SC, Goldman H, eds. Pathology of the gastrointestinal tract. Philadelphia: WB Saunders, 1992:570–83.

88. Hirota T, Ming SC, Itabashi M. Pathology of early gastric cancer. In: Nishi M, Ichikawa H, Nakajima T, Maruyama K, Tahara E, eds. Gastric cancer. Tokyo: Springer Verlag, 1993:66–87.

89. Hirota T, Ochiai A, Itabashi M, Maruyama K. Significance of histological type of gastric carcinoma as a prognostic factor. Stom Intest 1991;26:1149–58.

90. Hirota T, Okada T, Itabashi M, Kitaoka H. Histogenesis of human gastric cancer—with special reference to the significance of adenoma as a precancerous lesion. In: Ming SC, ed. Precursors of gastric cancer. New York: Praeger, 1984:233–52.

91. Hisamichi S, Shirane A, Sugawara N, et al. Early endoscopic features of stomach cancer and its mode of growth. Tohoku J Exp Med 1978;126:239–46.

92. Hole DJ, Quigley EM, Gillis CR, Watkinson G. Peptic ulcer and cancer: an examination of the relationship between chronic peptic ulcer and gastric carcinoma. Scand J Gastroenterol 1987;22:17–23.

93. Hornig D, Hermanek P, Gall FP. The significance of the extent of proximal margins of clearance in gastric cancer surgery. Scand J Gastroenterol 1987;22:69–71.

94. Houldsworth J, Cordon-Cardo C, Ladanyi M, Kelsen DP, Chaganti RS. Gene amplification in gastric and esophageal adenocarcinomas. Cancer Res 1990;50:6417–22.

95. Hurlimann J, Saraga EP. Expression of p53 protein in gastric carcinomas: association with histologic type and prognosis. Am J Surg Pathol 1994;18:1247–53.

96. Ichikura T, Tomimatsu S, Okusa Y, Uefuji K, Tamakuma S. Comparison of the prognostic significance between the number of metastatic lymph nodes and nodal stage based on their location in patients with gastric cancer. J Clin Oncol 1993;11:1894–900.

97. Iishi H, Tatsuta M, Okuda S. Endoscopic diagnosis of minute gastric cancer of less than 5 mm in diameter. Cancer 1985;56:655–9.

98. Isaacson P. Biopsy appearances easily mistaken for malignancy in gastrointestinal endoscopy. Histopathology 1982;6:377–89.

99. Ishikura H, Kirimoto K, Shamoto M, et al. Hepatoid adenocarcinoma of the stomach. An analysis of 7 cases. Cancer 1986;58:119–26.

100. Ito H, Masuda H, Shimamoto F, Inokuchi C, Tahara E. Gastric carcinoma with lymphoid stroma: pathological, immunohistochemical analysis. Hiroshima J Med Sci 1990;39:29–37.

101. Ito H, Tahara E. Human chorionic gonadotropin in human gastric carcinoma. A retrospective immunohistochemical study. Acta Pathol Jpn 1983;33:287–96.

102. Jass JR. A classification of gastric dysplasia. Histopathology 1983;7:181–93.

103. Jass JR, Filipe MI. A variant of intestinal metaplasia associated with gastric carcinoma: a histochemical study. Histopathology 1979;3:191–9.

104. Jass JR, Filipe MI. The mucin profiles of normal gastric mucosa, intestinal metaplasia and its variants and gastric carcinoma. Histochem J 1981;13:931–9.

105. Jass JR, Strudley T, Faludy J. Histochemistry of epithelial metaplasia and dysplasia in human stomach and colorectum. Scand J Gastroenterol Suppl 1984;104:109–30.

106. Johansen AA. Early gastric cancer. Curr Top Pathol 1976;63:1–47.

107. Kampschoer GH. The surgical treatment of gastric cancer—an appeal for lymph node dissection. Leiderdorp: BV Ouwehand, 1989.

108. Kampschoer GH, Maruyama K, van de Velde CJ, Sasako M, Kinoshita T, Okabayashi K. Computer analysis in making preoperative decisions: a rational approach to lymph node dissection in gastric cancer patients. Br J Surg 1989;76:905–8.

109. Katoh K, Hattori Y, Yokokura N, Suzuki H. Borrmann 3 type advanced gastric cancer followed up for 10 years and 6 months from the first histologically confirmed IIc lesion, report of a case. Stom Intest 1992;27:91–7.

110. Katoh M, Terada M. Oncogenes and tumor suppressor genes. In: Nishi M, Ichikawa H, Nakajima T, Maruyama K, Tahara E, eds. Gastric cancer. Tokyo: Springer-Verlag, 1993:196–208.

111. Kawai K, Nakagome A, Mochizuki H, Takasou K, et al. Type I early gastric carcinoma developing from a lesion followed up as adenoma. Report of a case. Stom Intest 1992;27:83–90.

112. Kazzaz BA, Eulderink F. Paneth cell-rich carcinoma of the stomach. Histopathology 1989;15:303–5.

113. Keller E, Stutzer H, Heitmann K, Bauer P, Gebbensleben B, Rohde H. Lymph node staging in 872 patients with carcinoma of the stomach and the presumed benefit of lymphadenectomy. German Stomach Cancer TNM Study Group. J Am Coll Surg 1994;178:38–46.

114. Kennedy BJ. The unified international gastric cancer staging classification system. Scand J Gastroenterol 1987;22:11–3.

115. Kidokoro T. Frequency of resection, metastasis, and five year survival rate of early gastric carcinoma in a surgical clinic. In: Murakami T, ed. Early gastric cancer. Gann Monogr Cancer Res no. 11. Tokyo: University of Tokyo, 1971:11:45–9.

116. Kihana T, Tsuda H, Hirota T, et al. Point mutation of c-Ki-*ras* oncogene in gastric adenoma and adenocarcinoma with tubular differentiation. Jpn J Cancer Res 1991;82:308–14.

117. Kim JP, Jung SE. Patients with gastric cancer and their prognosis in accordance with number of lymph node metastases. Scand J Gastroenterol 1987;22:33–5.

118. Kim JP, Yang HK, Oh ST. Is the new UICC staging system of gastric cancer reasonable? (Comparison of 5-year survival rate of gastric cancer by old and new UICC stage classification). Surg Oncol 1992;1:209–13.

119. Kobayashi S, Kusagai T, Yomazaki H. Endoscopic differentiation of early gastric cancer from benign peptic ulcer. Gastrointest Endosc 1979;25:55–7.

120. Kodama Y, Inokuchi K, Soejima K, Matsusaka T, Okamura T. Growth patterns and prognosis in early gastric carcinoma. Superficially spreading and penetrating growth types. Cancer 1983;51:320–6.

121. Kojima O, Ikeda E, Uehara Y, Majima T, Fujita Y, Majima S. Correlation between carcinoembryonic antigen in gastric cancer tissue and survival of patients with gastric cancer. Jpn J Cancer Res 1984;75:230–6.

122. Korenaga D, Okamura T, Saito A, Baba H, Sugimach K. DNA ploidy is closely linked to tumor invasion, lymph node metastasis, and prognosis in clinical gastric cancer. Cancer 1988;62:309–13.

123. Kraus B, Cain H. Is there a carcinoma in situ of the gastric mucosa? Pathol Res Pract 1979;164:342–55.

124. Kremer B, Henne-Bruns D, Weh HJ, Effenberger T. Advanced gastric cancer: a new combined surgical and oncological approach. Hepatogastroenterology 1989;36:23–6.

125. Lansdown M, Quirke P, Dixon M, et al. High-grade dysplasia of the gastric mucosa: a marker for gastric carcinoma. Gut 1990;31:977–83.

126. Larsen B, Tarp U, Kristensen E. Familial giant hypertrophic gastritis (Menetrier's disease). Gut 1987;25:1517–21.

127. Lauren P. The two histological main types of gastric carcinoma: diffuse and so-called intestinal-type carcinoma. An attempt at a histo-clinical classification. Acta Pathol Microbiol Scand 1965;64:31–49.

128. Lauren P, Nevalainen TJ. Epidemiology of intestinal and diffuse type of gastric carcinoma. A time-trend study in Finland with comparison between studies from high and low-risk areas. Cancer 1993;71:2926–33.

129. Laxen F, Sipponen P, Ihamaki T, Hakkiluoto A, Dortscheva Z. Gastric polyps: their morphological and endoscopical characteristics and relation to gastric carcinoma. Acta Path Microbiol Immunol Scand [A] 1982;90:221–8.

130. Lehnert T, Erlandson RA, Decosse JJ. Lymph and blood capillaries of the human gastric mucosa. A morphologic basis of metastases in early gastric carcinoma. Gastroenterology 1985;89:939–50.

131. Lertprasertsuke N, Tsutsumi Y. Gastric carcinoma with lymphoid stroma. Analysis using mucin histochemistry and immunohistochemistry. Virchows Arch [A] 1989;414:231–41.

132. Lev R, Siegel HI, Jerzy-Glass GB. The enzyme histochemistry of gastric carcinoma in man. Cancer 1969;23:1086–93.

133. Lewin KJ, Riddell RH, Weinstein WM. Dialogue, handling of biopsies and resected specimens. In: Lewin KJ, Riddell RH, Weinstein WM, eds. Gastrointestinal pathology and its clinical implications. New York: Igaku-Shoin, 1992:3–30.

134. Lewin KJ, Riddell RH, Weinstein WM. Immunodeficiency disorders. In: Lewin KJ, Riddell RH, Weinstein WM, eds. Gastointestinal pathology and its clinical implications. New York: Igaku-Shoin, 1992:104–50.

134a. Livingstone JI, Yasui W, Tahara E, Wastell C. Are Japanese and European gastric cancer the same biological entity? An immunohistochemical study. Br J Cancer 1995;72:976–80.

135. Mai M, Mibayashi Y, Okumura Y, Takahashi Y. The natural history of gastric carcinoma viewed from prospective or retrospective follow-up studies—in relation to histological type and growth patterns. Stom Intest 1991;27:39–50.

136. Majima S, Yamaguchi I, Yoshida K, Karube J, Teshima T. Duodenal extension of carcinoma of the stomach. Tohoku J Exp Med 1964;83:159–67.

137. Majmudar B, Dillard R, Susann PW. Collision carcinoma of the gastric cardia. Hum Pathol 1978;9:471–3.

138. Martin IG, Dixon MF, Sue-Ling H, Axon AT, Johnston D. Goseki histological grading of gastric cancer is an important predictor of outcome. Gut 1994;35:758–63.

139. Maruyama K. Results of surgery correlated with staging. In: Preece PE, Cuschieri A, Wellwood JM, eds. Cancer of the stomach. London: Grune and Stratton, 1986:145–63.

140. Maruyama K. The most important prognostic factors for gastric cancer patients: a study using univariate and multivariate analyses. Scand J Gastroenterol 1987;22 (Suppl 133):63–8.

141. Maruyama K, Gunven P, Okabayashi K, Sasako M, Kinoshita T. Lymph node metastases of gastric cancer: growth pattern in 1931 patients. Ann Surg 1989;210:596–602.

142. Maruyama K, Okabayashi K, Kinoshita T. Progress in gastric cancer surgery in Japan and its limits of radicality. World J Surg 1987;11:418–25.

143. Maruyama K, Sasako M, Kinoshita T, Okajima K. Effectiveness of systematic lymph node dissection in gastric cancer surgery. In: Nishi M, Ichikawa H, Nakajima T, Maruyama K, Tahara E, eds. Gastric cancer. Tokyo: Springer-Verlag, 1993:293–305.

144. Matsukura N, Suzuki K, Kawachi T, et al. Distribution of marker enzymes and mucin in intestinal metaplasia in human stomach and relation of complete and incomplete types of intestinal metaplasia to minute gastric carcinomas. JNCI 1980;65:231–40.

145. Matsusaka T, Kodama Y, Soejima K, et al. Recurrence in early gastric cancer: a pathologic evaluation. Cancer 1980;46:168–72.

146. Meister H, Holubarsch CH, Haferkamp O, Schlag P, Herfarth C. Gastritis, intestinal metaplasia and dysplasia versus benign ulcer in stomach and duodenum and gastric carcinoma: a histographical study. Pathol Res Pract 1979;164:259–69.

147. Menucle LS, Amber JR. Metastatic disease involving the stomach. Am J Dig Dis 1975;20:903–13.

148. Meyers WC, Damiano RJ Jr, Rotolo FS, Postlethwait RW. Adenocarcinoma of the stomach. Changing patterns over the last 4 decades. Ann Surg 1987;205:1–8.

149. Miller TA. Cancer of the stomach in the United States: some progress but mainly bad news. Gastroenterology 1994;107:314–6.

150. Min KW, Holmquist S, Peiper SC, O'Leary TJ. Poorly diffentiated adenocarcinoma with lymphoid stroma (lymphoepithelioma-like carcinomas) of the stomach. Report of three cases with Epstein-Barr virus genome demonstrated by the polymerase chain reaction. Am J Clin Pathol 1991;96:219–27.

151. Ming PL. Genetic and cytogenetic aspects. In: Ming SC, Goldman H, eds. Pathology of the gastrointestinal tract. Philadelphia: WB Saunders, 1992:81–97.

152. Ming SC. Gastric carcinoma. A pathobiological classification. Cancer 1977;39:2475–85.

153. Ming SC. Pathologic features and significance of gastric dysplasia. In: Ming SC, ed. Precursors of gastric cancer. New York: Praeger, 1984:9–27.

154. Ming SC. Significance of epithelial dysplasia in the esophagus and stomach. Endoscopy 1989;21:385–95.

155. Ming SC. Epithelial polyps of the stomach. In: Ming SC, Goldman H, eds. Pathology of the gastrointestinal tract. Philadelphia: WB Saunders, 1992:547–69.

156. Ming SC, Bajtai A, Correa P, et al. Gastric dysplasia: significance and pathologic criteria. Cancer 1984; 54:1794–801.

157. Miwa K. Evaluation of the TMN classification of stomach cancer and proposal for its rational stage grouping. Jpn J Clin Oncol 1984;14:385–410.

158. Mochizuki T. Method for histopathological examination of early gastric cancer. In: Murakami T, ed. Early gastric cancer. Gann Monogr Cancer Res, no 11. Tokyo: University of Tokyo Press, 1971:57–65.

159. Monufo WW Jr, Krause GL, Medina JG. Carcinoma of the stomach: morphological characteristics affecting survival. Arch Surg 1962;85:754–63.

160. Mori M, Ambe K, Adachi Y, et al. Prognostic value of immunohistochemically identified CEA, SC, AFP, and S-100 protein-positive cells in gastric carcinoma. Cancer 1988;62:534–40.

161. Mori M, Sugimachi K. Clinicopathologic studies of gastric carcinoma. Semin Surg Oncol 1990;6:19–27.

162. Morishita Y, Tanaka T, Kato K, et al. Gastric collision tumor (carcinoid and adenocarcinoma) with gastritis cystica profunda. Arch Pathol Lab Med 1991;115:1006–10.

163. Morson BC, Jass JR, Sobin LH. Precancerous lesions of the gastrointestinal tract. London: Bailliere Tindall, 1985.

164. Morson BC, Sobin LH, Grundmann E, Johansen A, Nagayo T, Serck-Hanssen A. Precancerous conditions and epithelial dysplasia in the stomach. J Clin Pathol 1980;33:711–21.

165. Murakami T. Early cancer of the stomach. World J Surg 1979;3:685–92.

166. Murakami T. Pathomorphological diagnosis. Definition and gross classification of early gastric cancer. In: Murakami T, ed. Early gastric cancer. Gann Monogr Cancer Res, no 11. Tokyo: University of Tokyo Press, 1971:53–5.

167. Murayama H, Imai T, Kikuchi M. Solid carcinomas of the stomach. A combined histochemical, light and electron microscopic study. Cancer 1983;51:1673–81.

168. Murayama H, Kamio A, Imai T, Kikuchi M. Gastric carcinoma with psammomatous calcification: report of a case, with reference to calculogenesis. Cancer 1982;49:788–96.

169. Nagai E, Ueyama T, Yao T, Tsuneyoshi M. Hepatoid adenocarcinoma of the stomach. A clinicopathologic and immunohistochemical analysis. Cancer 1993; 72:1827–35.

170. Nagayo T. Precursors of human gastric cancer: their frequencies and histological characteristics. In: Farber EE, ed. Pathophysiology of carcinogenesis in digestive organs. Baltimore: University Park Press, 1977:151–60.

171. Nagayo T. Histogenesis and precursors of human gastric cancer. Berlin: Springer-Verlag, 1986.

172. Nagayo T. Histopathology of gastric dysplasia. In: Filipe MI, Jass JR, eds. Gastric carcinoma. Edinburgh: Churchill Livingstone, 1986:116–31.

173. Nakamura K, Sugano H. Microcarcinoma of the stomach measuring less than 5 mm in the largest diameter and its histogenesis. Prog Clin Biol Res 1983;132D:107–16.

174. Nakamura T. Pathohistologische Einteilung der Magenpolypen mit spezifischer Betrachtung ihrer malignen Entartung. Chirurgie 1970;41:122–30.

175. Nakano K, Honda I, Majima H, Fujimoto S. A case of calcifying carcinoma of the stomach with long-term postoperative survival. Jpn J Surg 1991;21:335–40.

176. Nakano M, Matsusaki O, Fujimoto M, Matsushita T, Ohnishi T. Borrmann 2 type gastric carcinoma, resected 6 years and 2 months after the detection of cancer cells by biopsy, report of a case. Stom Intest 1992;27:77–82.

177. Nanus DM, Kelsen DP, Mentle IR, Altorki N, Albino AP. Infrequent point mutations of ras oncogenes in gastric cancers. Gastroenterology 1990;98:955–60.

178. Neuman WL, Wasylyshyn ML, Jacoby R, et al. Evidence for a common molecular pathogenesis in colorectal, gastric, and pancreatic cancer. Genes Chromosom Cancer 1991;3:468–73.

179. Nihei K, Terashima K, Avyama K, Imai Y, Sato H. Benign histiocytosis X of stomach. Previously undescribed lesion. Acta Pathol Jpn 1983; 33:577–88.

180. Nishi M, Nakajima T, Kajitani T. The Japanese Research Society for Gastric Cancer—the general rules for the gastric cancer study and an analysis of treatment results based on the rules. In: Preece PE, Cuschieri A, Wellwood JM, eds. Cancer of the stomach. London: Grune and Stratton, 1986:107–21.

181. Nishizawa M, Nomoto K, Ueno M, et al. Natural history of gastric cancer in a fixed population with emphasis on depressed submucosal cancer. Stom Intest 1992;27:16–24.

182. Nomura A, Stemmermann GN, Chyou PH, Kato I, Perez-Perez GI, Blaser MJ. Helicobacter pylori infection and gastric carcinoma among Japanese Americans in Hawaii. N Engl J Med 1991;325:1132–6.

183. Oda N, Tahara E, Taniyama K. Cytophotometric analysis on nuclear DNA contents of human scirrhous gastric carcinoma. Pathol Res Pract 1989;184:390–401.

184. Oehlert W. Preneoplastic lesions of the stomach. In: Ming SC, ed. Precursors of gastric cancer. New York: Praeger, 1984:73–82.

185. Oehlert W, Keller P, Henke M, Strauch M. Gastric mucosal dysplasia: what is its clinical significance? Front Gastrointest Res 1979;4:173–82.

186. Ogawa H, Kato I, Tominaga S. Family history of cancer among cancer patients. Jpn J Cancer Res 1985;76:113–8.

187. Oguro Y. Endoscopic treatment of early gastric cancer. Dig Endosc 1991;3:3–15.

188. Ohman U, Wetterfors J, Moberg A. Histologic grading of gastric cancer. Acta Chir Scand 1972;138:384–90.

189. Okabe H. Growth of early gastric cancer. Clinical study of growth and invasion patterns of early gastric cancer. Its position in the natural history of gastric cancer. In: Murakami T, ed. Early gastric cancer. Gann Monogr Cancer Res, no 11. Tokyo: University of Tokyo Press, 1971;11:67–79.

190. Okamura T, Korenaga D, Haraguchi M, et al. Growth mode and DNA ploidy in mucosal carcinomas of the stomach. Cancer 1987;59:1154–60.

191. Ooi A, Nakanishi I, Itoh T, Ueda H, Mai M. Predominant Paneth cell differentiation in an intestinal type gastric cancer. Pathol Res Pract 1991;187:220–5.

192. Pagnini CA, Rugge M. Advanced gastric carcinoma and prognosis. Virchows Arch [A] 1985;406:213–21.

193. Parsonnet J, Friedman GD, Vandersteen DP, et al. Helicobacter pylori infection and the risk of gastric carcinoma. N Engl J Med 1991;325:1127–31.

194. Penn I. Occurrence of cancer in immune deficiencies. Cancer 1974;34:858–66.

195. Planteydt HT, Willighagen RG. Enzyme histochemistry of gastric carcinoma. J Pathol Bacteriol 1965;90:393–8.

196. Priestman TJ. Adjuvant chemotherapy. In: Preece PE, Cuschieri A, Wellwood JM, eds. Cancer of the stomach. London: Grune and Stratton, 1986:231–42.

197. Qizilbash AH, Castelli M, Kowalski MA, Churly A. Endoscopic brush cytology and biopsy in the diagnosis of cancer of the upper gastrointestinal tract. Acta Cytol 1980;24:313–8.

198. Reid BJ, Haggitt RC, Rubin CE, et al. Observer variation in the diagnosis of dysplasia in Barrett esophagus. Hum Pathol 1988;19:166–78.

199. Ribeiro MM, Sarmento JA, Simoes S, Bastos J. Prognostic significance of Lauren and Ming classifications and other pathologic parameters in gastric carcinoma. Cancer 1981;47:780–4.

200. Riddell RH, Goldman H, Ransohoff DF, et al. Dysplasia in inflammatory bowel disease: standardized classification with provisional clinical applications. Hum Pathol 1983;14:931–68.

201. Ringertz N. The pathology of gastric carcinoma. Natl Cancer Inst Monogr 1967;25:275–85.

202. Robey-Cafferty SS, Ro JY, McKee EG. Gastric parietal cell carcinoma with an unusual, lymphoma-like histologic appearance: report of a case. Mod Pathol 1989;2:536–40.

203. Rollag A, Jacobsen CD. Gastric ulcer and risk of cancer. A five year follow-up study. Acta Med Scand 1984;216:105–9.

204. Rothery GA, Day DW. Intestinal metaplasia in endoscopic biopsy specimens of gastric mucosa. J Clin Pathol 1985;38:613–21.

205. Ruck P, Wehrmann M, Campbell M, Horny HP, Breucha G, Kaiserling E. Squamous cell carcinoma of the gastric stump. A case report and review of the literature. Am J Surg Pathol 1989;13:317–24.

206. Rugge M, Farinati F, Baffa R, et al. Gastric epithelial dysplasia in the natural history of gastric cancer: a multicenter prospective follow-up study. Interdisciplinary Group on Gastric Epithelial Dysplasia. Gastroenterology 1994;107:1288–96.

207. Saito K, Shimoda T. The histogenesis and early invasion of gastric cancer. Acta Pathol Jpn 1986;36:1307–18.

208. Sakinta T, Ogura Y, Takusu S, Fukutomi H, Miwa T, Yoshimori M. Observations on the healing of ulcerations in early gastric cancer. The life cycle of the malignant ulcer. Gastroenterology 1971;60:835–44.

209. Sakita T, Yoshimori M. Early diagnosis of gastric cancer. In: Hirayama R, ed. Cancer in Asia. Gann Monogr Cancer Res, no 18. Baltimore: University Park Press 1976:85–93.

210. Sano R. Pathological analysis of 300 cases of early gastric cancer with special reference to cancer associated with ulcer. Jpn J Cancer Res 1971;11:81–9.

211. Saraga EP, Gardiol D, Costa J. Gastric dysplasia: a histologic follow-up study. Am J Surg Pathol 1987;11:788–96.

212. Sasaki K, Takahashi M, Hashimoto T, Kawachnino K. Flow cytometric DNA measurement of gastric cancers: clinico-pathological implication of DNA ploidy. Pathol Res Pract 1989;184:561–6.

213. Sasako M, Kinoshita T, Maruyama K, et al. Local excision for early gastric cancers. Japanese Gastrointestinal Surgical Association 1990;23:2191–5.

214. Sasano N, Nakamura K, Arai M, Akazaki K. Ultrastructural cell patterns in human gastric carcinoma compared with nonneoplastic gastric mucosa—histogenetic analysis of carcinoma by mucin histochemistry. JNCI 1969;43:783–802.

215. Schafer LW, Larson DE, Melton LJ III, Higgins JA, Ilstrup DM. The risk of gastric carcinoma after surgical treatment for benign ulcer disease. A population-based study in Olmsted County, Minnesota. N Engl J Med 1983;309:1210–3.

216. Scharschmidt BF. The natural history of hypertrophic gastropathy (Menetrier's disease). Report of a case with 16 year follow-up and review of 120 cases from the literature. Am J Med 1977;63:644–52.

217. Schlag P, Bockler R, Peter M. Nitrite and nitrosamines in gastric juice: risk factors for gastric cancer? Scand J Gastroenterol 1982;17:145–50.

218. Schmitz-Moormann NP, Pohl C, Huttich C, Himmelman GW. Prediction of prognosis in patients with gastric cancer by quantitative morphology and multivariate analysis. Scand J Gastroenterol 1987;22:58–62.

219. Schrumpf E, Serck-Hanssen A, Stradaas J, Aune S, Myren J, Osnes M. Mucosal changes in the gastric stump 20-25 years after partial gastrectomy. Lancet 1977;2:467–9.

220. Scott N, Quirke P, Dixon MF. ACP Broadsheet 130: November 1992. Gross examination of the stomach. J Clin Pathol 1992;45:952–5.

221. Serck-Hanssen A, Osnes M, Myren J. Epithelial dysplasia in the stomach: the size of the problem and some preliminary results of a follow-up study. In: Ming SC, ed. Precursors of gastric cancer. New York: Praeger, 1984:53–71.

222. Shennib H, Lough J, Klein HW, Hampson LG. Gastric carcinoma: intestinal metaplasia and tumor growth patterns as indicators of prognosis. Surgery 1986;100:774–80.

223. Shibata D, Tokunaga M, Uemura Y, Sato E, Tanaka S, Weiss LM. Association of Epstein-Barr virus with undifferentiated gastric carcinomas with intense lymph infiltration. Lymphoepithelioma-like carcinoma. Am J Pathol 1991;139:469–74.

224. Shibata D, Weiss LM. Epstein-Barr virus-associated gastric adenocarcinoma. Am J Pathol 1992;140:769–74.

225. Siewert JR, Bottcher K, Roder JD, Busch R, Hermanek P, Meyer HJ. Prognostic relevance of systematic lymph node dissection in gastric carcinoma. German Gastric Carcinoma Study Group. Br J Surg 1993;80:1015–8.

226. Silverberg E, Boring CC, Squires TS. Cancer statistics. CA Cancer J Clin 1990;40:9–26.

227. Sipponen P. Gastric dysplasia. Curr Top Pathol 1990;81:61–76.

228. Sipponen P. Helicobacter pylori infection—a common worldwide environmental risk factor for gastric cancer? [Editorial] Endoscopy 1992;24:424–7.

229. Sipponen P. Long-term evaluation of Helicobacter pylori-associated chronic gastritis. Eur J Gastroenterol Hepatol 1993;5(Suppl 1):93–7.

230. Sipponen P, Kosunen TU, Valle J, Riihela M, Seppala K. Helicobacter pylori infection and chronic gastritis in gastric cancer. J Clin Pathol 1992;45:319–23.

231. Siurala M. Gastritis, its fate and sequelae. Ann Clin Res 1981;13:111–3.

232. Sjostedt S, Pieper R. Gastic cancer: factors influencing long term survival and postoperative mortality. Acta Chir Scand Suppl 1986;530:25–9.

233. Smith MJ, Kini SR, Watson E. Fine needle aspiration and endoscopic brush cytology: comparison of direct smears and rinsings. Acta Cytol 1980;24:456–9.

234. Sowa M, Yoshino H, Kano K, Nishimura M, Kamino K, Umeyama K. An analysis of the DNA ploidy patterns of gastric cancer. Cancer 1988;62:1325–30.

235. Stael von Holstein C, Hammar E, Eriksson S, Huldt B. Clinical significance of dysplasia in gastric remnant biopsy specimens. Cancer 1993;72:1532–5.

236. Stemmermann GN. Comparative study of histochemical patterns in non-neoplastic and neoplastic gastric epithelium. A study of Japanese in Hawaii. JNCI 1967;39:375–83.

236a. Stemmermann GN. Intestinal metaplasia of the stomach. A status report. Cancer 1994;74:556–64.

237. Stemmermann GN, Brown C. A survival study of intestinal diffuse types of gastric cancer. Cancer 1974;33:1190–5.

238. Stemmermann GN, Mower H. Gastritis, nitrosamines and gastric cancer. J Clin Gastroenterol 1981;3:23–7.

239. Sue-Ling HM, Martin I, Griffith J, et al. Early gastric cancer: 46 cases treated in one surgical department. Gut 1992;33:1318–22.

240. Sugano H, Nakamura K, Takagi K. An atypical epithelium of the stomach: a clinicopathological entity. Gann Monogr Cancer Res 1971;11:257–69.

241. Sugihara H, Hattori T, Fugita S, Hirose K, Fukuda M. Regional ploidy variations in signet ring cell carcinomas of the stomach. Cancer 1990;68:122–9.

242. Tada M, Karita M, Yanai H, Kawano H, Takemoto T. Evaluation of endoscopic strip biopsy therapeutically used for early gastric cancer. Stom Intest 1988;23:371–85.

243. Tahara E. Growth factors and oncogenes in human gastrointestinal carcinomas. J Cancer Res Clin Oncol 1990;116:121–31.

244. Tahara E, Sumiyoshi H, Hata J, et al. Human epidermal growth factor in gastric carcinoma as a biologic marker of high malignancy. Jpn J Cancer Res 1986;77:145–52.

245. Tahara E, Yasui W, Taniyama K, et al. Ha-ras oncogene product in human gastric carcinoma: correlation with invasiveness, metastasis or prognosis. Jpn J Cancer Res 1986;77:517–22.

246. Takekoshi T, Fujii A, Takagi K, Baba Y, Kato Y, Yanagisawa A. The indication for endoscopic double snare polypectomy of gastric lesions. Stom Intest 1988;23:386–98.

247. Talbot IC. Pathology and natural history of gastric carcinoma. In: Preece PE, Cuschieri A, Wellwood JM, eds. Cancer of the stomach. London: Grune and Stratton, 1986:73–87.

248. Talley NJ, Zinsmeister AR, Weaver A, et al. Gastric adenocarcinoma and Helicobacter pylori infection. JNCI 1991;83:1734–9.

249. Teglbjaerg PS, Nielsen HO. Small intestinal type and colonic type intestinal metaplasia of the human stomach and their relationship to the histogenetic types of gastric adenocarcinoma. Acta Pathol Microbiol Scand 1978;86A:351–5.

250. Timothy AR. Radiotherapy in gastric cancer. In: Preece PE, Cuschieri A, Wellwood JM, eds. Cancer of the stomach. London: Grune and Stratton, 1986:249–60.

251. Tsukuma H, Mishima T, Oshima A. Prospective study of early gastric cancer. Int J Cancer 1983;31:421–6.

252. Ueyama T, Nagai E, Yao T, Tsuneyoshi M. Vimentin-positive gastric carcinomas with rhabdoid features. A clinicopatholoic and immunohistochemical study. Am J Surg Pathol 1993;17:813–9.

253. Ulich TR, Kollin M, Lewin KJ. Composite gastric carcinoma. Report of a tumor of the carcinoma-carcinoid spectrum. Arch Pathol Lab Med 1988;112:91–3.

254. Viste A, Bjornestad E, Opheim P, et al. Risk of carcinoma following gastric operations for benign disease. A historical cohort study of 3470 patients. Lancet 1986;2:502–5.

255. Votte A, Sevestre H, Dupas JL, et al. Hepatoid adenocarcinoma of the stomach. Gastroenterol Clin Biol 1991;15:437–40.

256. Waldum HL, Haugen OA, Isaksen C, Mecsei R, Sardvik AK. Enterochromaffin-like tumor cells in the diffuse but not the intestinal type of gastric carcinomas. Scand J Gastroenterol Suppl 1991;180:165–9.

257. Wanebo HJ, Kennedy BJ, Chmiel J, Steele G Jr, Winchester D, Osteen R. Cancer of the stomach. A patient care study by the American College of Surgeons. Ann Surg 1993;218:583–92.

258. Watanabe H, Enjoji M, Imai T. Gastric carcinoma with lymphoid stroma: its morphologic characteristics and prognostic correlations. Cancer 1976;38:232–43.

259. Watanabe H, Jass JR, Sobin LH. Histological typing of oesophageal and gastric tumours. Berlin: Springer-Verlag, 1990.

260. Weisburger JH, Marquardt H, Mower HF, Hirota N, Mori H, Williams G. Inhibition of carcinogenesis; vitamin C and the prevention of gastric cancer. Prev Med 1980; 9:352–61.

261. Weiss LM, Gaffey MJ, Shibata D. Lymphoepithelioma-like carcinoma and its relationship to Epstein-Barr virus [Editorial]. Am J Clin Pathol 1991;96:156–8.

262. Wilke H, Preusser P, Fink U, et al. New developments in the treatment of gastric carcinoma. Semin Oncol 1990;17 (Suppl 2):61–70.

263. Wood GM, Bates C, Brown RC, et al. Intramucosal carcinoma of the gastric antrum complicating Menetrier's disease. J Clin Pathol 1983;36:1071–5.

264. Wright PA, Quirke P, Attanoos R, Williams GT. Molecular pathology of gastric carcinoma: progress and prospects. Hum Pathol 1992;23:848–59.

265. Xu ZC. Value of gastroscopy in postoperative patients with gastric cancer. Chung Hua Chung Liu Tsa Chih 1991;13:43–5.

266. Yamamoto T, Yasui W, Ochiai A. Immunohistochemical detection of c-myc oncogene product in human gastric carcinomas: expression in tumor cells and stromal cells. Jpn J Cancer Res 1987;78:1169–74.

266a. Yamao T, Shirao K, Ono H, et al. Risk factors for lymph node metastasis from intramucosal gastric carcinoma. Cancer 1996;77:602–6.

267. Yap P, Pantangco E, Yap A, Yap R. Surgical management of gastric carcinoma. Folllow-up results in 465 consecutive cases. Am J Surg 1982;143:284–7.

268. Yonemura Y, Ooyama S, Sugiyama K, et al. Retrospective analysis of the prognostic significance of DNA ploidy patterns and S-phase fraction in gastric carcinoma. Cancer Res 1990;50:509–14.

269. Yonemura Y, Sugiyama K, Fujimura T, et al. Correlation of DNA ploidy and proliferative activity in human gastric cancer. Cancer 1988;62:1497–502.

269a. Yoshikawa K, Maruyama K. Characteristics of gastric cancer invading to the propria muscle layer—with spacial reference to mortality and cause of death. Jpn J Clin Oncol 1985;15:499–503.

269b. Zamboni G, Franzin G, Scarpa A, et al. Carcinoma-like signet-ring cells in gastric mucosa associated lymphoid tissue (MALT) lymphoma. Am J Surg Path 1996;588–98.

270. Zhang Y. Epithelial dysplasia of the somach and its relationship with gastric cancer. In: Ming SC, ed. Precursors of gastric cancer. New York: Praeger, 1984:41–52.

### Adenocarcinoma of the Gastric Cardia and Proximal Stomach

271. Aikou T, Shimazu H. Difference in main lymphatic pathways from the lower esophagus and gastric cardia. Jpn J Surg 1989;19:290–5.

272. Kalish RJ, Clancy PE, Orringer MB, Appelman HD. Clinical, epidemiologic, and morphologic comparison between adenocarcinomas arising in Barrett's esophageal mucosa and in the gastric cardia. Gastroenterology 1984;6:461–7.

273. Kumagai K, Yasui A, Nishida Y, et al. Prognosis of gastric carcinoma sited in the cardiac part determined by the type of esophageal invasion. Gan No Rinsho 1990;36:1979–84.

274. Li L, Pan GL. Pathology of carcinoma of the gastric cardia. In: Huang GJ, Wu YK, eds. Carcinoma of the esophagus and gastric cardia. Berlin: Springer-Verlag, 1984:117–54.

275. MacDonald WC. Clinical and pathologic features of adenocarcinoma of the gastric cardia. Cancer 1972;29:724–32.

276. MacDonald WC, MacDonald JB. Adenocarcinoma of the esophagus and/or gastric cardia. Cancer 1987;60:1094–8.

277. Maehara Y, Moriguchi S, Kakeji Y, et al. Prognostic factors in adenocarcinoma in the upper one-third of the stomach. Surg Gynecol Obstet 1991;173:223–6.

278. Misumi A, Murakami A, Harada K, Baba K, Akagi M. Definition of carcinoma of the gastric cardia. Langenbecks Arch Chir 1989;374:221–6.

279. Mori M, Kitagawa S, Iida M, et al. Early carcinoma of the gastric cardia. A clinicopathologic study of 21 cases. Cancer 1987;59:1758–66.

280. Nishimata H, Setoyama S, Nishimata Y, et al. Natural history of gastric cancer in cardia. Stom Intest 1992;27:25–38.

281. Okamura T, Tsujitani S, Marin P, et al. Adenocarcinoma in the upper third part of the stomach. Surg Gynecol Obstet 1987;165:247–50.

282. Sons HU, Borchard F. Cancer of the distal esophagus and cardia. Incidence, tumorous infiltration and metastatic spread. Ann Surg 1986;203:188–95.

283. Tang GX, Wang ZS, Liu DG, Liu SS. Gastroesophageal anastomotic leakage following resection of carcinoma of the esophagus and gastric cardia: analysis of ten cases. J Surg Oncol 1990;43:50–2.

284. Wang HH, Antonioli DA, Goldman H. Comparative features of esophageal and gastric adenocarcinomas: recent changes in type and frequency. Hum Pathol 1986;17:482–7.

### Other Carcinomas

285. Aoki Y, Tabuse K, Wada M, Katsumi M, Uda H. Primary adenosquamous carcinoma of the stomach: experience of 11 cases and its clinical analysis. Gastroenterol Jpn 1978;13:140–5.

286. Bonnheim DC, Sarac OK, Fett W. Primary squamous cell carinoma of the stomach. Am J Gastroenterol 1985;80:91–4.

287. Chejfec G, Gould VE. Malignant gastric neuroendocrinomas. Ultrastructural and biochemical characterization of their secretory activity. Hum Pathol 1977;8:433–40.

288. Donald KL. Adenocarcinoma of the pyloric antrum with extensive squamous differentiation. J Clin Pathol 1967;20:136–8.

289. Eimoto T, Hayakawa H. Oat cell carcinoma of the stomach. Pathol Res Pract 1980;168:229–36.

290. French WE, Affolter H, Hurteau WW. Squamous cell carcinoma of the pylorus with diffuse metaplastic gastritis. Arch Surg 1957;74:322–6.

291. Fukuda T, Ohnishi Y, Nishimaki T, Ohtani H, Tachikawa S. Early gastric cancer of the small cell type. Am J Gastroenterol 1988;83:1176–9.

292. Garcia RL, Ghali VS. Gastric choriocarcinoma and yolk sac tumor in a man: observations about its possible origin. Hum Pathol 1985;16:955–8.

293. Guillou L, Nordback P, Gerber C, Schneider RP. Ductal adenocarcinoma arising in a heterotopic pancreas situated in a hiatal hernia. Arch Pathol Lab Med 1994;118:568–71.

293a. Herold G, Kraft K. Adenocarcinoma arising from ectopic gastric pancreas: two case reports with a review of the literature. Z Gastroenterol 1995;33:260–4.

294. Hussein AM, Otrakji CL, Hussein BT. Small cell carcinoma of the stomach. Case report and review of the literature. Dig Dis Sci 1990;35:513–8.

295. Krulewski T, Cohen LB. Choriocarcinoma of the stomach: pathogenesis and clinical characteristics. Dig Dis Sci 1988;83:1172–5.

296. Matsui K, Kitagawa M, Miwa A, Kuroda Y, Tsuji M. Small cell carcinoma of the stomach: a clinicopathologic study of 17 cases. Am J Gastroenterol 1991;86:1167–74.

297. Mori H, Soeda O, Kamano T, et al. Choriocarcinomatous change with immunocytochemically HCG-postive cells in the gastric carcinoma of the males. Virchows Arch [A] 1982;396:141–53.

298. Mori M, Iwashita A, Enjoji M. Adenosquamous carcinoma of the stomach. A clinicopathologic analysis of 28 cases. Cancer 1986;57:333–9.

299. Mori M, Fukuda T, Enjoji M. Adenosquamous carcinoma of the stomach. Histogenetic and ultrastructural studies. Gastroenterology 1987;92:1078–82.

300. Mori M, Iwashita A, Enjoji M. Squamous cell carcinoma of the stomach: report of three cases. Am J Gastroenterol 1986;81:339–42.

301. Ozaki H, Ito I, Sanao R, Hirota T, Shimosato Y. A case of choriocarcinoma of the stomach. Jpn J Clin Oncol 1971;1:83–94.

302. Ramponi A, Angeli G, Arceci F, Pozzuoli R. Gastric choriocarcinoma: an immunohistochemical study. Pathol Res Pract 1986;181:390–6.

303. Regan JF, Cremin JH. Chorioepithelioma of the stomach. Am J Surg 1960;100:224–33.

304. Saigo PE, Brigati DJ, Sternberg SS, Rosen PP, Turnbull AD. Primary gastric choriocarcinoma. An immunohistological study. Am J Surg Pathol 1981;5:333–42.

305. Unakami M, Hirota T, Itabashi M, et al. Three cases of choriocarcinoma of the stomach. Jpn J Cancer Clin 1982;28:204–10.

306. Won OH, Farman J, Krishnan MN, Iyer SK, Vulletin JC. Squamous cell carcinoma of the stomach. Am J Gastroenterol 1978;69:594–8.

❖❖❖

# 12

# ENDOCRINE CELL PROLIFERATIONS OF THE STOMACH

Endocrine cells are widely distributed throughout the entire length of the gastrointestinal tract, interspersed between other epithelial cells. They outnumber cells produced by any endocrine organ. As is true for endocrine organs, gastrointestinal endocrine cells can undergo hyperplasia and neoplasia (15,28,29,31,43,48,49, 56,59,63,70,71,73,79,92). However, in the gastrointestinal tract, there is a spectrum of epithelial proliferation ranging from pure endocrine cells to endocrine cells admixed with other epithelial cells to pure glandular epithelium (Table 12-1).

This chapter focuses on gastric endocrine cell proliferations. However, a brief discussion of the gastrointestinal endocrine system, of which the stomach is an integral part, is presented first.

## Normal Anatomy of the Gastric Endocrine Cells

There are many different types of endocrine cells in the gastrointestinal tract, most of which are restricted in distribution (22,48), but a few specific types, such as the serotonin-producing enterochromaffin cells (EC) and somatostatin D cells occur throughout the length of the stomach and intestines (Table 12-2). In the stomach, in addition to the EC and D cells, there are gastrin-producing G cells in the antrum and proximal duodenum and enterochromaffin-like cells (ECL) which produce histamine. There are several other cells, namely D1, P, and X cells, whose exact secretory products are as yet unclear.

The endocrine cells are wedged between the epithelial cells and basement membrane and, with the exception of the ECL cells, communicate with the glandular lumen by apical microvilli. The ECL cells function as autocrine cells, their secretions diffusing into the lamina propria, probably into the closely applied capillaries. In the gastric fundus and body the endocrine cells are found between the parietal and chief cells and in the antrum they occur primarily at the junction of the gastric pits and dhe pyloric glands (fig. 12-1). A few endocrine cells are also found in the lamina propria throughout the gastrointestinal tract (Table 12-3) (60,97) and in mucosa showing metaplastic change.

The many types of endocrine cells are characterized ultrastructurally by their dense core secretion granules. These are composed of a core of variable density, surrounded by a single limiting membrane, which is frequently separated from the core by a translucent halo (22,48). In the stomach, there is fairly good correlation between granule morphology and hormone product, in contrast to other parts of the gastrointestinal tract. In neoplasms there may be even greater heterogeneity of granules (22,48).

Two types of endocrine cells are stained by hematoxylin and eosin in routine sections; these can be difficult to visualize microscopically. The first type is the basigranulated cell, characterized by small eosinophilic granules beneath the nucleus; most of these are enterochromaffin cells. The second type is the so-called clear cell, which is typically round with a centrally located, vesicular nucleus surrounded by clear cytoplasm. Most of the other endocrine cells are this type; they are not easily detected in routine sections.

The most common methods for identifying gastric endocrine cells in routine sections are the

Table 12-1

## CLASSIFICATION OF GASTRIC ENDOCRINE CELL PROLIFERATIONS

Endocrine Cell Hyperplasia
  Primary
  Secondary to gastric disease

Carcinoid Tumors
  Carcinoid
  Poorly differentiated carcinoid
  Oat cell carcinoma

Mixed Endocrine and Nonendocrine
  Epithelial Tumors
  Carcinoma with interspersed endocrine cells
  Carcinoid with interspersed nonendocrine
    epithelial cells

Composite Glandular-Endocrine Cell Carcinoma

Collision Tumors

Amphicrine Tumors

Table 12-2

**GASTROINTESTINAL ENDOCRINE CELLS: CELL TYPE, DISTRIBUTION, AND LOCALIZATION**

| Cell Type | Location in GIT* | Silver Stains Argen | Silver Stains Argyro** | Secretory Products |
|---|---|---|---|---|
| G | Antrum, duodenum | - | + | Gastrin |
| ECL | Stomach | - | + | Histamine |
| D | Stomach, SI, and LI | - | - | Somatostatin |
| D1 | Stomach, SI, and LI | - | + | Unknown |
| EC | Stomach, SI, and LI | +++ | ++++ | Serotonin, motilin, substance P |
| P | Stomach, SI | - | + | ?GRP |
| X | Stomach | - | + | Unknown |
| I | Duodenum, jejunum | - | +/- | CCK |
| K | Duodenum, jejunum | - | +++ | GIP |
| M | Duodenum, jejunum | - | + | Motilin |
| S | Duodenum, jejunum | - | + | Secretin |
| PP | Duodenum | - | + | Pancreatic polypeptide |
| L | SI, LI | - | ++ | Enteroglucagon peptide YY |
| N | SI, LI | - | + | Neurotensin |

*GIT = gastrointestinal tract; SI = small intestine; LI = large intestine.
** Argen = argentaffin; argyro = argyrophil.

Table 12-3

**GASTROINTESTINAL ENDOCRINE CELLS: GRANULE MORPHOLOGY**

| Cell Type | Size (nm) | Shape | Electron Density | Limiting Membrane Close* | Limiting Membrane Halo |
|---|---|---|---|---|---|
| G | 180-300 | Round | Flocculent, highly variable density | + | |
| ECL | Variable | Round or oval | Dense eccentric core | | Wide |
| D | 300-400 | Round | Medium | | Narrow |
| D1 | 160 | Round | Dense | + | |
| EC | 200-400 | Round, oval, or pleomorphic | Dense | + | |
| P | 100-150 | Round | Medium | + | |
| X | 250 | Round | Medium | + | |
| I | 250-300 | Round to slightly irregular | Medium | + | |
| K | 200-350 | Irregular | Dense eccentric core | | Variable |
| M | 180 | Round | Moderate | + | |
| S | 180-220 | Round/irregular | Dense | | Narrow |
| PP | 150-170 | Round | Dense | + | |
| L | 250-300 | Round | Dense | + | |
| N | 300 | Round | Moderate | + | |

*Closely applied to core; separated from core by a space or halo.

argentaffin and argyrophil stains, although these are being superseded by immunostains for chromogranin A (fig. 12-1A). The argentaffin stain identifies mainly the basigranulated serotonin-producing EC cells, whereas the argyrophil stain identifies most endocrine cells. A few endocrine cells, such as gastrin cells, stain inconsistently with the silver stains. A variety of argyrophil stains are available for the demonstration of endocrine cells, such as Grimelius, Churukian-Schenk, Sevier-Munger, and Hellman-Hellerman. The most widely used is the Grimelius stain although the Churukian-Schenk stain is probably the most sensitive (89).

In searching for a universal marker for gastrointestinal endocrine cells a number of immunohistochemical stains have been developed. These include neuron-specific enolase (NSE), protein gene product (PGP) 9.5, chromogranin, secretogranin, and synaptophysin (17,30,51–53,78,108, 110). NSE is a soluble glycolytic enzyme, originally isolated from brain. It is made of two gamma subunits, and it is the most acidic form of the enolase isoenzyme (54). It has been identified immunohistochemically both in neurons and neuroendocrine cells and their corresponding tumors, such as gastric carcinoid. However, this antibody is not specific for gastric carcinoma since other tumors, such as carcinomas of the breast, ovary, and kidney, are also sometimes positive. Conversely, the absence of NSE in a tumor makes a diagnosis of carcinoid tumor unlikely (45,105). PGP 9.5 is another distinct cytoplasmic protein found in neurons that also stains gastrointestinal endocrine cells (78,104). Synaptophysin is a 38-kD hydrophobic glycoprotein of the membrane of presynaptic vesicles. It is also found in small clear vesicles in most neuroendocrine cells, such as in the anterior pituitary; in chromaffin cells of the adrenal medulla; C cells of the thyroid; pancreatic islet cells; and gastrointestinal endocrine cells, as well as their malignant counterparts (109). The demonstration of synaptophysin in paraffin sections of gastric carcinoid tumors is not as sensitive an indicator of endocrine cells as NSE since only about half of the tumors are reactive to synaptophysin. The stain is probably more sensitive if frozen tissue is used (32,61,110). The chromogranins are hydrophilic acidic proteins present in the granule matrix. There are three major types: chromogranin A,

chromogranin B (also known as secretogranin I), and chromogranin C (also known as secretogranin II). Of all the chromogranins, chromogranin A has been the most extensively studied and is the most widely used and useful antibody. It is the stain of choice in our laboratory because of the ease of immunohistologic preparation and interpretation. It should be noted however, that because chromogranin antibodies react with the protein within the granule matrix, tumors with few dense core granules, usually the poorly differentiated ones, may show a false-negative reaction for this marker.

The most definitive way to characterize gastric endocrine cells is to demonstrate their hormonal products immunohistochemically, for example, by the demonstration of gastrin in the G cells, somatostatin in the D cells, and serotonin in the EC cells (fig. 12-1C).

## ENDOCRINE CELL HYPERPLASIA

Most gastric endocrine cell hyperplasias are secondary to hypochlorhydria (3,6,9,13,19,25,37, 42,46,72,74,81,82,85,87,100), but a few are part of the multiple endocrine neoplasia syndrome (93). The major significance of these hyperplasias is their association with carcinoid tumors, albeit rare. In rare cases of primary hyperplasia, no underlying cause has been found (26,27,47,50,75,80,107).

Accurate quantitation of the absolute number of endocrine cells or the cellular content of peptide in the gastric mucosa is difficult because of technical factors relating to fixation, section thickness, pretreatment of tissues, absence of a universal marker, quality of antibodies, difficulty in estimating total mucosal volume, and difficulty in obtaining normal tissues for exact comparisons. In practice, however, in most of the recognized gastric endocrine cell hyperplasias, the magnitude of the hyperplasia is such that it is readily recognized by low-power microscopy and quantitation is unnecessary (47,48,50). Hyperfunction, with regards to gastrin cells, can easily be determined by gastrin levels in the serum.

### Primary G-Cell Hyperplasia

This condition is clinically indistinguishable from the Zollinger-Ellison syndrome due to gastrinoma. It is characterized by peptic ulcers, which may be single or multiple; basal hypergastrinemia; exaggerated gastrin response to

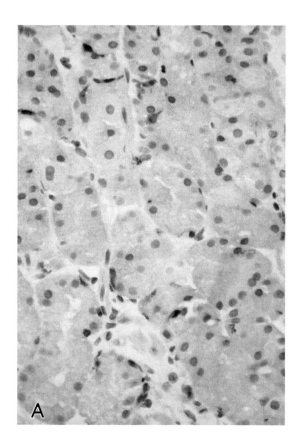

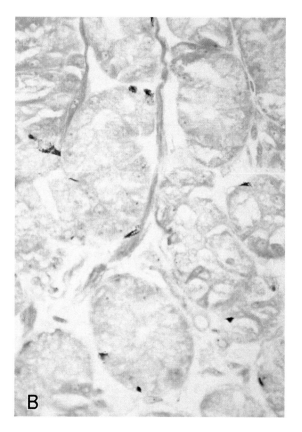

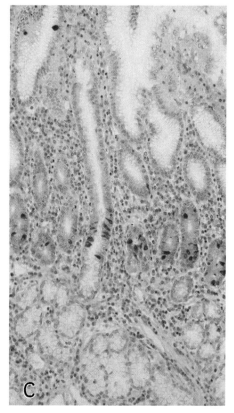

Figure 12-1
NORMAL ENDOCRINE CELLS
OF THE STOMACH IDENTIFIED BY SILVER
STAIN AND IMMUNOHISTOCHEMISTRY

A: In the fundic mucosa, the cells are scattered between parietal and chief cells and wedged between them and the basement membrane. (PAP stain for chromogranin)

B: Fundic mucosa stained for argyrophilia by the Grimelius method.

C: These are gastrin-producing cells (G cells) in the antrum, and are located at the junction of the foveolae and the mucous glands. (PAP stain for gastrin)

feeding; and absence of any known ectopic source of gastrin secretion. It should be considered in the differential diagnosis of patients with duodenal ulcers in whom there is no evidence of associated *Helicobactor pylori* infection or nonsteroidal anti-inflammatory disease medication. Patients often have a strong family history of ulcer disease, suggestive of an autosomal dominant inheritance pattern (26,27,47,50,75,80,102,107).

The cause of primary G-cell hyperplasia is unknown and since most of the cases reported were described before the discovery of *H. pylori,* its association with *H. pylori* gastritis is uncertain. In the cases that we have seen personally, there was no significant atrophic gastritis of the gastric body and fundus.

A number of tests have been developed to aid in differentiating primary gastrin endocrine cell hyperplasia from gastrinoma (106). In G-cell hyperplasia, fasting gastrin levels are modestly elevated but the response to a meal is greatly exaggerated, in contrast to gastrinoma in which there is a higher basal gastrin level but little or no increase in serum gastrin since the tumor is already secreting at maximum capacity. Also, gastrinomas, for reasons that are not understood, show a paradoxical increase in serum gastrin following secretin injection compared to G-cell hyperplasia.

The gross features are typical of Zollinger-Ellison syndrome, namely, multiple erosions and ulcers primarily in the first part of the duodenum (about 75 percent of cases). Ulcers are also found in the second and third parts of the duodenum, and in the proximal jejunum in 11 percent of cases.

Microscopically, there is hyperplasia of the antral G cells. Normally G cells are present in the antrum at the junction of the gastric pits and mucous glands as scattered single cells. In primary G-cell hyperplasia they migrate in both an upward and downward direction in a sleeve-like manner. G cells are not usually visible in hematoxylin and eosin–stained sections, but hyperplastic cells may be apparent (figs. 12-2, 12-3). The Grimelius stain usually demonstrates the increased number of G cells but the unpredictability of the silver stain makes it unreliable. The most consistent method for demonstrating G cells is by immunohistochemical staining for gastrin or chromogranin A (fig. 12-3). Only rarely is quantitation required to confirm the diagno-

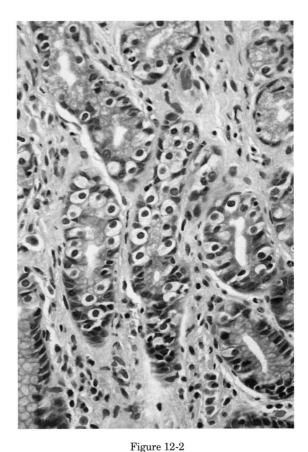

Figure 12-2
G-CELL HYPERPLASIA OF THE PYLORIC ANTRUM
The G cells, which are not normally readily visualized in hematoxylin and eosin–stained sections, are characterized by a centrally located, round, dense nucleus surrounded by clear cytoplasm. Normally, G cells occur singly and are relatively sparse but in this case they are clustered together and extend up to the foveolar gland interface.

sis, although comparison of the number of G cells with normal controls is essential (50).

G-cell hyperplasia has been treated in the past by antral resection. However, excellent responses have also been obtained with H2 receptor antagonists (107), which will almost certainly be replaced by proton pump inhibitors.

### Endocrine Cell Hyperplasia Secondary to Gastric Disease

**Pathogenesis.** The major pathogenetic mechanisms of gastric endocrine cell hyperplasia are hypochlorhydria secondary to atrophic gastritis, partial gastrectomy with resection of the body and fundic mucosa, or rarely, the Zollinger-Ellison syndrome (3,6,9,13,19,21,25,37,42,46,72, 74,81,82,85,87,93,100). Gastric acid normally

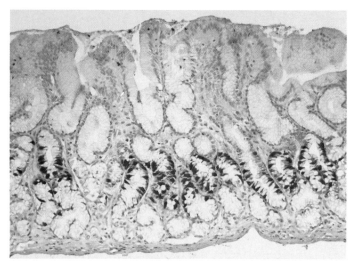

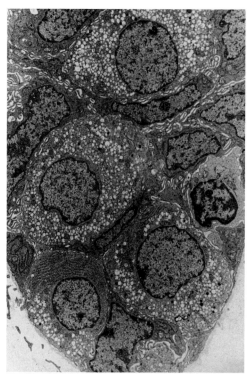

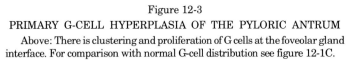

Figure 12-3
PRIMARY G-CELL HYPERPLASIA OF THE PYLORIC ANTRUM
Above: There is clustering and proliferation of G cells at the foveolar gland interface. For comparison with normal G-cell distribution see figure 12-1C.
Right: Electron micrograph shows a cluster of four gastrin cells containing numerous endocrine cell granules. The latter are much more translucent, a feature indicative of active secretion.

suppresses gastrin production; hypochlorhydria results in gastrin cell hyperplasia and hypergastrinemia (fig. 12-4A). The latter is trophic for the fundic endocrine cells and results in a predominantly argyrophil cell hyperplasia (fig. 12-4B–D). A number of distinctive cell types have been demonstrated in endocrine cell hyperplasia by immunohistochemistry and electron microscopy, such as enterochromaffin-like (ECL) (which are by far the most common), enterochromaffin (EC), gastrin, pancreatic polypeptide (PP), somatostatin (D), and D1 cells (13,37,39,72).

The major cause of hypochlorhydria is severe atrophic gastritis of the fundus, for example, in pernicious anemia and partial gastrectomy (4,19, 42,74). Hypochlorhydria may also be induced iatrogenically with acid-suppressing drugs such as the H2 blockers or the newer proton pump inhibitors such as omeprazole, which suppress gastric acid secretion by specific inhibition of the H+/K+ ATPase enzyme system. In animals, omeprazole has been shown to result in endocrine cell hyperplasia and even carcinoid tumors. Hyperplasia of ECL cells, but not tumors, have also been demonstrated in humans treated with proton pump inhibitors although the clinicopathologic

evidence suggests that the hyperplasia is more likely related to the atrophic gastritis than the acid suppressors (4,44,95,96). A rare cause of hypergastrinemia is a gastrinoma.

A recent study has shown that hyperplastic endocrine cells express BCL-2 oncoprotein which may expose them to oncogenic factors, leading to further proliferation of these cells (4a).

**Clinical Features.** There are no significant clinical symptoms related to endocrine cell hyperplasia (7,18). Occasionally, fundic endocrine cell hyperplasia progresses to dysplasia or, rarely, carcinoid tumors. Regular gastroscopic screening for carcinoid tumor in the stomach is not considered worthwhile other than in high-risk groups, namely, those with juvenile pernicious anemia and those with multiple endocrine neoplasia (MEN) (8,88).

**Microscopic Findings.** The histologic findings in endocrine cell hyperplasia secondary to gastric disease are G-cell hyperplasia of the antrum and endocrine cell proliferations of the gastric body and fundus (fig. 12-4). In our experience, the latter usually originate from the atrophic glands (often showing features of pseudopyloric metaplasia or mucous cell metaplasia) rather

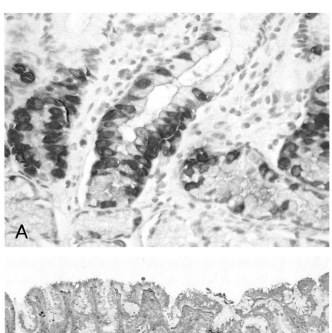

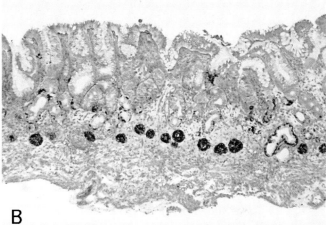

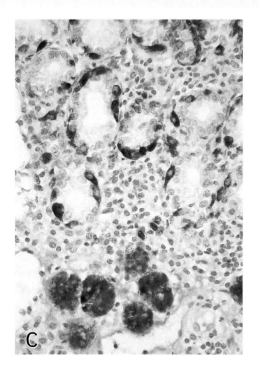

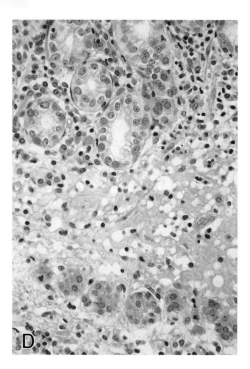

Figure. 12-4
ENDOCRINE CELL HYPERPLASIA OF
GASTRIC ANTRUM AND BODY, IN
PERNICIOUS ANEMIA

A: Antral mucosa stained for gastrin demonstrates the gastrin cells (G cells).

B: Scanning view of mucosa, showing marked atrophic gastritis and black-staining endocrine cell nests.

C: Higher power view of mucosa to show endocrine cell nests and proliferations in a sleeve-like manner around gastric glands. (Grimelius stain)

D: Low-power view of lower half of mucosa showing indistinct epithelial nodules with pale basophilic cytoplasm, resembling gastric chief cells.

than from areas of intestinal metaplasia. Proliferation of the fundic endocrine cells may occur in a diffuse manner, most commonly in Zollinger-Ellison syndrome associated with the MEN syndrome, in a sleeve-like manner around gastric glands (fig. 12-5), or as small balls or nests of cells budding from the base of glands and often lying free within the lamina propria (fig. 12-4B–D). These proliferations are best appreciated with silver stains or immunostains for chromogranin (figs. 12-4D, 12-5). In hematoxylin and eosin–stained sections, the endocrine cells are not readily apparent; the nodular proliferations appear pale with a somewhat basophilic cytoplasm and are often confused with gastric chief cells (fig. 12-4D). The G-cell proliferations secondary to atrophic gastritis may be as numerous as those in primary G-cell hyperplasia but clinically the two entities differ since the gastric fundus and body are atrophic and patients do not develop symptoms due to excess acid production (3,19,74).

## GASTRIC CARCINOID TUMORS

Carcinoid tumors of the stomach constitute approximately 4 percent of all gastrointestinal carcinoids (29,57,83) and 0.3 percent of gastric neoplasms (57). There is some geographic variation in incidence: gastric carcinoids represent 30 percent of all gastrointestinal carcinoids in Japan, which may be related to the high incidence of gastritis in that country (65).

There are two major variants: one in which the tumors are commonly multiple and associated with atrophic gastritis and endocrine cell hyperplasia; the other unassociated with endocrine cell proliferations and usually single (74a). Rarely, gastric carcinoids are associated with endocrinopathies such as Zollinger-Elllison syndrome, MEN 1 syndrome, or hyperparathyroidism and there is one report of a carcinoid tumor arising in a gastric stump (11–12,14,20,77). In general, the pathology and clinical behavior of these tumors, with minor exceptions, is similar to that of other intestinal carcinoids.

**Pathogenesis and Clinical Features.** The two major variants of gastric carcinoids show distinctive clinicopathologic and pathogenetic characteristics that are identified on the basis of presence or absence of associated chronic atrophic gastritis. The relationship of endocrine

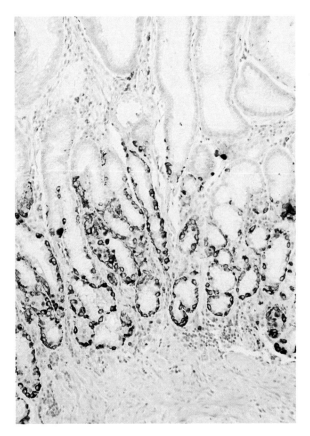

Figure 12-5
ENDOCRINE CELL HYPERPLASIA OF
GASTRIC BODY IN PERNICIOUS ANEMIA
There is marked proliferation of endocrine cells in a sleeve-like manner around gastric glands. Similar changes may be seen in hypergastrinemia secondary to gastrinomas. (PAP for chromogranin)

cell hyperplasia with severe atrophic fundic gland gastritis has already been discussed (6,10, 11,29,37,38,66,67,98,111). In a few cases, the endocrine cell hyperplasia is associated with endocrine dysplasia and carcinoid tumor, suggesting an evolution from normal to neoplastic growth (91). However, the risk of neoplastic transformation is very small and hypergastrinemia alone probably has very little, if any, neoplastic potential. It is likely that other yet unidentified factors, such as those inherent in pernicious anemia, or genetic factors as are present in the MEN syndrome, are necessary for neoplasia to develop (62,90). The carcinoid tumors associated with atrophic gastritis are usually multiple, small, and limited to the mucosa and submucosa. They are usually benign in behavior and may regress following antrectomy.

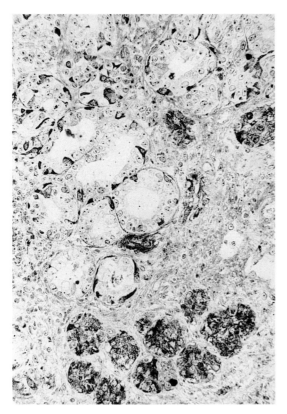

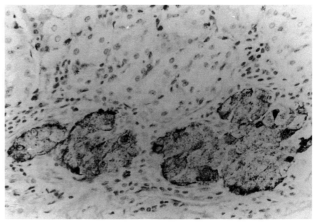

Figure 12-6
ADENOMATOID ENDOCRINE CELL HYPERPLASIA
AND DYSPLASIA

These sections from patients with chronic atrophic gastritis and hypergastrinemia associated with pernicious anemia were stained by the Sevier-Munger silver stain. (Courtesy of Drs. E. Solcia and C. Bordi, Pavia, Italy.)

Left: Adenomatoid hyperplasia characterized by more than five micronodules of endocrine cells in close proximity to one another.

Right: Endocrine cell dysplasia showing enlargement and fusion of micronodules.

The second variant of gastric carcinoid tumor is usually single, unassociated with endocrine cell proliferation, and has a more aggressive behavior. This tumor appears to arise from the gastric epithelial renewal zone at the base of the gastric pits, and does not benefit from antrectomy (14). These tumors present in one of two ways: 1) as a mass lesion with clinical features similar to carcinoma, namely, with gastrointestinal hemorrhage, obstruction, or metastases and no evidence of endocrine symptoms; 2) as an endocrinopathy whose clinical features depend on the hormonal secretion products. Some patients have an atypical carcinoid syndrome characterized by a red rather than cyanotic flushing of the skin. These tumors differ from the usual carcinoids by producing primarily 5 hydroxytryptophan rather than serotonin, as well as histamine. Other modes of presentation are with the Zollinger-Ellison syndrome due to gastrin production (it should be noted that most gastrinomas arise from the pancreas or duodenum) or with Cushing's syndrome due to adrenocorticotrophic hormone (ACTH) production (35,58). Gastric carcinoids have also been associated with the multiple endocrine adenopathy syndrome and there is a case report of another familial syndrome characterized by flushing, gastric obstruction, hyperparathyroidism, exophthalmos, and acromegaly (77).

Gastrointestinal endocrine cell proliferations have been classified by Solcia et al. (90) into hyperplasia, adenomatoid hyperplasia, dysplasia, and neoplasia. We use this classification here. However, as previously stated, only rarely have all intermediate patterns between hyperplasia and carcinoid tumor been observed (91). Hyperplasia is defined as micronodular clusters of five or more cells, not exceeding the diameter of gastric glands, present either within gastric glands or lying in the lamina propria of the mucosa. The clusters are surrounded by a thin basement membrane (fig. 12-4B,C). Adenomatoid hyperplasia is defined as five or more micronodules lying close to each other widh interspersed basement membrane, lying deep in the mucosa (fig. 12-6, left). Endocrine cell dysplasia consists of enlargement and fusion of the micronodules (greater than 150 mm but less than 0.5 mm) with disappearance of intervening basement membrane (figs. 12-6, right; 12-7).

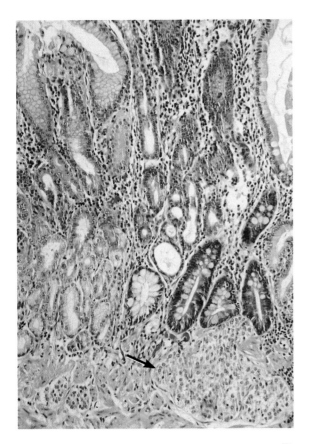 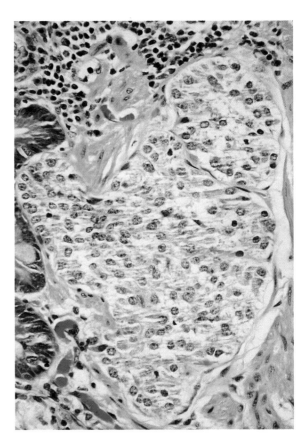

Figure 12-7
ENDOCRINE CELL DYSPLASIA OF THE STOMACH

A: Endocrine cell dysplasia consisting of a large nodule of endocrine cells resulting from fusion of endocrine cell micronodules (arrow).

B: High-power view of figure A shows the fused endocrine cell nodules.

Microinvasion of the lamina propria between glands may also occur, resulting in nodules with newly formed stroma. The cytology of these cells tends to be somewhat atypical, with irregular cells and reduced argyrophilia.

Carcinoid tumors are divided into intramucosal and invasive types (figs. 12-8, 12-9). Intramucosal lesions consist of infiltrative or solid endocrine growths greater than 0.5 mm in diameter but confined to the mucosa. Endocrine cell proliferations penetrating beyond the muscularis mucosae are invasive carcinoids.

**Endoscopic and Gross Findings.** Gastric carcinoids may be single or multiple and are mostly submucosal, measuring less than 2 cm in maximum diameter. They may project into the lumen and cause attenuation of the overlying mucosa but rarely ulceration. Endoscopically, they appear as smooth, rounded, submucosal, yellow masses covered by mucosa of normal appearance (fig. 12-10). As they enlarge they develop a characteristic, irregularly shaped, erythematous depression or ulceration (68). The larger lesions are generally deeply invasive and are often associated with extensive fibrosis. Metastases from these large tumors are common and are frequently larger than the primary (59,64,103).

Carcinoid tumors associated with atrophic gastritis and endocrine cell hyperplasia often consist of multiple, small, mucosal, tan nodules in the gastric body, measuring 1 to 3 mm in diameter and only rarely accompanied by a larger tumor (fig. 12-10, left).

**Microscopic Findings.** Gastric carcinoids have the typical histologic features of foregut carcinoids: ribbon or trabecular patterns, with occasional rosette formation and mucin production (fig. 12-11). Although this pattern is different

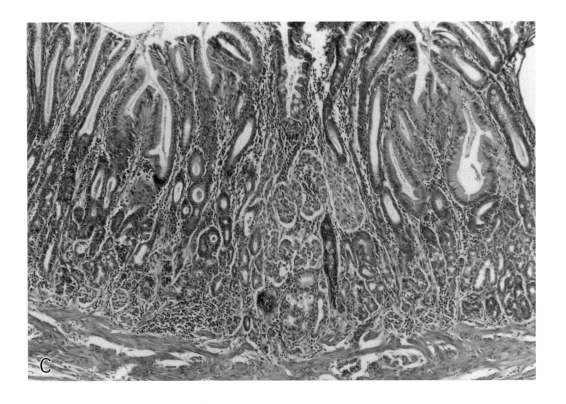

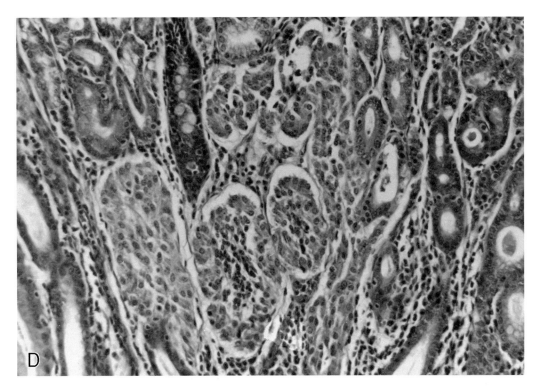

Figure 12-7 (Continued)

C: Low-power view of gastric mucosa showing chronic atrophic gastritis with intestinal metaplasia. In the center of the field several endocrine cell nests of variable size can be seen in the mid-portion of the mucosa.

D: Higher magnification showing several micronodules of endocrine cells infiltrating the lamina propria.

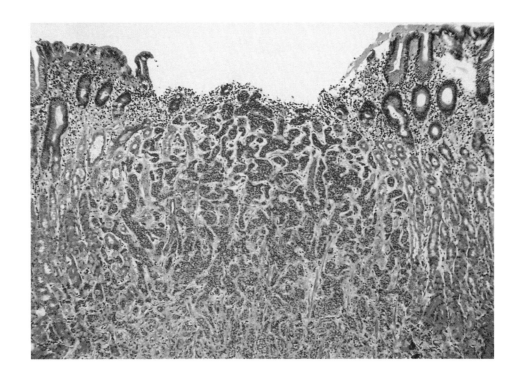

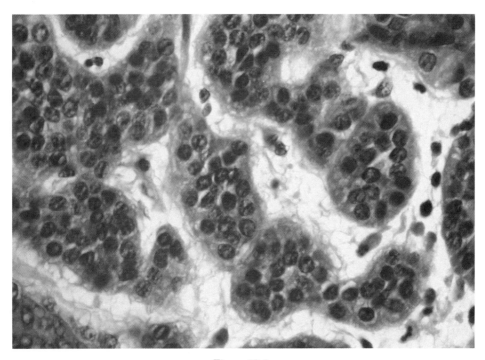

Figure 12-8
INTRAMUCOSAL CARCINOID TUMOR OF THE STOMACH
Top: Low-power view of a small tumor confined to the mucosa.
Bottom: Higher magnification of the tumor above shows the typical trabecular pattern of the carcinoid.

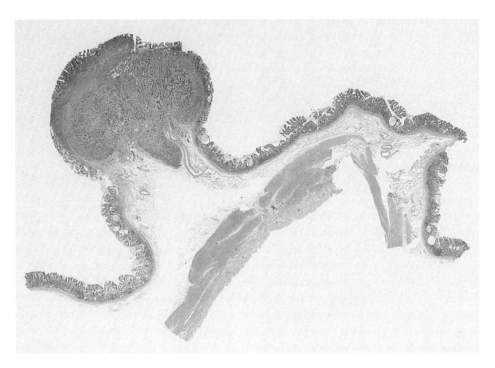

Figure 12-9
SOLITARY PEDUNCULATED CARCINOID TUMOR
The tumor is located mostly in the superficial submucosa.

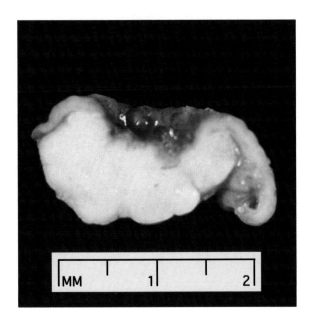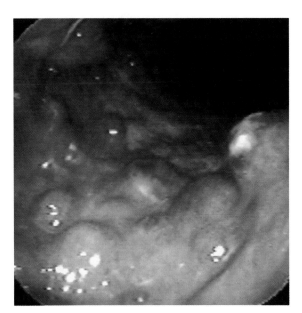

Figure 12-10
ENDOSCOPIC AND GROSS APPEARANCES OF GASTRIC CARCINOIDS
Left: Longitudinal section of a solitary carcinoid involving the full thickness of the stomach and a depressed ulcerated surface.
Right: Endoscopic appearance of the gastric body in a patient with pernicious anemia demonstrating multiple small, smooth, rounded mucosal nodules.

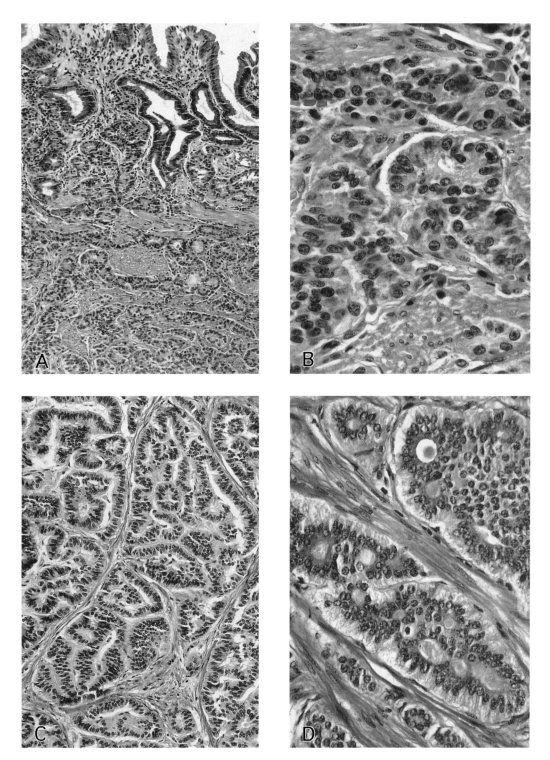

Figure 12-11
GASTRIC CARCINOID: HISTOLOGIC SPECTRUM

A: Low-power view of gastric carcinoid demonstrating tumor within the mucosa and infiltrating the muscularis mucosa and submucosa. The tumor has a trabecular pattern with rosette formation.

B: High-power view of the infiltrating cords and nests of tumor.

C: High-power view demonstrating a ribbon-like pattern.

D: High-power view demonstrating glandular profiles with mucin in the lumens.

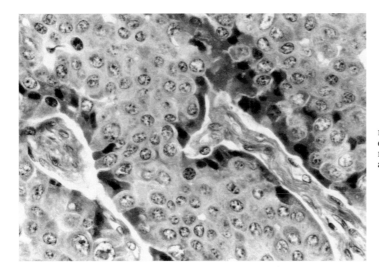

Figure 12-12
GASTRIC CARCINOID TUMOR
High-power magnification illustrating the monotonous-appearing sheets of tumor cells with centrally located nuclei and indistinct cytoplasmic borders. Note the darkly staining cytoplasm at the periphery of the tumor nests.

Figure 12-13
GASTRIC CARCINOID TUMOR
High-power magnification illustrating densely packed cords of tumor.

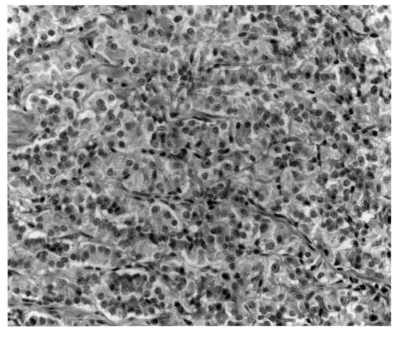

from the usual midgut carcinoids (small intestine and proximal colon), which have an insular pattern, these histologic differences cannot be relied upon to determine the site of origin of gastrointestinal carcinoids or even extraintestinal carcinoids and pancreatic islet cell tumors. The individual tumor cells are round or polygonal, with ill-defined cell outlines. They have monotonous-appearing, round, centrally located nuclei with finely stippled chromatin, small nucleoli, and infrequent mitoses. The cytoplasmic appearance is variable: in some tumors it is faintly eosinophilic, while in others it is coarsely

granular and eosinophilic, especially at the periphery of the tumor nests (figs. 12-12, 12-13).

Occasionally, gastric carcinoid tumors display a wide variety of histologic appearances. They may have a plasmacytoid-like appearance, a spindle cell configuration, or rhabdoid features; they may become anaplastic (fig. 12-14), sometimes to the point of being difficult to differentiate from other poorly differentiated tumors of the stomach such as carcinoma or lymphoma. The increasing atypia of carcinoid tumors is accompanied by cytologic atypia, increased mitotic activity, and necrosis (fig. 12-14A). Another variant

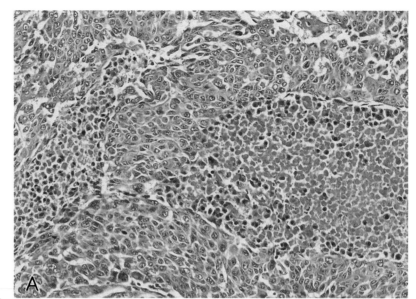

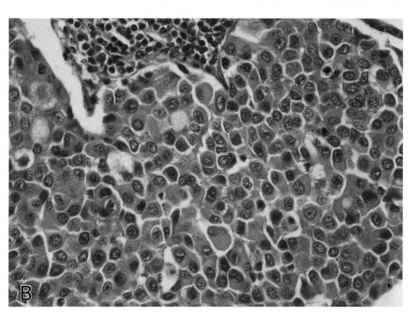

Figure 12-14
POORLY DIFFERENTIATED
CARCINOID TUMOR

A: Low-power view showing sheets
of tumor cells with central necrosis.

B: High-power magnification showing
tumor cells with a plasmacytoid-like appearance with enlarged nuclei and basophilic cytoplasm.

of poorly differentiated carcinoid tumor is the oat
cell tumor which is discussed separately.

Special stains reveal that gastric carcinoids
are usually argyrophilic and rarely argentaffinic
(fig. 12-15A) (9). The tumors stain immunohistochemically for chromogranin A (fig. 12-15B) but
not usually chromogranin B; for synaptophysin
in about 50 percent of formalin-fixed tumors; and
for a variety of secretory products such as serotonin, pancreatic polypeptide, histamine, gastrin, and rarely ACTH, B-MSH, epinephrine and
parathyroid hormone related protein. By elec-

tron microscopy the majority show features of
ECL cells (5,14,35,84,94,100a).

**Differential Diagnosis.** As already indicated, carcinoid tumors display a wide variety of
atypical histologic appearances that may mimic
other tumors, such as poorly differentiated adenocarcinomas, lymphoma, and mesenchymal
neoplasms. In general, poorly differentiated endocrine tumors tend to have a relatively uniform
cell population compared to similarly poorly differentiated adenocarcinomas, which tend to be pleomorphic. Lymphomas can normally be excluded by

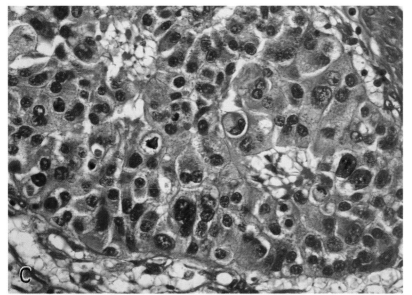

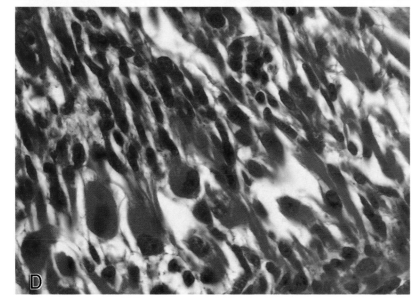

Figure 12-14 (Continued)
C: High-power view demonstrates marked nuclear pleomorphism and hyperchromasia.
D: A poorly differentiated carcinoid with rhabdoid-like features.

the immunohistochemical demonstration of common leucocyte antigen. Any unusual gastric tumor showing spindled, organoid, or ribbon-like patterns should raise the suspicion of a carcinoid. This should prompt further studies such as silver stains; immunohistochemistry for the demonstration of chromogranin, synaptophysin, and specific peptides; and the search for dense core granules by electron microscopy. Unfortunately, the silver stains and immunohistochemical markers for poorly differentiated endocrine tumors are often not sufficiently sensitive to make a diagnosis of carcinoid tumor. Furthermore, the

usual markers for nonendocrine epithelial cells, such as keratin and carcinoembryonic antigen, are not helpful because they may also be present in carcinoid tumors (69). To date, the demonstration of dense core granules by electron microscopy remains the most definitive method of diagnosis of poorly differentiated carcinoids. However, as already stated in the section on gastric adenocarcinomas, carcinomas frequently contain scattered endocrine cells. Thus, in order to diagnose a poorly differentiated carcinoid tumor and differentiate it from carcinoma, the majority of tumor cells should contain dense core

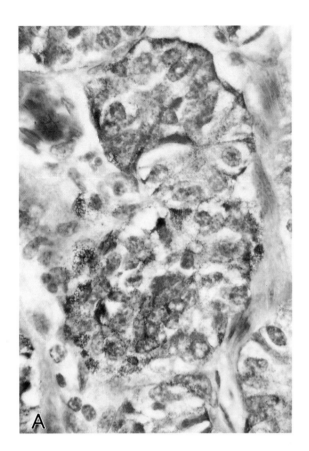

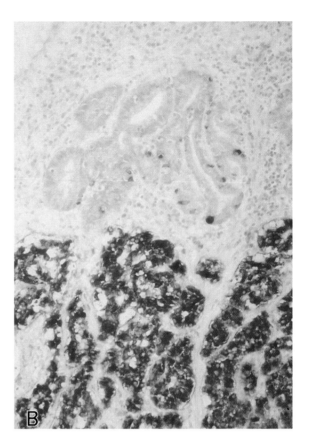

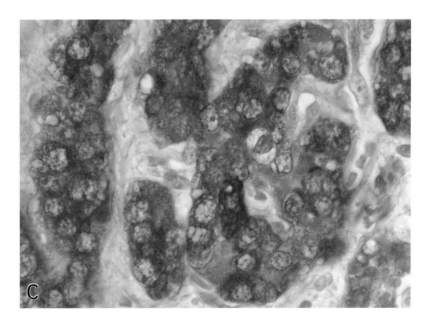

Figure 12-15
DEMONSTRATION OF GASTRIC CARCINOID TUMOR BY SPECIAL STAINS

A: Grimelius stain demonstrating argyrophilia of the tumor.

B: Chromogranin immunohistologic reaction shows the diffuse-staining tumor cells and the normal endocrine cells in the overlying mucosa.

C: Immunohistochemical stain for neuron-specific enolase showing diffuse staining of all tumor cells.

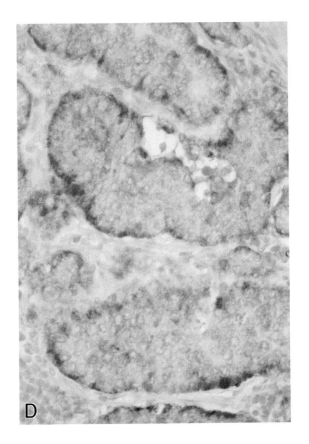

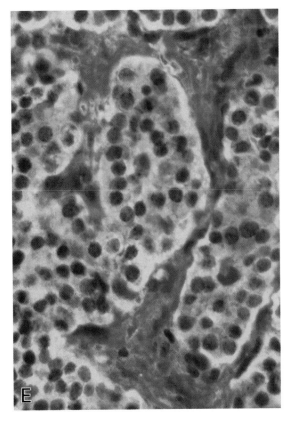

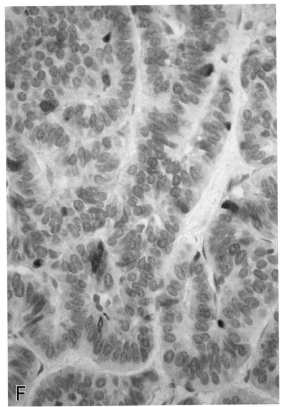

Figure 12-15 (Continued)

D: Immunohistologic stain for chromogranin to show another reaction pattern characterized mainly by peripheral staining of the tumor nests.

E: A gastrinoma stained for gastrin by immunofluorescence to show diffuse staining of all tumor cells.

F: A solitary, clinically silent gastric carcinoid tumor stained for pancreatic polypeptide. Scattered positive tumor cells are seen.

granules as evidence of endocrine differentiation. It could also be argued that the expense of electron microscopy is not justified presently, since the treatment of poorly differentiated carcinoma and carcinoid is similar.

Occasionally, glomus tumors of the stomach (2,16) mimic carcinoids, especially on frozen section, since both have an organoid pattern. However, the characteristic features of glomus tumors, namely, vascular channels, negative silver stains, and absence of dense core granules and smooth muscle differentiation ultrastructurally, should help in separating the two (for a detailed description see chapter 14) (1,16,33).

**Spread and Metastases.** The tumors grow and spread in a fairly predictable pattern. As they enlarge they extend directly into the muscle coat, serosa, and mesentery, often accompanied by extensive fibrosis. There is also lymphatic permeation. Larger lesions metastasize locally to regional lymph nodes and liver and also to distant sites such as bone and skin. Tumor growth is usually slow and metastases may be present for many years before leading to the death of the patient.

**Prognosis and Treatment.** The management of gastric endocrine cell hyperplasia with associated small carcinoids is still arbitrary, primarily because of the insufficient number of cases studied. For smaller, multiple lesions less than 1.0 cm in diameter surgery is probably unnecessary because of their very slow growth (34,75a). These patients should be followed endoscopically and probably have their lesions removed through the endoscope (34,86,99). However, if there are many small lesions, endoscopic removal may not be practical, and a decision between a major gastric resection and periodic endoscopic surveillance is necessary (9–11,14, 28a,67,99). There are also reports that antrectomy, by abolishing hypergastrinemia, causes the arrest or regression of hyperplastic lesions of the gastric fundus, and in one report also of carcinoid tumors (8,20a,24,36,41,55,67).

As previously stated, solitary gastric carcinoids are not usually associated with atrophic gastritis or the Zollinger-Ellison or MEN syndrome. However, because of the clinical implications, it is probably worthwhile for the clinician to confirm this either by obtaining biopsies of the gastric antrum and body or testing the serum for hypergastrinemia. The clinical behavior of solitary gastric carcinoids unassociated with severe atrophic gastritis and endocrine cell hyperplasia is that of carcinoids in general and their management is the same as in other sites. The overall 5-year survival rate for patients with stomach lesions is 70 to 80 percent (23,28,64,75a,76).

No absolute criteria exist by which to judge the malignant potential of the larger carcinoid tumors. Size and invasiveness correlate best with the probability of metastasis. If the tumors exceed 2 cm in diameter, there is a significant potential for metastasis, while those that are less than 2 cm have a very low risk (103a). Tumors less than 1 cm in diameter may remain stable for many years, often with no progression in size, although exceptions occur (34,86,88,99). On the basis of these findings, it is recommended that lesions larger than 2 cm in diameter be resected; lesions of 1 to 2 cm should be treated by polypectomy or circumscribed local resection (67,86).

Less well-differentiated carcinoid tumors appear to have a greater potential for metastasis, although at present there is insufficient follow-up data to be certain (40,101). Poorly differentiated lesions, such as the rare small cell (oat cell) carcinoids, are highly invasive and have a poor prognosis: most patients die of metastasis within 6 months (see Small Cell Carcinoma).

There is also a suggestion that histologic type of tumor affects prognosis. In one study tumors with an insular, trabecular, or mixed pattern were less aggressive than those with a glandular or undifferentiated pattern (40).

## SMALL CELL (OAT CELL) CARCINOMA

These are similar to the oat cell cancers of the lung and only a few cases have been reported in the stomach. The prognosis of these tumors is poor, and most patients die within 1 year of diagnosis (112–116a).

Grossly, early lesions are polypoid and advanced lesions are fleshy and may develop deep ulcerations (116). Microscopically, these tumors are identical to those found in the esophagus and other parts of the gastrointestinal tract (for illustrations see Small Cell Carcinoma of the Esophagus). In the stomach they tend to grow in sheets, cords, and trabecular or alveolar-like patterns, separated by thin bands of vascularized connective tissue, similar to oat cell carcinoma of the lung. The tumor cells may be small lymphocyte–like or of intermediate cell type, characterized by small polygonal or fusiform cells with scant cytoplasm. The nuclei are hyperchromatic, with a "salt and pepper" chromatin pattern, frequently exhibiting nuclear moulding. A number of these tumors have foci of adenocarcinomatous or squamous differentiation (114,116). Lymphatic and vascular invasion are common (116,116a).

Most of the small cell carcinomas of the stomach are reported to be argyrophilic, often stain positively for chromogranin and neuron-specific enolase, and do not usually contain carcinoembryonic antigen. The hallmark of these tumors is the presence of dense core granules, albeit sometimes few, as demonstrated by electron microscopy. As is true for the oat cell tumors of the lung, not all the reported small cell tumors of the stomach have features of endocrine cells, namely argyrophilia, immunoreactivity to chromogranin, or the presence of dense-core granules (5). In some cases this may be because the tumors are so poorly differentiated that the endocrine cell markers are not sufficiently sensitive. However, it is probable that some poorly differentiated carcinomas and lymphomas are indistinguishable from small cell carcinomas. From a practical point of view the behavior and treatment of these tumors is the same, irrespective of their cell of origin.

## MIXED ENDOCRINE AND NON-ENDOCRINE EPITHELIAL TUMORS

Many epithelial tumors of the gastrointestinal tract are not pure and contain admixtures of different epithelial cells, including glandular epithelium, endocrine cells, and Paneth cells. These findings are not surprising since embryologic studies have shown that gastrointestinal epithelial cells and endocrine cells are derived from a common stem cell (118,125,128). The behavior of these tumors, in general, depends upon their predominant cellular component.

Epithelial tumors of mixed cell types, listed in Table 12-1, can be classified as follows (48,126): 1) carcinomas with interspersed endocrine cells; 2) carcinoids with interspersed nonendocrine cells; 3) composite glandular-endocrine cell carcinomas, defined as tumors consisting of discrete areas of carcinoma (with any degree of differen-

tiation) and of carcinoid (also of any degree of differentiation); 4) collision tumors in which endocrine tumors and adenocarcinomas are closely juxtaposed but not admixed; 5) amphicrine tumors composed predominantly of cells that exhibit dual differentiation, for example, mucus and dense core granules within the cytoplasm of the same cell; and 6) combination tumors of the above types. Amphicrine tumors are extremely rare and have been described primarily in the pancreas and lung (117,121,132). We are aware of only one amphicrine lesion in the stomach in which the amphicrine tumor constituted one component of a combination tumor which also contained adenocarcinoma and carcinoid.

There are two reasons for subclassifying these tumors. First, the behavior and treatment may differ from other neoplasms at that site. For example, a composite tumor made up of a poorly differentiated carcinoma and carcinoid tumor behaves more like a carcinoma than a carcinoid. Second, the recognition of histologically distinctive patterns might cause diagnostic problems, even though their clinical behavior does not necessarily differ from the corresponding carcinomas. The mixed glandular-endocrine cell carcinoma of scirrhous argyrophil cell type falls into this category.

## Carcinoid Tumors with Interspersed Nonendocrine Cells

Some carcinoid tumors have an acinar or glandular architecture with mucicarminophilic or Alcian blue–positive material within their lumina and in scattered, albeit rare, tumor cells (fig. 12-11D) (120,123). Clinically, no evidence exists that mucin-secreting carcinoids are more aggressive than their nonmucinous counterparts. Oat cell carcinomas of the gastrointestinal tract can also occur in association with nonendocrine tumors such as squamous carcinoma or adenocarcinoma (see Oat Cell Carcinoma).

## Adenocarcinoma with Interspersed Endocrine Cells

These are gastric adenocarcinomas that may be well or poorly differentiated, and contain varying proportions of endocrine cells interspersed among nonendocrine and mucin-secreting cells (119,122,124,127). They are characterized by the same architectural pattern as usual adenocarcinomas. In some cases the interspersed endocrine cells may be identifiable in hematoxylin and eosin–stained sections by the presence of fine, basally situated, eosinophilic granules that are not as coarse as the similarly eosinophilic but apically situated granules of Paneth cells. These tumors behave as adenocarcinomas.

## Composite Glandular-Endocrine Cell Carcinomas and Gastric Collision Tumors

About 20 of these tumors have now been described (117,133,134). The age incidence and sex distribution are the same as for gastric carcinoma, as is the prognosis (134).

Histologically, either component of the tumor may vary from well to poorly differentiated; in one report roughly half the tumors showed well-differentiated carcinoma and the other half poorly differentiated carcinoma. Sometimes, these lesions may be difficult or impossible to differentiate from collision tumors which consist of two distinct neoplasms arising next to one another and then growing into one another (65). Metastatic lesions may clarify which tumor one is dealing with, in that metastases from composite tumors show both components of the tumor, whereas only one type is seen in collision tumor metastases (133). Another rare condition considered in the differential diagnosis of these mixed tumors is the very occasional primary gastric tumor that contains a metastasis within it.

## Poorly Differentiated (Signet-Ring Cell) Carcinoma with Interspersed Endocrine Cells

A number of poorly differentiated or signet-ring cell adenocarcinomas have been described that contain a large proportion of argyrophilic cells (124,129–131). They may occur as diffusely infiltrating lesions associated with marked desmoplasia and resembling linitis plastica, or as localized lesions found mainly in the antrum and confined to the mucosa and submucosa (131).

Microscopically, they are characterized by infiltrating nests or cords of poorly differentiated

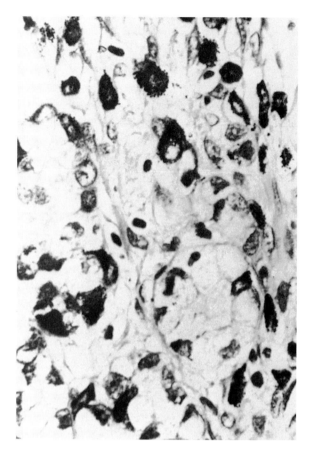

Figure 12-16
"SCIRRHOUS" ARGYROPHIL CELL
CARCINOMA OF THE STOMACH
High-power magnification of infiltrating signet-ring cells and admixed argentaffin cells with black granules. (Masson Fontana stain) (Courtesy of Dr. E. Tahara, Hiroshima, Japan.)

adenocarcinoma or signet-ring cell carcinoma admixed with endocrine cells, which may not be immediately apparent on hematoxylin and eosin stain. Silver stains show that the majority of tumor cells are argyrophilic, and only a few are argentaffinic (fig. 12-16). The tumor cells can produce multiple polypeptide hormones as well as amines, human chorionic gonadotropin, and carcinoembryonic antigen (113) but are not accompanied by any recognizable hormonal syndromes. The behavior of these tumors appears to be similar to their adenocarcinomatous counterpart (124) and they should be treated in a similar manner.

# REFERENCES

## Endocrine Cell Hyperplasia and Carcinoid Tumors

1. Almagro UA, Schulte WJ, Norback DH, Turcotte JK. Glomus tumor of the stomach. Histologic and ultrastructural features. Am J Clin Path 1981;75:415–9.

2. Appelman MD, Helwig EB. Glomus tumors of the stomach. Cancer 1969;23:203–13.

3. Arnold R, Hulst MV, Neuhof CH, Schwarting H, Becker HD, Creuzfeldt W. Antral gastrin producing G-cells and somatostatin-producing D-cells in different states of gastric acid secretion. Gut 1982;23:285–91.

4. Arnold R, Koop H. Omeprazole: long-term safety. Digestion 1989;44:77–86.

4a. Azzoni C, Doglioni C, Viale G, et al. Involvement of BCL-2 oncoprotein in the development of enterochromaffin-like cell gastric carcinoids. Am J Surg Pathol 1996;20:433–41.

5. Bader LV, Lykke AW, Hinterberger H. Multiple biogenic amine-secreting "carcinoid" tumour of the stomach: a case report. Pathology 1977;9:353–8.

6. Black WC, Haffner HE. Diffuse hyperplasia of gastric argyrophil cells and multiple carcinoid tumors. Cancer 1968;21:1080–99.

7. Bloom SR, Polak JM. Hormone profiles. In: Bloom SR, Polak JM, eds. Gut hormones. Edinburgh: Churchill Livingstone, 1981:555–60.

8. Borch K. Atrophic gastritis and gastric carcinoid tumours. Ann Med 1989;21:291–7.

9. Borch K, Renvall H, Kullman E, Eilander E. Gastric carcinoid associated with the syndrome of hypergastrinemic atrophic gastritis. A prospective analysis of 11 cases. Am J Surg Pathol 1987;11:435–44.

10. Borch K, Renvall H, Liedberg G. Gastric endocrine cell hyperplasia and carcinoid tumors in pernicious anemia. Gastroenterology 1985;88:638–48.

11. Borch K, Renvall H, Liedberg G. Endocrine cell proliferation and carcinoid development: a review of new aspects of hypergastrinaemic atrophic gastritis. Digestion 1986;35(suppl 1):106–15.

11a. Bordi C. Endocrine tumors of the stomach. Pathol Res Pract 1995;191:373–80.

12. Bordi C, Cocconi G, Togni R, Vezzadini P, Missale C. Gastric endocrine cell proliferation associated with Zollinger-Ellison syndrome. Arch Pathol 1974;98:274–9.

13. Bordi C, Ferrari C, D'Adda T, et al. Ultrastructural characterization of fundic endocrine cell hyperplasia associated with atrophic gastritis and hypergastrinemia. Virchows Arch [A] 1986;409:335–47.

14. Bordi C, Yu JY, Baggi MT, et al. Gastric carcinoid and their precursor lesions: a histologic and immunohistochemical study of 23 cases. Cancer 1991;67:663–72.

15. Brown GA, Kollin J, Rajan PH. The coexistence of carcinoid tumor and Crohn's disease. J Clin Gastroenterol 1986;8:286–9.

16. Caccamo D, Kaneko M, Gordon RE. Glomus tumor of the stomach. Mt Sinai J Med 1987;54:344–7.

17. Chejfec G, Falkmer S, Grimelius L, et al. Synaptophysin. A new marker for pancreatic neuroendocrine tumors. Am J Surg Pathol 1987;11:241–7.

18. Creutzfeldt W. Gut hormones and disease: a perspective. In: Bloom SR, Polak JM, eds. Gut hormones. Edinburgh: Churchill Livingstone, 1981:533–40.

19. Creutzfeldt W, Arnold R, Creutzfeldt C, Feurle G, Ketterer H. Gastrin and G-cells in the antral mucosa of patients with pernicious anemia, acromegaly, and hyperparathyroidism and in a Zollinger-Ellison tumor of the pancreas. Eur J Clin Invest 1971;1:461–79.

20. D'Adda T, Azzoni C, Franze A, Bordi C. Malignant enterochromaffin-like cell carcinoid of the gastric stump: an ultrastructural study. Ultrastruct Pathol 1991;15:257–65.

20a. D'Adda T, Pilato FP, Sivelli R, Azzoni C, Sianesi M, Bordi C. Gastric carcinoid tumor and its precursor lesions. Ultrastructural study of a case before and after antrectomy. Arch Pathol Lab Med 1994;118:658–63.

21. Dayal Y. Endocrine cells of the gut and their neoplasms. In: Norris TH, ed. Pathology of the colon, small intestine and anus. New York: Churchill Livingstone, 1983:267–302.

22. Dobbins WO, Austin LL. Electron microscopic definition of intestinal endocrine cells. Ultrastruct Pathol 1991;15:15–39.

23. Dockerty MB. Carcinoids of the gastrointestinal tract [Editorial]. Am J Clin Pathol 1955;25:794–6.

24. Eckhauser FE, Lloyd RV, Thompson NW, Raper SE, Vinik AI. Antrectomy for multicentric, argyrophil gastric carcinoid: a preliminary report. Surgery 1988;104:1046–53.

25. Feldman AJ, Weinberg M, Raess D, Richardson ML, Fry WJ. Gastric carcinoid tumor: its occurrence with ossification and diffuse argyrophil cell hyperplasia. Arch Surg 1980;116:118–21.

26. Frieson SR, Schimke RN, Pearse AG. Genetic aspects of the Z-E syndrome: prospective studies in two kindred; antral gastrin cell hyperplasia. Ann Surg 1972;176:370–83.

27. Ganguli PC, Polak JM, Pearse AG, Elder JB, Hegarty M. Antral "G" cell hyperplasia with peptic ulcer disease: a new clinical entity. Gut 1973;14:822–3.

28. Gardiner GW, Van Patter T, Murray D. Atypical carcinoid tumor of the small bowel complicating celiac disease. Cancer 1985;56:2716–22.

28a. Gilligan CJ, Lawton GP, Tang LH, West AB, Modlin IM. Gastric carcinoid tumors: the biology and therapy of an enigmatic and controversial lesion. Am J Gastroenterol 1995;90:338–52.

29. Godwin JD. Carcinoid tumors—an analysis of 2837 cases. Cancer 1975;36:560–9.

30. Gould VE. Synaptophysin. A new and promising pan-neuroendocrine marker. Arch Pathol Lab Med 1987;111:791–4.

31. Gould VE, DeLellis RA. The neuroendocrine cell system: its tumors, hyperplasias and dysplasias. In: Silverberg SC, ed. Principles and practice of surgical pathology. New York: John Wiley and Sons, 1983:1487–501.

32. Gould VE, Wiedenmann B, Lee I, et al. Synaptophysic expression in neuroendocrine neoplasms as determined by immunocytochemistry. Am J Pathol 1987;126:243–57.

33. Hamilton CW, Shelburne JD, Bossen EH, Lowe JE. A glomus tumor of the jejunum masquerading as a carcinoid tumor. Hum Pathol 1982;13:859–61.

34. Harvey RF, Bradshaw MJ, Davidson CM, Wilkinson SP, Davies PS. Multifocal gastric carcinoid tumours, achlorhydria, and hypergastrinemia. Lancet 1985;1:951–4.

35. Hirata Y, Sakamoto N, Yamamoto H, Matsukura S, Imura H, Okada S. Gastric carcinoid with ectopic production of ACTH and beta-MSH. Cancer 1976;37:377–85.

36. Hirschowitz BI, Griffith J, Pellegrin D, Cummings OW. Rapid regression of enterochromaffinlike cell gastric carcinoids in pernicious anemia after antrectomy. Gastroenterology 1992;102:1409–18.

37. Hodges JR, Isaacson P, Wright R. Diffuse enterochromaffin-like (ECL) cell hyperplasia and multiple gastric carcinoids: a complication of pernicious anaemia. Gut 1981;22:237–41.

38. Imura H, Matsukura S, Yamamoto H, Hirata Y, Nakai Y. Studies on ectopic ACTH-producing tumors. II. Clinical and biochemical features of 30 cases. Cancer 1975;35:1430–7.

39. Ito H, Yokozaki H, Hata J, Mandai K, Tahara E. Glicentin containing cells in intestinal metaplasia, adenoma and carcinoma of the stomach. Virchows Arch [A] 1984;404:17–29.

40. Johnson LA, Lavin P, Moertel CG, et al. Carcinoids: the association of histologic growth pattern and survival. Cancer 1983;51:882–9.

41. Kern SE, Yardley JH, Lazenby AJ, et al. Reversal by antrectomy of endocrine cell hyperplasia in the gastric body in pernicious anemia: a morphometric study. Mod Pathol 1990;3:561–6.

42. Korman MG, Scott DF, Hansky J, Wilson H. Hypergastrinemia due to an excluded gastric antrum: a proposed method for differentiation from Zollinger-Ellison syndrome. Aust N Z Med 1972;2:266–71.

43. Kuiper DH, Gracie WA, Jr, Pollard HM. Twenty years of gastrointestinal carcinoids. Cancer 1970;25:1424!9630.

44. Lamberts R, Creutzfeldt W, Struber HG, Brunner G, Solcia E. Long-term omeprazole therapy in peptic ulcer disease: gastrin, endocrine cell growth, and gastritis. Gastroenterology 1993;104:1356–70.

45. Leader M, Collins M, Patel J, Henry K. Antineuron specific enolase staining reactions in sarcomas and carcinomas: its lack of neuroendocrine specificity. J Clin Pathol 1986;39:1186–92.

46. Lehy T, Mignon M, Cadiot G, et al. Gastric endocrine cell behavior in Zollinger-Ellison patients upon long-term potent antisecretory treatment. Gastroenterology 1989;96:1029–40.

47. Lewin KJ. The endocrine cells of the gastrointestinal tract. The normal endocrine cells and their hyperplasias, Part 1. Pathol Annu 1986;21:1–27.

48. Lewin KJ, Riddell RH, Weinstein WM. Endocrine cells. In: Lewin KJ, Riddell RH, Weinstein WM, eds. Gastrointestinal pathology and its clinical implications. New York: Igaku-Shoin, 1992:97–257.

49. Lewin KJ, Ulich T, Yang K, Layfield L. The endocrine cells of the gastrointestinal tract. Tumors Part II. Pathol Annu 1986:21;181–215.

50. Lewin JK, Yang K, Ulich T, Elashoff JD, Walsh J. Primary gastrin cell hyperplasia: report of five cases and a review of the literature. Am J Surg Pathol 1984;8:821–32.

51. Lloyd RV. Immunohistochemical localization of chromogranins in polypeptide hormone producing cells and tumors. In: Lechago J, Kamey T, eds. Endocrine pathology update. New York: Field and Wood, 1990:259–75.

52. Lloyd RV, Cano M, Rosa P, Hille A, Huttner WB. Distribution of chromogranin A, secretogranin 1 (chromogranin B) in neuroendocrine cells and tumors. Am J Pathol 1988;130:296–304.

53. Lloyd RV, Mervak T, Schmidt K, Warner TF, Wilson BS. Immunohistochemical detection of chromogranin and neuron specific enolase in pancreatic endocrine neoplasm. Am J Surg Pathol 1984;8:607–14.

54. Lloyd RV, Warner TF. Immunohistochemistry of neuron-specific enolase. In: DeLellis RA, ed. Advances in immunohistochemistry. New York: Masson, 1984:127–40.

55. Lundell L, Olbe L, Sundler F, Simonsson M, Hakanson R. Reversibility of multiple ECL-cell gastric carcinoids by antrectomy in a pernicious anemia patient. Hepatogastroenterology 1989;36:43–4.

56. Lundqvist M, Wilander E. A study of the histopathogenesis of carcinoid tumors of the small intestine and appendix. Cancer 1987;60:201–6.

57. MacDonald RA. A study of 356 carcinoids of the gastrointestinal tract. Report of four new cases of the carcinoid syndrome. Am J Med 1956;21:867–78.

58. Mallinson CN, Bloom SR, Warin AP, Salmon PR, Cox B. A glucagonoma syndrome. Lancet 1974;2:1–5.

59. Martin ED, Potet F. Pathology of endocrine tumours of the GI tract. Clin Gastroenterol 1974;3:511–32.

60. Masson P. La glande endocrine de l'intestine chez l'homme. C R Acad Sci 1914;158:59–61.

61. Miettinen M. Synaptophysin and neurofilament proteins as markers for neuroendocrine tumors. Arch Pathol Lab Med 1987;111:813–8.

62. Modlin IM, Nangia AK. The pathobiology of the human enterochromaffin-like cell. Yale J Biol Med 1992;65:775–92; discussion 827–9.

63. Moertel CG, Sauer WG, Dockerty MB, Baggenstoss AH. Life history of the carcinoid tumor of the small intestine. Cancer 1961;14:901–12.

64. Morgan JG, Marks C, Hearn D. Carcinoid tumors of the gastrointestinal tract. Ann Surg 1974;180:720–7.

65. Morishita Y, Tanaka T, Kato K, et al. Gastric collision tumor (carcinoid and adenocarcinoma) with gastritis cystica profunda. Arch Pathol Lab Med 1991;115:1006–10.

66. Moses RE, Frank BB, Leavitt M, Miller R. The syndrome of type A chronic atrophic gastritis, pernicious anemia, and multiple gastric carcinoids. J Clin Gastroenterol 1986;8:61–5.

67. Muller J, Kirchner T, Muller-Hermelink HK. Gastric endocrine cell hyperplasia and carcinoid tumors in atrophic gastritis type A. Am J Surg Pathol 1987;11:909–17.

68. Nakamura S, Iida M, Yao T, Fujishima M. Endoscopic features of gastric carcinoids. Gastrointest Endosc 1991;37:535–8.

69. Nash SV, Said JW. Gastroenteropancreatic neuroendocrine tumors. A histochemical and immunohistochemical study of epithelial (keratin proteins, carcinoembryonic antigen) and neuroendocrine (neuron-specific enolase, bombesin, and chromogranin) markers in foregut, midgut and hindgut tumors. Am J Clin Pathol 1986;86:415–22.

70. Norheim I, Oberg K, Theodorsson-Norheim E, et al. Malignant carcinoid tumors. An analysis of 103 patients with regard to tumor localization, hormone production and survival. Ann Surg 1987;206:115–25.

71. Oberndorfer S. Karzinoide tumoren des Dunndarms. Frankfurt Ztschr Pathol 1907;1:426–32.

72. Ogata T. An electron microscopic study on the endocrine cells in the atypical epithelial lesion of the stomach. In: Fugita T, ed. Gastro-entero-pancreatic endocrine system. A cell-biological approach. Tokyo: Igaku-Shoin, 1973:120–4.

73. Pearse AG. The APUD cell concept and its implications in pathology. Pathol Annu 1974;9:27–41.

74. Polak JM, Hoffbrand AV, Reed PI, Bloom S, Pearse AG. Qualitative and quantitative studies of antral and fundic G-cells in pernicious anemia. Scand J Gastroenterol 1973;8:361–7.

74a. Perry RR, Vinik AI. Endocrine tumors of the gastrointestinal tract. Ann Rev Med 1996;47:57–68.

75. Polak JM, Stagg B, Pearse AG. Two types of Zollinger-Ellison syndrome: immunofluorescent, cytochemical, and ultrastructural studies of the antral and pancreatic gastrin cells in different clinical states. Gut 1972; 13:501–12.

75a. Rappel S, Altendorf-Hofmann A, Stolte M. Prognosis of gastric carcinoid tumors. Digestion 1995;56:455–62.

76. Ritchie AC. Carcinoid tumors. Am J Med Sci 1956;232:311–28.

77. Rode J, Dhillon AP, Cotton PB, Woolf A, O'Riordan JL. Carcinoid tumour of the stomach and primary hyperparathyroidism: a new association. J Clin Pathol 1987;40:546–51.

78. Rode J, Dhillon AP, Doran JF, Jackson PJ, Thompson RJ. PGP 9.5. A new marker for human neuroendocrine tumors. Histopathology 1985;9:147–58.

79. Rosai J, Higa E. Mediastinal endocrine neoplasm, of probably thymic origin, related to carcinoid tumor. Clinicopathologic study of 8 cases. Cancer 1972;29:1061–74.

80. Royston CM, Polak JM, Bloom SR, et al. G cell population of gastric antrum, plasma gastrin and gastric acid secretion in patients with and without duodenal ulcer. Gut 1978;19:689–98.

81. Rubin W. Proliferation of endocrine-like (enterochromaffin) cells in atrophic gastric mucosa. Gastroenterology 1969;57:641–8.

82. Rubin W. A fine structural characterization of the proliferated endocrine cells in atrophic gastric mucosa. Am J Pathol 1973;70:109–18.

83. Sanders RJ, Axtel HK. Carcinoids of the gastrointestinal tract. Surg Gynecol Obstet 1964;119:369–80.

84. Sandler M, Snow PJ. An atypical carcinoid tumour secreting 5-hydroxy tryptophan. Lancet 1958;1:137–9.

85. Shimoda T, Tanoue S, Ikegami M, Fujii Y, Muroya T, Ishikawa E. A histopathological study of diffuse hyperplasia of gastric argyrophil cells. Acta Pathol Jpn 1983;33:1259–67.

86. Sjoblom SM, Haapiainen R, Miettinen M, Jarvinen H. Gastric carcinoid tumors and atrophic gastritis. Acta Chir Scand 1987;153:37–439.

87. Sjoblom SM, Sipponen P, Karonen SL, Jarviren HJ. Mucosal argyrophil endocrine cells in pernicious anaemia and upper gastrointestinal carcinoid tumours. J Clin Pathol 1989;42:371–7.

88. Sjoblom SM, Sipponen P, Miettinen M, Karonen SL, Jarvinen HJ. Gastroscopic screening for gastric carcinoids and carcinoma in pernicious anemia. Endoscopy 1988;20:52–6.

89. Smith DM Jr, Haggitt RC. A comparative study of generic stains for carcinoid secretory granules. Am J Surg Pathol 1983;7:61–8.

90. Solcia E, Bordi C, Creutzfeldt W, et al. Histopathologic classification of nonantral gastric endocrine growths in man. Digestion 1988;41:185–200.

91. Solcia E, Capella C, Buffa R, et al. Endocrine cells of the gastrointestinal tract and related tumors. Pathobiol Annu 1979;9:163–204.

92. Solcia E, Capella C, Fiocca R, Cornaggia M, Bosi F. The gastroenteropancreatic endocrine system and related tumors. Gastroenterol Clin North Am 1989;18:671–93.

93. Solcia E, Capella C, Fiocca R, Rindi G, Rosai J. Gastric argyrophil carcinoidosis in patients with Zollinger-Ellison syndrome due to type 1 multiple endocrine neoplasia. A newly recognized association. Am J Surg Pathol 1990;14:503–13.

94. Solcia E, Capella C, Sessa F, et al. Gastric carcinoids and related endocrine growths. Digestion 1986;35:3–22.

95. Solcia E, Fiocca R, Havu N, Dalvag A, Carlsson R. Gastric endocrine cells and gastritis in patients receiving long-term omeprazole treatment. Digestion 1992;51(Suppl 1):82–92.

96. Solcia E, Rindi G, Havu N, Elm G. Qualitative studies of gastric endocrine cells in patients treated long-term with omeprazole. Scand J Gastroenterol 1989;24:129–37.

97. Stachura J, Krause WJ, Ivey KJ. Ultrastructure of endocrine-like cells in lamina propria of human gastric mucosa. Gut 1981;22:534–41.

98. Stockbrugger RW, Menon GG, Beilby JO, Mason RR, Cotton PB. Gastroscopic screening in 80 patients with pernicious anaemia. Gut 1983;24:1141–7.

99. Stolte M, Ebert D, Seifert E, Schulte F, Rode J. The prognosis of carcinoid tumors of the stomach. Leber Magen Darm 1988;18:246–56.

100. Stremple JF, Watson CG. Serum calcium, serum gastrin, and gastric acid secretion before and after parathyroidectomy for hyperparathyroidism. Surgery 1974;75:841–52.

100a. Sugishita K, Tanno M, Kijima M, Kamoshita H, Mitamura T, Hayakawa K. Malignant hypercalcemia due to gastric endocrine cell carcinoma. Intern Med 1995;34:104–7.

101. Sweeney EC, McDonnell L. Atypical gastric carcinoids. Histopathology 1980;4:215–24.

102. Tahara E, Haizuka S, Kodama T, Yamada A. The relationship of gastrointestinal endocrine cells to gastric epithelial changes with special reference to gastric cancer. Acta Pathol Jpn 1975;25(2):161–77.

103. Teitelbaum SL. The carcinoid, a collective review. Am J Surg 1972;123:564–72.

103a. Thomas RM, Baybick JH, Elsayed AM, Sobin LH. Gastric carcinoids. An immunohistochemical and clinicopathologic study of 104 patients. Cancer 1994;73:2053–8.

104. Thompson RJ, Doran JF, Jackson P, Dhillon AP, Rode J. PGP 9,5—a new marker for vertebrate neurons and neuroendocrine cells. Brain Res 1983;278:224–8.

105. Vyberg M, Horn T, Francis D, Askaa J. Immunohistochemical identification of neuron-specific enolase, synaptophysin, chromogranin and endocrine granule constituent in neuroendocrine tumors. Acta Histochemica 1990;38:179–81.

106. Walsh JH. Functional and provocative tests for gastroduodenal disorders. J Clin Gastroenterol 1981; 3(Suppl 2):73–8.

107. Walsh JH, Nair PK, Kleibeuker J, et al. Pathological acid secretion not due to gastrinoma. Scand J Gastroenterol 1983;82:45–58.

108. Weiler R, Fisher-Colbrie R, Schmid KW, et al. Immunological studies on the occurrence and properties of chromogranin A and B and secretogranin II in endocrine tumors. Am J Surg Pathol 1988;12:877–84.

109. Wiedenmann B, Huttner WB. Synaptophysin and chromogranins/secretogranins—widespread constituents of distinct types of neuroendocrine vesicles and new tools in tumor diagnosis. Virchows Arch [Cell Pathol] 1989; 58:95–121.

110. Weidenmann B, Waldherr R, Buhr H, Hille A, Rosa P, Huttner WB. Identification of gastroenteropancreatic neuroendocrine cells in normal and neoplastic human tissue with antibodies against synaptophysin, chromogranin A, secretogranin I (chromogranin B) and secretogranin II. Gastroenterology 1988;95:1364–74.

111. Wilander E, El-Salhy M, Pitkanen P. Histopathology of gastric carcinoids: a survey of 42 cases. Histopathology 1984;8:183–93.

## Small Cell (Oat Cell) Carcinoma

112. Bader LV, Lykke AW, Hinterberger H. Multiple biogenic amine-secreting "carcinoid" tumour of the stomach: a case report. Pathology 1977;9:353–8.

112a. Chejfec G, Gould VE. Malignant gastric neuroendocrinomas. Ultrastructural and biochemical characterization of their secretory activity. Hum Pathol 1977;8:433–40.

113. Eimoto T, Hayakawa H. Oat cell carcinoma of the stomach. Pathol Res Pract 1980;168:229–36.

114. Fukuda T, Ohnishi Y, Nishimaki T, Ohtani H, Tachikawa S. Early gastric cancer of the small cell type. Am J Gastroenterol 1988;83:1176–9.

115. Hussein AM, Otrakji CL, Hussein BT. Small cell carcinoma of the stomach. Case report and review of the literature. Dig Dis Sci 1990;35:513–8.

116. Matsui K, Kitagawa M, Miwa A, Kuroda Y, Tsuji M. Small cell carcinoma of the stomach: a clinicopathologic study of 17 cases. Am J Gastroenterol 1991;86: 1167–75.

116a. Wilander E, El-Salhy M, Pitkanen P. Histopathology of gastric carcinoids: a survey of 42 cases. Histopathology 1984;8:183–93.

## Mixed Endocrine and Nonendocrine Epithelial Tumors

117. Ali MH, Davidson A, Azzopardi JG. Composite gastric carcinoid and adenocarcinoma. Histopathology 1984;8:529–36.

118. Andrew A. Further evidence that enterochromaffin cells are not derived from the neural crest. J Embryol Exp Morphol 1974;31:589–98.

119. Azzopardi JG, Pollock DJ. Argentaffin and argyrophil cells in gastric carcinoma. J Pathol Bacteriol 1963;86:443–51.

120. Gibbs NM. Incidence and significance of argentaffin and paneth cells in some tumours of the large intestine. J Clin Pathol 1967;20:826–31.

121. Gould VE, Memoli VA, Dardi LE, Sobel HJ, Somers SC, Johannessen JV. Neuroendocrine carcinomas with multiple immunoreactive peptides and melanin production. Ultrastruct Pathol 1981;2:199–217.

122. Hamperl H. Uber die argyrophile Zellen. Virchows Arch A Pathol Anat 1951;321:482–507.

123. Horn RC. Carcinoid tumors of the colon and rectum. Cancer 1949;2:819–37.

124. Kubo T, Watanabe H. Neoplastic argentaffin cells in gastric and intestinal carcinomas. Cancer 1971;27:447–54.

125. LeDouarin NM. The embryological origin of the endocrine cells associated with the digestive tract: experimental analysis based on the use of a stable cell marking technique. In: Bloom SR ed. Gut hormones. Edinburgh: Churchill Livingstone, 1978: 49–56.

126. Lewin K. Carcinoid tumors of the mixed (composite) glandular-endocrine cell carcinomas. Am J Surg Pathol 1987;11(Suppl 1):71–86.

127. Ooi A, Mai M, Ogino T, et al. Endocrine differentiation of gastric adenocarcinoma. The prevalence as evaluated by immunoreactive chromogranin A and its biologic significance. Cancer 1988;62:1096–104.

128. Pictet RL, Rall LB, Phelps P, Rutter WJ. The neural crest and the origin of the insulin-producing and other gastrointestinal hormone-producing cells. Science 1976;191:191–2.

129. Prade M, Bara J, Gadenne C, et al. Gastric carcinoma with argyrophilic cells: light microscopic, electron microscopic, and immunochemical study. Hum Pathol 1982;13:588–92.

130. Soga J, Tazawa K, Aizawa O, Wada K, Tuto O. Argentaffin cell adenocarcinoma of the stomach: an atypical carcinoid? Cancer 1971;28:999–1003.

131. Tahara E, Ito H, Nakagami K, Shimamoto F, Yamamoto M, Sumii K. Scirrhous argyrophil cell carcinoma of the stomach with multiple production of polypeptide hormones, amine, CEA, lysozyme, and HCG. Cancer 1982;49:1904–15.

132. Ulich T, Cheng L, Lewin KJ. Acinar-endocrine cell tumor of the pancreas. Report of a pancreatic tumor containing both zymogen and neuroendocrine granules. Cancer 1982;50:2099–105.

133. Ulich T, Kollin M, Lewin KJ. Composite gastric carcinoma. Report of a tumor of the carcinoma-carcinoid spectrum. Arch Pathol Lab Med 1988;112:91–3.

134. Yang GC, Rotterdam H. Mixed (composite) glandular-endocrine cell carcinoma of the stomach. Report of a case and review of literature. Am J Surg Pathol 1991;15:592–8.

## 13

# LYMPHOPROLIFERATIVE DISORDERS OF THE STOMACH

The gastrointestinal tract is a common site for lymphoproliferative disorders: about 50 percent of all primary extranodal lymphomas occur here (51,86). Gastrointestinal involvement is found at autopsy in 50 percent of patients with disseminated nodal lymphoma or lymphocytic leukemia (23,48,59,85,93,121,128,137). Although more than half of all primary and secondary gastrointestinal lymphomas in the United States are of gastric origin, overall these tumors are uncommon, representing only about 5 percent of all gastric tumors (85). However, there are indications that the incidence of primary gastric lymphoma is increasing. In one study based on data from the Surveillance, Epidemiology and End Results (SEER) program the incidence of gastric lymphoma in patients over the age of 60 years increased two-fold between 1973 and 1986. Whether this was due to better endoscopic diagnosis, more accurate separation of gastric lymphoid hyperplasias from lymphoma, or other factors is not known (23,57,127,134). There is also marked geographic variation in incidence of gastrointestinal lymphomas: in the Middle East, Iran, and South Africa there is a greater incidence of intestinal lymphoma (about 35 percent) than gastric lymphoma because of the high incidence of Mediterranean lymphoma and alpha-chain disease (59,85). Advances in immunophenotyping of gastric lymphomas (as well as other gastrointestinal lymphomas) has led to a better understanding of the pathogenesis, pathology, and clinical behavior of many of these lymphomas. For example, low-grade B-cell gastric lymphomas possess many histologic similarities to normal mucosa-associated lymphoid tissue (MALT) and differ significantly morphologically and immunophenotypically from primary nodal lymphomas. However, despite these advances there are still problems with the classification of gastric lymphomas. The Working Formulation and Kiel classification systems, which were devised for nodal lymphomas, are difficult to apply to many of gastrointestinal lymphomas. Consequently Isaacson (71) and Hall (52) have proposed alternative classifications for gastrointestinal dis-

orders based on current knowledge of MALT. However, these classifications are not entirely satisfactory either, as will be discussed.

Gastric lymphoid hyperplasia (pseudolymphoma) is a controversial lesion. Some authorities question whether these lesions indeed exist or are actually low-grade lymphomas. This problem is partially linked to the question of whether monoclonality occurs in lymphoid hyperplasia or whether it automatically denotes lymphoma (18,142,148).

## LYMPHOMA

**Definition.** Primary gastric lymphomas are defined in the same way as primary gastrointestinal lymphomas, namely, as lymphomas presenting in the stomach and in which there is no evidence of liver, spleen, peripheral or mediastinal lymph node, and bone marrow involvement at the time of presentation. Problems in definition arise in those cases of lymphoma presenting with gastric manifestations but which on work-up are found to be microscopically disseminated. Are these cases of primary gastric lymphoma with secondary dissemination (which we know can occur in roughly 50 percent of cases) or do they represent nodal lymphomas with gastric involvement? We and others prefer to regard them as gastrointestinal lymphomas with dissemination, although it is possible that some cases may be disseminated nodal lymphoma (86,87,162). This question may well be resolved in the future, since MALTomas appear to be immunophenotypically distinct from the nodal types of lymphoma (see Classification). From a practical point of view the question is somewhat moot as these lymphomas need to be managed as disseminated lymphomas. Another interesting distinction between low-grade MALTomas and nodal lymphomas is that the former appear to remain localized to the gastrointestinal tract for a long time. However, this has been disputed by some (162) and, if on definitional grounds one excludes all gastrointestinal lymphomas which on presentation show evidence of dissemination, because of the difficulty of excluding disseminated nodal lymphoma, then it is not surprising that these "early" lymphomas behave in a relatively less aggressive manner and remain localized.

**Incidence.** Figures on the incidence of gastric lymphoma are given in the introductory paragraph. However, because of the definitional problems in separating primary gastric lymphoma from secondary lymphomatous involvement of the stomach these figures may not be entirely correct. The recently described genetic and immunohistochemical differences between nodal lymphomas and MALTomas, such as the lack of *bcl*-2 rearrangement, CD5 and CD10 negativity, and KB61 positivity in gastric lymphomas (73), may help in determining the true incidence of primary lymphomas in future studies.

**Clinical Features.** Primary gastric lymphomas involve predominantly middle-aged and elderly patients of either sex, and with the exception of the "Mediterranean lymphomas," which are very rare in the stomach, show no significant racial distribution (2,7,36,42,43,48,86,156). Low-grade lymphomas are typically slow growing, with a low incidence of mesenteric node involvement and extraintestinal dissemination. Small foci of lymphoma at distances remote from the main tumor mass and consisting of a single reactive lymphoid follicle surrounded by tumor have been reported (66,169). If they recur, they tend to involve other parts of the gastrointestinal tract or Waldeyer's ring. There are indications that the incidence of these tumors is increasing for reasons that are unclear but possibly due to changes in diagnostic criteria (23,57,134). Patients with high-grade lymphomas present with signs and symptoms similar to those of gastric cancer, such as early satiety, weight loss, and anemia, or peptic ulcer symptoms. In advanced cases there may be frank obstruction, sometimes accompanied by a palpable mass.

**Pathogenesis.** The majority of gastric lymphomas are of B-cell origin; only a few gastric T-cell lymphomas have been described (9,49,96, 173). The precise cell of origin of gastrointestinal B-cell lymphomas is uncertain but genetic and immunophenotypic studies have shown that many lymphomas, especially low-grade MALTomas, are homologous with normal mucosa-associated lymphoid tissue; others (probably a minority) are identical to nodal lymphomas (55,70). In one study, Isaacson (20) found the coexistence of low- and high-grade lymphoma in 28 percent of cases, suggesting that some if not most high-grade lymphomas originate from low-grade MALTomas. Isaacson and others have reported that the low-grade B-cell lymphomas are phenotypically similar to B lymphocytes of the marginal zones of the spleen and lymph nodes (104, 107,163). These findings suggest that at least low-grade gastrointestinal lymphomas arise from the outer mantle zone region (the marginal zone) of intestinal lymphoid follicles rather than from germinal center cells. Of further interest is the fact that monocytoid B-cell lymphomas and some cases of MALToma appear to be morphologically and phenotypically indistinguishable, and in one report a number of patients with nodal monocytoid B-cell lymphoma had concomitant gastric and other extranodal lesions. However, it remains to be determined whether these two tumors are in fact the same but arising in different tissues (3,80,104).

The pathogenesis of gastric lymphoma remains uncertain, although a number of associations are emerging such as with *Helicobacter pylori* infection (47,66,110); gastric lymphoid hyperplasia; immunodeficiency disorders, both primary and acquired; and occasionally, familial tendency (58). Celiac sprue, which usually predisposes to intestinal lymphoma, may occasionally be associated with gastric lymphoma.

It has been shown that the frequency of *H. pylori* infection in patients with low-grade lymphoma is similar to that found in gastric carcinoma (80 to 90 percent) and substantially higher than that found in the background population (50 to 60 percent) (110,170). It has been shown that some strains of *H. pylori* appear to be more virulent and more likely to predispose the host to neoplasia. These strains include *CagA,* a gene found in approximately 60 percent of *H. pylori* strains, and *VacA* (vacuolating cytoxin) genotype (14a,25a, 113a). Wotherspoon and colleagues (170) hypothesized that *H. pylori*–induced gastritis induces a lymphoid infiltrate with associated lymphoid follicles, similar to the mucosa-associated lymphoid tissue of the intestines, and provides the background on which other yet unidentified factors, for example mutagens in the diet, act to produce lymphoma in a small proportion of cases (69).

Much of the recent literature on diffuse, superficial, benign-appearing lymphoproliferative lesions of the stomach, often containing admixed plasma cells and lymphoid follicles, has been devoted to discussing whether these lesions are lymphoid hyperplasias or low-grade lymphomas (15,18,33,65,95,126,130,132,142,166). Is there such a thing as a benign gastric lymphoproliferative lesion, the lymphoid equivalent of adenoma/dysplasia of the stomach, which has a propensity toward malignancy? It is noteworthy that the above-mentioned features of lymphoid hyperplasia are not unique to the stomach and similar infiltrations have been described at other sites of the gastrointestinal tract, the orbit, salivary glands, skin, lung, and breast (40,130,148).

Since many diffuse lymphoproliferative lesions of the stomach are monotypic and have gene rearrangements, does monoclonality always denote lymphoma? In the past, monoclonality was considered the sine qua non of malignancy or at least an intermediary stage in the evolution of lymphoma (142,148), but the biologic significance of monoclonality is no longer so clear. A number of clonal but benign lymphocytic proliferations have been described at other sites, including benign monoclonal gammopathy and idiopathic cold hemaglutinin disease, which have an increased but not absolute risk of malignant transformation (46). This would suggest that monoclonality might be an intermediate stage in the evolution of lymphoma although representing two separate events.

The following hypothesis, a modification of one put forward by Sigal (142), best summarizes our current understanding of the pathogenesis of lymphoid hyperplasia and its relationship to gastric lymphoma. Mucosal ulceration or *H. pylori* gastritis leads to chronic antigenic stimulation, which results in follicular gastritis composed of a dense polyclonal lymphoid infiltrate. Continued antigenic stimulation, coupled with mutagens in the diet, may give rise to one or more clones of lymphoid cells. Initially the clones are dependent on antigenic and environmental factors and are at least under limited control. In the stomach for example, as detailed above, MALTomas may regress with antibiotic therapy (10a,64,150,167,168) and the same has been reported in cases of immunoproliferative small intestinal disease (IPSID) and IPSID-associated lymphomas (presumably by reducing the antigenic stimuli). However, with time, the lesion becomes autonomous, although this may not be recognizable morphologically (18a). At this point the lesion may be viewed as a benign neoplasm with limited growth potential. With further passage of time, malignant lymphoma may ensue, characterized by increase in lesion size, cytologic atypia, and metastasis (142).

From a practical viewpoint, however, since we cannot at this stage differentiate morphologically benign-behaving lymphoid lesions from low-grade lymphomas, all these lesions are best considered low-grade lymphomas.

**Classification.** Gastric lymphomas have histologic features in common with other gastrointestinal lymphomas. Therefore, the classification of all gastrointestinal lymphomas is presented, since all types of lymphoma may occur in the stomach, although the frequency of the specific types varies greatly from one site to another. With the current availability of many monoclonal antibodies and molecular biology techniques such as gene rearrangement analysis, it is now possible to determine the cell lineage of most gastric lymphomas. With the exception of a few cases of T-cell lymphoma, all gastric lymphomas are of B-cell derivation. The majority are *diffuse lymphomas; follicular lymphomas* are rare (probably around 10 percent). Sometimes diffuse lymphomas mimic nodular lymphomas; for example, *multiple lymphomatous polyposes* (many of which are disseminated mantle zone lymphomas) usually appear as nodular aggregates throughout the gut. Also, *diffuse low-grade B-cell lymphomas (low-grade MALTomas)* have been reported to colonize hyperplastic lymphoid follicles and mimic nodular lymphoma (72). *Primary Hodgkin's disease* (144) of the stomach and *true histiocytic lymphomas* are rare, and most cases are misdiagnosed *immunoblastic lymphoma* or the occasional *Ki-1 (CD-30) lymphoma:* the scattered pleomorphic cells containing multilobed nuclei and prominent nucleoli resemble Reed-Sternberg cells (29, 86,112,122,144). *Immunoproliferative small intestinal disease (IPSID)* and associated lymphoma (considered a subtype of MALToma by Isaacson) is a unique B-cell lymphoma of the gastrointestinal tract (116), although rare in the stomach. *Burkitt's lymphoma* is another tumor often originating in the gut, although rare in the stomach (84,89). A number of lymphomas are

Table 13-1

## CLASSIFICATION OF GASTROINTESTINAL LYMPHOMAS

| | Working Formulation Equivalent | Updated Kiel Classification Equivalent |
|---|---|---|
| **B-Cell** | | |
| *LOW GRADE* | | |
| **Gut Type** | | |
| MALToma (marginal) | Small lymphocytic, plasmacytoid | Low-grade lymphoma of MALT |
| IPSID and α-chain disease* (Mediterranean lymphoma) | | α-chain disease |
| Plasmacytoma | | Immunocytoma |
| **Nodal Type** | | |
| Follicular center cell lymphoma | Diffuse small or mixed | Centoblastic/centrocytic |
| Follicular and diffuse | Follicular | |
| Diffuse | | |
| Multiple lymphomatous polyposis (MLP)/Mantle cell lymphoma | | Centrocytic with MLP |
| *HIGH GRADE* | | |
| **Gut Type** | | |
| High-grade MALToma | Diffuse large cell and | |
| IPSID-associated lymphoma | immunoblastic | |
| **Nodal Type** | | |
| Diffuse large cell and other types of nodal lymphoma | Diffuse large cell and immunoblastic | Centroblastic (classic, polymorphic, centrocytoid, multilobulated) |
| Burkitt and Burkitt type | Burkitt and Burkitt type | Burkitt and Burkitt type |
| Large cell anaplastic (Ki=1) | Large cell anaplastic (Ki=1) | Large cell anaplastic (Ki=1) |
| *UNCLASSIFIABLE* | | |
| Post-transplant lymphoproliferative disorder | | |
| Polyclonal | | |
| Monoclonal | | |
| **T-Cell** | | |
| Enteropathy associated | | |
| Nonenteropathy associated | | |

*IPSID = immunoproliferative small intestinal disease.

impossible to subclassify beyond their lymphoid derivation and are designated as "unclassified."

Although the cell lineage of most gastric lymphomas can be readily determined, there is currently still no universally accepted classification system for gastric or gastrointestinal lymphomas. Some authorities have used phenotypic data as the basis for classifying these tumors but unfortunately the phenotype of the lymphoma, the morphology, and the clinical outcome do not always correlate.

The major classification systems currently used are the Working Formulation, the Kiel classification, one proposed by Isaacson, and the World Health Organization (WHO) modification of the Working Formulation (Table 13-1). The problem with the Working Formulation is that it was originally developed for nodal lymphomas, and many gastrointestinal lymphomas are histologically distinctive and appear to be derived from gut-associated lymphoid tissue. Many gastrointestinal lymphomas, such as low-grade lymphomas (MALTomas), multiple lymphomatous polyposis, Mediterranean lymphomas (IPSID-associated lymphomas), and enteropathy-associated T-cell lymphomas, show histologic features distinct from nodal lymphomas.

Because of these problems with the Working Formulation classification, Isaacson (68,70,71) proposed an alternative classification for gastrointestinal tumors based on their unique clinicopathologic features, morphogenesis (derivation of many from the normal mucosa-associated lymphoid tissue), histology, and phenotype. His classification, however, is not entirely satisfactory because not all gastrointestinal lymphomas fit into neat morphologic categories. Low-grade lymphomas (MALTomas) have histologic features resembling normal mucosa-associated lymphoid tissue, namely, prominent reactive-appearing lymphoid follicles with neoplastic cells occupying the mantle or marginal zones, plasma cells distributed in distinct subepithelial or interfollicular zones, and lymphoepithelial lesions (see Histology) (99). However, on closer examination, there is a great variability of morphology ranging from mature-appearing lymphocytes to larger somewhat cleaved cells (Isaacson's centrocyte-like cells) to monocytoid (clear) cells to plasmacytoid cells (99). Furthermore, some of the described MALTomas are monomorphous, whereas others are polymorphous with admixed inflammatory cells which are sometimes so prominent that they partially obscure the malignant infiltrate. Also, not all mucosal lymphomas are MALT-type lymphomas. Furthermore, several tissues with large normal lymphoid structures, such as Peyer's patches and Waldeyer's ring, probably give rise to nodal-type lymphomas rather than MALTomas. In contrast, low-grade B-cell MALTomas are most common in the stomach where there is no normal lymphoid tissue (55). In Isaacson's classification, MALTomas are subdivided into low grade and high grade, on the presumption that many, if not most, high-grade tumors are derived from low-grade MALTomas, based on the finding of mixed patterns such as high-grade lymphomas with foci of low-grade MALToma (20). While this is probably true, it might be asked whether by classifying MALTomas into high and low grades, the term MALToma is just being substituted for gastrointestinal

lymphoma, since high-grade tumors of nodal and MALT type cannot be distinguished morphologically; the unique clinicopathologic characteristics of low-grade tumors are then not identified. While the concept of MALToma is attractive and provides a useful framework for understanding gastrointestinal lymphomas, it does not explain everything about these tumors. The most practical value of this concept is the realization that the low-grade tumors may have characteristic histologic features and, frequently, a benign course.

The ideal classification of gastrointestinal lymphomas is one that recognizes all histologic varieties of non-Hodgkin's lymphomas. At the present time no satisfactory scheme has been developed. Nevertheless, it is important to strive toward a uniform classification so that treatment protocols and prognostic factors in studies from different centers can be compared.

A number of principles regarding classification of gastrointestinal lymphomas have been generally accepted. These are: determining whether the lymphoma is primary or secondary (immunohistochemistry may help to differentiate); determining whether it is of B- or T-cell origin; determining whether it is of mucosal or nodal type; and categorizing it as low or high grade.

The classification we have adopted is a modification of Isaacson's and Kiel's (30); we have found this to be of greatest practical value (Table 13-1). Gastric lymphomas are subdivided into low and high grades rather than low, intermediate, and high grades as in the Working Formulation, because several recent publications have indicated that this more accurately predicts their clinical behavior.

**Radiologic and Endoscopic Findings.** At endoscopy or barium X-ray examination, gastric lymphomas exhibit three main patterns: ulceration, polypoid mass, or diffuse growth (14,41, 133,154). The small lesions appear as roughened hyperemic patches or small erosions with prominent margins. Larger diffuse lesions are characterized by thickened, stiff, sometimes nodular mucosal folds that may or may not be ulcerated and involve the entire body or antrum. These lesions may be indistinguishable from advanced carcinoma. The localized lesions are less common, and consist of a tumorous raised lesion with a central stellate ulcer and a sharp margin between the lesion and the normal mucosa (fig. 13-1).

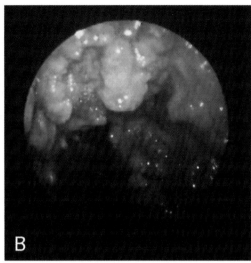

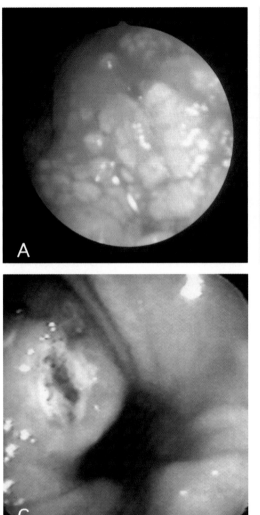

Figure 13-1
MALIGNANT LYMPHOMA OF THE
STOMACH: ENDOSCOPIC APPEARANCE
A: Slightly raised nodular mucosal lesions.
B: Irregular mucosal masses which are indistin-
guishable from carcinoma. (Fig. 5-23 from Lewin
KJ, Riddell RH, Weinstein WM. Gastrointestinal
pathology and its clinical implication. New York:
Igaku Shoin, 1992:171.)
C: Raised, centrally ulcerated nodule with
smooth mucosal margins.

**Gross Findings.** Like carcinomas, gastric lymphomas may occur in any part of the stomach but are most common in the antrum. Occasionally they present as exaggerated mucosal folds and may look like Menetrier's disease. They are usually single although several studies have found tiny, often microscopic, mucosal tumor foci, distinct from the main mass, throughout the stomach (37, 67,158,169). Multiple gross lesions occur in up to 20 percent of cases but are usually found in the same general area (27,36,86).

At the time of diagnosis, the tumors vary greatly in size. Early lesions average less than 1 cm in largest diameter and are increasingly being recognized; large lesions average about 8 cm in diameter, and were previously the most frequently seen gastric lymphomas (86).

Generally, the gross appearance is related to the grade of the tumor. Low-grade tumors tend to be superficial with minimal ulceration; high-grade tumors are diffusely infiltrative nodular masses with extensive ulceration and which sometimes perforate.

The small lesions have a flat, irregular, granular or nodular appearance, sometimes associated with surface erosions (fig. 13-2A). They are often localized to the mucosa and submucosa.

Large gastric lymphomas may mimic gastric ulcers or carcinomas (fig. 13-2B,C). They may form multiple polypoid masses or infiltrative lesions with localized mucosal ulceration. The tumor margins are typically wide, raised, and well defined. There may be uniform thickening of the gastric wall, extending anywhere from the

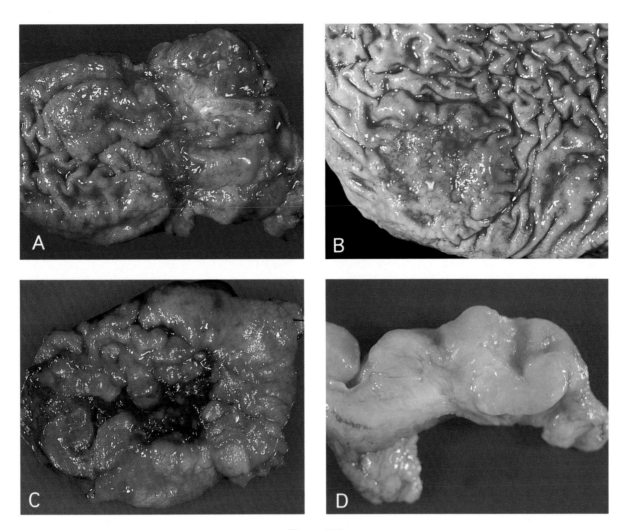

Figure 13-2
MALIGNANT LYMPHOMA OF THE STOMACH: GROSS APPEARANCE
A: A small nodular lesion.
B: An elevated tumor mass with an irregular granular surface and well-defined margin.
C: A tumor mass with an ulcerated nodular surface.
D: Cut surface of a gastric lymphoma showing the characteristic "fish-flesh" appearance involving the full thickness of the stomach wall.

submucosa through the muscularis propria to the serosa and sometimes to the adjacent viscera. Sometimes, annular, napkin ring–like lesions are formed which mimic carcinoma. On cut section they have a characteristic white-yellow appearance and a "fish flesh" consistency (fig. 13-2D). Since lymphomas of the gastrointestinal tract in general, including gastric lymphoma, are at times associated with destruction of the full thickness of the bowel wall without an associated desmoplastic reaction, it is not surprising that some may perforate (7,84,88).

Multiple lymphomatous polyposis (mantle cell lymphoma) is an uncommon form of gastrointestinal lymphoma and is exceedingly rare in the stomach (25,27,105,124). Grossly, it is characterized by numerous tiny, tan mucosal nodules, about 2 to 3 mm in diameter, often occurring throughout the gut. It should be stressed that secondary involvement of the gastrointestinal tract by leukemia and other nodal lymphomas may also result in multiple intestinal polyps and is more common than multiple lymphomatous polyposis (38,96a, 176). In our experience, the lymphomatous polyps due to secondary involvement by nodal lymphoma are usually much larger (often greater than 5 mm in diameter) than those found in multiple lymphomatous polyposis. The leukemic lesions on the other hand, which are commonly a terminal event, consist of multiple, small, bluish mucosal nodules usually measuring less than 5 mm in diameter (for a detailed discussion see Subtypes of Gastric Lymphoma and Leukemic Involvement of the Stomach).

**Microscopic Findings.** Low-grade lymphomas tend to be limited to the mucosa and superficial submucosa (fig. 13-3). The infiltrate causes expansion and thickening of the mucosa, frequently replacing the glandular compartment. The gastric pits or glands are pushed apart from one another and from the underlying muscularis mucosae and there is transmigration of atypical lymphocytes through the gastric pits or glands and surface epithelium, often with destruction of epithelium. The destructive epithelial lymphoid infiltrates have been called lymphoepithelial lesions and are sometimes difficult to find (fig. 13-4). Keratin stains highlight the epithelial destruction and lymphoid infiltration (fig. 13-4J). The more advanced gastric lymphomas are commonly associated with mucosal ulceration and more extensive infiltration of the viscus. Invasion may occur in a band-like manner, with a pushing border (fig. 13-3B), sometimes associated with underlying fibrosis. In other cases the lymphoma has an irregular infiltrating margin (fig. 13-3D) which sometimes elicits a dense desmoplastic reaction; in our experience this occurs most commonly when there is perigastric extension.

The lymphoma commonly invades the muscle coats in a single-file pattern, separating individual muscle fibers (fig. 13-3E). A similar invasion of muscle fibers may be seen involving the vasculature. Eventually the muscle undergoes atrophy or lysis.

Histologically, gastric lymphomas are typically composed of a dense monomorphous infiltrate of mature-appearing or atypical lymphocytes (fig. 13-4G). Low-grade tumors are frequently polymorphous and often peppered with numerous inflammatory cells that consist primarily of mature lymphocytes, plasma cells, histiocytes, eosinophils, and lymphoid follicles (fig. 13-4A). Sometimes the admixed inflammatory infiltrate is so dense that it obscures the underlying

lymphoma and is confused with lymphoid hyperplasia (86). Differentiation of gastric lymphoma from the latter is discussed under differential diagnosis. Another rare histologic variant of lymphoma is accompanied by marked eosinophilia and may mimic eosinophilic gastroenteritis. This appears to be a T-cell lymphoma that is usually found in the small intestine but has also been described in the stomach (135).

The precise incidence of the different subtypes of gastric lymphoma varies from one study to another because of the different classifications used and because of geographic variation. However, the main histologic subtypes often have characteristic microscopic and behavioral features and these are described below.

*Low-Grade Mucosal Type Lymphomas.* 1) The MALTomas (Marginal). Low-grade lymphomas frequently have histologic features in common with normal mucosa-associated lymphoid tissue, namely, prominent reactive-appearing lymphoid follicles, plasma cells, and transmigrating epithelial lymphocytes. The lymphoid follicles are frequently partially or totally surrounded by a sheath of neoplastic cells occupying the mantle or marginal zones (fig. 13-4A,B); plasma cells (which may be reactive or monotypic) are distributed below the surface epithelium or the interfollicular zones (fig. 13-4F). Lymphoepithelial lesions (fig. 13-4H–J) are characterized by clusters of at least three or more atypical lymphocytes infiltrating and destroying the foveolar or glandular epithelium. They differ from the normal transmigrating epithelial lymphoctyes which consist of scattered single mature lymphocytes, usually of T-cell type, lying between the epithelial cells. Occasionally, the lymphoid follicles may be colonized by lymphomatous cells.

Cytologically, an admixture of lymphocytic cell types is commonly found within MALTomas, although one cell type may predominate. MALTomas are characteristically CD5, CD10, and bcl-2 negative and CD22 and 43 positive (fig. 13-5). The commonly found types of lymphocytes are small lymphocytes, lymphoplasmacytoid cells, Isaacson's centrocyte-like cells, and mixtures of the three (figs. 13-4, 13-6). The small lymphocytes often resemble normal mature lymphocytes. However, careful cytologic examination often reveals slightly abnormal cells characterized by somewhat enlarged, irregular or wrinkled nuclei with

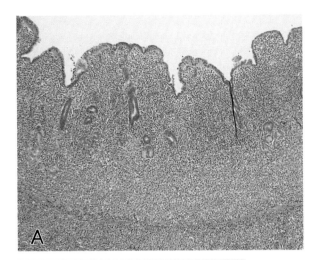

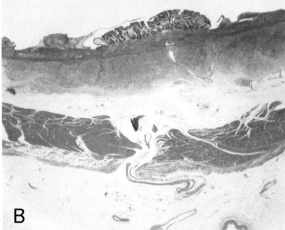

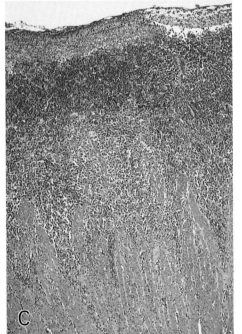

### Figure 13-3
### LOW-GRADE GASTRIC LYMPHOMA:
### ARCHITECTURAL CHARACTERISTICS

A: Low-power view of mucosa showing a dense lymphocytic infiltrate pushing apart the gastric pits and glands and elevating them away from the muscularis mucosae.

B: Scanning-power view of a dense lymphoid infiltrate of mucosa and superficial submucosa with a pushing margin. Although there are mucosal erosions, the typical features of a chronic gastric ulcer with destruction of muscle coats and fibrosis are absent.

C: Lymphomatous infiltrate showing an irregular lower margin, infiltrating the muscularis propria.

D: Higher magnification of B demonstrating mucosal erosion and a dense submucosal lymphoid infiltrate.

E: Malignant lymphoma showing separation of the muscle fibers of the muscularis propria by the lymphomatous infiltrate.

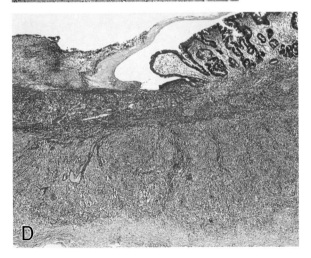

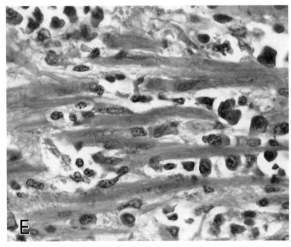

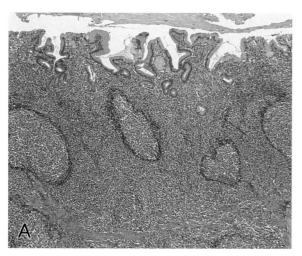

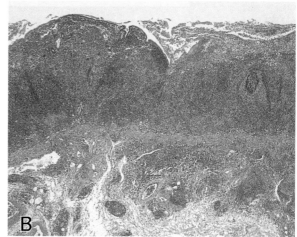

Figure 13-4

GASTRIC LYMPHOMA, LOW-GRADE MALTOMA:
HISTOLOGIC CHARACTERISTICS

A: Mucosa showing a diffuse infiltrate with several well-defined lymphoid follicles in the center.

B: Section of gastric mucosa and submucosa showing a diffuse lymphoid infiltrate. There are numerous ill-defined lymphoid follicles both within the lymphoid infiltrate and in the submucosa at the periphery of the infiltrate.

C: Lymphoid follicle colonized by the lymphomatous infiltrate.

D: Higher magnification of the germinal center showing the diffuse infiltrate consisting of small lymphocytes. (C,D courtesy of Dr. B. Schnitzer, Ann Arbor, MI.)

E: High-power magnification showing a diffuse monomorphous lymphoid infiltrate composed of mature-appearing lymphocytes. Some of the cells appear somewhat larger than normal lymphocytes and have an irregular outline. Several larger mononuclear cells can also be seen in the center of the field.

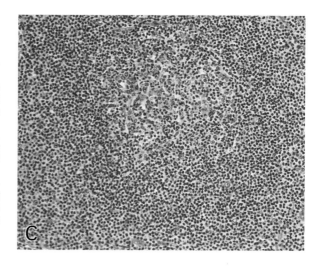

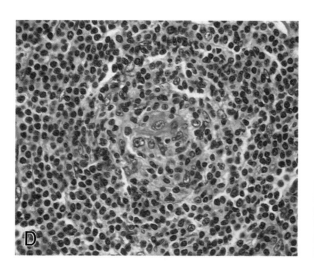

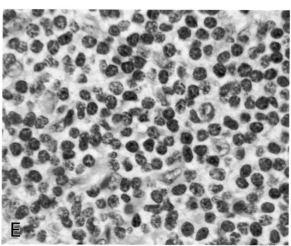

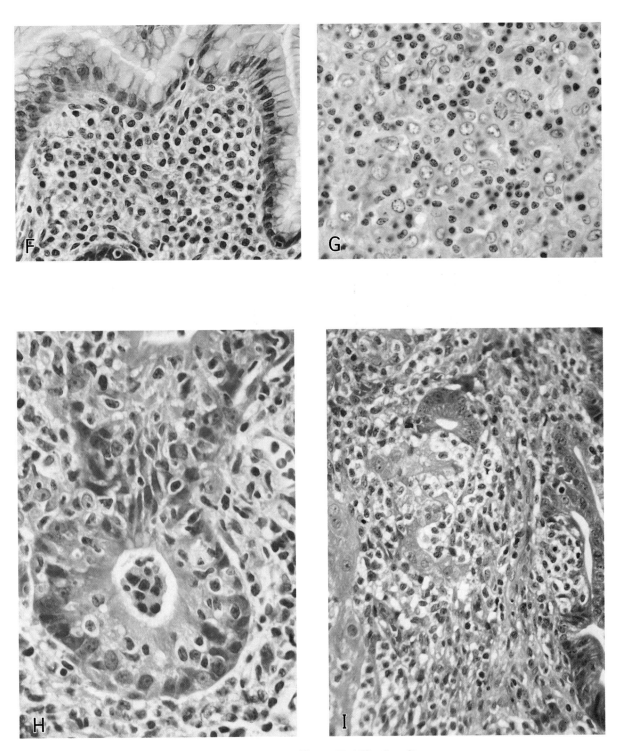

Figure 13-4 (Continued)

F: High-power magnification of the superficial mucosa shows the monomorphous infiltrate which is composed of plasmacytoid cells.

G: Malignant lymphoma of the stomach with a lymphomatous infiltrate admixed with mature-appearing lymphocytes.

H: High-power magnification of a lymphoepithelial lesion showing a gastric gland infiltrated by the atypical small cleaved lymphocytes.

I: A lymphoepithelial lesion causing destruction of gastric glands. There is a diffuse lymphoid infiltrate in the center of which are several lymphoepithelial lesions that have partially destroyed the glands.

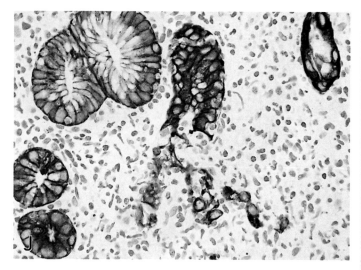

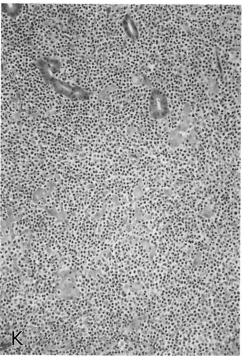

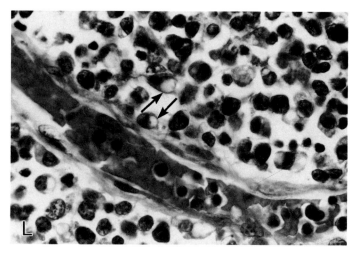

Figure 13-4 (Continued)
GASTRIC LYMPHOMA, LOW-GRADE
MALTOMA: HISTOLOGIC CHARACTERISTICS

J: Immunoperoxidase reaction with anti-cytokeratin antibody demonstrating the infiltration and destruction of the gastric glands.

K: Low-power view of gastric mucosa shows massive substitution of gastric glands by the lymphomatous infiltrate.

L: Malignant lymphoma, diffuse small cell type (well-differentiated lymphocytic). Note the diffuse monomorphous infiltrate composed of mature-looking lymphocytes, some of which show cytoplasmic vacuolation and produce a signet-ring cell pattern (arrows).

less dense chromatin. These MALTomas are sometimes difficult to differentiate from lymphoid hyperplasia, disseminated nodal small lymphocytic cell lymphoma, and gastric involvement by chronic lymphocytic leukemia. The latter, which is exceedingly rare in the stomach, can be excluded by examining blood and bone marrow smears. Nodal small lymphocytic cell lymphoma, which is most unusual in the stomach, can be differentiated immunohistochemically since these lesions are virtually always CD5 positive compared to MALTomas which are CD5, CD10, and *bcl*-2 negative, and CD22 positive.

Lymphoplasmacytoid cells (fig. 13-4F) often contain intracytoplasmic immunoglobulin, commonly of the IgM class, with light chain restriction and Dutcher's bodies (intranuclear periodic acid–Schiff [PAS] inclusions). The cytoplasmic immunoglobulin has a perinuclear distribution that can be demonstrated in formalin-fixed tissues; in some cases it is so abundant that it produces a signet-ring–like cell which may mimic carcinoma (fig. 13-4L) (60,160,174a). Since the immunoglobulin in these cells is PAS positive, it may be confused with signet-ring cell carcinoma. Rarely, some cases are associated with Waldenstrom's macroglobulinemia.

Isaacson's centrocyte-like cells are lymphocytes intermediate between cells of small lymphocytic and small cleaved cell lymphoma. They

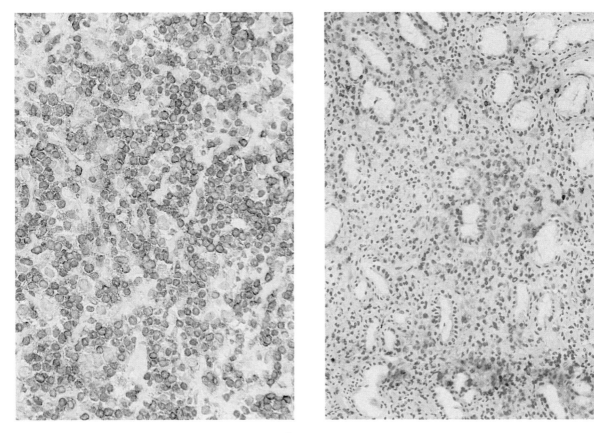

Figure 13-5
CD5 IMMUNOHISTOCHEMISTRY OF A PRIMARY NODAL LYMPHOMA
AND A PRIMARY GASTRIC LYMPHOMA OF MUCOSAL TYPE
There is diffuse staining of the lymph node (left) compared to the stomach (right) which shows only rare immunostaining of mature lymphocytes. (Courtesy of Dr. J. Said, Los Angeles, CA.)

have a dense nucleus which is irregular in shape but not as cleaved as in the cell of classic cleaved cell lymphoma. Variants of centrocyte-like cells are common and seem to have more abundant clear cytoplasm and well-defined cell margins resembling monocytoid B-cell nodal lymphoma (fig. 13-6E). The relationship of these lymphomas to monocytoid B-cell lymphoma is still unclear; the typical cases of monocytoid B-cell lymphoma appear to have unique features and only rarely has extranodal involvement been described (68,70,73,74,94,148).

It is not uncommon for there to be admixtures of the above described three cell types. In addition, large noncleaved lymphocytes may be scattered in between the small lymphocytes.

In summary, MALTomas consist of a dense, commonly heterogenous infiltrate of lymphocytes varying from almost normal-appearing cells to

cells somewhat similar but smaller than small cleaved lymphocytes; of plasma cells and lymphoplasmacytoid cells sometimes containing Dutcher's bodies; and of admixed reactive lymphoid follicles and pathognomonic lymphoepithelial lesions.

2) Immunoproliferative Small Intestinal Disease (IPSID). This is a disease of teenagers or young adults who usually present with symptoms of malabsorption and abdominal pain. It occurs primarily in developing nations with poor socioeconomic conditions. It affects mainly the small bowel but occasionally involves the stomach. Histologically, it is characterized by a dense lymphoid infiltrate of the mucosa composed of mature plasma cells and less commonly of lymphocytes. It is usually associated with alpha-heavy chain production, although the serum concentrations may be very low and it may be

369

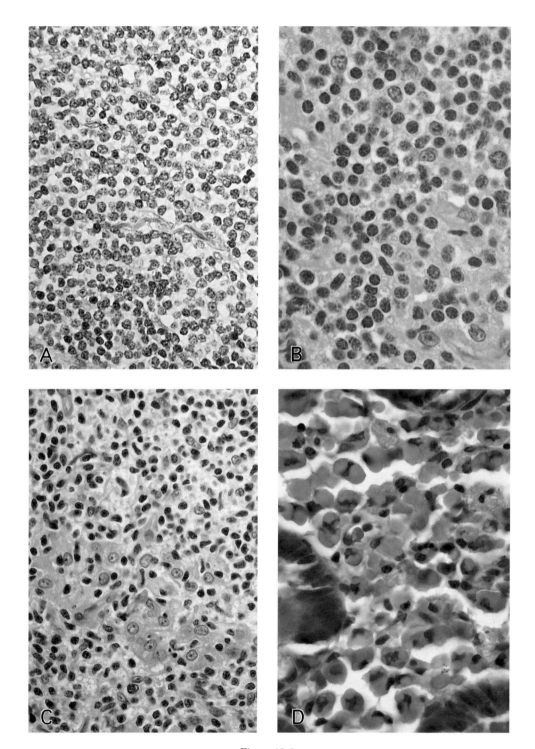

Figure 13-6
LOW-GRADE MALTOMA: HISTOLOGIC SPECTRUM

A: There is a diffuse monomorphous infiltrate composed of small lymphocytes.

B: The lymphoid infiltrate is composed primarily of small lymphocytes. Scattered larger lymphoid cells are also present.

C: The lymphoid infiltrate in this lymphoma is composed of small, elongated, cleaved lymphocytes some of which are seen infiltrating an oxyntic gland.

D: Maltoma with marked plasma cell differentiation. The cytoplasm is markedly distended by immunoglobulin globules (Russell bodies) which have also displaced the mildly atypical nuclei, to the periphery of the cell.

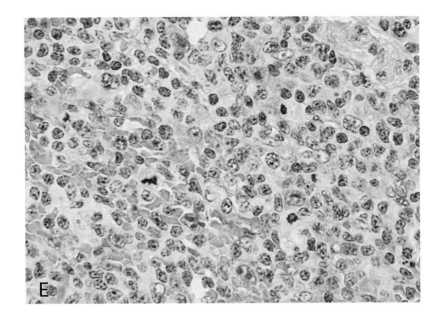

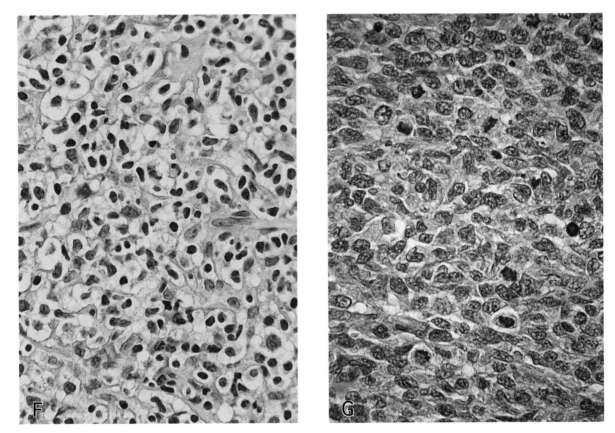

Figure 13-6 (Continued)

E: In this MALToma there is an admixture of small and large lymphocytes indicating transformation from low- to high-grade MALToma.

F: MALToma composed of lymphocytes with abundant clear cytoplasm and well-defined cell margins resembling intermediate cell lymphoma (Isaacson's centrocytic-like cells).

G: This MALToma is composed predominantly of larger oblong wrinkled lymphocytes. The cytologic features favor those of a high-grade MALToma. However, lymphoma of nodal type needs to be excluded.

necessary to demonstrate this product within the cytoplasm of the plasma cells. The latter cases, which are indistinguishable from IPSID, have been called alpha-chain disease. Lymphoma, usually of B-cell immunoblastic type, develops in the majority of cases after many years (87). However, Price (116) believes all cases of IPSID represent lymphoma that dedifferentiates into high-grade lymphoma with time.

*Low-Grade Nodal Type Lymphomas.* 1) Follicular Center Cell Lymphomas, Follicular and Diffuse. These lymphomas are rare in the stomach and may be either follicular or follicular and diffuse (fig. 13-7) (86). Histologically and phenotypically they resemble their counterparts in lymph nodes. The nodular tumors may be morphologically indistinguishable from MALTomas, with follicular colonization of hyperplastic lymphoid follicles, and may only be differentiated by immunohistochemical markers such as CD5 and CD10 (see Table 13-1) (72). Follicular lymphoma must not be confused with multiple lymphomatous polyposis which is a diffuse lymphoma characterized by nodular infiltrates (see below).

2) Multiple Lymphomatous Polyposis. The literature on this subject is confusing. The entity of multiple lymphomatous polyposis was first introduced by Cornes in 1961 (25) to describe an intestinal lymphoma that presented as multiple polyps affecting long segments of the gastrointestinal tract. Since then only 24 cases have been reported (25,105). However, it is apparent that multiple lymphomatous polyps of the gastrointestinal tract can be part of a primary lesion or part of disseminated nodal lymphoma. As already indicated, disseminated nodal lymphoma is the most common cause of lymphomatous polyposis; terminal leukemia also results in multiple nodular deposits throughout the gastrointestinal tract.

The term multiple lymphomatous polyposis is currently restricted to a fairly distinctive form of diffuse lymphomatous polyps with immunophenotypic features of mantle cell lymphoma. What is still unclear about this condition is whether it is a primary disorder of the gastrointestinal tract or representative of disseminated mantle cell lymphoma in which the lymph node lesions are initially clinically inapparent.

Clinically, this is a disease of the middle aged and elderly, the mean age being about 60 years, and is more common in males. Patients usually present with nonspecific generalized symptoms such as weight loss, fatigue, and iron deficiency anemia. Any part of the gastrointestinal tract may be involved including the stomach; however, the ileocecal region is the most common site of involvement. Barium studies and endoscopy reveal multiple polyps.

Grossly, the lesions consist of small, fleshy, sessile or pedunculated, superficially umbilicated polyps, measuring 2 to 3 mm in diameter but occasionally are as large as 2 cm. The lesions may be multiple, producing a studding or a cobblestone effect of the mucosa, or they may be more widely spaced with normal intervening mucosa.

Microscopically, the polyps straddle the muscularis mucosae, and involve the mucosa and superficial submucosa (fig. 13-7C). They consist of nodular aggregates of intermediate type lymphocytes (intermediate between small lymphocytic and cleaved cell lymphomas), sometimes surrounding lymphoid follicles, with nuclei that are round to slightly or moderately irregular which resemble those of mantle zone lymphocytes (fig. 13-7D). Because of the polypoid nature of the lesions, they may be confused with nodular lymphoid hyperplasia or follicular lymphoma. However, the diffuse nature of the infiltrate, the distinctive cytology, and the characteristic phenotype, namely, CD5,19,20,22,24 positive, Leu-8 positive, and HLA-DR positive, should help in the differential diagnosis.

3) Gastric Plasmacytomas. These are described separately later in this chapter.

*High-Grade Lymphomas.* 1) Diffuse Large Cell Lymphoma including High-Grade MALToma and Immunoblastic Lymphoma. These are tumors of adults (average age 60 years) (85) and account for 40 to 60 percent of all gastric lymphomas (43,85, 86,161). They are often advanced at the time of presentation and have an aggressive clinical course. Grossly, they characteristically show marked mucosal nodularity, extensive ulceration, and destructive invasion of the muscularis propria. Lymph node involvement is common.

Microscopically, the gut type and nodal type are usually indistinguishable; in some instances there is evidence of low-grade MALToma adjacent to the high-grade tumor, characterized by the presence of lymphoepithelial lesions and admixed lymphoid follicles; this indicates transformation of low-grade lymphoma to high grade

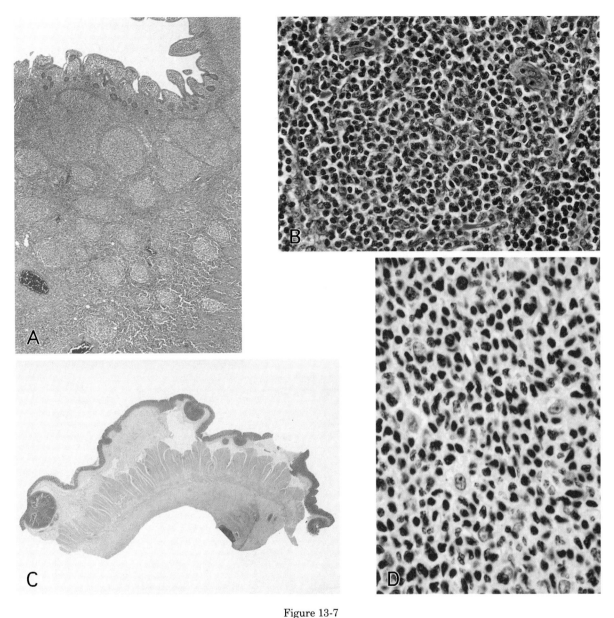

Figure 13-7
FOLLICULAR LYMPHOMA OF THE STOMACH AND MULTIPLE LYMPHOMATOUS POLYPOSIS

A: Scanning-power view of a follicular lymphoma. Note the nodular infiltration of the mucosa and submucosa.

B: Higher magnification shows the irregular small lymphocytes morphologically similar to those found in follicular lymphoma of lymph nodes.

C: Scanning-power view of diffuse lymphomatous polyposis. Compared to follicular lymphoma, these tiny mucosal polyps consist of scattered circumscribed nodules each of which is composed of a uniform population of lymphocytes of mantle zone type. (Courtesy of Dr. B. Schnitzer, Ann Arbor, MI.)

D: Higher magnification of C shows a diffuse infiltrate of intermediate-type lymphocytes.

(fig. 13-6D). The lymphomatous infiltrate is composed of sheets of large noncleaved cells with large, round, vesicular nuclei and many nucleoli (fig. 13-8). Immunoblastic lymphomas are a variant of large cell lymphomas but contain ample purple cytoplasm. In addition, many are polymorphous and pleomorphic, often containing large, bizarre, atypical lymphocytes, some of which resemble Reed-Sternberg cells (see Anaplastic Large Cell Lymphoma [Ki-1 Lymphoma]) and admixed mature lymphocytes, plasma cells, histiocytes, and sometimes eosinophils (86). Immunophenotypically,

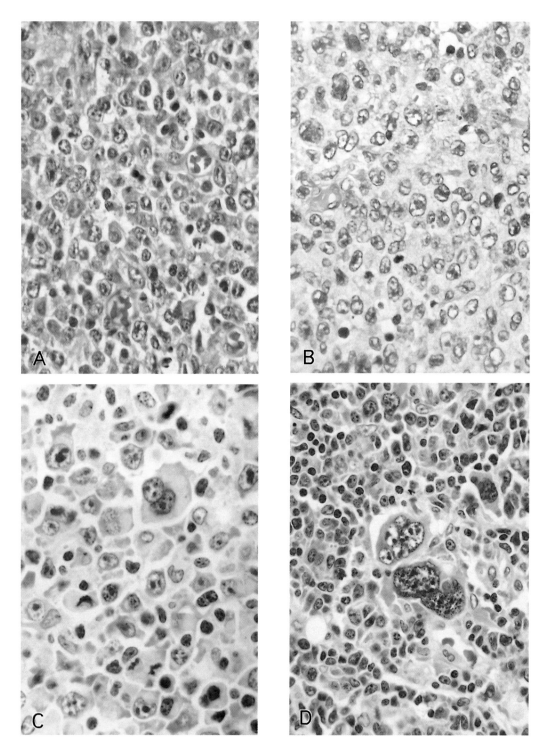

Figure 13-8
HISTOLOGIC SPECTRUM OF HIGH-GRADE GASTRIC LYMPHOMA

A: Diffuse large cell lymphoma consisting of atypical, mitotically active lymphocytes with vesicular nuclei and ample cytoplasm.

B: Diffuse large cell type characterized by a monomorphous infiltrate of atypical large lymphoid cells containing ample cytoplasm and large round vesicular nuclei with many prominent nucleoli.

C: Large cell immunoblastic type. In contrast to figure 13-8A, the tumor cells are pleomorphic, many are binucleated and others are plasmacytoid in appearance.

D: Pleomorphic large cell lymphoma. Note the two large bizarre multinucleated cells.

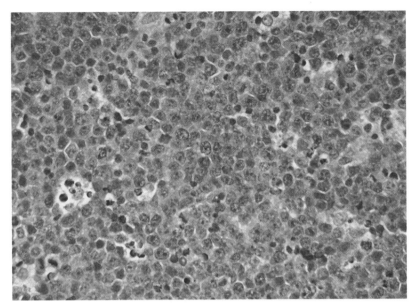

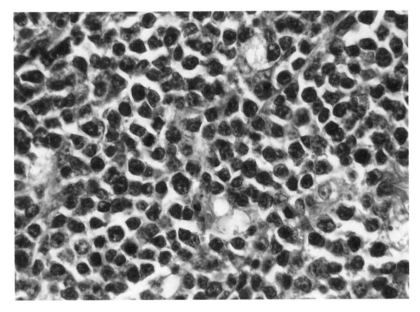

Figure 13-9
BURKITT'S LYMPHOMA
Top: Low-power view illustrating the "starry-sky" pattern which results from interspersed macrophages containing phagocytosed nuclear debris.
Bottom: High-power magnification of the lymphoid infiltrate which consists of undifferentiated lymphocytes with scant cytoplasm, regular round nuclei, and small nucleoli.

the majority of these tumors are of B-cell type. In one study the tumor cells frequently and strongly expressed the lymphocyte adhesion molecules CD44, CD45, and LFA-1; monotypic cytoplasmic immunoglobulin, which is often absent in small lymphocytic lymphomas, was present in one third of cases (161).

2) Burkitt's Lymphoma. Typically this tumor involves children and rarely adults (85). It is usually found around the ileocecal region, but rare cases of gastric involvement have been reported (84–86). The lymphomas are usually advanced at

the time of diagnosis, with extensive involvement of all layers of the stomach wall but little mucosal ulceration. Following excision local recurrence is common with widespread peritoneal dissemination.

Histologically, the tumors characteristically have a "starry sky" pattern and consist of sheets of monotonous-appearing, medium-sized lymphoblasts (12 to 15 mm) with regular round nuclei, finely dispersed chromatin, numerous small nucleoli, and scant cytoplasm (fig. 13-9). Mitoses are prominent, as are numerous apoptotic cells and reactive histiocytes containing phagocytosed nuclear debris. The latter account for the characteristic starry sky pattern. There is usually diffuse infiltration of the stomach wall with a tendency to permeate between, but not destroy, muscle fibers. In the terminal ileum these tumors may have a nodular pattern, supporting evidence that nonendemic Burkitt's lymphoma is of B-cell origin and may selectively involve B-cell areas such as Peyer's patches and solitary lymphoid follicles (89).

3) AIDS-Associated Lymphoma. Lymphomas are the second most common neoplasms in patients with acquired immunodeficiency syndrome (AIDS), occurring most frequently in the gastrointestinal tract. About half of the gastrointestinal lesions are gastric and present with symptoms related to ulcer, tumor mass, hemorrhage, or perforation. The prognosis of these tumors is poor due to the very aggressive course (12,19,44,80). Histologically, most AIDS-associated gastric lymphomas are composed of either noncleaved or blast cells similar to Burkitt's lymphoma, and almost all are of B-cell phenotype.

4) Hodgkin's Disease of the Stomach. One percent of all primary gastric lymphomas are reported to be due to Hodgkin's disease but this figure should be regarded with skepticism since many of the previously reported cases were probably other types of lymphoma such as immunoblastic and large cell anaplastic lymphomas (29). Hodgkin's disease of the lymph nodes may also secondarily involve the stomach (174), and there is a reported composite lymphoma with a component of non-Hodgkin's diffuse large cell lymphoma. No cases of esophageal Hodgkin's lymphoma have been reported to date (29).

Most patients are in their fifties or sixties; there appears to be a slight male predominance. The modes of presentation are similar to those of other gastric lymphomas, with signs and symptoms similar to gastric cancer, such as early satiety, weight loss, and anemia, or with symptoms of peptic ulceration.

Grossly, Hodgkin's lymphoma is a tumorous mass or an ulcerating lesion (144). The tumor may be confined to the mucosa and submucosa or extend into the muscle coats, serosa, and the regional lymph nodes.

On histologic examination there is frequent mucosal ulceration. The tumor may focally infiltrate between the gastric glands or replace them. The histologic features of Hodgkin's disease of the stomach are similar to those of lymph nodes: Reed-Sternberg and atypical mononuclear cells in a background of inflammatory cells composed of small mature lymphocytes, eosinophils, plasma cells, and histiocytes. The usual subtypes of Hodgkin's disease of lymph nodes, mixed cellularity, nodular sclerosis, or lymphocyte predominant types are also found in the stomach (24,29). Lymphocyte-depleted Hodgkin's disease is rare and most of the reported cases were probably large cell lymphoma (see below). The mucosa adjacent to the lymphoma frequently shows chronic gastritis and intestinal metaplasia (29).

The differential diagnosis of Hodgkin's disease of the stomach includes inflammatory conditions and other forms of lymphoma. The reactive inflammatory processes include Crohn's disease, histiocytosis X, eosinophilic gastritis, and inflammatory fibroid polyp. These conditions all have a polymorphous infiltrate containing numerous eosinophils and large lymphocytes or immunoblasts which should not be confused with Reed-Sternberg cells. In problematic cases careful examination of the clinical setting, the background histologic features, and immunohistochemical studies (see below) are usually helpful in diagnosis.

Differentiating immunoblastic lymphoma and other diffuse large cell lymphomas may be more difficult since they may all have a polymorphous infiltrate and contain cells resembling Reed-Sternberg cells. Careful study of the background lymphocytes is usually helpful: in Hodgkin's disease the lymphocytes are typically small whereas in non-Hodgkin's lymphomas there is usually a broader spectrum in size of lymphocytes, ranging from small to large (29). Lymphocyte-depleted Hodgkin's lymphoma may be difficult to differentiate from Ki-1 (CD30)-positive anaplastic large cell lymphoma as the latter frequently contains large bizarre cells with huge nucleoli that mimic Reed-Sternberg cells. Although the typical immunohistochemical features of both these tumors differ, they may overlap in some cases. Thus, the only way to distinguish the two entities is by finding a significant admixture of reactive components in Hodgkin's disease (83). Differentiating between the two diseases may be more of an academic exercise at this time since both conditions behave aggressively.

Immunohistochemical studies further aid in the confirmation or exclusion of the diagnosis of gastric Hodgkin's disease. The large, atypical mononuclear and typical Reed-Sternberg cells are Leu-M1 (CD15) positive and leukocyte common antigen (CD45) negative. In contrast Ki-1 (CD30)-positive anaplastic large cell lymphoma is CD15 negative and CD45 positive. However, as already stated, there may be overlap and some cases of Hodgkin's disease have been shown to be CD30 positive (fig. 13-10) (29,83,144).

Because of the rarity of gastric Hodgkin's disease and the frequent confusion with other large cell non-Hodgkin's lymphomas it is recommended that the diagnosis of Hodgkin's disease be based on adequate histology and confirmed by immunohistochemistry.

5) Anaplastic Large Cell Lymphoma (Ki-1 Lymphoma). This is a rare heterogeneous group of lymphomas characterized by sheets of large noncleaved lymphocytes, immunoblasts, and undifferentiated lymphocytes containing large, often binucleated nuclei with huge nucleoli frequently resembling Reed-Sternberg cells. There are relatively few admixed inflammatory cells (fig. 13-10C) (112,122). Because of their reactivity with monoclonal anti-Ki-1 antibody they are called Ki-1 lymphomas. Phenotypically, these tumors may be of B- or T-cell type and are also typically CD30 and CD45 positive (fig. 13-10D). Histologically, these tumors may be confused with Hodgkin's disease of the stomach and other undifferentiated tumors. The clinical presentation, behavior, and prognosis of these tumors is similar those of other large cell lymphomas of the stomach (112).

6) Post-Transplant Lymphoproliferative Disorders. Post-transplant lymphoproliferative disorder (PTLD) is a term used to describe a family of tumors that arise in organ allograft recipients and is one of the most dreaded complications of orthotopic transplantation (26,100). The reported incidence varies according to the type of transplant: it is 1 percent in renal transplants, 3 percent in liver transplants, 2 to 3 percent in heart transplants, and 5 percent in heart/lung transplants. It is rare in bone marrow transplants (21,92,100–102,153).

PTLD usually develops within 6 months of transplantation, but can occur as early as 4 or 6 weeks after surgery (100,102). There appears to be a relationship between PTLD and increased immu-nosuppression for rejection episodes; the typical scenario is that of a transplant patient with a rejection episode that either does not respond to steroids or recurs after the steroids are decreased. Treatment with one or two courses of OKT3 or antilymphocyte globulin is then necessary. Shortly thereafter the patient develops PTLD.

Clinically, PTLD presents either as a fulminant, rapidly progressive polyclonal disease; as a lymphadenopathy that resembles infectious mononucleosis; or most commonly, as single or metastatic polyclonal or clonal tumors. The latter occur most frequently in extranodal locations, usually involving the brain, gastrointestinal tract including the stomach, or allograft organ. The fulminant form of PTLD is characterized by a combination of peripheral lymphadenopathy, severe metabolic acidosis, organ failure, or allograft dysfunction (92,102). There is also evidence of a close association of active Epstein-Barr virus (EBV) infection, either primary or by reactivation, in almost all patients. EBV genomic DNA can be detected in up to 100 percent of patients depending on the sensitivity of the methods used (50,61,82,119).

Grossly, PTLD presents either as a tumorous mass or as an infiltrative lesion indistinguishable from usual lymphomas. The lesion is superficially ulcerated and covered with a greenish yellow fibrinous exudate. On cut surface the tumor has a grayish color and a soft consistency. It may extend to the serosa and sometimes perforate (92,100,102).

Although the gastrointestinal tract is one of the common sites of extranodal involvement of PTLD, most of the histologic reports in the literature describe the general features of this disorder in tissues outside the lymph nodes rather than in specific sites such as the stomach. However, in our experience, the histologic features of PTLD in the stomach are no different from those described in the literature. PTLD is characterized by a dense inflammatory infiltrate, with a histologic spectrum ranging from that found in infectious mononucleosis to that of lymphoma. It is either polymorphous or monomorphous, and may be associated with extensive necrosis (fig. 13-11). The polymorphous infiltrate consists of a spectrum of mature or immature lymphocytes including one or several of the following types: small mature cells; small and large cleaved or

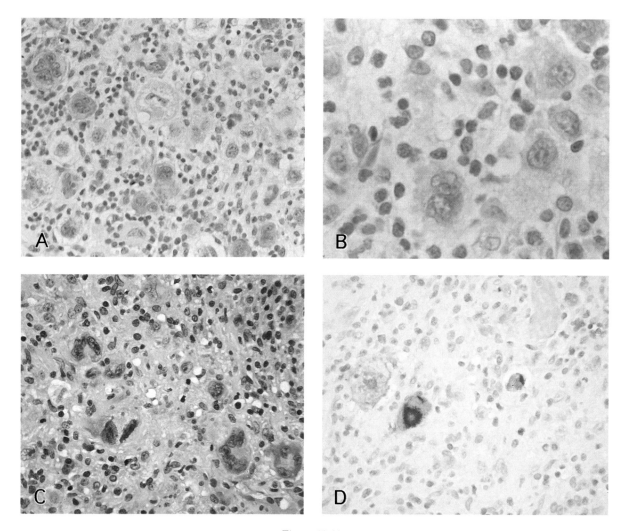

Figure 13-10

HODGKIN'S DISEASE AND ANAPLASTIC LARGE CELL (Ki-1) LYMPHOMA OF THE STOMACH

A: Hodgkin's disease of the stomach stained for CD15. Note the stained (red cytoplasm) atypical mononuclear cells and Reed-Sternberg cells scattered among the unstained inflammatory cells.

B: Hodgkin's disease stained for CD30 to show positive Reed-Sternberg cells. It should be noted that not all cases of Hodgkin's disease are CD30 positive. (A,B courtesy of Dr. E. Jaffe, Bethesda, MD.)

C: Anaplastic large-cell (Ki-1) lymphoma showing an atypical lymphoid infiltrate composed of an admixture of large multinucleated cells, some of which resemble Reed-Sternberg cells, and poorly defined lymphocytes. These tumors frequently resemble Hodgkin's disease but differ from the latter in that they commonly contain atypical lymphocytes and have different immunohistochemical markers.

D: Anaplastic large cell (Ki-1) lymphoma stained for CD 30. Note the positive cytoplasmic stain (red) in two enlarged cells. In contrast to Hodgkin's disease this tumor was positive for CD45 but negative for CD15.

noncleaved cells; immunoblasts, some of which may be atypical; and plasma and plasmacytoid cells (fig. 13-11). Mitotic figures are commonly present. There may be extensive necrosis and in these cases numerous neutrophils and histiocytes are commonly seen. The monomorphous infiltrate consists primarily of atypical lymphocytes but may also show extensive necrosis (102).

Almost all cases of PTLD are of B-cell origin, although rare T-cell proliferations have been reported (79). It has also been shown that in some instances the proliferating B lymphocytes were of donor origin, apparently originating from "passenger" lymphocytes within the donor organ (102). EBV has been implicated as a cofactor in most cases. In nonimmunosuppressed individuals,

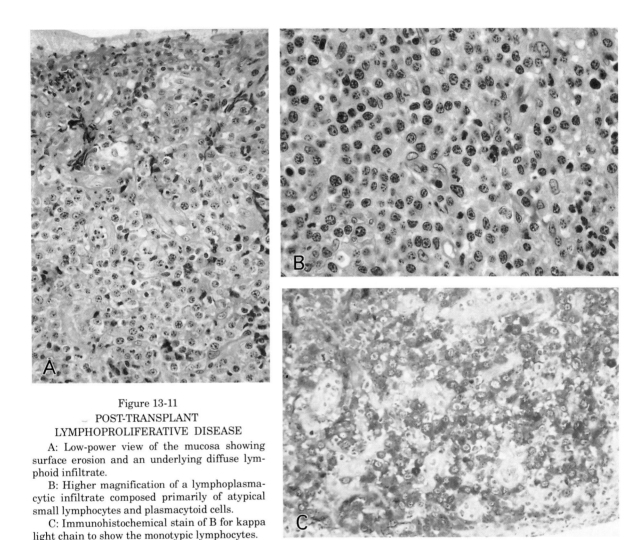

Figure 13-11
POST-TRANSPLANT
LYMPHOPROLIFERATIVE DISEASE

A: Low-power view of the mucosa showing surface erosion and an underlying diffuse lymphoid infiltrate.

B: Higher magnification of a lymphoplasmacytic infiltrate composed primarily of atypical small lymphocytes and plasmacytoid cells.

C: Immunohistochemical stain of B for kappa light chain to show the monotypic lymphocytes.

T lymphocytes play a central role in the coordinated host response to EBV-induced B-cell proliferation; interference with this control in the allograft recipient is thought to be an important factor in producing an environment suitable for the development of PTLD (100). PTLD can be either monoclonal or polyclonal. Polyclonal PTLD is commonly polymorphous but may have a monoclonal component, seen with genotypic analysis. In some cases different monoclonal and polyclonal populations are present in the affected organs or sites (102,153). Unfortunately, analysis of clonality cannot be used to reliably predict behavior in individual patients. For example, Nalesnik et al. (100) have shown that polymorphous polyclonal proliferations developing shortly after transplantation often have a

fulminant and fatal course. Nevertheless, although some reported cases of monoclonal PTLD regress completely after discontinuation of all immunosuppressive therapy, there is evidence that monoclonal PTLD, especially involving multiple sites, has a worse prognosis and usually does not regress with discontinuance of immunosuppression alone (101,145,149).

Reduction of immunosuppression is the primary treatment of choice, although as stated above, some tumors are unresponsive to this. This therapy is usually coupled with the administration of Acyclovir and surgical treatment of symptomatic and resectable lesions such as those that perforate the intestine. In most centers, antilymphoma chemotherapy is used only in cases in which there is tumor progression despite a reduction of immunosuppression (100). Tumor regression can often be striking in its speed and extent. Disappearance of tumors within 1 to 2 weeks is not unusual and in some instances the regression appears to be accompanied by maturation of the clonal PTLD cells into mature plasma cells, concurrent with a reduction in their numbers. In other instances, tumor regression results in progressively more malignant clones and ultimately death (100,102).

*Primary Gastric T-Cell Lymphoma.* Primary T-cell lymphomas are rare neoplasms: only nine cases have been reported up to 1994. However, this underestimates the true incidence since it does not include some lymphomas with distinctive morphology, such as anaplastic large cell Ki-1 lymphomas, some of which are phenotypically T-cell lymphomas (see Ki-1 Lymphomas) (9, 78,81,96,173). In addition, the stomach may be secondarily involved in rare cases of enteropathy-associated T-cell lymphoma (68) and in node-based adult T-cell leukemia/lymphoma.

Grossly, primary gastric T-cell lymphomas present as multiple polypoid lesions or as a localized protuberant, polypoid, or deeply ulcerated mass.

Histologically, these tumors may resemble node-based peripheral T-cell lymphomas. They are typically polymorphous, consisting of a diffuse infiltration of atypical lymphocytes admixed with histiocytes, eosinophilic granulocytes, clusters of epithelioid histiocytes, and occasional stromal fibrosis (9,78,81,173). The lymphocytic infiltration is typically polymorphous (fig 13-12). It may consist of small lymphocytes with somewhat wrinkled nuclei; lymphocytes with features of large cell immunoblastic T-cell lymphoma, characterized by plasmacytoid cells containing peripherally located cerebriform vesicular nuclei with prominent eosinophilic nucleoli; or as blast cells with deeply indented or gyriform vesicular nuclei, indistinct nucleoli, and abundant clear cytoplasm. Multinucleated giant cells have also been described (81,135). It should be stressed that the previously described histologic features are not distinctive of T-cell lymphoma and that a definitive diagnosis can only be made immunohistochemically.

*Malignant lymphoma with eosinophilia* is an unusual variant of T-cell lymphoma. It is most common in the small intestine but a few cases have been described in the stomach (135). There is such extensive necrosis and eosinophilic infiltration that the lesion may be misdiagnosed as eosinophilic gastroenteritis. However, careful examination reveals blast-like cells admixed with the inflammatory cells (13).

The majority of T-cell lymphomas are phenotypically of the helper-inducer type but occasional suppressor-cytotoxic phenotypes have been described (9). There have been too few cases to predict the clinical behavior of these lymphomas. In one report of four cases, one patient died within 6 months of diagnosis and the others were in remission, two patients at 3 years and one patient at 4 years after surgical resection (9,96). Overall, more than half the patients reported to date are in remission following treatment. However, the length of the follow-up in some cases is short and tumor stage is not always clear.

*Miscellaneous Lymphomas.* There are unusual varieties of gastrointestinal lymphomas. We have seen a lymphoma that was composed of areas of follicular small cleaved cell lymphoma, follicular small and large cell lymphoma, and diffuse large cell lymphoma with areas of pleomorphism. In addition there are reports of lymphomas associated with other tumors such as early gastric cancers (157).

A number of gastric lymphomas are unclassifiable. In some cases this is because of poor fixation. Many of these specimens are large and fixed en masse resulting in considerable variation in cytologic preservation. Preservation is usually best near the mucosal or serosal surfaces, where the tissue is most rapidly exposed to the fixative. Some of the difficulties can be circumvented by promptly fixing thin slices of neoplasm when lymphoma is suspected.

**Differential Diagnosis.** The major problems in diagnosis are in differentiating low-grade lymphomas from lymphoid hyperplasia and some high-grade lymphomas from poorly differentiated adenocarcinoma. The main distinguishing microscopic features are the chronic peptic ulceration in lymphoid hyperplasia and the nature of the lymphoid infiltrate (5). The form of gastric lymphoid hyperplasia most familiar to pathologists is that present at the margins of a typical chronic peptic ulcer. However, sometimes a similar distribution of the lymphoid infiltrate is seen in lymphoma, presumably in cases of gastric lymphoma arising from ulcer-associated lymphoid

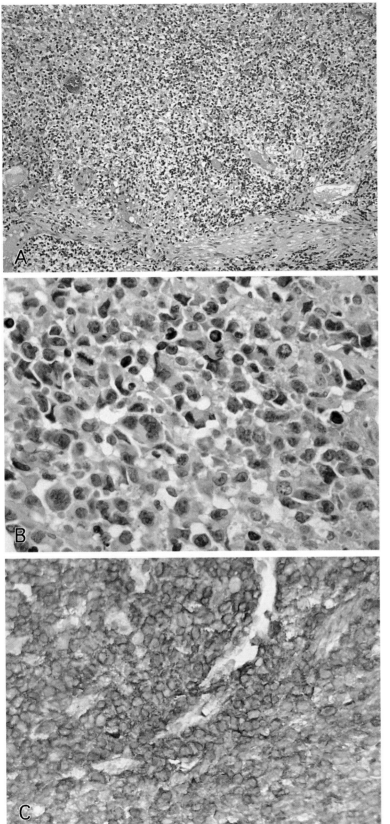

Figure 13-12
GASTRIC T-CELL LYMPHOMA

A: Mucosa showing loss of glands and a diffuse lymphocytic infiltration.

B: Higher magnification of the lymphoid infiltrate which is composed of variably sized lymphocytes ranging from small lymphocytes with round or wrinkled nuclei to cells with large, irregular, hyperchromatic nuclei.

C: Immunohistochemical stain for CD3, a pan-T-cell marker, shows that the majority of lymphocytes are of T-cell phenotype.

hyperplasia. This is not surprising since *H. pylori* infection is known to be associated with peptic ulceration and in some cases to predispose to MALToma. A further problem in distinguishing between lymphoid hyperplasia and gastric lymphoma is that lymphomas are frequently superficially ulcerated. Thus, while it is fairly easy to distinguish between erosions and ulcers in resection specimens, it is often impossible to distinguish between ulcers and erosions endoscopically or on biopsy. The depth of lymphoid infiltration of the gastric wall is of no aid in distinguishing between lymphoid hyperplasia and malignant lymphoma (166). Although the lymphoid infiltrate in gastric lymphoid hyperplasia is commonly confined to the mucosa and submucosa, in many cases it may involve the full thickness of the gastric wall. Conversely, a significant number of gastric lymphomas have a uniform "pushing" margin with involvement of the mucosa and submucosa only. Because of these problems, careful examination of the lymphoid infiltrate is essential in distinguishing between benign and malignant lymphoid proliferations (15,118).

Histologically, low-grade malignant lymphoma is the most difficult lesion to differentiate from lymphoid hyperplasia; other lymphomas are easier to differentiate because of the cytologic atypia and frequent monomorphous nature of the lymphoid infiltrate (5,118,177). If the lymphoid infiltrate is monomorphous, then there is usually not much of a problem in diagnosing the low-grade lymphomas. The major problem arises with low-grade lymphomas that have a polymorphous infiltrate consisting of mature-appearing lymphocytes, admixed plasma cells, other inflammatory cells, and lymphoid follicles, all of which are also typical of lymphoid hyperplasia (177). For this reason, it is important to determine the setting in which the lymphoid infiltrate occurs, such as peptic ulceration, and to search for other subtle histologic features that are indicative of lymphoma. In low-grade lymphoma, the lymphoid infiltrate is often denser, more monomorphous, and mildly atypical (somewhat larger than normal lymphocytes and showing nuclear clefts) than in lymphoid hyperplasia; Dutcher's bodies are more frequent; and plasma cells tend to lie superficially in the mucosa, between the lymphoid infiltrate and the surface epithelium. Sometimes focal nests of mono-

morphous atypical lymphocytes, consisting of small cleaved or monocytoid cells, are found distributed within the polymorphous infiltrate, often adjacent to the mantle zone of the lymphoid follicles. Immunohistochemistry on frozen and formalin-fixed tissue has shown these lymphoid aggregates to be monotypic B cells; there is also evidence of gene rearrangement (37,143).

Other features indicative of lymphoma are the massive substitution of the gastric glands by lymphoma and the presence of prominent lymphoepithelial lesions (5). On rare occasions, lymphoepithelial lesions have been reported in lymphoid hyperplasia. However, these are sparse, usually consisting of collections of three or fewer mature lymphocytes, characteristically similar to mature intraepithelial lymphocytes, and do not cause epithelial destruction (5,177). Lymphomas are CD20 positive in contrast to lymphoid hyperplasia in which lymphocytes are usually T cells (5,177). Large cell lymphoma, poorly differentiated carcinoma, and undifferentiated tumors of the stomach can on occasion be almost indistinguishable from one another. It is important to differentiate between them because treatment protocols and prognoses are different. Multiple sections (taken especially from the margins of the tumor) should be examined for evidence of glandular differentiation and stained with diastase PAS for mucin production. In the last few years the problem of differentiating lymphoma from other malignancies has been almost eliminated by the immunohistochemical demonstration of keratins and carcinoembryonic antigen in carcinomas (fig. 13-13), S-100 in metastatic malignant melanoma, and common leukocyte antigen in lymphomas. Rarely, tumors show aberrant markers that cause diagnostic confusion: a case of lymphoma showed focal keratin positivity and absent common leukocyte antigen on biopsy and in the resection specimen (28). Medullary carcinoma of the stomach can sometimes be confused with large cell lymphoma because of the dense admixture of lymphocytes and plasma cells which may overshadow the carcinoma. Mucin stains and the demonstration of epithelial cell markers, such as keratin and carcinoembryonic antigen, help differentiate these two tumors.

Differentiating between the various subtypes of lymphoma depends in many instances on their characteristic cytology, as described before

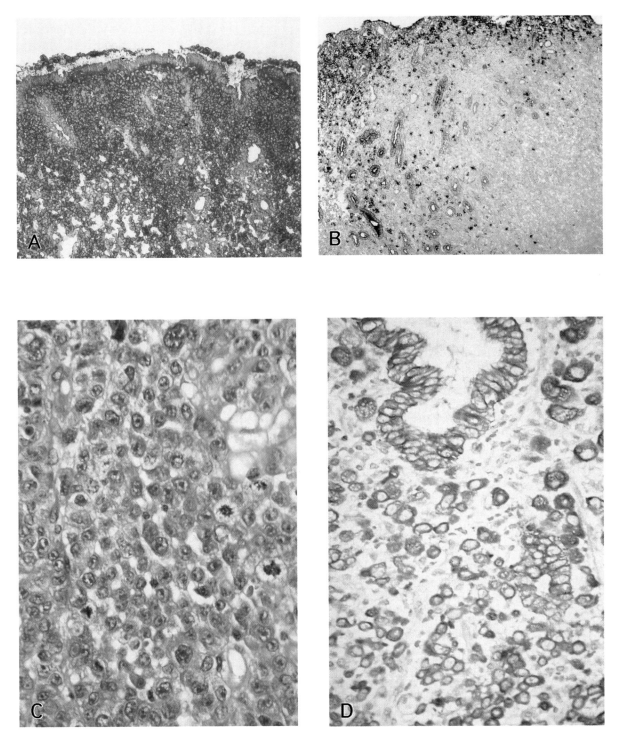

Figure 13-13
IMMUNOHISTOCHEMISTRY OF LYMPHOMA AND
UNDIFFERENTIATED GASTRIC CARCINOMA OF THE STOMACH

Biopsy of a gastric lymphoma of B-cell type to illustrate monoclonality.

A: Diffusely positive immunoreactivity for kappa light chain.

B: Negative reaction for lambda light chain except for mature lymphocytes at the periphery of the lymphoma.

C: High-power magnification of the carcinoma showing a resemblance to large cell lymphoma.

D: Cytokeratin immunoreactivity in the tumor cells present in C establish the epithelial nature of the tumor.

under histologic subtypes. In addition, the immunophenotypic characteristics of the various subtypes are helpful, and these are summarized in Table 13-2.

Multiple lymphomatous polyposis, although rare, needs to be distinguished from diffuse nodular lymphoid hyperplasia (25,27,86,124). This distinction can usually be easily made with careful histologic examination, since the nodules in nodular lymphoid hyperplasia are small, largely confined to the lamina propria, and often contain prominent, reactive germinal centers, whereas multiple lymphomatous polyposis is monomorphous. However, some cases have the typical mantle zone pattern with residual germinal centers; careful examination of the mantle zone region is important and if frozen tissue is available, it can be shown to be monotypic.

**Immunohistochemical Findings and Genetic Analysis.** Immunohistochemistry and genetic analysis are often of great help in the differential diagnosis of malignant lymphoma and lymphoid hyperplasia. As previously stated, the majority of gastric lymphomas are of B-cell origin (9,49,96,173). They usually express surface and cytoplasmic immunoglobulins and show light chain restriction. However, surface immunoglobulin, which is the dominant immunoglobulin in MALTomas, is difficult to demonstrate in formalin-fixed tissue sections. In contrast, cytoplasmic immunoglobulin, which is strongly expressed in those lymphomas with plasmacytoid differentiation, is well preserved in formalin (161). Most tumors express IgM, a few express IgA, but IgG is rare. Kappa or lambda light chains are equally expressed. Genotype analysis of MALTomas using Southern blot techniques or polymerase chain reaction (PCR) confirm the presence of both clonal heavy and light chain expression and light chain restriction (1,37,148). The latter studies can be done on formalin-fixed, paraffin-embedded tissue. The *bcl*-2 oncogene is not rearranged in MALTomas in contrast to follicular lymphomas (109). However, low-grade MALTomas are positive for *bcl*-2 protein, suggesting that the MALTomas may regulate *bcl*-2 gene expression differently from nodal lymphoma (103b).

The major differences between low-grade gut-associated lymphomas, nodal lymphomas, and chronic lymphocytic leukemia is reactivity to CD5, CD10, CD20, CD22, CD23, and KB61. In most primary low-grade gastrointestinal lymphomas CD5 and CD10 are both negative, whereas CD20, CD22, and CDW32 (KB61) are positive; in other lymphomas CD5 or CD10 may be positive and KB61 negative. Frozen section tissues are necessary for many of the above studies. If only paraffin sections are available, determination of cell lineage (B versus T) and assessment of clonality with light chain restriction and CD43 expression are usually only possible. These studies in association with morphology usually help differentiate benign from malignant lesions. For detailed phenotypic features of the various lymphomas see Table 13-2 (55,67,103a,136,147,151). Immunohistochemical studies of gastric and gastrointestinal lymphomas are limited to date and their practical value remains to be confirmed.

The *bcl*-2 gene is not rearranged in gut-type lymphomas (73). Cytogenetic studies on MALTomas have shown abnormalities but have failed to show a unifying karyotypic aberration. One study found certain recurring abnormalities, particularly involving chromosomes 1, 3, and 7 (171), and another an acquired translocation, t(11;18)(q21;q21.1) (62). The majority of the primary T-cell gastric lymphomas are of helper/inducer type but suppressor/cytotoxic types have also been described.

Electron microscopy is rarely, if ever, of value in the differential diagnosis of malignant lymphoma; it is of no help in differentiating lymphoma subtypes. In the differential diagnosis of lymphoma versus undifferentiated tumors, immunohistochemical markers such as leukocyte common antigen, keratin, carcinoembryonic antigen, and S-100 are more helpful than electron microscopy.

**Work-Up of Gastric Lymphomas.** *Clinical Evaluation.* The prognosis of gastric lymphomas is related to the stage of the disease at the time of diagnosis. Consequently, a proper staging procedure should be undertaken to determine whether the lymphoma is localized to the stomach or secondarily involved in disseminated nodal disease (59,86,165). The clinical work-up (Table 13-3) should include a careful physical examination for peripheral adenopathy and hepatosplenomegaly; computerized tomography (CT) scanning for abdominal, retroperitoneal, and mediastinal adenopathy; and bone marrow aspiration (51). Endoscopic ultrasound is a newly introduced procedure for the staging of

Table 13-2

## IMMUNOPHENOTYPING AND GENETIC ALTERATIONS IN GASTROINTESTINAL LYMPHOMAS

| | Light Chain Restrictions (kappa, lambda) | Ig Expression | CD Expression — CD3* | 5** | 10* | 20* / L26 | CDw32 / 30 | KB61 / 35 | 35 | 45 | 45RO* / UCHL-1 | Other | Genetic Alterations — Ig chains | bcl-2 | Cytogenetics |
|---|---|---|---|---|---|---|---|---|---|---|---|---|---|---|---|
| **B CELL** | | | | | | | | | | | | | | | |
| **LOW GRADE** | | | | | | | | | | | | | | | |
| **MUCOSAL TYPE** | | | | | | | | | | | | | | | |
| Maltoma (20,67,69,71,99,147,148,151,177) | +(k/l) | M,A,G,D | –ve | –ve | –ve | +ve | –ve | +ve | +/– | NA+ | –ve | CD5&7– CD43+ | HC,LC‡ | –ve | translocation (11;18)(q21;q21.1) rearr. chromosomes 1,3,7 |
| IPSID lymphoma and alpha-chain disease (69,116) | +/– | A | –ve | –ve | –ve | +ve | NA | +ve | NA | NA | NA | NA | NA | NA | NA |
| Plasmacytoma (189,191)§ | +(k/l) | M,G,A | NA | NA | NA | +ve | NA | +ve | +ve | +ve | NA | NA | NA | NA | NA |
| **NODAL TYPE** | | | | | | | | | | | | | | | |
| Follicular center cell lymphoma (67,71,177) follicular and diffuse, diffuse | +(k/l) | NA | NA | +ve | +ve | +ve | –ve | NA | NA | NA | NA | NA | HC | +/– | t(14;18),t(2;8), t(8;22)17 and 21 |
| Multiple lymphomatous polyposis (MLP) (67,105,147) | +(k/l) | D,M | NA | +ve | +/– | +ve | NA | NA | +ve | +ve | NA | NA | NA | NA | t(11;14) |
| **HIGH GRADE** | | | | | | | | | | | | | | | |
| **MUCOSAL TYPE** | | | | | | | | | | | | | | | |
| High-grade MALToma (20,67,161)§ | +(k/l) | M,G,A | –ve | –ve | NA | +ve | NA | NA | NA | NA | –ve | NA | HC,LC | –ve | NA |
| IPSID-associated lymphoma (116) | +/–k | A | NA | NA | NA | NA | NA | NA | NA | NA | NA | NA | NA | NA | NA |
| **NODAL TYPE** | | | | | | | | | | | | | | | |
| Diffuse large cell and other types of nodal lymphoma (5,156,161) | +/–(k/l) | M,D,M,G | –ve | –ve | NA | +ve | NA | NA | NA | NA | –ve | NA | HC,LC | +/– | trisomy3,2p21-p23 14q32,del5q |
| Burkitt and Burkitt type (156,161) | +/–(k/l) | M,A,D | –ve | –ve | NA | +ve | NA | NA | NA | NA | –ve | NA | HC,LC | –ve | translocation of c-myc locus |
| Large cell anaplastic (Ki-1) (112,122) | NA | NA | NA | NA | NA | NA | +ve | NA | NA | NA | NA | NA | NA | NA | NA |
| **T CELL** | | | | | | | | | | | | | | | |
| Nonenteropathy associated (9,77,96,117,173) | –ve | –ve | +/– | +ve | NA | –ve | +/– | NA | NA | +/– | +ve | CD7+/– | NA | NA | NA |
| Enteropathy associated (67,147) | –ve | –ve | +/– | NA | NA | NA | +/– | NA | NA | NA | NA | CD7+ | NA | NA | T-cell receptor-beta rearrangement |
| **HODGKIN'S** (24,29,144) | NA | +ve | NA | NA | NA | –ve | +ve | NA | NA | –ve | –ve | CD15+ | NA | NA | NA |
| **POST-TRANSPLANT LYMPHOPROLIFERATIVE DISORDER** | | | | | | | | | | | | | | | |
| Monoclonal (50)§ | +(k) | A | NA | NA | NA | +ve | NA | NA | NA | NA | –ve | NA | NA | NA | NA |
| Polyclonal | k+l | NA | NA | NA | NA | NA | NA | NA | NA | NA | NA | NA | NA | NA | NA |

*Will work on formalin-fixed tissue.
**Frozen tissue necessary.
†NA = Studies not available.
§Demonstrated on gastric tissue.
‡HC = heavy chain; LC = light chain

Table 13-3

## GASTRIC LYMPHOMAS: DIAGNOSIS AND WORK-UP

1. History and clinical findings
   Are there extraintestinal manifestations, such as lymphadenopathy?

2. Endoscopic findings
   Ulceration?
   Site of lesion?
   Multiple?

3. Histologic features
   Character of infiltrate
   Diffuse, nodular, or perifollicular
   Monomorphous or polymorphous
   Low-grade or high-grade
   Lymphoepithelial lesions
   Lymphoid follicles
   Depth of infiltrate
   Perigastric node involvement

4. Immunohistochemical findings
   Monoclonality or polyclonality of the immuno-globulin light chains by immunoperoxidase or flow cytometry (for lymphoma versus lymphoid hyperplasia)
   CD5, CD10 to determine mucosal versus nodal type
   Common leukocyte antigen, keratin, carcino-embryonic antigen, S-100 protein (to differentiate lymphoma from undifferentiated carcinoma and melanoma)

5. Gene rearrangement studies (lymphoma versus lymphoid hyperplasia if immunohistochemistry results are unsatisfactory)

6. If lymphoma is diagnosed, staging is critical before treatment is started

---

esophageal and gastric tumors; preliminary studies suggest it is more accurate in local staging of lymphomas than CT scan particularly in assessing the depth of intramural invasion and extension into surrounding gastric structures (45,108,129,159).

*Endoscopic Biopsy.* If the endoscopic biopsy is adequate in size, not crushed, and not from a deeply ulcerated area, a definite or presumptive diagnosis of malignant lymphoma can be made from it in most cases (fig. 13-14) (5,154). One exception is the rare low-grade small lymphocytic lymphoma in which differentiation from gastritis and lymphoid hyperplasia may be difficult (see Lymphoid Hyperplasia) (5,177). Problems arise if biopsies are small, crushed, or sub-

optimally fixed; difficulty in interpretation may also occur in those biopsies showing necrosis and a mixed inflammatory infiltrate, since these findings may be seen in superficial biopsies of ulcerated lymphomas and in those of gastric lymphoid hyperplasia associated with peptic ulceration. In cases in which the biopsy is nondiagnostic, it is important to repeat the biopsies from multiple sites. In order to minimize crush artifact, a larger endoscope should be used (therapeutic endoscope) which contains a larger diameter channel capable of taking a large cup; these yield superior specimens with much less distortion (fig. 13-14). Another endoscopic procedure that is now available, and produces even larger biopsy specimens, is the large particle electrocautery snare biopsy. In problematic cases, marker studies such as immunohistochemistry, flow cytometry with or without frozen section, and gene rearrangement studies may be diagnostic (37,143). Immunohistochemistry for the demonstration of immunoglobulins, especially surface immunoglobulins, is best done on frozen tissue and is generally unreliable when formalin-fixed, Bouin-fixed, or B5-fixed paraffin-embedded tissue is used. However, in our experience, the demonstration of monotypic immunoglobulins in fresh frozen tissue is often difficult to interpret due to high background staining and distortion artifact. In some of these cases the coexpression of CD20 and CD43 helps diagnose gastric lymphomas. If repeat biopsies do not resolve the issue of lymphoma versus lymphoid hyperplasia, laparotomy may be necessary (Tables 13-3, 13-4).

*Laparotomy.* Before laparotomy is undertaken, lymphoma staging is essential to determine the extent of the disease. This should include sampling perigastric and para-aortic lymph nodes; careful inspection of the spleen (8,76,87); and studies of touch preparations, immunohistochemistry, flow cytometry, or gene rearrangement for determination of the type of lymphoma, or in the case of undifferentiated tumors, for diagnosis (11,55,67,151).

Frozen sections are indicated for two reasons. The first is for evaluation of resection margins for tumor. This may be difficult in *H. pylori* gastritis since it is not easy to differentiate a lymphoid infiltrate associated with *H. pylori* and lymphoma on frozen section. The second reason is to obtain adequate tissues for special studies.

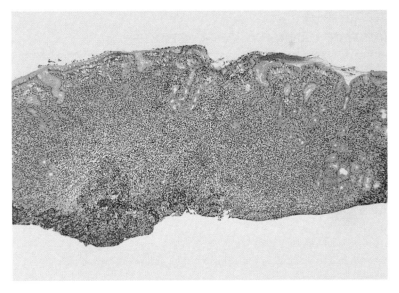

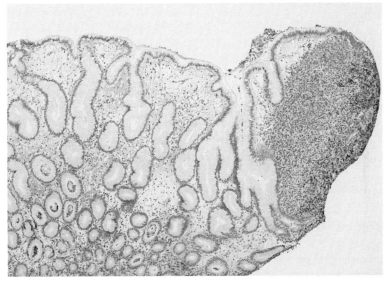

Figure 13-14
GASTRIC LYMPHOMA
Endoscopic biopsy specimen of gastric lymphoma shows a diffuse lymphoid infiltrate of the entire mucosa on the top and a focal infiltrate on the bottom to the right.

**Staging.** The staging system almost universally adopted for gastric lymphomas and the one used here is a modification of the Ann-Arbor classification (98). This classification subdivides gastric lymphomas according to depth of invasion (superficial or deeply invasive tumors), regional node metastases, more widespread local nodal metastases, and widespread extraintestinal dissemination (Table 13-5). A recent report applying the TNM staging system to gastric lymphomas has shown it to be equally effective in determining prognosis (140).

**Spread of Disease.** Low-grade gastric lymphomas are slow growing, remain localized to the stomach for long periods, and have a low incidence of extraintestinal spread. Recurrence depends upon the stage of disease (see Prognosis) and has been reported to occur up to 14 years following treatment. In half the cases, recurrence involves the previous primary site, regional lymph nodes, other parts of the gastrointestinal tract, or occasionally Waldeyer's ring (113,117); the remainder develop into generalijed disease with involvement of the bone marrow, liver, peripheral lymph nodes, and other viscera.

High-grade lymphomas are aggressive and spread beyond the stomach in 40 to 60 percent of cases (23,35,48,53,77,86). Often, there is local

Table 13-4

## GASTRIC LYMPHOMAS: HANDLING OF SPECIMENS*

1. Touch Imprints

   Air dry touch imprints and stain with hematoxylin and eosin; alternatively, smears may be fixed in formalin and stained with hematoxylin and eosin or in alcohol for Papanicolau staining

2. Tissue Fixation

   a. Formalin

      Fix for 1 hour, then slice thinner and fix overnight

      Routine processing

   b. B5 fixation

      Fix for 1 hour, then slice thinner and fix for 4 hours

      Transfer to formalin and fix overnight

      Wash in water for 1 hour before routine processing

      B5 should be made up immediately prior to use by adding 3 ml of 40 percent formalin to 27 ml of B5 reagent

3. Frozen Tissue

   a. Immunohistochemistry

      Place slice of tissue ($1 \text{ cm}^2$ by 0.3 cm ) on a plastic mold for frozen sections and cover with OCT compound embedding medium; snap freeze in isopentane/dry ice or liquid nitrogen; if immunostaining cannot be done right away store in freezer, preferentially at minus 70 degrees

   b. Gene rearrangement studies

      Freeze 1 g of tissue in liquid nitrogen, wrap in foil and store at minus 70 degrees until study is performed; alternatively, multiple 100 μm sections of frozen material can be obtained from the immunohistochemistry laboratory for these studies (In our experience the latter method is easier and more reliable)

   c. Flow cytometry

      Mince 1-2 $\text{mm}^3$ into RPMI (Roswell Park Memorial Institute) medium; refrigerate

   d. Cytogenetics

      Mince 3 $\text{mm}^3$ into RPMI medium; refrigerate; tissue needs to be sterile

*When tissue is limited, hematoxylin and eosin staining, immunohistochemistry, and touch preparations should have priority.

Table 13-5

## MODIFIED ANN ARBOR STAGING SYSTEM FOR PRIMARY GASTRIC LYMPHOMAS*

IE   Localized involvement of the stomach without lymph node metastases
     IE-1  Early gastric lymphoma; tumor confined to the mucosa and submucosa
     IE-2  Lymphoma extends beyond the submucosa

IIE   Gastric lymphoma of any depth of infiltration with lymph node metastases
     IIE-1 Gastric lymphoma with regional node metastases
     IIE-2 Gastric lymphoma with lymph node metastases beyond regional nodes

IIIE  Localized involvement of the stomach with lymph nodes on both sides of the diaphragm (from a practical point almost never applies to the stomach)

IVE  Gastric lymphoma with or without associated lymph node metastases with diffuse lymphomatous dissemination beyond the gastrointestinal tract

*Table obtained from reference 98.

extension of tumor to adjacent soft tissues and involvement of draining lymph nodes, such as the perigastric and para-aortic nodes. Other abdominal viscera may also be involved (7,53,86, 162). Extra-abdominal spread occurs in up to 50 percent of cases, involving most commonly the peripheral lymph nodes, lung, brain, and meninges (86), although almost any organ can be affected (75,86). The majority of relapses occur within 1 year of diagnosis, and most patients die within 1 year of relapse.

**Prognosis.** Low-grade gastrointestinal lymphoma tends to remain localized for a long time and if it recurs, which may happen after a long disease-free interval, the recurrence usually involves regional lymph nodes, other parts of the gastrointestinal tract, or Waldeyer's ring. The prognosis of this lymphoma is better than that of low-grade nodal lymphoma. Some gastrointestinal lymphomas develop within specific clinical settings peculiar to the gastrointestinal tract, such as alpha heavy chain disease.

The overall survival of patients with gastric lymphoma is good: the 5-year survival rate is 40 to 60 percent (16,32,77,86,106,120,141). Data on prognosis and response to treatment are not detailed in the literature for a number of reasons. First, many cases are not adequately staged at the time of diagnosis. Also, most series are relatively small (100 or less cases) and comprise different histologic types, sites, stages, and treatment protocols, so that statistical analysis becomes impossible. There has been no uniformity in the classification of gastric lymphomas, and patient selection in various studies has differed: some include all lymphomas whereas others restrict to stages IE (lymphoma localized to the viscus) and IIE (accompanying involvement of regional lymph nodes), thus making comparisons between different studies difficult.

Nevertheless, some trends are becoming apparent. Prognosis appears to correlate best with the stage of the disease at the time of presentation (16,23,59,77,90,91,117,120,125,139,140,155). The survival for resectable tumors localized to the viscus and regional nodes is remarkably good, with 5-year survival rates ranging from 43 to 75 percent and 10-year rates from 46 to 58 percent; the range is probably related to the grade of the tumor (23,77, 90,117,120). This contrasts with a 30 to 35 percent 5-year survival rate in patients who have residual

Table 13-6

**PROGNOSTIC FACTORS FOR GASTRIC LYMPHOMAS**

| | Survival Figures (%) | |
|---|---|---|
| | 5 Year | 10 Year |
| All gastric lymphomas | 43-75 | 46-58 |
| Prognosis according to stage (23,117) | | |
| IE | 60-87 | 40-60 |
| EI-1 | 90 | 70 |
| EI-2 | 54 | 47 |
| IIE | 41-61 | 41 |
| IIE-1 | 47 | 47 |
| IIE-2 | 30 | 0 |
| Prognosis according to grade | | |
| Irrespective of stage (23) | | |
| Low-grade | 91 | |
| Low-grade with high-grade | 73 | |
| High-grade | 56 | |
| According to stage | | |
| IE | | |
| Low-grade | 95 | |
| Low-grade with high-grade | 78 | |
| High-grade | 74 | |
| IIE | | |
| Low-grade | 82 | |
| Low-grade with high-grade | 65 | |
| High-grade | 39 | |
| Prognosis according to size of tumor (117) | | |
| Less than 5 cm in diameter | 65 | 53 |
| More than 5 cm in diameter | 43 | 0 |

tumor following surgery or who have unresectable tumor at the time of presentation (77,120). Tumor resectability is associated with increased patient survival independent of other prognostic factors (120). However, this is clearly a reflection of tumor stage. Those patients who have widely disseminated disease at the time of presentation rarely survive (86). There is also increasing evidence that patients with stage IE lesions have a better survival rate (60 to 87 percent) than those with stage IIE (40 to 60 percent) (4,6,16,31, 32,39,77,86,88,90,103,120,123,139,155,165). One study showed that progressive extension of tumor worsens the prognosis, although prognosis for tumors that extend beyond the gastric confines is no better than for those that metastasize to the immediate draining lymph nodes (Table 13-6) (117).

The size of the gastric lymphoma also appears to affect prognosis, although this is probably a reflection of tumor stage and not a truly independent prognostic factor. Tumors less than 5 cm in diameter have a much better prognosis than larger tumors.

It was previously thought that histologic type did not affect survival. However, recent reports indicate that low-grade lymphomas do better than such high-grade lymphomas as diffuse large cell and immunoblastic lymphomas (4,23,39,139): the overall 5-year survival rates are 65 to 90 percent for low-grade lymphomas and 40 to 55 percent for high grade (Table 13-6) (23,32). Whereas low-grade lymphomas of the stomach have a much better prognosis than their nodal counterparts, this is not true for high-grade lymphomas, which appear to behave in a manner similar to primary nodal lymphomas (125).

A number of papers have reported the development of gastric cancers in patients treated for gastric lymphoma. These have occurred up to 8 years following resection of the gastric lymphoma. It has been suggested that the cause of these tumors is probably similar to gastric stump tumors that occur following gastrectomy, and are further aggravated by postoperative radiation and chemotherapy (10,175). Finally, there are rare case reports in which spontaneous regression of primary gastric lymphoma appears to have occurred (138).

**Treatment.** The treatment of choice for primary gastric lymphoma remains to be determined. The most exciting development in the treatment of low-grade lymphomas is the current preliminary reports of tumor remission following the eradication of *H. pylori* infection (10a,50,54,64,119a,167, 168). However, reports are now appearing describing relapse of MALT lymphomas after antibiotic treatment (63). Controlled studies and long-term follow-up are needed to determine whether these initial findings hold up, which type of lymphoma will respond to this treatment, and whether the remissions are temporary or long term.

In the past most studies indicated that for localized disease, surgery was the primary mode of treatment. Some studies found that radiotherapy and adjuvant chemotherapy produced no benefit in survival (23,120). However, recent reports show that patients treated with surgery and postoperative radiotherapy or chemotherapy do significantly better than those treated

with surgery only, especially when the lymphoma involves the serosa and lymph nodes (6,8, 32,77,111,139,140,146,154). A few studies have shown that patients with early or aggressive gastric lymphoma do as well when treated with chemotherapy, radiotherapy, or a combination of both as patients treated with surgery alone (91, 125,154); the feared complications of radiotherapy and chemotherapy, such as bleeding and perforation, did not occur. This latter treatment may resolve the problem of residual tumor or inoperability, which occurs in about one third of patients undergoing surgery.

## SECONDARY MALIGNANT LYMPHOMAS

Secondary involvement of the gastrointestinal tract, including the stomach, by disseminated nodal lymphoma is common. In most instances the secondary tumor deposits are incidental findings at autopsy, occurring in up to 20 percent of cases. The clinical features of these tumors do not differ significantly from those of primary intestinal lymphoma ($8,59,121): about 20 percent of patients have palpable abdominal masses; the sites of involvement by tumor are similar, with 56 percent in the stomach, 25 percent in the small intestine, and 10 percent in the large intestine. Pathologically, secondary lymphomas tend to produce punched-out ulcers in the stomach and involve multiple gastrointestinal sites more frequently.

## GASTRIC LYMPHOID HYPERPLASIA (PSEUDOLYMPHOMA)

This lesion is currently rare because of the effective treatment of peptic ulceration. When the older literature on lymphoid hyperplasia is reviewed, it is clear that two major histologic patterns were described. The most common, reported to occur in about 80 percent of gastric lymphoid hyperplasias (17,22,34,35,76,114,115, 118,164,172), was a lesion which was occasionally tumorous and always associated with peptic ulceration. The second lesion was characterized by a diffuse, frequently superficial, mature-appearing lymphoid infiltrate often admixed with lymphoid follicles and unassociated with gastric ulceration. Much of the recent literature on lymphoid hyperplasia has revolved around the latter cases and the majority opinion now is that they are low-grade lymphomas. These lesions are now being diagnosed more frequently than before, and whether this is because they are being recognized more readily on endoscopy or because the frequency of gastric lymphoma is increasing is not certain. These lesions are discussed under gastric lymphoma; in this section lymphoid hyperplasia associated with peptic ulceration is discussed.

Chronic gastric inflammation associated with prominent lymphoid follicles may also be found accompanying a number of gastric disorders such as *H. pylori* gastritis, especially in children in whom it is associated with fine nodularity of the gastric mucosa (56); chronic gastric ulceration; Crohn's disease; and infections such as gastric tuberculosis. In practice, however, the term gastric lymphoid hyperplasia is confined to chronic nonspecific gastric inflammations in which the proliferation of lymphoid tissue presents as a tumorous mass.

**Pathogenesis.** Because of the association of gastric lymphoid hyperplasia with peptic ulceration of long duration, it has been speculated that it is a reactive inflammatory process that develops as a result of longstanding antigenic stimulation (65, 142). A number of reports have suggested that gastric lymphoid hyperplasia predisposes to gastric lymphoma (15,97,132,166). Sigal (142) has hypothesized that the development of lymphoma is the result of chronic antigenic stimulation in chronic peptic ulceration which ultimately leads to clonal lymphoid proliferation and lymphoma in some individuals. (For further details see Low-Grade Gastric Lymphomas.)

**Clinical Features.** Gastric lymphoid hyperplasia is an uncommon condition of the stomach which occurs in adults, most frequently during the fourth to sixth decades, and affects males about twice as commonly as females. Patients usually present with longstanding symptoms of peptic ulcer disease.

**Radiologic and Endoscopic Findings.** The radiologic and endoscopic features are usually those of a plaque-like thickening of the rugal gastric folds or gastric ulceration, and it is only on histologic examination that the excessive lymphoid infiltrate causes concern (fig. 13-15) (22). Sometimes lymphoid hyperplasia looks like an ulcerating mass lesion mimicking carcinoma or lymphoma (17,22,34,35,76,114,115,118,172). There is

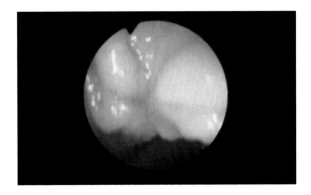

Figure 13-15
ENDOSCOPIC APPEARANCE OF
GASTRIC LYMPHOID HYPERPLASIA
Plaque-like thickening of rugal folds radiating from a central erosion.

thickening of the gastric wall and the mucosa is elevated with central ulceration; the latter is sometimes surrounded by overhanging margins.

**Gross Findings.** Lesions are usually solitary, measuring up to 5 cm in diameter (118) but occasionally may be as large as 14 cm. On cut section, in addition to the features of chronic gastric ulceration, lymphoid hyperplasia is characterized by a localized mass with a fish-flesh consistency due to the lymphoid infiltrate. The lesion may be confined to the mucosa and submucosa but often extends to the muscularis propria or into the serosa.

**Microscopic Findings.** Histologically, lymphoid hyperplasia is characterized by chronic peptic ulceration, a dense inflammatory infiltrate invariably accompanied by *H. pylori* infection, and fibrosis (figs. 13-16–13-18). The inflammatory infiltrate may be associated with thickened mucosal folds. Sometimes the infiltrate is localized to the margin of the ulcer or confined to the mucosa and submucosa and has a smooth "pushing" border; often it is transmural and has an "infiltrative" pattern (fig. 13-16).

The inflammation consists of a polymorphous infiltrate, composed predominantly of small mature lymphocytes, admixed with fewer histiocytes, immunoblasts, plasma cells, eosinophils, and neutrophils; the latter is especially prominent near the ulcerated surface (fig. 13-17). Lymphoid follicles are scattered throughout the lymphoid infiltrate, and in our experience, are most distinct and most abundant superficially in the mucosa

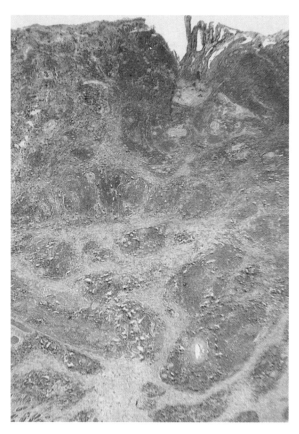

Figure 13-16
LOW-POWER APPEARANCE OF GASTRIC
LYMPHOID HYPERPLASIA ASSOCIATED
WITH CHRONIC PEPTIC ULCERATION

Gastric lymphoid hyperplasia in an area overlying and adjacent to chronic peptic ulceration. There is mucosal ulceration, dense lymphoid infiltration, fibrosis, and destruction of the muscularis propria. Note the prominent lymphoid follicles in the submucosa.

and submucosa (118). Clumps of intraepithelial lymphocytes superficially resembling lymphoepithelial lesions may occasionally be found, but as already stated, they differ from the latter in that they consist of mature lymphocytes, are usually no more than three in number, and do not cause epithelial destruction. The latter is best demonstrated by keratin stains.

Fibrosis is a common accompaniment of lymphoid hyperplasia, especially beneath the ulcerated areas. It is often characterized by dense acellular collagen bundles separating columns of intact lymphocytes in a single file pattern (fig. 13-17B), a pattern which differs from the fibrosis accompanying malignant lymphoma (15).

Two variants of lymphoid hyperplasia, *diffuse nodular lymphoid hyperplasia* and *angiofollicular hyperplasia,* have on rare occasion been reported in the stomach (15,76). However unlike the usual gastric lymphoid hyperplasias, these lesions are not associated with ulceration or fibrosis. Diffuse nodular lymphoid hyperplasia involves primarily the small bowel and is frequently associated with hypogammaglobulinemia and parasitic infestation of the bowel, in most instances with giardia. Histologically, it is usually confined to the mucosa, and consists of several lymphoid follicles heaped up on one another. Gastric angiofollicular lymphoid hyperplasia is morphologically similar to its nodal counterpart: both have a lymphoid infiltrate with numerous lymphoid follicles containing hyalinized germinal centers and vascular structures (15).

**Immunohistochemical and Ultrastructural Findings.** The lymphoid infiltrate in gastric lymphoid hyperplasia shows a polyclonal pattern of immunoglobulin light chains. The ultrastructural findings reflect the type of lymphoid infiltrate and are noncontributory to the diagnosis.

**Differential Diagnosis.** Malignant lymphoma is the most important lesion to exclude and is discussed under gastric lymphoma.

**Endoscopic Biopsy and Immunohistochemistry.** A presumptive diagnosis of lymphoid hyperplasia is aided by the availability of jumbo punch biopsy forceps, large particle snare biopsy, fine-needle aspirates, and immunohistochemistry (fig. 13-18). In many cases, however, diagnosis cannot be made for a number of reasons.

Some gastric carcinomas and lymphomas may be obscured by necrosis and a severe inflammatory reaction in the overlying and adjacent tissues. Since endoscopic biopsies sample only the superficial tissues, the finding of a polymorphous infiltrate does not exclude an underlying neoplasm (14). Sometimes it may just be very difficult to differentiate between lymphoid hyperplasia and lymphoma, for example, in suboptimally fixed specimens or in cases of low-grade lymphoma. Repeat biopsy with careful fixation may sometimes help if previous biopsies were poorly fixed and distorted. For some of the problem cases, immunohistochemistry and gene rearrangement studies are useful since lymphoid hyperplasia shows a polyclonal pattern in contrast to

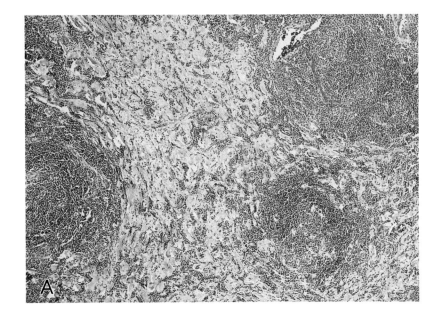

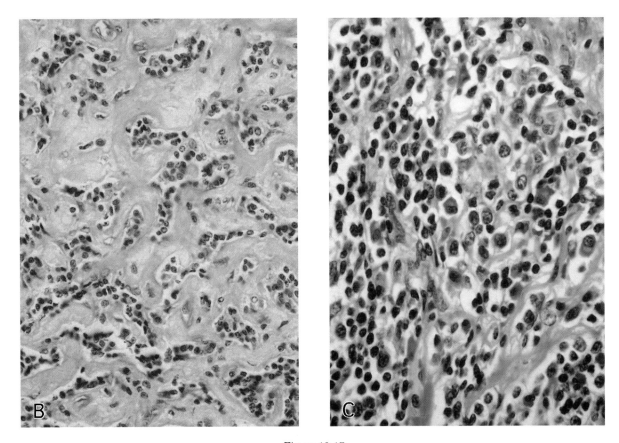

Figure 13-17
GASTRIC LYMPHOID HYPERPLASIA

A: Low-power view showing dense lymphoid infiltration, admixed lymphoid follicles, and fibrosis.

B: Area of dense collagenous fibrosis and intervening single file columns of mature lymphoid cells.

C: High-power view of a polymorphous infiltrate composed of mature lymphocytes, larger activated lymphocytes, plasma cells, eosinophils, and histiocytes.

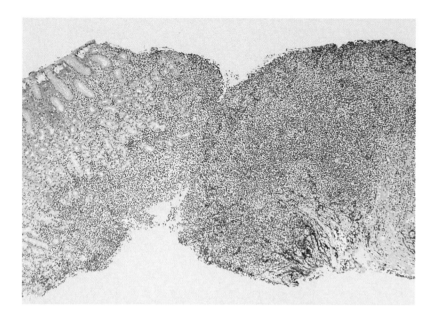

Figure 13-18
ENDOSCOPIC BIOPSY
SPECIMEN OF GASTRIC
LYMPHOID HYPERPLASIA

Top: Low-power view showing dense mucosal and submucosal inflammatory infiltrate.

Bottom: High-power view of the mucosal surface showing active gastritis.

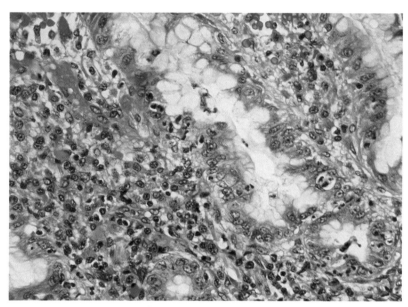

lymphoma which shows monoclonality and, frequently, gene rearrangement.

**Treatment and Risk of Developing Lymphoma.** Many of the cases of gastric lymphoid hyperplasia diagnosed in the past and now less frequently are first seen in gastrectomy specimens resected for intractable peptic ulceration or a suspicion of malignancy. For cases diagnosed by endoscopy and biopsy, management may be by repeat endoscopy and follow-up or limited gastric resection. The risk of lymphoma developing in cases of lymphoid hyperplasia is difficult to assess but it appears to be low (131,152). Up to 1989, only 12 cases of lymphoma developed secondary to lymphoid hyperplasia of the stomach; six of them occurred 2 to 8 years following diagnosis of lymphoid hyperplasia (131). However, we concur with Scoazec et al. (132) that surgical removal is indicated because of the uncertainty of excluding malignant lymphoma in unsampled areas (especially areas that are deep). The only exception would be for the small, bland-appearing lesions, associated with chronic gastric ulcers.

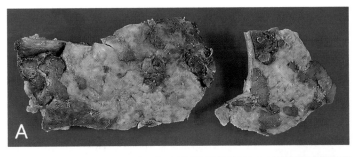

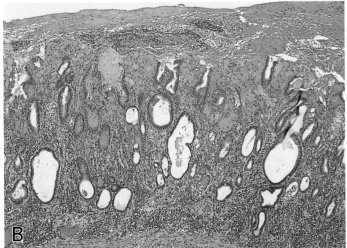

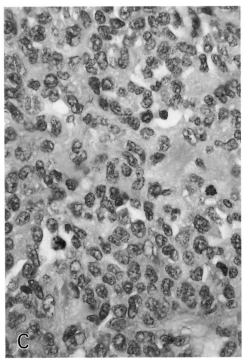

Figure 13-19
GROSS AND HISTOLOGIC FEATURES OF GASTRIC LEUKEMIA
A: Gross appearance of the opened stomach, showing marked thickening and nodularity of the mucosa due to diffuse lymphomatous infiltration. Part of the mucosa is purplish due to diffuse hemorrhage.
B: Low-power view of mucosa showing hemorrhage and superficial necrosis. The deeper areas of the mucosa show leukemic infiltration.
C: Higher magnification of B shows leukemic infiltration of the lamina propria. The infiltrate is composed of small lymphocytes with somewhat irregular nuclei.

## GASTRIC INVOLVEMENT IN LEUKEMIA

Clinical gastrointestinal complications of leukemia are common, occurring in up to 25 percent of cases (181,182,197), although most reports date from 1960 to 1980. Whether the lack of recent reports is a reflection of a decrease in incidence of gastric complications of leukemia is not certain. Complications are most frequent in the acute leukemias, especially during the inductive phase of therapy for remission. The majority of the lesions occur in the intestines, however, the stomach is also involved. Rarely, granulocytic sarcomas of the stomach may precede leukemia (178).

The major gastric complications of leukemia are mucosal hemorrhage and necrosis, leukemic infiltration, and opportunistic infection (178, 181,190,197); these are found in 75 percent of cases at autopsy (figs. 13-19, 13-20) (197).

Gastric mucosal hemorrhage has been reported in 60 percent of cases of leukemia at autopsy. It may be severe and associated with large quantities of blood within the stomach. About 10 percent of these cases are associated with mucosal necrosis (figs. 13-19, 13-20). Massive hemorrhage may be associated with thrombocytopenia.

Leukemic infiltration of the stomach occurs in 25 percent of cases (197). Half of these cases are associated with gross lesions consisting of multiple, bluish, mucosal nodules that are superficially ulcerated or thickened in a plaque-like manner. In rare instances the gastric mucosa has a convoluted "brain-like" appearance due to

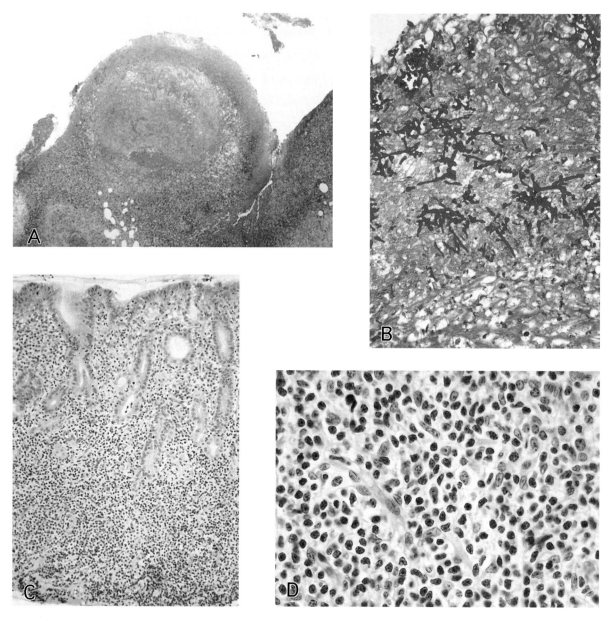

Figure 13-20
GROSS AND HISTOLOGIC FEATURES OF GASTRIC LEUKEMIA

A: Low-power view of the mucosa showing a circumscribed necrotic lesion.

B: Higher magnification of A stained with PAS to demonstrate fungal hyphae.

C: Low-power view of gastric mucosal biopsy from a patient with hairy cell leukemia. Note diffuse lymphoid infiltrate of the mucosa.

D: High-power magnification shows that the lymphoid infiltrate is composed of rather bland cells with clear cytoplasm and small, bland, round to oval nuclei with smudgy chromatin and indistinct nucleoli.

diffuse leukemic infiltration. Leukemic infiltration of the stomach must be differentiated from diffuse small cell lymphocytic lymphoma (well-differentiated lymphocytic lymphoma) which it can resemble. If there is any doubt as to the nature of the infiltrate, differentiation can be achieved by searching for eosinophilic myelocytes using the chloracetate esterase stain. Examination of blood smears and bone marrow will usually confirm the leukemia.

Opportunistic infections of the stomach consist primarily of *Candida,* which may become disseminated (197), and sometimes other fungi

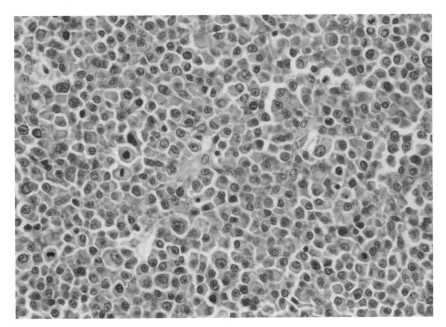

Figure 13-21
GASTRIC PLASMACYTOMA
A monomorphous infiltrate of atypical large plasma cells with enlarged nuclei and prominent nucleoli resembling immunoblasts is seen.

such as mucor. It results in irregular small ulcers covered by a fibrinohemorrhagic exudate. In one case of gastric mucor infection, there was extensive hemorrhagic necrosis due to vascular infiltration by the organism (fig. 13-20A,B). These lesions may perforate and give rise to Gram-negative sepsis (197). They are similar to the more commonly found lesions of neutropenic enterocolitis (181).

## SOLITARY PLASMACYTOMAS

Solitary plasmacytomas of the stomach are uncommon: they account for approximately 5 percent of extramedullary plasmacytomas (183, 188,189,196,202). They have many of the features of myelomas, since they are more common in middle-aged and elderly men (204) and sometimes associated with a monoclonal protein spike in the serum or urine (196). They commonly present with ulcer symptoms.

**Gross Findings.** At endoscopy the lesions grossly resemble lymphomas. They commonly present as ulcerated masses but may appear as single or multiple polypoid masses (186,193, 200). The tumors may be large, measuring as much as 15 cm in diameter, and extend from the mucosa to serosa (196). On cut section they have a rubbery consistency and are grey-white or pink, similar to lymphomas.

**Histologic Findings.** Solitary plasmacytomas are composed of a monomorphous infiltrate of plasma cells and often involve the full thickness of the stomach, although occasionally they may be confined to the mucosa or mucosa and submucosa (191). The plasmacytic infiltrate may be mature or immature; giant cells are sometimes seen in the latter (figs. 13-21, 13-22) (189, 200). The lesions may contain extracellular amyloid deposition. Gastric plasmacytomas must be differentiated from localized extramedullary manifestations of multiple myeloma and inflammatory pseudotumors (plasma cell granulomas) (195,204). Histologically, plasmacytomas demonstrate a monomorphic population of plasma cells with little admixture of inflammatory cells or granulomatous change (in contrast to the polymorphous infiltrate of the pseudotumors) (195,204). The plasma cells may contain crystalline inclusions (183,184) and we have seen a pleomorphic plasmacytoma which contained numerous bizarre Russell bodies (fig. 13-22). Those cases are invariably associated with dysproteinemia. The neoplastic nature of the lesion can be shown immunohistochemically by the demonstration of a single immunoglobulin in the plasma cells (184,189). The lack of bone marrow plasmacytosis indicates that the tumor is not a localized manifestation of multiple myeloma. Bone marrow aspirates from several sites and a reasonable

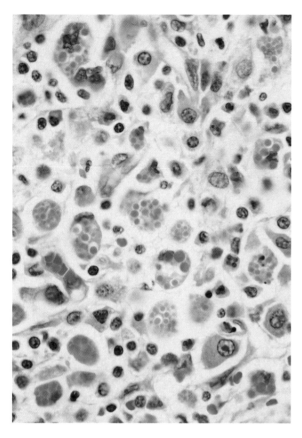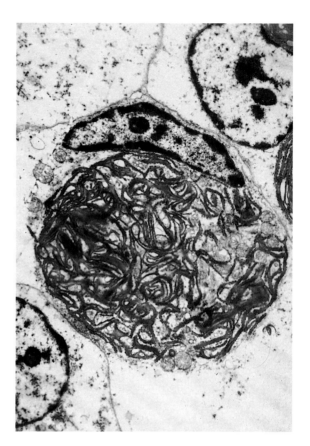

Figure 13-22
PLEOMORPHIC GASTRIC PLASMACYTOMA

Left: High-power magnification showing infiltrate composed of mature and immature plasma cells. Some of the atypical plasma cells contain numerous bizarre Russell bodies.

Right: Electron micrograph of Russell bodies. These consist of numerous cytoplasmic granules composed of aggregates of membranes.

period of follow-up should differentiate these two diseases (204). Plasmacytomas are distinguished from lymphomas morphologically. Although these tumors may be related histogenetically, they have sufficiently characteristic clinicopathologic features to warrant distinction from lymphomas with plasmacytoid features (192).

Data on the long-term prognosis of gastric plasmacytomas are limited (189,193,195,202). Surgery, with or without local radiotherapy, appears to be the treatment of choice, although some authorities advocate chemotherapy. In one study of five cases of primary gastric plasmacytoma, four of which were of early type confined to the mucosa and submucosa, there was no tumor recurrence with surgery alone after 12 years of follow-up (189).

## ANGIOCENTRIC LYMPHOPROLIFERATIVE LESION (LYMPHOMATOID GRANULOMATOSIS) INVOLVING THE STOMACH

This lesion is a rare T-lymphocyte proliferative disorder characterized by an angiocentric, angiodestructive, polymorphous infiltrate of atypical lymphocytes (small or large cleaved), abundant histiocytes, plasma cells, and neutrophils. It is associated with extensive destruction and necrosis of arterioles and venules. It affects primarily the lung but extrapulmonary disease has been noted in 83 percent of cases (180,187,199,201). Gastric involvement appears to be rare. Rubin (201) reported two patients with lymphomatoid granulomatosis with gastrointestinal involvement, one of whom had gastric lesions. This patient had severe gastrointestinal hemorrhage and numerous gastric erosions. Subsequently he developed a large gastric ulcer which histologically showed transmural infiltration with lymphomatoid granulomatosis.

## MYCOSIS FUNGOIDES INVOLVING THE STOMACH

Mycosis fungoides is a distinctive T-cell lymphoma of the skin that subsequently may involve lymph nodes and viscera (188,194,198,203). Gastric involvement is rare, usually asymptomatic, and associated with microscopic infiltration of the stomach by mycosis fungoides. However, there is one report of a patient who presented with severe gastrointestinal hemorrhage and was found to have an ulcerated nodule in the stomach which histologically showed the typical features of mycosis fungoides, namely, a dense monomorphous infiltrate of large atypical mononuclear cells, many of which retain the features of the mycosis cell with its characteristic cerebriform (irregularly cleaved) nucleus and scant cytoplasm (179). Histologically, mycosis fungoides may be confused with other lymphomas, especially immunoblastic sarcoma and Hodgkin's disease, because of the admixed eosinophils, plasma cells, and lymphocytes. A previous history of mycosis fungoides usually aids in the diagnosis. Also, mycosis cells are not found in immunoblastic sarcoma and Hodgkin's disease.

## REFERENCES

### Lymphoid Hyperplasia and Lymphoma

1. Algara P, Martinez P, Sanchez L, et al. The detection of B-cell monoclonal populations by polymerase chain reaction: accuracy of approach and application in gastric endoscopic biopsy specimens. Hum Pathol 1993;24:1184–8.
2. Allen AW, Donaldson G, Sniffen RC, Goodale F Jr. Primary malignant lymphoma of the gastrointestinal tract. Ann Surg 1954;140:428–38.
3. Aozasa K, Matsumoto M, Katagiri S, et al. Monocytoid B-cell lymphoma arising in extranodal organs. Cancer 1991;67:2305–10.
4. Aozasa K, Ueda T, Kurata A, Kum CW, Inoue M, Matsuura N. Prognostic value of histologic and clinical factors in 56 patients with gastrointestinal lymphomas. Cancer 1988;61:304–15.
5 Arista-Nasr J, Jimenez A, Keirns C, Larraza O, Larriva-Sahd J. The role of the endoscopic biopsy in the diagnosis of gastric lymphoma. Hum Pathol 1991;22:339–48.
6. Azab MB, Henry-Amar M, Rougier P, et al. Prognostic factors in primary gastrointestinal non-Hodgkin's lymphoma. A multivariate analysis, report of 106 cases and review of the literature. Cancer 1989;64:1208–17.
7. Azzopardi JG, Menzies T. Primary malignant lymphoma of the alimentary tract. Br J Surg 1960;47:358–66.
8. Bailey RL, Laws HL. Lymphoma of the stomach. Am Surg 1989;55:665–8.
9. Banerjee D, Walton JC, Jory TA, Crukley C, Meek M. Primary gastric T-cell lymphoma of suppressor-cytotoxic (CD8+) phenotype: discordant expression of T-cell receptor subunit beta F1, CD7 and CD3 antigens. Hum Pathol 1990;21:872–4.
10. Baron BW, Bitter MA, Baron JM, Bostwick DG. Adenocarcinoma after gastric lymphoma. Cancer 1987;60:1876–82.
10a.Bayerdorffer E, Neubauer A, Rudolph B, et al. Regression of primary gastric lymphoma of mucosa-associated lymphoid tissue type after cure of Helicobacter pylori infection. MALT Lymphoma Study Group. Lancet 1995;345:1591–4.
11. Berger F, Coiffier B, Bonneville C, Scoazec JY, Magaud JP, Bryon PA. Gastrointestinal lymphomas. Immunohistologic study of 23 cases. Am J Clin Pathol 1987;88:707–12.
12. Bernal A, del Junco GW. Endoscopic and pathologic features of esophageal lymphoma: a report of four cases in patients with acquired immune deficiency syndrome. Gastrointest Endosc 1986;32:96–9.
13. Blackshaw AJ, Levison DA. Eosinophilic infiltrates of the gastrointestinal tract. J Clin Pathol 1986;39:1–7.
14. Blackstone MO. Endoscopic interpretation. Normal and pathologic appearances of the gastrointestinal tract. Raven Press: New York, 1985.
14a.Blaser MJ. Helicobacter pylori phenotypes associated with peptic ulceration. Scan J Gastroenterol 1994;205:1–5.
15. Brooks JJ, Enterline HT. Gastric pseudolymphoma: its three subtypes and relation to lymphoma. Cancer 1983;51:476–86.
16. Brooks JJ, Enterline HT. Primary gastric lymphomas. Clinicopathological study of 58 cases with long-term follow-up and literature review. Cancer 1983;51:701–11.
17. Buchholz RR, Reid RA. Pseudolymphoma of the stomach. Surg Clin North Am 1972;2:485–91.
18. Burke JS, Sheibani K, Nathwani BN, Winberg CD, Rappaport H. Monoclonal small (well-differentiated) lymphocytic proliferations of the gastrointestinal tract resembling lymphoid hyperplasia: a neoplasm of uncertain malignant potential. Hum Pathol 1987;18:1238–45.

18a. Calvert R, Randerson J, Evans P, et al. Genetic abnormalities during transition from Helicobacter-pylori-associated gastritis to low-grade MALToma. Lancet 1995;345:26–7.

19. Cappell MS, Botros N. Predominantly gastrointestinal symptoms and signs in 11 consecutive AIDS patients with gastrointestinal lymphoma: a multicenter, multiyear study including 763 HIV-seropositive patients. Am J Gastroenterol 1994;89:545–9.

20. Chan JK, Ng CS, Isaacson PG. Relationship between high-grade lymphoma and low-grade B-cell musosa-associated lymphoid tissue lymphoma (MALToma) of the stomach. Am J Pathol 1990;136:1153–64.

21. Chen JM, Barr ML, Chadburn A, et al. Management of lymphoproliferative disorders after cardiac transplantation. Ann Thorac Surg 1993;56:527–38.

22. Chiles JT, Platz CE. The radiographic manifestations of pseudolymphoma of the stomach. Radiology 1975;116:551–6.

23. Cogliatti SB, Schmid U, Schumacher U, et al. Primary B-cell gastric lymphoma: a clinicopathological study of 145 patients. Gastroenterology 1991;1:1159–70.

24. Colucci G, Giotta F, Maiello E, Fucci L, Caruso ML. Primary Hodgkin's disease of the stomach. A case report. Tumori 1992;78:280–2.

25. Cornes JS. Multiple lymphomatous polyposis of the gastrointestinal tract. Cancer 1961;14:249–57.

25a. Cover TL, Tummuru MK, Cao P, Thompson SA, Blaser MJ. Divergence of genetic sequences for the vacuolating cytotoxin among Helicobacter pylori strains. J Biol Chem 1994;269:10566–73.

26. Craig FE, Gulley ML, Banks PM. Posttransplantation lymphoproliferative disorders. Am J Clin Pathol 1993;99:265–76.

27. Dawson IM, Cornes JS, Morson BC. Primary malignant lymphoid tumors of the intestinal tract. Report of 37 cases with a study of factors influencing prognosis. Br J Surg 1961;49:80–9.

28. de Mascarel A, Merlio JP, Coindre JM, Goussot JF, Broustet A. Gastric large cell lymphoma expressing cytokeratin but no leukocyte common antigen. A diagnostic dilemma. Am J Clin Pathol 1989;91:478–81.

29. Devaney K, Jaffe ES. The surgical pathology of gastrointestinal Hodgkin's disease. Am J Clin Pathol 1991;95:794–801.

30. Domizio P, Owen RA, Shepherd NA, Talbot IC, Norton AJ. Primary lymphoma of the small intestine. A clinicopathological study of 119 cases. Am J Surg Pathol 1993;17:429–42.

31. Dragosics B, Bauer P, Radaszkiewicz T. Primary gastrointestinal non-Hodgkin's lymphomas. A retrospective clinicopathologic study of 150 cases. Cancer 1985;55(5):1060–73.

32. Dworkin B, Lightdale CJ, Weingrad DN, et al. Primary gastric lymphoma. A review of 50 cases. Dig Dis Sci 1982;27:986–92.

33. Eimoto T, Futami K, Naito H, Takeshita M, Kikuchi M. Gastric pseudolymphoma with monotypic cytoplasmic immunoglobulin. Cancer 1985;55:788–93.

34. Eras P, Winawer SJ. Benign lymphoid hyperplasia of the stomach simulating gastric malignancy. Am J Dig Dis 1969;14:510–5.

35. Faris TD, Saltzstein SL. Gastric lymphoid hyperplasia: a lesion confused with lymphosarcoma. Cancer 1964;17:207–12.

36. Faulkner JW, Docherty MB. Lymphosarcoma of the small intestine. Surg Gynecol Obstet 1952;95:76–84.

37. Fend F, Schwaiger A, Weyrer K, et al. Early diagnosis of gastric lymphoma: gene rearrangement analysis of endoscopic biopsy samples. Leukemia 1994;8:35–9.

38. Fernandes BJ, Amato D, Goldfinger M. Diffuse lymphomatous polyposis of the gastrointestinal tract. A case report with immunohistochemical studies. Gastroenterology 1985;88:1267–70.

39. Filippa DA, Lieberman PH, Weingrad DN, Decosse JJ, Bretsky SS. Primary lymphomas of the gastrointestinal tract. Analysis of prognostic factors with emphasis on histological type. Am J Surg Pathol 1983;7:363–72.

40. Fishleder A, Tubbs R, Hesse B, Levine H. Uniform detection of immunoglobulin-gene rearrangement in benign lymphoepithelial lesions. N Engl J Med 1987;316:1118–21.

41. Fork FT, Haglund U, Hogstrom H, Wehlin L. Primary gastric lymphoma versus gastric cancer. An endoscopic and radiographic study of differential diagnostic possibilities. Endoscopy 1985;17:5–7.

42. Frazer JW Jr. Malignant lymphomas of the gastrointestinal tract. Surg Gynecol Obstet 1959;108:182–90.

43. Freeman C, Berg JW, Cutler SJ. Occurrence and prognosis of extranodal lymphomas. Cancer 1972;29:252–60.

44. Friedman SL. Gastrointestinal and hepatobiliary neoplasms in AIDS. Gastroenterol Clin North Am 1988;17:465–86.

45. Fujishima H, Misawa T, Maruoka A, Chijiiwa Y, Sakai K, Nawata H. Staging and follow-up of primary gastric lymphoma by endoscopic ultrasonography. Am J Gastroenterol 1991;86:719–24.

46. Galton DA, Catovsky D, Wiltshaw E. Clinical spectrum of lymphoproliferative diseases. Cancer 1978;42:901–10.

47. Genta RM, Hamner HW, Graham DY. Gastric lymphoid follicles in Helicobacter pylori infection: frequency, distribution, and response to triple therapy. Hum Pathol 1993;24:577–83.

48. Gray GM, Rosenberg SA, Cooper AD, Gregory PB, Stein PT, Herzenberg H. Lymphomas involving the gastrointestinal tract. Gastroenterology 1982;82:143–52.

49. Grody WW, Magidson JG, Weiss LM, Hu E, Warnke RA, Lewin KJ. Gastrointestinal lymphomas. Immunohistochemical studies on the cell of origin. Am J Surg Pathol 1985;9:328–37.

50. Guettier C, Hamilton-Dutoit S, Guillemain R, et al. Primary gastrointestinal malignant lymphomas associated with Epstein-Barr virus after heart transplantation. Histopathology 1992;20:21–8.

51. Haber DA, Mayer RJ. Primary gastrointestinal lymphoma. Semin Oncol 1988;2:154–69.

52. Hall PA, Jass JR, Levison DA, et al. Classification of primary gut lymphomas [Letter]. Lancet 1988;2:1317.

53. Hande KR, Fisher RI, DeVita VT, Chabner BA, Young RC. Diffuse histiocytic lymphoma involving the gastrointestinal tract. Cancer 1978;41:1984–9.

54. Harris AW, Misiewicz JJ. Antibiotic treatment for low-grade gastric MALT lymphoma [Letter]. Lancet 1994;343:1503.

55. Harris NL. Extranodal lymphoid infiltrates and mucosa-associated lymphoid tissue (MALT). A unifying concept. Am J Surg Pathol 1991;15:879–84.

56. Hassall E, Dimmick JE. Unique features of Helicobacter pylori disease in children. Dig Dis Sci 1991;36:417–23.

57. Hayes J, Dunn E. Has the incidence of primary gastric lymphoma increased? Cancer 1989;63:2073–6.

58. Hayoz D, Extermann M, Odermatt BF, Pugin P, Regamey C, Knecht H. Familial primary gastric lymphoma. Gut 1993;34:136–40.

59. Herrmann R, Panahon AM, Barcos MP, Walsh D, Stutzman L. Gastrointestinal involvement in non-Hodgkin's lymphoma. Cancer 1980;46:215–22.

60. Hernandez JA, Sheehan WW. Lymphomas of the mucosa-associated lymphoid tissue. Signet-ring lymphomas presenting in mucosal lymphoid organs. Cancer 1985;35:592–7.

61. Ho M, Miller G, Atchinson RW, et al. Epstein-Barr virus infections and DNA hydridization studies in posttransplantation lymphoma and lymphoproliferative lesions: the role of primary infection. J Infect Dis 1985;152:876–86.

62. Horsman D, Gascoyne R, Klasa R, Coupland R. t(11;18)(q21;q21.1): a recurring translocation in lymphomas of mucosa-associated lymphoid tissue (MALT)? Genes Chromosom Cancer 1992;4:183–7.

63. Horstmann M, Erttmann R, Winkler K. Relapse of MALT lymphoma associated with Helicobacter pylori after antibiotic treatment [Letter]. Lancet 1994;343:1098–9.

64. Hussell T, Isaacson PG, Crabtree JE, Spencer J. The response of cells from low-grade B-cell gastric lymphomas of mucosa-associated lymphoid tissue to Helicobacter pylori. Lancet 1993;342:571–4.

65. Hyjek E, Kelenyi G. Pseudolymphomas of the stomach: a lesion characterized by progressively transformed germinal centres. Histopathology 1982;6:61–8.

66. Isaacson PG. Gastric lymphoma and Helicobacter pylori [Editorial]. N Engl J Med 1994;330:1310–1.

67. Isaacson PG. Gastrointestinal lymphomas and lymphoid hyperplasias. In: Knowles DM, ed. Neoplastic hematopathology. Williams and Wilkens: Baltimore, 1992:953–78.

68. Isaacson PG. Lymphomas of mucosa-associated lymphoid tissue (MALT). Histopathology 1990;16:617–9.

69. Isaacson PG, Spencer J. The biology of low grade MALT lymphoma. J Clin Pathol 1995;48:395–7.

70. Isaacson PG, Spencer J. Malignant lymphoma of mucosa-associated lymphoid tissue. Histopathology 1987;11:445–62.

71. Isaacson PG, Spencer J, Wright DH. Classifying primary gut lymphomas [Letter]. Lancet 1988;2:1148–9.

72. Isaacson PG, Wotherspoon AC, Diss T, Pan LX. Follicular colonization in B-cell lymphoma of mucosa-associated lymphoid tissue. Am J Surg Pathol 1991;15:819–28.

73. Isaacson PG, Wotherspoon AC, Diss TC, Pan LX. Bcl-2 expression in lymphomas [Letter]. Lancet 1991;337:175–6.

74. Isaacson PG, Wright DH. Malignant lymphoma of mucosa-associated lymphoid tissue: a distinctive type of B-cell lymphoma. Cancer 1983;52:1410–6.

75. Isaacson PG, Wright DH. Extranodal malignant lymphoma arising from mucosa associated lymphoid tissue. Cancer 1984;53:2515–24.

76. Jacobs DS. Primary gastric malignant lymphoma and pseudolymphoma. Am J Clin Pathol 1963;40:379–94.

77. Jones RE, Willis S, Innes DJ, Wanebo HJ. Primary gastric lymphoma. Problems in staging and management. Am J Surg 1988;155:118–23.

78. Kanavaros P, Lavergne A, Galian A, Houdart R, Bernard JF. Primary gastric peripheral T-cell malignant lymphoma with helper/inducer phenotype. First case report with a complete histological ultrastructural and immunochemical study. Cancer 1988;61:1602–10.

79. Kemnitz J, Cremer J, Gebel M, Uysal A, Haverich A, Georgii A. T-cell lymphoma after heart transplantation. Am J Clin Pathol 1990;94:95–101.

80. Knowles DM. Chamulak GA, Subar M, et al. Lymphoid neoplasia associated with the acquired immunodeficiency syndrome (AIDS). The New York University Medical Center experience with 105 patients (1981-1986). Ann Intern Med 1988;108:744–53.

81. Kurihara K, Mizuseki K, Ichikawa M, Kohno H, Okanoue T. Primary gastric T-cell lymphoma with manifold histologic appearances. Acta Pathol Jpn 1991;41:824–8.

82. Lamy ME, Favart MA, Cornu S, et al. Epstein-Barr virus infection in 59 orthotopic liver transplant patients. Med Microbiol Immunol 1990;179:137–44.

83. Leoncini L, Del Vecchio MT, Kraft R, et al. Hodgkin's disease and CD30-positive anaplastic large cell lymphomas—a continuous spectrum of malignant disorders. A quantitative morphometric and immunohistologic study. Am J Pathol 1990;137:1047–57.

84. Levine PH, Kamaraja LS, Connelly RR, et al. The American Burkitt's Lymphoma Registry: eight years' experience. Cancer 1982;49:1016–22.

85. Levison DA, Shepherd NA. Pathology of gastric lymphomas and smooth muscle tumours. In: Preece PE, Cuschieri A, Welwood JM, eds. Cancer of the stomach. Grune and Stratton: London, 1986:47–72.

86. Lewin KJ, Ranchod M, Dorfman RF. Lymphomas of the gastrointestinal tract: a study of 117 cases presenting with gastrointestinal disease. Cancer 1978;42:693–707.

87. Lewin KJ, Riddell RH, Weinstein WM. Lymphoproliferative disorders. In: Lewin KJ, Riddell RH, Weinstein WM, eds. Gastrointestinal pathology and its clinical implications. Igaku-Shoin: New York, 1992:151–96.

88. Lim FE, Hartman AS, Tan EG, Cady B, Meissner WA. Factors in the prognosis of gastric lymphoma. Cancer 1977;39:1715–20.

89. Mann RB, Jaffe ES, Braylan RC, Frank MM, Ziegler JL, Berard CW. Non-endemic Burkitt's lymphoma. A B-cell tumor related to germinal centers. N Engl J Med 1976;295:685–91.

90. Maor MH, Maddux B, Osborne BM, et al. Stages IE and IIE non-Hodgkin's lymphomas of the stomach. Comparison of treatment modalities. Cancer 1984;54:2330–7.

91. Maor MH, Velasquez WS, Fuller LM, Solvermintz KB. Stomach conservation in stages IE and IIE gastric non-Hodgkin's lymphoma. J Clin Oncol 1990;8:266–71.

92. McAlister V, Grant D, Roy A, Yilmaz Z, Ghent G, Wall W. Posttransplant lymphoproliferative disorders in liver recipients treated with OKT3 or ALG induction immunosuppression. Transplant Proc 1993;25:1400–1.

93. McNeer G, Berg JW. The clinical behavior and management of primary malignant lymphoma of the stomach. Surgery 1959;46:829–40.

94. Moore I, Wright DH. Primary gastric lymphoma—a tumor of mucosa-associated lymphoid tissue. A histological and immunohisdochemical study of 36 cases. Histopathology 1984;8:1025–39.

95. Mori S, Mohri N, Shimamine T. Reactive lymphoid hyperplasia of the stomach. An immunohistochemical study. Acta Pathol Jpn 1980;30:671–80.

96. Moubayed P, Kaiserling E, Stein H. T-cell lymphomas of the stomach: morphological and immunological studies characterizing two cases of T-cell lymphoma. Virchows Arch [A] 1987;411:523–9.

96a. Moynihan MJ, Bast MA, Chan WC, et al. Lymphomatous polyposis. A neoplasm of either follicular mantle or germinal center cell origin. Am J Surg Pathol 1996;20:442–52.

97. Murayama H, Kikuchi M, Eimoto T, Doki T, Doki K. Early lymphoma coexisting with reactive lymphoid hyperplasia of the stomach. Acta Pathol Jpn 1984;34:679–86.

98. Musshoff K. Klinische Stadieneinteilung der nicht-Hodgkin Lymphome. Strahlentherapie 1977;153:218–21.

99. Myhre MJ, Isaacson PG. Primary B-cell gastric lymphoma–a reassessment of its histogenesis. J Pathol 1987;152:1–11.

100. Nalesnik MA. Lymphoproliferative disease in organ transplant recipients. Springer Semin Immunopathol 1991;13:199–216.

101. Nalesnik MA, Demetris AJ, Fung JJ, Starzl TE. Lymphoproliferative disorders arising under immunosuppresion with FK-506: initial observations in a large transplant population. Transplant Proc 1991;23:1108–10.

102. Nalesnik MA, Jaffe R, Starzl TE, et al. The pathology of posttransplant lymphoproliferative disorders occurring in the setting of cyclosporine A-prednisone immunosuppression. Am J Pathol 1988;133:173–92.

103. Naqvi MS, Burrows L, Kark AE. Lymphosarcoma of the gastrointestinal tract: prognostic guides based on 162 cases. Ann Surg 1969;170:221–31.

103a. Nathwani B, Brynes RK, Linola T, Hansmann ML. Classifications of non-Hodgkin's lymphoma. In: Knowles DM, ed. Neoplastic hematopathology. Baltimore: Williams & Wilkins, 1992:554–601.

103b. Navratil E, Gaulard P, Kanavaros P, et al. Expression of the bcl-2 protein in B cell lymphomas arising from mucosa associated lymphoid tissue. J Clin Pathol 1995;48:18–21.

104. Nizze H, Cogliatti SB, von Schilling C, Feller AC, Lennert K. Monocytoid B-cell lymphoma: morphological variants and relationship to low-grade B-cell lymphoma of the mucosa-associated lymphoid tissue. Histopathology 1991;18:403–14.

105. O'Briain DS, Kennedy MJ, Daly PA, et al. Multiple lymphomatous polyposis of the gastrointestinal tract. A clinicopathologically distinctive form of non-Hodgkin's lymphoma of B-cell centrocytic type. Am J Surg Pathol 1989;13:691–9.

106. Orlando R, Pastuszak W, Preissler PL, Welch JP. Gastric lymphoma: a clinicopathological reappraisal. Am J Surg 1982;143:450–5.

107. Ortiz-Hidalgo C, Wright DH. The morphologic spectrum of monocytoid B-cell lymphoma and its relationship to lymphomas of mucosa-associated lymphoid tissue. Histopathology 1992;21:555–61.

108. Palazzo L, Roseau G, Ruskone-Fourmestraux A, et al. Endoscopic ultrasonography in the local staging of primary gastric lymphoma. Endoscopy 1993;25:502–8.

109. Pan L, Diss TC, Cunningham D, Isaacson PG. The bcl-2 gene in primary B-cell lymphoma of mucosa-associated lymphoid tissue (MALT). Am J Pathol 1989;135:7–11.

110. Parsonnet J, Hansen S, Rodriguez L, et al. Helicobacter pylori infection and gastric lymphoma. N Engl J Med 1994;330:1267–71.

111. Pasini F, Ambrosetti A, Sabbioni R, et al. Postoperative chemotherapy increases the disease-free survival rate in primary gastric lymphomas stage IE and IIE. Eur J Cancer 1994;30A:33–6.

112. Paulli M, Rosso R, Kindl S, et al. Primary gastric CD30 (Ki-1)-positive large cell non-Hodgkin's lymphomas. A clinicopathologic analysis of six cases. Cancer 1994;73:541–9.

113. Paulsen J, Lennert K. Low-grade B-cell lymphoma of mucosa-associated lymphoid tissue type in Waldeyer's ring. Histopathology 1994;24:1–11.

113a. Peek RM Jr, Miller GG, Tham KT, et al. Detection of Helicobacter pylori gene expression in human gastric mucosa. J Clin Microbiol 1995;33:28–32.

114. Perez CA, Dorfman RF. Benign lymphoid hyperplasia of the stomach and the duodenum. Radiology 1966;57:505–10.

115. Perrillo RP, Tedesco FJ. Gastric pseudolymphoma. A spectrum presenting features and diagnostic considerations. Am J Gastroenterol 1976;65:226–30.

116. Price SK. Immunoproliferative small intestinal dicease: a study of 13 cases with alpha heavy-chain disease. Histopathology 1990;17:7–17.

117. Radaszkiewicz T, Dragosics B, Bauer P. Gastrointestinal malignant lymphomas of the mucosa-associated lymphoid tissue: factors relevant to prognosis. Gastroenterology 1992;102:1628–38.

118. Ranchod M, Lewin KJ, Dorfman RF. Lymphoid hyperplasia of the gastrointestinal tract. A study of 26 cases and review of the literature. Am J Surg Pathol 1978;2:383–400.

119. Randhawa PS, Jaffe R, Demetris AJ, et al. The systemic distribution of Epstein-Barr virus genomes in fatal posttransplantation lymphoproliferative disorders. An in situ hybridization study. Am J Pathol 1991;138:1027–33.

119a. Roggero E, Zucca E, Pinotti G, et al. Eradication of Helicobacter pylori infection in primary low-grade gastric lymphoma of mucosa-associated lymphoid tissue. Ann Intern Med 1995;122:767–9.

120. Rosen CB, van Heerden JA, Martin JK, Wold LE, Ilstrup DM. Is an aggressive surgical approach to the patient with gastric lymphoma warranted? Ann Surg 1987;205:634–20.

121. Rosenfelt F, Rosenberg SA. Diffuse histiocytic lymphoma presenting with gastrointestinal tract lesions. The Stanford experience. Cancer 1980;45:2188–93.

122. Ross CW, Hanson CA, Schnitzer B. CD30 (Ki-1)-positive, anaplastic large cell lymphoma mimicking gastrointestinal carcinoma. Cancer 1992;70:2517–23.

123. Rudders RA, Ross ME, De Lellis RA. Primary extranodal lymphoma: response to treatment and factors influencing prognosis. Cancer 1978;42:406–16.

124. Ruppert GB, Smith VM. Multiple lymphomatous polyposis of the gastrointestinal tract. Gastrointest Endosc 1979;25:67–9.

125. Salles G, Herbrecht R, Tilly H, et al. Aggressive primary gastrointestinal lymphomas: review of 91 patients treated with the LNH-84 regimen. A study of the Groupe d'Etude des Lymphomes Agressifs. Am J Med 1991;90:77–84.

126. Salzstein SL. Extranodal malignant lymphomas and pseudolymphomas. In: Anonymous. Pathology annual. Vol 4. New York:Appleton-Century-Crofts, 1969:159–84.

127. Sandler RS. Has primary gastric lymphoma become more common? J Clin Gastroenterol 1984;6:101–7.

128. Schmidt U, Gloor U, Schildknecht O. Das maligne Nicht-Hodgkin-Lymphom des Magens. Dtsch Med Wochenschr 1980;105:1147–52.

129. Schuder G, Hildebrandt U, Kreissler-Haag D, Seitz G, Feifel G. Role of endosonography in the surgical management of non-Hodgkin's lymphoma of the stomach. Endoscopy 1993;25:509–12.

130. Schulman H, Sickel J, Kleinman M, Adams JT. Gastric pseudolymphoma with restricted light chain expression in a patient with obscure gastrointestinal blood loss. Dig Dis Sci 1991;36:1495–9.

131. Schwartz MS, Sherman H, Smith T, Janis R. Gastric pseudolymphoma and its relationship to malignant gastric lymphoma. Am J Gastroenterol 1989;84:1555–9.

132. Scoazec JY, Brousse N, Potet F, Jeulain JF. Focal malignant lymphoma in gastric pseudolymphoma. Histologic and immunohistochemical study of a case. Cancer 1986;57:1330–6.

133. Seifert E, Schulte F, Weismuller J, de Mas CR, Stolte M. Endoscopic and bioptic diagnosis of malignant non-Hodgkin's lymphoma of the stomach. Endoscopy 1993;25:497–501.

134. Severson RK, Davis S. Increasing incidence of primary gastric lymphoma. Cancer 1990;66:1283–7.

135. Shepherd NA, Blackshaw AJ, Hall PA, et al. Malignant lymphoma with eosinophilia of the gastrointestinal tract. Histopathology 1987;11:115–30.

136. Shepherd NA, McCarthy KP, Hall PA. 14;18 translocation in primary intestinal lymphoma: detection by polymerase chain reaction in routinely processed tissue. Histopathology 1991;18:415–9.

137. Sherlock P. The gastrointestinal manifestations and complications of malignant lymphoma. Schweiz Med Wochenschr 1980;110:1031–6.

137. Shigematsu A, Iida M, Lien GS, et al. Spontaneous regression of primary malignant lymphoma of the stomach in two nontreated Japanese. J Clin Gastroenterol 1989;11:511–7.

139. Shimm DS, Dosoretz DE, Anderson T, Linggood RM, Harris NL, Wang CC. Primary gastric lymphoma. An analysis with emphasis on prognostic factors and radiation therapy. Cancer 1983;52:2044–8.

140. Shimodaira M, Tsukamoto Y, Niwa Y, et al. A proposed staging system for primary gastric lymphoma. Cancer 1994;73:2709–15.

141. Shiu MH, Nisce LZ, Pinna A, et al. Recent results of multimodal therapy of gastric lymphoma. Cancer 1986;58:1389–99.

142. Sigal SH, Saul SH, Auerbach HE, Raffensperger E, Kant JA, Brooks JJ. Gastric small lymphocytic proliferation with immunoglobulin gene rearrangement in pseudolymphoma versus lymphoma. Gastroenterology 1989;97:195–201.

143. Smith WJ, Price SK, Isaacson PG. Immunoglobulin gene rearrangement in immunoproliferative small intestinal disease (IPSID). J Clin Pathol 1987;40:1291–7.

144. Soderstrom KO, Joensuu H. Primary Hodgkin's disease of the stomach. Am J Clin Pathol 1988;89:806–9.

145. Sokal EM, Caragiozoglou T, Lamy M, Reding R, Otte JB. Epstein-Barr virus serology and Epstein-Barr virus-associated lymphoproliferative disorders in pediatric liver transplant recipients. Transplantation 1993;56:1394–8.

146. Solidoro A, Payet C, Sanchez-Lihon J, Montalbetti JA. Gastric lymphomas: chemotherapy as a primary treatment. Semin Surg Oncol 1990;6:218–25.

147. Spencer J, Cerf-Bensussan N, Jarry A, et al. Enteropathy-associated T cell lymphoma (malignant histiocytosis of the intestine) is recognized by a monoclonal antibody (HML-1) that defines a membrane molecule on human mucosal lymphocytes. Am J Pathol 1988;132:1–5.

148. Spencer J, Diss TC, Isaacson PG. Primary B cell gastric lymphoma. A genotypic analysis. Am J Pathol 1989;135:557–64.

149. Starzl TE, Porter KA, Iwatsuki S. Reversibility of lymphomas and lymphoproliferative lesions developing under cyclosporine-steroid therapy. Lancet 1984;1:583–7.

150. Stolte M, Eidt S. Healing gastric MALT lymphomas by eradicating H pylori? Lancet 1993;342:568.

151. Sundeen JT, Longo DL, Jaffe ES. CD5 expression in B-cell small lymphocytic malignancies. Correlations with clinical presentation and sites of disease. Am J Surg Pathol 1992;16:130–7.

152. Sweeney JF, Muus C, McKeown PP, Rosemurgy AS. Gastric pseudolymphoma. Not necessarily a benign lesion. Dig Dis Sci 1992;37:939–45.

153. Swerdlow SH. Post-transplant lymphoproliferative disorders: a morphologic, phenotypic and genotypic spectrum of disease. Histopathology 1992;20:373–85.

154. Taal BG, Burgers JM, van Heerde P, Hart AA, Somers R. The clinical spectrum and treatment of primary non-Hodgkin's lymphoma of the stomach. Ann Oncol 1993;4:839–46.

155. Taal BG, den Hartog Jager FC, Burgers JM, van Heerde P, Tio TL. Primary non-Hodgkin's lymphoma of the stomach: changing aspects and therapeutic choices. Eur J Cancer Clin Oncol 1989;25:439–50.

156. Takahashi H, Hansmann ML. Primary gastrointestinal lymphoma in childhood (up to 18 years of age). A morphological, immunohistochemical and clinical study. J Cancer Res Clin Oncol 1990;116:190–6.

157. Takenaga T, Sakano T, Kitahara T, Kitaoka H, Watanabe S, Hirota T. Five cases of malignant lymphoma associated with early gastric cancer. Jap J Clin Oncol 1978;8:209–18.

158. Takeshita K, Ashikawa T, Watanuki S, et al. Endoscopic and clinicopathological features of primary gastric lymphoma. Hepatogastroenterology 1993;40:485–90.

159. Tio TL, Tytgat GN. Endoscopic ultrasonography in analysing peri-intestinal lymph node abnormality. Preliminary results of studies in vitro and in vivo. Scand J Gastroenterol 1986;21:158–63.

160. Tungeker MP. Gastric signet-ring cell lymphoma with alpha heavy chains. Histopathology 1986;10:725–33.

161. Van Krieken JH, Medeiros LJ, Pals ST, Raffeld M, Kluin PM. Diffuse aggressive B-cell lymphomas of the gastrointestinal tract. An immunophenotypic and gene rearrangement analysis of 22 cases. Am J Clin Pathol 1992;97:170–8.

162. Van Krieken JH, Otter R, Hermans J, et al. Malignant lymphoma of the gastrointestinal tract and mesentery: a clinico-pathologic study of the significance of histologic classification. Am J Pathol 1989;135:281–9.

163. Van Krieken JH, von Schilling C, Kluin M, Lennert K. Splenic marginal zone lymphocytes and related cell in the lymph nodes. Human Pathology 1989;20:320–5.

164. Watson RJ, O'Brien MT. Gastric pseudolymphoma (lymphofollicular gastritis). Ann Surg 1970;171:98–106.

165. Weingrad DN, Decosse JJ, Sherlock P, et al. Primary gastrointestinal lymphoma: a thirty year review. Cancer 1982;49:1258–65.

166. Wolf JA, Spjut HJ. Focal lymphoid hyperplasia of the stomach preceding gastric lymphoma: a case report and review of the literature. Cancer 1981;48:2518–23.

167. Wotherspoon AC, Doglioni C, de Boni M, Spencer J, Isaacson PG. Antibiotic treatment for low-grade gastric MALT lymphoma [Letter]. Lancet 1994;43:1503.

168. Wotherspoon AC, Doglioni C, Diss TC, et al. Regression of primary low-grade B-cell gastric lymphoma of mucosa-associated lymphoid tissue type after eradication of Helicobacter pylori. Lancet 1993;342:575–7.

169. Wotherspoon AC, Doglioni C, Isaacson PG. Gastric B cell lymphoma of mucosa-associated lymphoid tissue is a multifocal disease [Abstract]. J Pathol 1990;161:345a.

170. Wotherspoon AC, Ortiz-Hidalgo C, Falzon MR, Isaacson PG. Helicobacter pylori-associated gastritis and primary B-cell gastric lymphoma. Lancet 1991;338:1175–6.

171. Wotherspoon AC, Pan LX, Diss TC, Isaacson PG. Cytogenetic study of B-cell lymphoma of mucosa-associated lymphoid tissue. Cancer Genet Cytogenet 1992;8:35–8.

172. Wright CJ. Pseudolymphoma of the stomach. Hum Pathol 1973;4:305–18.

173. Yatabe Y, Mori N, Oka K, Nakazawa M, Asai J. Primary gastric T-cell lymphoma. Morphological and immunohistochemical studies of two cases. Arch Pathol Lab Med 1994;118:547–50.

174. Zaloznik AJ, Giudice RO. Gastric Hodgkin's disease: recurrence after autologous bone marrow transplant. Mil Med 1992;157:617–9.

174a.Zamboni G, Franzin G, Scaroa A, et al. Carcinoma-like Signet-ring cells in gastric mucosa-associated lymphoid tissue (MALT) lymphoma Am J Surg Pathol 1996;20:588–98.

175. Zorlu AF, Atahan IL, Gedikoglu G, Ruacan S, Sayek I, Tekuzman G. Does gastric adenocarcinoma develop after the treatment of gastric lymphoma? J Surg Oncol 1993;54:126–31.

176. Zuckerman MJ, Pittman D, Bomar D, Farley PC. Multiple lymphomatous polyposis of the gastrointestinal tract with immunologic marker studies. J Clin Gastroenterol 1986;8:295–300.

177. Zukerberg LR, Ferry JA, Southern JF, Harris NL. Lymphoid infiltrates of the stomach. Evaluation of histologic criteria for the diagnosis of low-grade gastric lymphoma on endoscopic biopsy specimens. Am J Surg Pathol 1990;14:1087–99.

## Miscellaneous Lymphoproliferative Disorders

178. Brugo EA, Marshall RB, Riberi AM, Pautasso OE. Preleukemic granulocytic sarcomas of the gastrointestinal tract. Report of two cases. Am J Clin Pathol 1977;68:616–21.

179. Case Records of the Massachusetts General Hospital. Case 52-1971. N Engl J Med 1971;285:1526–32.

180. Chen KT. Abdominal form of lymphomatoid granulomatosis. Hum Pathol 1977;8:99–103.

181. Cornes JS, Jones TG, Fisher GB. Leukaemic lesions of the gastrointestinal tract. J Clin Pathol 1962;15:305–13.

182 Dewar GJ, Lim CN, Michalyshyn B, et al. Gastrointestinal complications in patients with acute and chronic leukemia. Can J Surg 1981;24:67–71.

183. Ferrer-Roca O. Primary gastric plasmacytoma with massive intracytoplasmic crystalline inclusions: a case report. Cancer 1982;50:755–9.

184. Funakoshi N, Kanoh T, Kobayashi Y, Miyake T, Uchino H, Ochi K. IgM-producing gastric plasmacytoma. Cancer 1984;54:638–43.

185. Ganz R, Olinger E, Variakojis D, Gordon L. Mycosis fungoides with gastrointestinal involvement. Gastrointest Endosc 1988;34:478–81.

186. Goeggel-Lamping C, Kahn SB. Gastrointestinal polyposis in multiple myeloma. JAMA 1978;239:1786–7.

187. Homma K, Umezu H, Nemoto K, Ohnishi Y, Sekine A, Yoshioka K. Angiocentric immunoproliferative lesion of the stomach. Case report. Virchows Arch [A] 1991;418:267–70.

188. Isaacson P, Buchanan R, Mepham BL. Plasma cell granuloma of the stomach. Hum Pathol 1978;9:355–8.

189. Ishido T, Mori N. Primary gastric plasmacytoma: a morphological and immunohistochemical study of five cases. Am J Gastroenterol 1992;87:875–8.

190. Katabami S, Hinoda Y, Ohe Y, et al. Adult T-cell leukemia/lymphoma (lymphoma type) with remarkable gastric lesions: a case report. Gastroenterol Jpn 1992;27:95–101.

191. Koyama S, Koike N, Saito T, Todoroki T, Mori N, Fukutomi H. Early extramedullary plasmacytoma confined to the lamina propria of the gastric mucosa: case report. Jpn J Clin Oncol 1992;22:136–41.

192. Lewin KJ, Kahn LB, Novis BH. Primary intestinal lymphoma of Western and Mediterranean type, alpha-chain disease and massive plasma cell infiltration: a comparative study of 37 cases. Cancer 1976;38:2511–28.

193. Line DH, Lewis RH. Gastric plasmacytoma. Gut 1969;10:230–3.

194. Long JC, Mihm MC. Mycosis fungoides with extracutaneous dissemination: a distinct clinicopathologic entity. Cancer 1974;34:1745–55.

195. McCaffrey J, Kingston CW, Hasker WE. Extramedullary plasmacytoma of the gastrointestinal tract. Aust N Z J Surg 1972;41:351–3.

196. Nakanishi I, Kajikawa K, Migita S, Mai M, Akimoto R, Mura T. Gastric plasmacytoma: an immunologic and immunohistochemical study. Cancer 1982;49:2025–8.

197. Prolla JC, Kirsner JB. The gastrointestinal lesions and complications of the leukemias. Ann Intern Med 1964;61:1084–103.

198. Rappaport H, Thomas LB. Mycosis fungoides: the pathology of extracutaneous involvement. Cancer 1974;34:1198–229.

199. Rattinger MD, Dunn TL, Christain D Jr, et al. Gastrointestinal involvement in lymphomatoid granulomatosis. Report of a case and review of the literature. Cancer 1983;51:694–700.

200. Remigio PA, Klaum A. Extramedullary plasmacytoma of stomach. Cancer 1971;27:562–8.

201. Rubin LA, Little AH, Kolin A, Keystone EC. Lymphomatoid granulomatosis involving the gastrointestinal tract. Two case reports and a review of the literature. Gastroenterology 1983;84:829–33.

202. Sharma KD, Shrivastav JD. Extramedullary plasmacytoma of gastrointestinal tract with a case report of plasmoma of the rectum and a review of the literature. Arch Pathol 1961;71:229–33.

203. Slater DN, Bleehen SS, Beck S. Gastrointestinal complications of mycosis fungoides. J R Soc Med 1984;77:114–9.

204. Wiltshaw E. The natural history of extramedullary plasmacytoma and its relation to solitary myeloma of bone and myelomatosis. Medicine 1976;55:217–38.

# MESENCHYMAL TUMORS AND TUMOR-LIKE PROLIFERATIONS

The stomach is the most common gastrointestinal site of origin for stromal or mesenchymal tumors, just as it is for lymphomas. Stromal neoplasms may be divided into two groups. The first group, the less common, consists of tumors that are identical to those that usually arise in the soft tissues throughout the body, including lipomas, hemangiomas, usual leiomyomas, and their malignant counterparts. The second group, the more common, is a collection of distinctive stromal tumors that arise within the gastric wall almost exclusively; that is, they are unlikely to arise elsewhere, even in other sites within the gastrointestinal tract. These common gastric stromal tumors have attracted the most interest because of uncertainties about their histogenesis (their cell or cells of origin), their differentiation (the type or types of cells they contain), and their behavior (how they act, and how to separate the benign ones from the malignant ones).

There are no established risk factors for gastric stromal tumors. Rare postirradiation sarcomas have been reported. Buffalo rats, who develop gastric adenocarcinomas and sarcomas when given the carcinogen N-methyl-N'-nitro-N-nitrosoguanidine in combination with stress, aspirin, or sodium taurocholate, are the animal model (19).

## COMMON STROMAL TUMORS COMPOSED OF UNDIFFERENTIATED, MINIMALLY DIFFERENTIATED, OR PECULIARLY DIFFERENTIATED CELLS/ LEIOMYOMAS AND LEIOMYOSARCOMAS

Traditionally, common or generic gastric stromal tumors have been designated as smooth muscle tumors, probably because many contain long spindled cells, and there is much smooth muscle in the stomach from which they could arise. There are three morphologic types: two homogeneous benign tumor types and one heterogeneous group of malignant tumors or sarcomas. The first benign type is a spindle cell tumor, also called *cellular leiomyoma,* although it is too often designated simply as *leiomyoma,* since it is assumed that it is a tumor composed of typical benign smooth muscle cells, which it is not. The second is a benign epithelioid cell tumor that has been given the name of *epithelioid leiomyoma.* The third type includes all the sarcomas whether they contain spindled cells, epithelioid cells, or both. Although all three of these tumor types have been and are still being referred to as smooth muscle proliferations, they are composed of cells with conflicting evidence of smooth muscle differentiation or any other differentiation, depending upon whether the analytic system is electron microscopy or immunohistochemistry, and if immunohistochemistry, what markers are used and which laboratory performs the studies. Furthermore, it is widely believed that the biologic behavior of the these tumors is unpredictable. As a consequence of these perceived peculiarities in differentiation and behavior, an impressive literature on gastric stromal tumors has accumulated over the past 30 years, and the results of studies using new analytic techniques are reported as they became available. Yet, little has been learned about their histogenesis or type of differentiation. Although the spindle cell tumors and the epithelioid cell tumors are histologically distinctive in most cases, there are tumors which contain areas of both cell types. Clinically and grossly, they are not significantly different: the sarcomas and the benign lesions often present with the same clinical features, and as is discussed later, the benign tumors may be the precursors of the sarcomas. Therefore, both the benign and the malignant varieties of the common gastric stromal tumor are discussed together rather than separately.

**Clinical Features.** Both benign and malignant gastric stromal neoplasms usually occur in the fifth through the seventh decades of life, the same age range as that for most other neoplastic diseases of the gastrointestinal tract, including most carcinomas. Some studies report a male predominance of as much as 2 to 1 for sarcomas, but other studies report a female predominance (8,10,34,56). Probably, there is no sex predilection except for the tumors of Carney's triad, nearly all of which occur in females (see Sarcomas) (17).

The presenting manifestations are similar to those of patients with other gastric neoplasms,

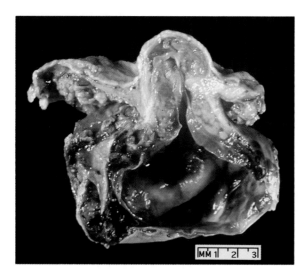

Figure 14-1
CYSTIC LEIOMYOMA/
CYSTIC BENIGN STROMAL TUMOR
The mucosa is the thick white layer at the top. This tumor is situated in the submucosa and muscularis propria, and it bulges the subserosa.

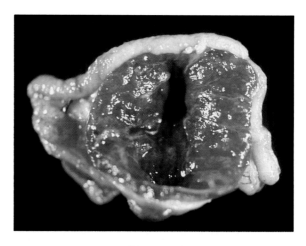

Figure 14-2
SUBMUCOSAL LEIOMYOMA/
BENIGN STROMAL TUMOR
The mucosa is the thick white layer covering the tumor. The muscularis propria is below the tumor.

with slight differences between the benign and malignant types. Upper gastrointestinal bleeding, the result of ulcers developing over the lesions, expressed as either hematemesis, melena, or slowly developing iron deficiency anemia, is the most common clinical expression. About 50 percent of patients have such bleeding. Upper abdominal ulcer-like pain is the second most common manifestation, and this occurs about twice as often in patients with sarcomas. Anorexia, nausea, and vomiting occur in about one quarter of patients. There is a palpable mass in about 10 percent of the benign cases but in over one third of the sarcomas; this reflects the greater overall size of sarcomas compared to their benign counterparts. Weight loss occurs in one quarter of sarcoma patients, but is uncommon in patients with benign tumors. Weight loss may be related to high tumor stage, including metastases; however, sarcomas rarely present with symptoms attributable to metastases in extragastric sites. Almost one third of patients with benign tumors are asymptomatic, possibly because of smaller lesion size, while patients with sarcoma are rarely asymptomatic.

The clinical diagnosis is often made endoscopically for tumors that cause bleeding, pain, weight loss, nausea, vomiting, and anorexia since these symptoms are common indications for upper endo-scopy. Since the tumors are intramural masses, the endoscopic findings are not specific. Tumors situated within the submucosa are likely to protrude into the lumen as smooth lumps covered by a mucosa that may be intact or ulcerated.

Radiographic imaging studies, including computed tomography (CT) and barium contrast examination present different views of these tumors, but both are capable of detecting them as masses. Their sensitivity is such that they can detect intramural masses as small as 1 cm in diameter, if the radiologist knows what is being sought. These techniques are more sensitive if the stomach is targeted using distention and variable angle views. If the radiologist has no indication that the stomach is the problem area, then intramural masses 2 or 3 cm across may be missed. In barium swallow studies the tumors appear as smooth filling defects indenting the barium column, and the contrast material may pool in ulcer craters. CT often can determine if the mass is solid or cystic; centrally necrotic tumors may appear cystic. Magnetic resonance imaging (MRI) is not a useful technique for gastrointestinal tract diseases.

**Gross Findings.** Most gastric stromal tumors, both benign and malignant, are situated within the submucosa and the muscularis propria in continuity, although smaller ones may be totally submucosal or intramuscular (figs. 14-1, 14-2). Bigger tumors extend into the perigastric tissues, and some of these appear dumbbell shaped, with a bulbous submucosal component, a constricted area in the muscularis propria, and a second bulbous component in the subserosa (fig. 14-3). Occasional tumors are predominantly extramural with very narrow attachments to the outer layer of the muscularis propria. Most of these are large, benign, and on the greater curvature, and often they project into the omentum where tumors 25 cm and more in maximal diameter have been observed.

Upon palpation, stromal tumors usually feel firm and seem to be well circumscribed, although some may be multinodular. Large intramural tumors commonly have overlying ulcers, and occasionally a tumor may have more than one ulcer on its surface (figs. 14-4, 14-5). When they are cut across, they do not have the bulging, whorled appearance and gristly consistency of uterine leiomyomas. Instead, the cut surface is flat, often granular, and pock-marked by vessels and foci of hemorrhage and necrosis (figs. 14-6, 14-7). This is true for benign tumors and many malignant ones as well. The tumors are firm and slightly rubbery. The amount of central necrosis is variable and does not help in differentiating benign from malignant. Some tumors have huge patches of necrosis and hemorrhage. This is especially true for ulcerated tumors in which the ulcers communicate with the necrotic foci. In fact some tumors may be so necrotic centrally that they look

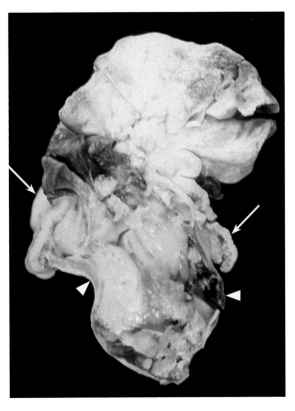

Figure 14-3
DUMBBELL-SHAPED LEIOMYOMA/
BENIGN STROMAL TUMOR

The arrows point to the mucosa and the arrowheads to the muscularis propria on either side of the tumor. There is a large tumor component protruding above the mucosal surface and another large component protruding through the muscularis propria into the subserosa.

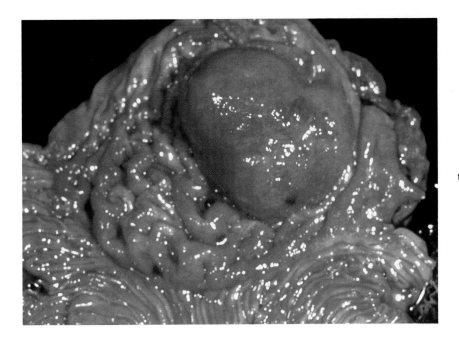

Figure 14-4
STROMAL TUMOR,
MUCOSAL ASPECT
The large bulging tumor has two small ulcers on its surface.

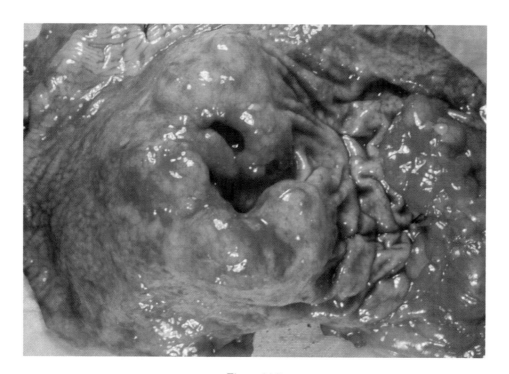

Figure 14-5
MUCOSAL VIEW OF A LEIOMYOSARCOMA/SARCOMA
There is a large, deep ulcer crater surrounded by nodules of tumor which elevate the mucosa.

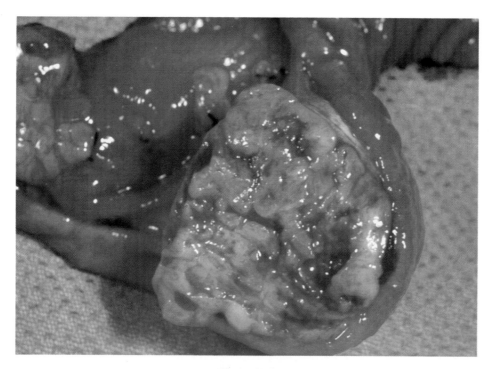

Figure 14-6
TYPICAL CROSS-SECTIONAL APPEARANCE OF MOST STROMAL TUMORS
The surface of the solid tumor is pale with small dark spots, some of which are vessels, and large dark areas which are necrosis and possibly hemorrhage.

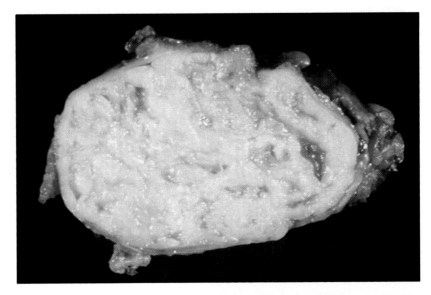

Figure 14-7
TYPICAL
WELL-CIRCUMSCRIBED
LEIOMYOMA/
BENIGN STROMAL TUMOR
The cut surface is mottled, pale, and nonwhorled. This is very different from the usual uterine leiomyoma.

Figure 14-8
CYSTIC LEIOMYOMA/
BENIGN STROMAL TUMOR
This well-circumscribed tumor has become cystic as a result of extensive necrosis.

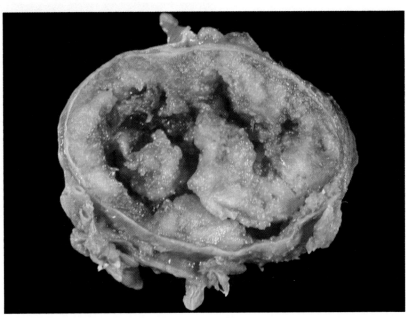

like cysts with irregularly thickened walls (figs. 14-1, 14-8). Tumor color depends upon whether examination occurs before, during, or after fixation, and how much blood and necrotic debris is present. Before fixation, tumors are likely to be pink, tan, or slightly yellow. After fixation, they look gray or brown. Benign tumors and sarcomas may look exactly the same; however, some sarcomas, especially the larger ones, have extensive areas that are homogeneous, firm, and white on cross section so that they look like sarcomas of the soft tissues (figs. 14-9, 14-10).

Benign tumors and small sarcomas usually are so well circumscribed with sharp peripheral boundaries that on cross section they appear to be encapsulated. There is no fibrous capsule, but the muscularis propria at the edges often becomes hypertrophied and partly envelopes the tumor (fig. 14-11). Most tumors form a single, round, perhaps slightly lobulated mass. In contrast, large sarcomas may be multinodular with several contiguous masses (figs. 14-9, 14-10). Even these sarcomas do not have infiltrative or indistinct edges. Only rarely will a sarcoma appear to invade

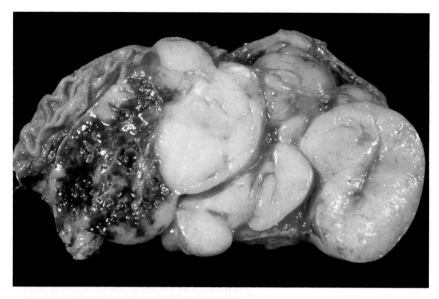

**Figure 14-9**
**LEIOMYOSARCOMA/**
**SARCOMA**

This multinodular tumor is solid and pale, except for a large area of necrosis and hemorrhage on the left which lays beneath a large ulcer that is not in this picture. The mucosa is at the far left.

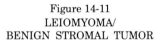

**Figure 14-10**
**LEIOMYOSARCOMA/**
**SARCOMA**

Beneath the mucosa is a nodular plaque-like neoplasm. Although it was 5 cm in maximal dimension, it was only about 1.5 cm thick.

**Figure 14-11**
**LEIOMYOMA/**
**BENIGN STROMAL TUMOR**

The mucosa is at the far left. The tumor is partly surrounded by the muscularis propria which seems to blend with the base of the mucosa, probably the muscularis mucosae, thus forming an almost acceptable capsule.

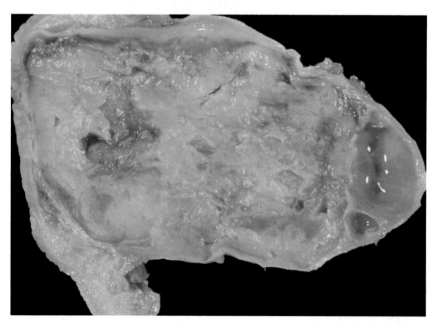

another organ, such as the liver, spleen, or pancreas. Benign tumors at times become adherent to these organs, although there is no invasion.

Specific tumor types tend to arise in specific sites within the stomach (5). Although the gastric body is the most common site for all tumors, about half of benign spindle cell tumors and one third of the epithelioid sarcomas arise in the proximal stomach (the fundus and cardia). In contrast, almost half of the benign epithelioid cell tumors arise in the antrum, but only one quarter of the epithelioid sarcomas arise there. We have no explanation for these site predilections.

In general, a large, multinodular, firm, white, dense, homogeneous tumor is probably a sarcoma. No other gross features are of much help in separating the benign from the malignant.

**Microscopic Findings.** The microscopic features of the three major types of generic gastric stromal tumors differ and are discussed separately. However, they share some features. At the periphery of many of the tumors, especially the smaller benign ones, the muscularis propria becomes hypertrophied and collagenized and partly surrounds the tumor, occasionally merging with the muscularis mucosae to form a partial muscular pseudocapsule, which may be appreciated grossly (fig. 14-11). Irregularly shaped lobules of tumor cells or even strands or clusters of tumor cells may interdigitate with hypertrophic smooth muscle bundles of the muscularis propria, imparting an appearance of invasion of the muscularis by the tumor (fig. 14-12). Lobulation is common and is most pronounced in the epithelioid cell variety (fig. 14-13). The lobules are separated by muscular septa or by thin collagenous septa, and the histologic patterns often differ from one lobule to another, especially in epithelioid cell tumors (figs. 14-14, 14-15). The large tumors frequently contain foci of liquefaction necrosis which appear as pools of acellular edema with tumor cell islands, often perivascular, separated by the fluid (figs. 14-16, 14-17). Areas of dense collagenization or hyalinization are also common and contain similar tumor cell islands (fig. 14-18). At times, the hyalinized foci calcify (fig. 14-19). Recent hemorrhage may be found, but it is probably operation induced in tumors that have central liquefaction. Old hemorrhage is also common and is manifested by hemosiderin-laden macrophages in the stroma or by large pools of frag-

mented erythrocytes. There may be occasional foci of infarction with ghosts or outlines of tumor.

*Common Benign Spindle Cell Stromal Tumors (Cellular Leiomyomas, Leiomyomas with Regimentation).* These tumors are composed almost entirely of long spindle cells with plentiful, longitudinally fibrillar, pale eosinophilic cytoplasm (figs. 14-20, 14-21) (7). The cells are usually uniform in size and shape. Only infrequently are there larger forms with bigger nuclei (fig. 14-22). The nuclei are elongated and may be straight or wavy, blunt-ended or tapered. Many cells contain single perinuclear vacuoles which indent the nuclei at one end (figs. 14-20, 14-22). These vacuoles may vary in size. They are probably artifacts of fixation since they do not appear in frozen sections but are present in the permanent sections. There is no ultrastructural equivalent of the vacuoles. Mitotic figures are often present but scattered widely, so that it is unusual to find more than 2 or 3 for every 50 high-power fields, regardless of the size of the field.

The tumor cells may be arranged in whorls and fascicles, sometimes interlacing, sometimes in a storiform pattern, or sometimes in a herringbone pattern (figs. 14-23–14-25). In many tumors, the spindled cells form spectacular palisades, some of which are unusually large, larger even than those that occur in schwannomas (fig. 14-26). Because of this palisaded pattern, many of these tumors have been reported as neural tumors of one type or another. In one classification scheme, they were called "leiomyomas with regimentation" (79).

In summary, a tumor composed of long, generally uniform spindle cells with perinuclear vacuoles and a growth pattern that is either palisaded or storiform is a benign spindle cell stromal tumor or cellular leiomyoma. However, these are not leiomyomas composed of typical mature smooth cells; those leiomyomas are discussed below under Tumors Composed of Mature Smooth Muscle Cells (Typical Leiomyomas).

*Benign Epithelioid Cell Tumors (Epithelioid Leiomyomas, Leiomyoblastomas, Bizarre Smooth Muscle Tumors).* Tumors composed mainly of round or epithelioid cells are the same tumors that Arthur Purdy Stout referred to as "leiomyoblastomas" or "bizarre smooth muscle tumors" in his classic paper in 1962 (87). Actually, 2 years earlier, six of these tumors were reported in France by Martin et al. (62).

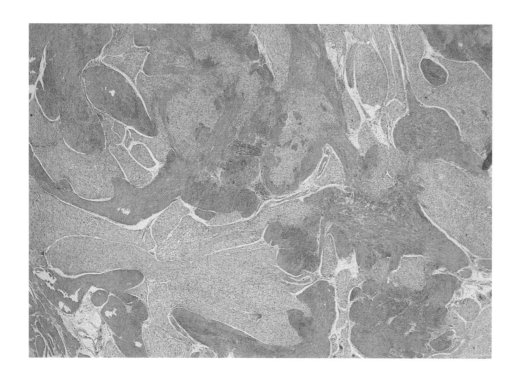

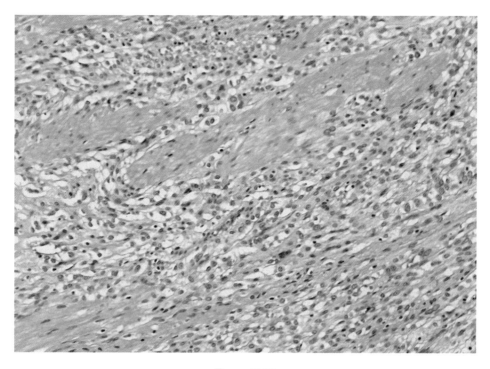

Figure 14-12
EPITHELIOID LEIOMYOMA/BENIGN EPITHELIOID CELL STROMAL TUMOR
Top: Low-power view of smooth muscle bundles of the muscularis propria, separated by paler tumor cells.
Bottom: High-power view.

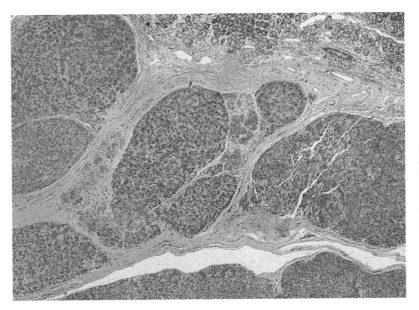

Figure 14-13
EPITHELIOID LEIOMYOMA/
BENIGN EPITHELIOID
CELL STROMAL TUMOR

This multinodular benign tumor is in the submucosa. Some of the more superficial nodules are separated by septa containing muscle fibers from the muscularis mucosae. The differences in staining intensity among the nodules result from different cell densities and amounts of intercellular stroma.

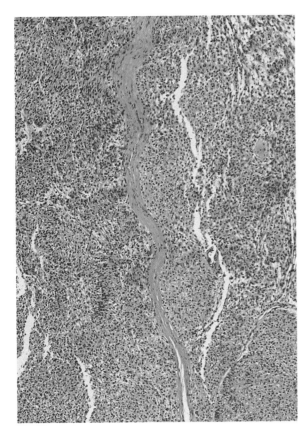

Figure 14-14
EPITHELIOID LEIOMYOMA/
BENIGN EPITHELIOID CELL STROMAL TUMOR

In the center, a thick muscular septum separates two tumor lobules. Even at this low magnification, different growth patterns in the two lobules can be appreciated.

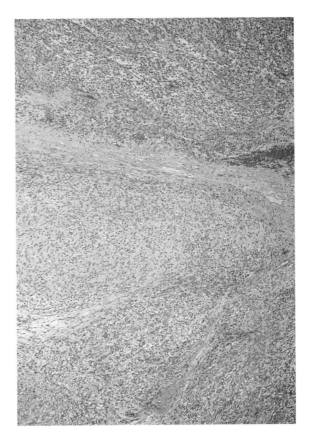

Figure 14-15
LEIOMYOMA/BENIGN STROMAL TUMOR

The tumor nodules on each side of the central horizontal septum differ in cell density and growth pattern. Such variation is common both in epithelioid and spindle cell tumors.

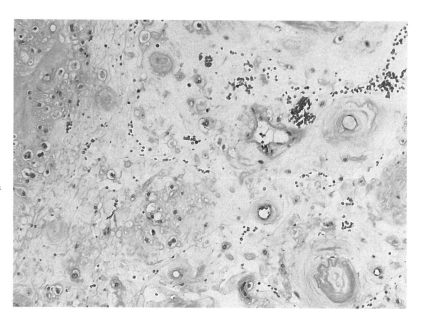

Figure 14-16
EPITHELIOID LEIOMYOMA/
BENIGN EPITHELIOID
CELL STROMAL TUMOR

A cluster of viable tumor cells is on
the far left. In the rest of the field,
there is a large area of liquefaction in
which there is no tumor, only vessels.

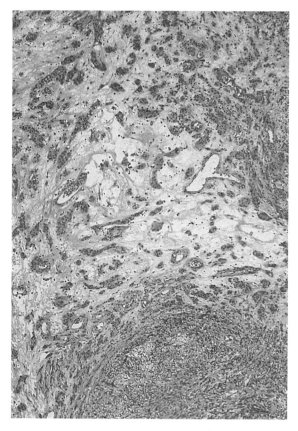

Figure 14-17
LEIOMYOMA/BENIGN SPINDLE
CELL STROMAL TUMOR

On the upper and lower right are solid nodules of tumor.
In the left center, there is a large area of liquefaction
containing small tumor nests.

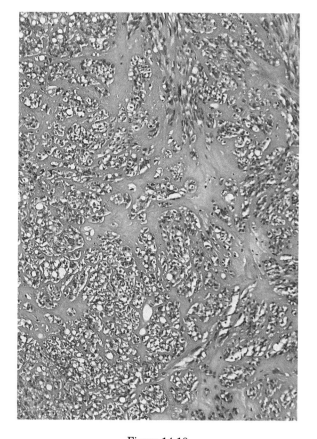

Figure 14-18
LEIOMYOMA/BENIGN SPINDLE
CELL STROMAL TUMOR

Tumor cell clusters are separated by stellate hyalinization.

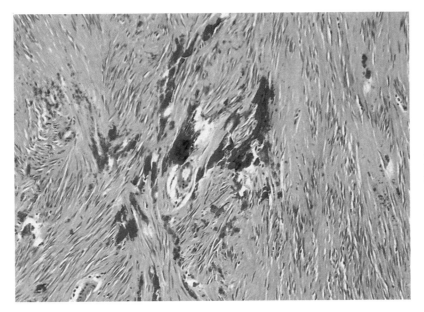

Figure 14-19
LEIOMYOMA/BENIGN SPINDLE
CELL STROMAL TUMOR
The dark material is dystrophic calcification, occurring in hyalinized areas
which probably formed in foci of liquefaction.

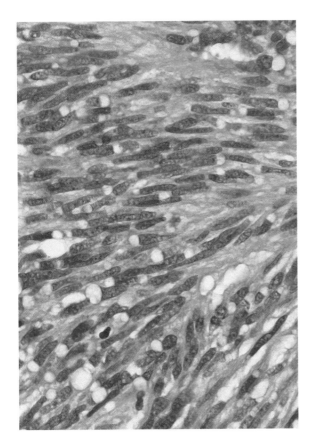

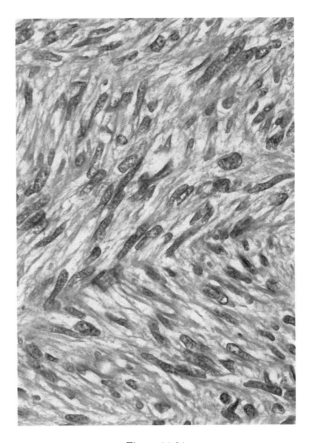

Figure 14-20
LEIOMYOMA/BENIGN SPINDLE
CELL STROMAL TUMOR
This is a high-power view of the characteristic spindle
cells with long nuclei and perinuclear vacuoles. Both the
cells and the vacuoles are uniform.

Figure 14-21
LEIOMYOMA/BENIGN SPINDLE
CELL STROMAL TUMOR
These spindle cells are uniform as are their nuclei, but
in this tumor the cells do not have perinuclear vacuoles.

415

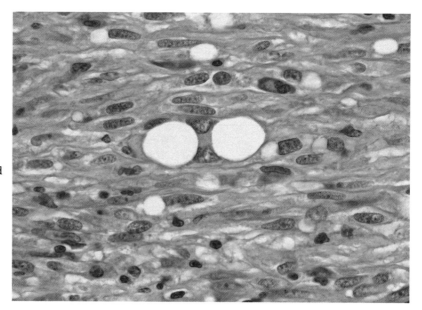

Figure 14-22
LEIOMYOMA/BENIGN SPINDLE
CELL STROMAL TUMOR
The spindle cells, their nuclei, and
their vacuoles vary in size and shape.

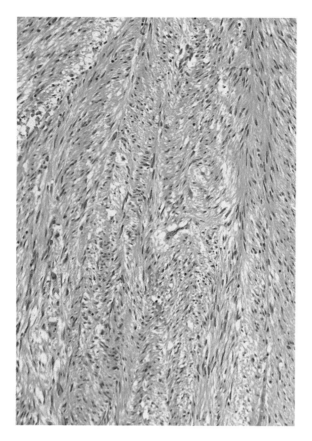

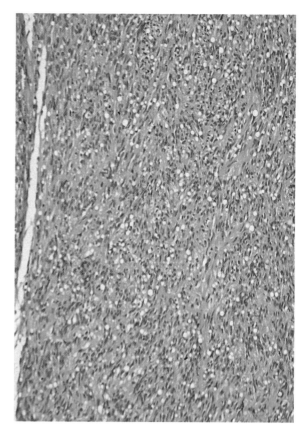

Figure 14-23
LEIOMYOMA/BENIGN SPINDLE
CELL STROMAL TUMOR
The spindle cells are in broad fascicles which are arranged
at right angles to each other, producing a herringbone pattern.

Figure 14-24
LEIOMYOMA/BENIGN SPINDLE
CELL STROMAL TUMOR
The spindle cells with their perinuclear vacuoles form a
large sheet with only a vague suggestion of fascicles.

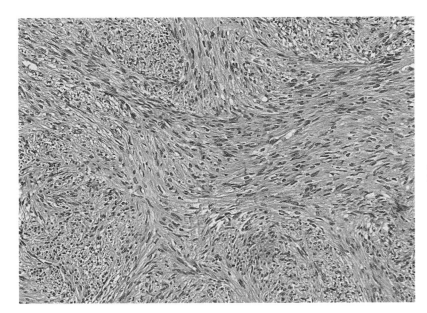

Figure 14-25
LEIOMYOMA/BENIGN SPINDLE
CELL STROMAL TUMOR
The spindle cells are arranged in short curving fascicles which abut each other, forming a typical storiform pattern.

Figure 14-26
LEIOMYOMA/BENIGN SPINDLE
CELL STROMAL TUMOR
The spindle cells are arranged in palisades with parallel nuclei. This pattern resembles that of a schwannoma.

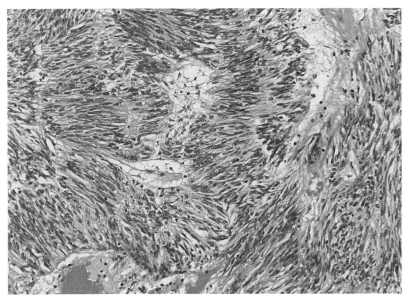

The epithelioid cells appear to have pale or clear cytoplasm, but on close scrutiny, a small rim of cytoplasm is seen adherent to the nuclei, with peripheral cytoplasmic clearing (figs. 14-27, 14-28). This clearing, much like the perinuclear vacuoles in spindle cell tumors, is also an artifact of processing, since it does not appear in frozen sections, does not contain any stainable material such as glycogen and lipid, and is not present in electron microscopic views (21,78). In a few tumors, the cleared cytoplasmic area is eccentric, with the nucleus pushed to one side, so that the cells resemble lipoblasts or signet-ring carcinoma cells (fig. 14-29). However, not all epithelioid cells have this peripheral cytoplasmic clearing; some have abundant eosinophilic cytoplasm (fig. 14-30). In fact, some tumors are composed almost entirely of cells with red cytoplasm. The nuclei are usually round and dense with a few small nucleoli. The size of the cells is about that of normal hepatocytes, and the spacing of the nuclei resembles that of liver. In some foci, however, especially near zones of liquefaction or hyalinization, the cells become pleomorphic, with the formation of

417

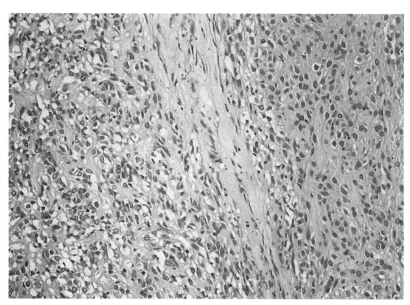

Figure 14-27
EPITHELIOID LEIOMYOMA/
BENIGN EPITHELIOID CELL
STROMAL TUMOR

The tumor cells are round and have abundant, frequently clear cytoplasm. The cells form sheets with scattered vessels.

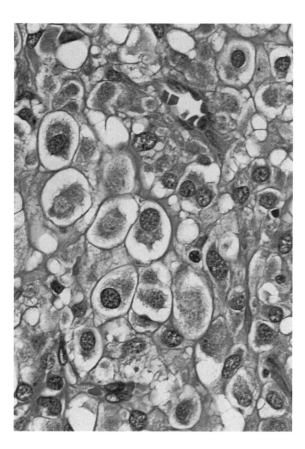

Figure 14-28
EPITHELIOID LEIOMYOMA/
BENIGN EPITHELIOID CELL STROMAL TUMOR

These are the characteristic round cells. There is artefactual peripheral cytoplasmic clearing and small amounts of cytoplasm adherent to the nuclei.

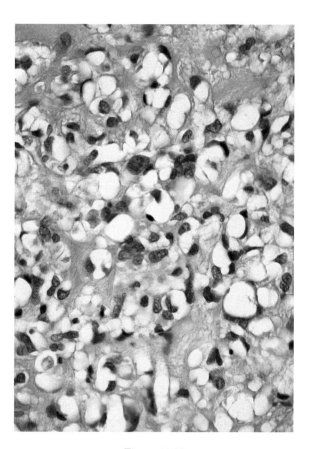

Figure 14-29
EPITHELIOID LEIOMYOMA/
BENIGN EPITHELIOID CELL STROMAL TUMOR

Many of the cells have central cytoplasmic clear areas. The nuclei are pushed to one side, so that the cells resemble signet-ring cells or even lipoblasts.

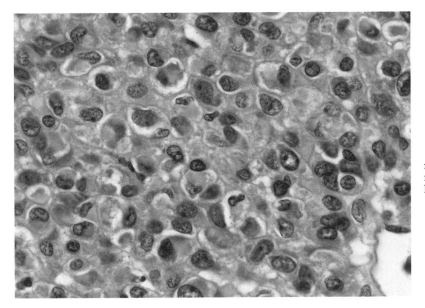

Figure 14-30
EPITHELIOID LEIOMYOMA/
BENIGN EPITHELIOID
CELL STROMAL TUMOR
These round cells have smaller, peripheral, clear cytoplasmic areas and more perinuclear cytoplasm. Some cells have no clear cytoplasm.

Figure 14-31
EPITHELIOID LEIOMYOMA/
BENIGN EPITHELIOID CELL
STROMAL TUMOR:
COMMON PLEOMORPHISM
Many of the cells are multinucleated, and the nuclei vary considerably in size and staining characteristics. The cells are separated by a hyalinized stroma.

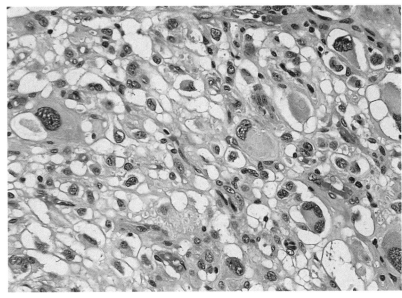

multinucleated giant cells and cells with single, large, often bizarre nuclei (figs. 14-31, 14-32) (8). Mitotic figures are sometimes found, but, as in the spindle cell tumors, they are infrequent.

Some tumors are composed almost totally of these epithelioid cells, arranged in sheets or imperfect nests, frequently surrounded by hyalinized or liquefied stroma. In reticulin-stained sections, clusters of cells and single cells are surrounded by delicate silver-staining material. Sometimes, the epithelioid tumor cells seem to surround small vessels in a perithelial pattern.

Many tumors or parts of tumors are composed of a mixture of epithelioid cells and plump spindle cells arranged in sheets (fig. 14-33). Occasional epithelioid cell tumors have lobules of the pure cellular spindle pattern (fig. 14-34).

*Sarcomas (Malignant Stromal Tumors, Leiomyosarcomas).* In general, gastric sarcomas contain smaller cells that are more densely crowded and that have more mitoses than benign tumors. The sarcomas may contain mostly epithelioid cells, mostly spindle cells, or any mixture. The growth patterns tend to be much like those found in benign

419

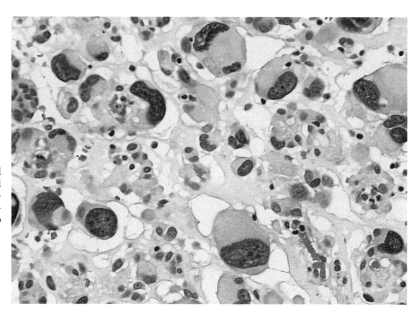

Figure 14-32
EPITHELIOID LEIOMYOMA/
BENIGN EPITHELIOID
CELL STROMAL TUMOR:
EXAGGERATED PLEOMORPHISM

There is great variation in cell and nuclear size, nuclear number and shape, and staining. This is not an indication of malignancy, but in an epithelioid cell tumor, it is more likely to be an indication of benign behavior.

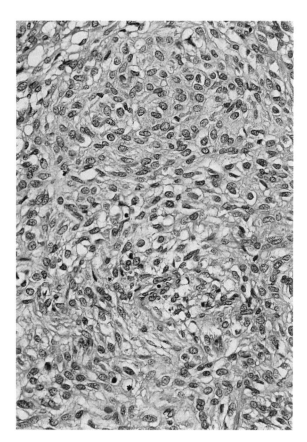

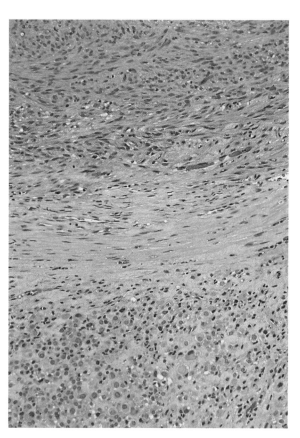

Figure 14-33
EPITHELIOID LEIOMYOMA/BENIGN
EPITHELIOID CELL STROMAL TUMOR

Many of the epithelioid cell tumors have areas that contain a mixture of round and plump spindle cells, as seen in this field. Some tumors are composed entirely of this mixture.

Figure 14-34
EPITHELIOID LEIOMYOMA/BENIGN
EPITHELIOID CELL STROMAL TUMOR

There are two tumor nodules separated by a horizontal fibromuscular septum. The nodule at the bottom contains epithelioid cells, while the nodule at the top is composed completely of spindled cells.

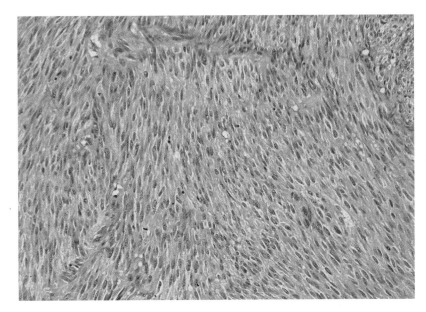

Figure 14-35
LEIOMYOSARCOMA/SARCOMA
This highly cellular spindled cell
tumor has a broad fascicular pattern.

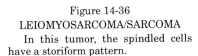

Figure 14-36
LEIOMYOSARCOMA/SARCOMA
In this tumor, the spindled cells
have a storiform pattern.

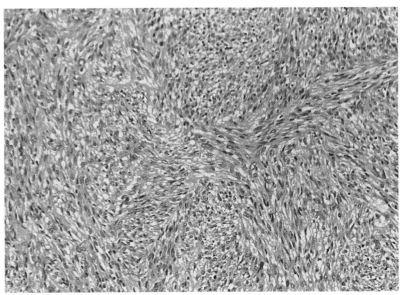

epithelioid and spindle cell tumors, except that there is more of a tendency for sarcoma cells to form large sheets. Thus, spindle cell sarcomas may have a variety of fascicular and storiform patterns (figs. 14-35, 14-36). In general, sarcoma cells tend to be smaller than those of benign tumors, while the nuclei are much the same size, so that there is greatly increased cell density (figs. 14-37, 14-38). In some sarcomas, especially those that contain mostly spindle cells, the nuclei are more vesicular and primitive looking. Mitotic figures are usually found with very little searching, but there are some

sarcomas, even some that have metastasized, that have very few mitoses (fig. 14-39). In general, any tumor that has 10 or more mitoses in 50 high-power fields will have other microscopic characteristics of malignancy (10).

In the predominantly epithelioid cell sarcomas, there is a tendency for different lobules or geographic areas to have different patterns. These patterns include epithelioid cells arranged in acinus-like clusters often resembling nests of carcinoma cells, and tight palisades of tiny spindle cells (figs. 14-40, 14-41). In these two

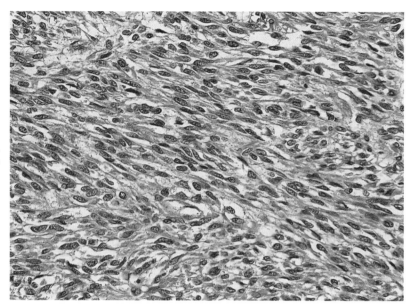

Figure 14-37
LEIOMYOSARCOMA/SARCOMA
This densely cellular tumor is composed of short spindled cells with large but generally uniform nuclei.

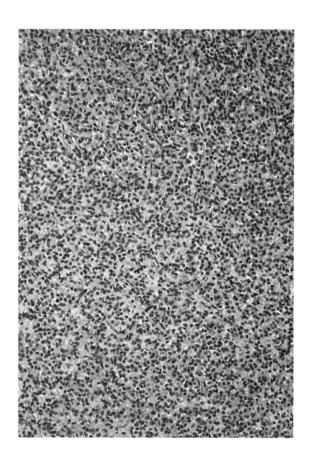

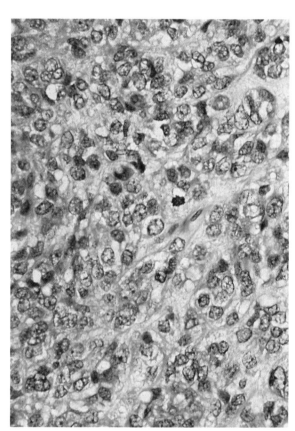

Figure 14-38
LEIOMYOSARCOMA/SARCOMA
Left: Low-power magnification shows a highly cellular tumor composed of epithelioid cells with relatively large nuclei and smaller cytoplasmic volume than in benign epithelioid cell tumors. Compare these cells with those in figure 14-28.
Right: High power details the cells.

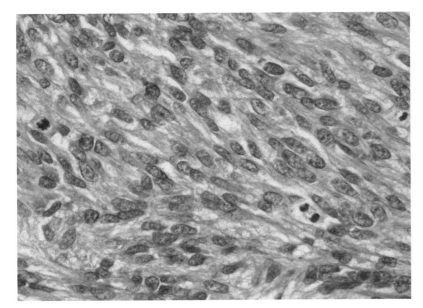

Figure 14-39
LEIOMYOSARCOMA/SARCOMA
These small spindled cells have relatively larger nuclei in relation to cytoplasmic volume than the benign counterparts, such as those in figures 14-20 and 14-21. There are two mitoses in this field.

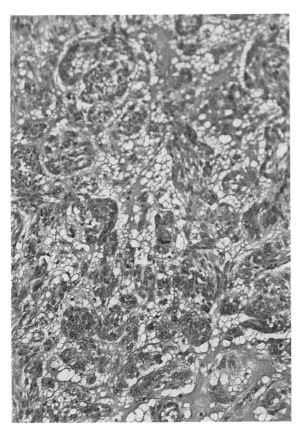

Figure 14-40
EPITHELIOID LEIOMYOSARCOMA/
EPITHELIOID CELL SARCOMA
The tumor cells are arranged in clusters or alveolar groups, separated by a mucin-rich stroma.

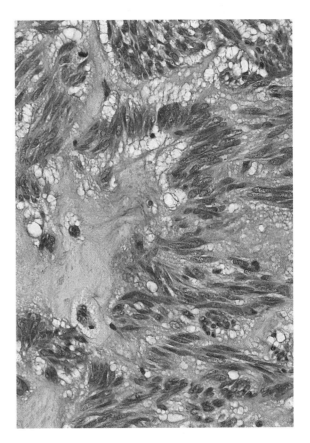

Figure 14-41
EPITHELIOID LEIOMYOSARCOMA/
EPITHELIOID CELL SARCOMA
In this pattern, the tumor cells are short and spindled, arranged in tight palisades, and separated by a mucin-rich stroma.

patterns, the cell clusters and tight palisades are frequently surrounded by an acid mucopolysaccharide-rich stroma. Sarcomas, especially the epithelioid cell varieties, commonly have lobules histologically identical to the benign epithelioid cell tumor.

Cellular and nuclear pleomorphism is not common, although very rare sarcomas have pleomorphic foci. In fact, when pleomorphism occurs in gastric stromal tumors, it is likely to appear in benign epithelioid cell tumors which have multinucleated and large bizarre uninucleated cells.

*Carney's Triad.* Cabney's triad is an unusual syndrome that occurs mostly in girls (14,17,61); the average age at presentation is about 16 years. The morphologic expressions of this syndrome include epithelioid cell gastric sarcomas; pulmonary chondromas that are pure cartilaginous tumors, not the mixed epithelial and stromal chondroid hamartomas; and functioning extra-adrenal paragangliomas that cause hypertension and are likely to be multifocal. Recently, intra-adrenal functioning pheochromocytomas have been reported in this syndrome (61). In Carney's triad, the gastric sarcomas are usually multifocal, forming small discrete nodules, although occasional large masses occur; some patients only have one large tumor (fig. 14-42). The entire gastric mesenchyme seems to be at risk to form these tumors, and, as a result, after they are resected, new tumors tend to develop in the gastric stump. The gastric tumors are usually pure epithelioid cell proliferations with small, tightly packed, uniform cells that may have clear peripheral cytoplasm. The cells have less cytoplasm than in benign tumors, and they have more mitoses. They may be arranged in an organoid pattern in which nests of tumor cells are separated by fine fibrovascular septa. Occasionally, small foci with benign histologic features may be found. Some sarcomas contain spindle cells. Ultrastructurally, the tumor cells have the same features as do other generic gastric stromal tumors, with most cells having no specific features, a few having imperfect smooth muscle characteristics, and a few looking neural (14,104).

In this syndrome, the metastatic risk of the sarcomas is low, possibly a manifestation of their small size, and once they metastasize, survival is still long. Sometimes the chondromas or paragangliomas become clinically apparent be-fore the gastric sarcomas. In such cases, the extragastric tumors are a marker of high risk for the development of a gastric sarcoma, particularly if they occur in a young female. A few patients have died of their disease, and death may be due to either metastatic sarcoma or unresectable paraganglioma with uncontrolled hypertension.

**Differentiation of Generic Gastric Stromal Tumors.** Many recent publications have analyzed the cells of generic gastric stromal tumors for differentiation characteristics. Perhaps these studies came about because the tumors had peculiar gross and microscopic features, as noted above, which were different from those usually encountered in typical differentiated smooth muscle tumors, the prototype of which is leiomyoma of the myometrium. When cut across, these gastric tumors do not bulge above the cut surface as a uterine leiomyoma would, and they are not whorled, white, and gristly. The spindled cells are not typical smooth muscle cells, and the arrangement of the spindle cells is often in Schwann cell–like palisades rather than in smooth muscle cell fascicles. Furthermore, many of the tumors contain epithelioid cells, and some are purely epithelioid cell tumors.

*Ultrastructural Findings.* Early studies used electron microscopy in an attempt to determine the type of cells within gastric stromal tumors. These studies reported that the tumor cells are largely undifferentiated (51,53,63,79,103), with occasional microfilaments that only rarely aggregate to form dense bodies. A cell here and there has a few pinocytotic vesicles or a subplasmalemmal linear density. Occasional cells have a basement membrane–like material plastered on their membranes, but continuous basement membrane is not found. All of these features, including microfilaments, cytoplasmic dense bodies, pinocytotic vesicles, subplasmalemmal densities, and continuous basement membrane are ultrastructural characteristics of smooth muscle cells. In some spindle cell tumors, the cells have long processes with microfilaments which interdigitate or overlap, somewhat like Schwann cells (63). Nevertheless, in virtually all studies, most, and sometimes all, of the tumor cells show no differentiation characteristics (58,104). In one study, some of the spindled cells contained large perinuclear, membrane-bound vesicles, supposedly corresponding

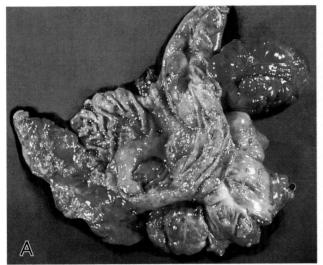

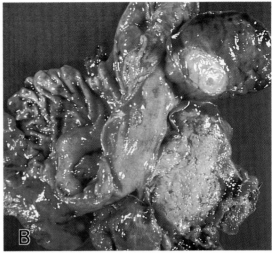

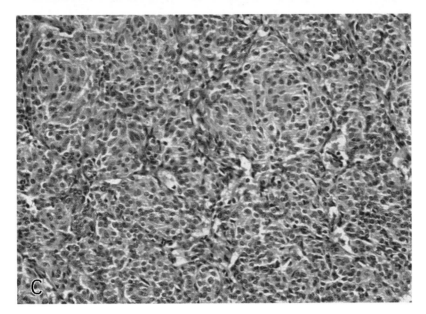

Figure 14-42
CARNEY'S SYNDROME

A: External view of the tumors. The gastric wall contains several small, well-circumscribed individual sarcomas. This multiplicity of tumors is characteristic of all components of the syndrome (see text).

B: Same view with the tumors cut across. The cross-sectional appearance is identical to that of the tumor in figure 14-6.

C: The epithelioid tumor cells are arranged in clusters and separated by fine fibrovascular septa in an organoid pattern. (A and B courtesy of Dr. R. Eckstein, St. Leonards, New South Wales, Australia.)

to the light microscopic perinuclear vacuoles, but this was not substantiated in all studies (63). The combined ultrastructural data suggest that occasional tumor cells have imperfect smooth muscle or Schwann cell features, but most cells are undifferentiated. These changes are found in both benign and malignant tumors.

*Immunohistochemical Findings.* Several antibodies have been developed against different cellular elements found in normal stromal cells. Most of these antibodies are commercially available. Some are directed against cytoplasmic filaments or proteins, such as actins, desmin, vimentin, myosin, and keratins. Normal smooth

muscle cells contain specific actins, desmin, specific myosin, and perhaps certain cytokeratins. S-100 protein is considered to be an excellent marker of Schwann cell differentiation, although it is common to a number of different cells, including adipocytes, chondrocytes, and myoepithelial cells. Recently, some investigators used antibodies against PGP 9.5 protein as a marker of neural differentiation (91). Details about this antibody are in the discussion of neural tumors. Vimentin is an intermediate filament protein that is not a specific marker of any particular stromal cell type. It occurs in fibroblasts and endothelial cells but not in normal smooth muscle (31). The newest

Table 14-1
## GASTRIC STROMAL TUMORS:
## IMMUNOHISTOCHEMICAL REACTIONS, USING FIXED TISSUE

| Author | Year | DES | MSA | Antibodies* SMM | VIM | S-100 |
|---|---|---|---|---|---|---|
| Mazur (63) | 1983 | ND** | ND | ND | ND | 1/28[†] |
| Donner (27) | 1983 | ND | ND | 1/17 | ND | ND |
| Hjermstad (46) | 1987 | ?1/31 | ND | ND | ?20/21 | 1/91 |
| Saul (81)[‡] | 1987 | 23/46 | ND | ND | 46/46 | 0/46 |
| Pike (74) | 1988 | 0/20 | 16/20[§] | ND | 19/20 | 1/20 |
| Tsutsumi (95) | 1988 | 2/15 | ND | ND | 13/15 | 0/15 |
| Miettinen (65) | 1988 | 14/29 | 17/29 | ND | ND | 4/29 |
| (over 10% cells positive) | | 3/29 | 6/29 | | | 2/29 |
| Ueyama (97) | 1992 | 18/57 | 50/57 | ND | 52/57 | 2/57 |
| (diffuse positive) | | 4/57 | 38/57 | | 40/57 | 0/57 |

*DES = desmin; MSA = muscle specific actin; SMM = smooth muscle myosin; VIM = vimentin; S-100 = S-100 protein.
**ND = not done.
[†]One tumor was strongly positive; 7 others were focally positive.
[‡]Bouin's fixative. All other studies used formalin fixation.
[§]Actin staining intensity much less than normal muscle of muscularis.

marker is the CD34 antigen, a surface glycoprotein found normally in hematopoietic cells, in endothelium, and in solitary fibrous pleural tumors. In one study this was found in 9 of 10 gastric stromal tumors, while in another study, it was detected in only 19 of 28 tumors considered to be of smooth muscle lineage and in 1 of 7 considered to be neural (65a,97a). The meaning of these results is not clear, since gastric stromal tumors are not hematopoietic or endothelial. Presumably, the presence of CD34 antigen in gastric stromal tumors indicates that this antigen is more widespread than was originally thought.

The results of immunostaining often depend upon whether the tissue is frozen or fixed and whether buffered formalin, Bouin's, or B5 is the fixative. New generations of antibodies with improved sensitivities and specificities continually appear on the market, so that those currently in use are likely to be supplanted by better reagents. As a result, it is difficult to determine if any immune marker studies of gastric stromal tumors have meaning. Studies using antibodies available in late 1994 may have little validity by the time this Fascicle is published. Table 14-1 is a list of the immunohistochemical studies of

gastric stromal tumors performed to date. Unfortunately, many studies have lumped gastric stromal tumors with stromal tumors arising in other gastrointestinal sites, as if they were all the same. This is not optimal, since it is likely that tumors that arise in different sites are different, much like carcinomas that arise in different gastrointestinal sites are different. Therefore, this discussion concentrates upon those studies that analyzed gastric tumors separately.

The studies are not comparable since they did not grade the staining intensity of the tumor cells in the same manner. In addition, there was variation in fixatives, and the studies were performed at different times over almost 10 years, in different laboratories, with different antibodies. In some studies, focal staining was defined as a cell here and there, while in others, the same focal designation referred to extensive but not total positivity. In several studies, faint, weak, or very focal staining of tumor cells by various antibodies was considered positive, but whether this was true positivity or nonspecific background staining is impossible to determine. Almost all of these studies lump benign and malignant tumors together, and there is no data to suggest that they have different staining reactions. Formalin-fixed tumor tissues were usually analyzed, but in one study, Bouin's fixation was used, and that study deviates most from the others (81). Whether Bouin's fixation produces increased sensitivity and specificity or simply increased sensitivity alone is not known. Some antibodies seem to work better with one fixative, whereas others do better with another. As an example, when Zenker's fixative was compared with buffered formalin on rhabdomyosarcomas, it was discovered that Zenker's decreased the intensity of staining and the number of stained cells with antibody to muscle specific actin while not affecting the staining with antibody to desmin (76).

In spite of these limitations, all these studies indicate that there is common staining of gastric stromal tumor cells with antibodies to vimentin, presumably a primitive differentiation marker of stromal cells which is also found in some lymphomas and carcinomas. On the other hand, smooth muscle markers, such as desmin, actin, and myosin are unpredictable and as often negative as positive. Furthermore, positivity with any of the muscle markers does not correlate well with ultrastructural evidence of smooth muscle differentiation, except possibly for desmin, which Mackay et al. (58) correlated with abundant ultrastructural myofilaments. It has also been reported that some of the tumor cells coexpress both neural and muscle markers, further clouding the differentiation issue (65,71).

Some investigators have found immunoreactive keratins in some gastric stromal tumors (89). Keratin immunoreactivity seems to be more demonstrable in frozen sections than in paraffin-embedded tissues. However keratins have been identified in a variety of tumorous and nontumorous stromal cells, including normal and neoplastic smooth muscle cells, synovial sarcoma epithelial cells, some cells of malignant fibrous histiocytoma, and epithelioid sarcoma cells. Such studies expand the spectrum of keratin-containing cells to include cells of a few generic gastric stromal tumors, but they add little in terms of defining differentiation (57).

**Predictors of Behavior.** There has been much debate in the literature about those morphologic features that separate benign tumors from sarcomas and those features that separate metastasizing from nonmetastasizing sarcomas.

Unfortunately, many published studies have analyzed combined tumors from all gastrointestinal sites rather than gastric tumors alone. The specific criteria of malignancy and predilection to metastasize may differ for tumors arising in different sites, so it is not clear if the information derived from studies combining tumors from all sites is applicable to gastric tumors specifically (4).

The most commonly analyzed criteria of malignancy include tumor size, usually defined as greatest or maximal diameter; mitotic counts; and microscopic cellularity. In one remarkable study in which stromal tumors from all over the gastrointestinal tract were analyzed together, the authors defined two types of benign tumors, three types of borderline tumors, and three types of malignant tumors based upon a combination of mitoses, cell shape, and pleomorphism or hyperchromasia (71).

*Size.* The risk of metastasis of a gastric stromal tumor is a function of the size of the tumor. The larger the tumor, the greater is the metastatic risk, although small tumors, even those as tiny as 2 cm in maximal diameter, metastasize on occasion. In one study, only 1 of 74 (1.5 percent) combined benign and malignant epithelioid cell tumors less than 5.5 cm across metastasized, while 9 of 36 (25 percent) tumors 6 cm across and larger metastasized (8). Since sarcomas as a group are larger tumors than benign tumors, it follows that bigger tumors are more likely to metastasize than smaller tumors because bigger tumors are more likely to be sarcomas. However, size as a determinant of metastatic risk becomes most useful for sarcomas that have been diagnosed by criteria other than size. In a study of 44 sarcomas, metastases occurred in 20 percent of those less than 6 cm across and in 85 percent of those that were larger (10). In a review of 211 reported gastric sarcomas coupled with an analysis of 30 cases of their own, Roy and Sommers (77) concluded that the feature most closely related to metastasis or death of the patient was tumor size: metastasis or death occurred in 15 percent of sarcomas under 2.5 cm, in 29 percent of those from 2.5 to 5 cm, in 65 percent of those from 5 to 10 cm, and in almost 100 percent of those larger than 10 cm. No other parameter, including invasion, necrosis, cellularity, cytologic atypia, tumor giant cells, or mitotic rate had such strong correlation with survival in this study. For unexplained reasons, in this analysis, there were more sarcomas 5 cm in diameter and less that metastasized than in any other series.

In other studies using different size ranges, patients with sarcomas 5 cm or less in diameter survived 5 years, whereas about half of those with bigger tumors survived; the mean postoperative survival rate for patients with sarcomas 10 cm or less was about twice that of patients with larger ones, and the 3-year survival for tumors over 8 cm across was much worse than for smaller tumors (34,56,84). In the last study, size as well as histologic grade and metastasis were independent prognostic factors, both in univariate and multivariate analyses.

*Mitotic Counts.* Every study that has analyzed mitotic counts as a prognostic parameter has shown that higher counts are associated with decreased survival. However, in these studies, there is no standardized way of counting so that the number of fields counted and the number of mitoses per field separating benign from malignant is inconsistent. In some studies, sarcomas are arbitrarily distinguished from benign tumors or high-grade from low-grade sarcomas by mitotic counts (75,84). However, counting mitoses is subject to great variability and lack of reproducibility, due to delays in fixation, type of fixative, and the criteria of different pathologists (11). Tables 14-2 and 14-3 are summaries of several studies that have used mitotic counts to separate benign tumors from sarcomas and very aggressive from less aggressive sarcomas. In spite of the variation in number of microscopic fields counted and the different counts used in separating one tumor from another, all of these studies came to the same conclusion: that mitotic counts do indeed help to distinguish less aggressive from more aggressive tumors. In one additional study, the authors found that 6 fatal gastric tumors had mitotic counts of 4 to 54 per 10 high-power fields, while 46 that were not fatal had counts of 0 to 7 per 10 high-power fields with a median of 0 mitoses (20). In general, the larger the tumor, the higher the mitotic count, although this correlation is not constant.

*Cellularity.* Of all the criteria used to determine whether a stromal tumor is benign or malignant, none is more frustrating for the pathologist than determining degree of cellularity. In those studies in which it is stressed, there is no quantitation of cellularity. Often different de-

Table 14-2

## STUDIES OF GASTRIC STROMAL TUMORS USING MITOTIC COUNTS TO SEPARATE BENIGN FROM MALIGNANT

| Author | Tumor | No. Fields* | No. MIT** | Percent Metastases |
|---|---|---|---|---|
| Appelman (8) | epithelioid | 50 | 0 | 2 |
| | | | 1-5 | 13 |
| | | | >10 | 100 |
| Byard (16) | epithelioid | 10[†] | <10 | 5 |
| | | | 10+ | 100 |
| Ranchod (75) | all | 10 | <5 | 10 |
| | | | 5+ | 100 |

*Number fields = the number of high-power microscopic fields counted for mitoses.
**Number MIT = the number of mitotic figures in the counted fields.
[†]150 fields counted and results expressed as mitoses/10 high-power fields.

grees of cellularity are identified simply by terms such as "mild, moderate, or dense" (20,56,75). It is the rare study in which cellularity is analyzed by counting the number of cells per unit area. Cellularity is the result of three microscopic phenomena: cell size, nuclear cytoplasmic ratio, and the amount of intercellular stroma. The smaller the cells, the more of them are packed into a given area; the smaller the cytoplasmic volume, the closer together are the nuclei. When little stroma separates the cells from each other, more cells can be compacted. As a result of these considerations, if cellularity is a valid criterion for the separation of benign from malignant, then smaller, more closely packed cells with little intervening stroma will likely be sarcoma cells, while large cells with plentiful cytoplasm and abundant pericellular stroma will be benign. In fact, this is exactly the situation, but quantitation of cellularity is tedious and time consuming, so there are no quantitative data on cellularity as a valid predictor of behavior. Furthermore, for different classes of tumor, normal cellularity differs. The cellular leiomyoma is a spindle cell tumor which is commonly densely cellular, while the typical benign epithelioid cell tumor has much larger cells with much more cytoplasm and more stroma between the cells (7,8). Nevertheless, for

Table 14-3

## STUDIES OF GASTRIC SARCOMAS, USING MITOTIC FIGURES TO SEPARATE VERY AGGRESSIVE OR HIGH-GRADE TUMORS FROM LESS AGGRESSIVE OR LOW-GRADE TUMORS

| Author | Number Fields | Number MIT | Outcome/Survival Period |
|---|---|---|---|
| Shiu (84) | 10 | 1–9 | 5-yr survival (81%) |
| | | 10+ | 5-yr survival (32%) |
| Evans* (33) | 10 | 1–5 | median survival (98 mos) |
| | | 10+ | median survival (25 mos) |
| Appelman (8) | 50 | 0 | metastases (0%) |
| | | 1–5 | metastases (57%) |
| | | 10+ | metastases (100%) |

* This study combined all gastrointestinal sarcomas, about 40% of which were gastric.

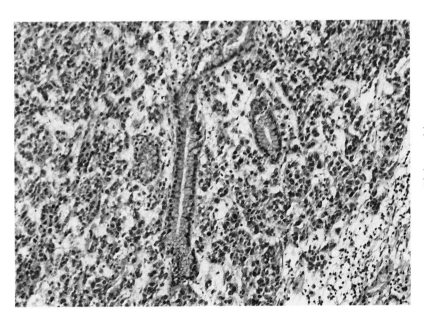

Figure 14-43
EPITHELIOID LEIOMYOSARCOMA/
EPITHELIOID CELL SARCOMA
This is a frozen section of a sarcoma which invaded the mucosa, extending between the gastric pits and glands.

both types of benign tumors, the malignant counterparts are composed of smaller cells that are even more closely packed together. It is not unusual for a gastric stromal tumor to have some areas of benign cellularity and other areas of malignant cellularity, and it is not known how much of the latter indicates that the whole tumor is malignant.

*Other Light Microscopic Parameters.* In one study, an infiltrating microscopic margin was an important indicator of malignancy in epithelioid cell tumors: 4 of 5 tumors with infiltrating margins metastasized, whereas none of 17 tumors with pushing margins did (16). However, the 4 tumors that metastasized also had high mitotic counts, so the status of the margins may not have been an independent predictor of malignancy. Microscopic invasion of the mucosa, with tumor cells infiltrating the lamina propria between the glands, is a useful indication of malignancy, but it is not a common finding, probably because such invasive foci lead to ulceration (fig. 14-43) (5). Invasion of adjacent organs appears to correlate with poor outcome: in one study, all 12 patients with such invasion died from their tumors (84). Tumor necrosis was judged to be a useful parameter for distinguishing malignant from benign tumors in one study (6), but in another study, it was useless (75). Any large tumor, whether benign or malignant, is likely to have necrotic foci, and these may be extensive.

*Nuclear DNA Content.* DNA content, as determined either by flow cytometry or by image analysis, may be an aid in the determination of stromal tumor malignancy. In a flow cytometric gastric tumor study using paraffin-embedded tissues, 55 percent of gastric sarcomas, 35 percent of benign epithelioid cell tumors, and 13 percent of tumors designated simply as "leiomyomas," probably cellular spindled cell tumors, had abnormal ploidy patterns which were either aneuploid or tetraploid/polyploid (94). Abnormal ploidy was related to tumor size and grade: 64 percent of sarcomas 5 cm or more in diameter had abnormal DNA content, while only 20 percent of smaller sarcomas did. Only 25 percent of the lowest grade sarcomas had abnormal ploidy, while 61 percent of the higher grade tumors did. Also, ploidy was related to survival for sarcomas, with the poorest survival for aneuploid tumors, slightly better survival for those that were tetraploid/polyploid, and close to 100 percent survival for those that were diploid. Unfortunately, the report did not include detailed histologic definitions of the various tumor categories.

Flint et al. (36) used image analysis on Feulgen-stained paraffin-embedded sections to study the DNA content of the nuclei of three groups of gastric stromal tumors. Aneuploidy was defined as a tumor cell population having nuclei that deviated more than 10 percent from the diploid standard. They found that 6 of 7 sarcomas were aneuploid, but so were 7 of 12 histologically benign epithelioid cell tumors and 13 of 16 benign cellular spindled cell tumors. When they analyzed their data using the 5c exceeding rate (5cER), that is, the number of nuclei that had more than the pentaploid value for DNA, they found that 4 of the 7 sarcomas had more than 10 percent of their nuclei with more than 5c, while only 1 of 12 benign epithelioid and 2 of 16 benign spindled cell tumors had this abnormality. Federspeil et al. (35) calculated the 5cER for 31 gastric stromal tumors and found that 3 of 16 tumors classified as sarcomas and 2 of 15 benign tumors had DNA exceeding the 5c amount in over 10 percent of cells. However, when they used 5 percent instead of 10 percent as the discriminating value, 10 of the 16 sarcomas but only

5 of the 15 benign tumors surpassed that value. The studies of Flint et al. and Federspeil et al. suggest that the method of calculation and the definition of what is or is not aneuploid are critical in the image analysis system, and the results vary considerably according to the type of calculation. In both studies, benign and malignant could be reasonably well separated by using one calculation or another, but there was still too much overlap for such analysis to be of diagnostic help.

Two other studies used flow cytometry on paraffin-fixed sections of stromal tumors from all gastrointestinal sites combined, so it is impossible to determine what contributions the gastric tumors made to the data. In one of these studies, Kiyabu et al. (29) studied 30 resection and 11 autopsy tumors of all sizes and separated them into benign, low-grade malignant, high-grade malignant, and uncertain malignant potential categories by a combination of criteria including symptoms, cellularity, size, mitotic rate, and necrosis. In the study of El-Naggar et al. (52) only resected tumors over 2 cm in diameter were studied. These were divided into three categories of indeterminate malignant potential and low- and high-grade sarcomas, based mostly on mitotic rate. However, the categories in these two studies were probably comparable, since indeterminate or uncertain tumors, by definition, had mitotic counts of less than 5 per 10 high-power fields, low-grade sarcomas had counts of 5 to 9 and high-grade sarcomas had counts of 10 or more. In both studies, the sarcomas were more frequently aneuploid than were the uncertain or indeterminate tumors. However, in the Kiyabu study, high-grade sarcomas were more commonly aneuploid than were low-grade sarcomas, with only half of the low-grade sarcomas being aneuploid. In contrast, in the El-Naggar study, both sarcoma grades were almost always aneuploid. Furthermore, ploidy was related to survival. In Kiyabu's series, the mean survival period of 10 patients with aneuploid tumors was 32 months, while that for 4 patients with diploid tumors was 51 months. In El-Naggar's study, the median survival period for 15 patients with diploid tumors was 200 months while that for 43 patients with aneuploid tumors was 24 months. The DNA content of the indeterminate and low-grade sarcoma groups differed considerably in these studies, but this may be related to the selection of tumors studied, such as the use of small tumors and autopsy material in the Kiyabu study and the exclusion of these tumors in the El-Naggar study. Nevertheless, these data indicate that for all stromal tumors from all gastrointestinal sites combined, including those arising in the stomach, there is a strong correlation between ploidy status as determined by flow cytometry on paraffin sections, and the class of tumor as defined by the mitotic count. Sarcomas are more frequently aneuploid than are borderline tumors. In addition, patients with diploid tumors are likely to survive longer than those with aneuploid tumors, whether the calculations are based upon mean or median survival periods.

*Cell Proliferation Measurements.* Two techniques have been used to evaluate cell proliferation in gastrointestinal stromal tumors: nucleolar organizer region (AgNOR) content and proliferating cell nuclear antigen (PCNA). AgNORs are silver-stained interphase nucleolar structures that are thought to relate to cellular proliferation in neoplasms. PCNA is a nuclear protein essential for DNA replication, against which a commercially available antibody has been raised for immunohistochemical use. Unfortunately, in the two published studies, tumors from all gut sites were mixed together, so it is not possible to evaluate the results for gastric tumors alone (13,109). However, two recent abstracts summarized the PCNA staining results for gastric stromal tumors only (3,40).

In all the studies, results of PCNA staining correlated well with tumors identified as benign and malignant based upon other criteria such as mitotic counts, although the counts were different in different studies. Sarcomas had greater PCNA staining than did benign and borderline tumors, and this was always statistically significant. Amin et al. (3) suggested that PCNA staining correlated with mitotic counts when the tumors were separated into those with 5 or fewer mitoses per 50 high-power fields and those with more than 5 mitoses. Goldblum et al. (40) found that PCNA staining tended to correlate with survival for gastric sarcomas, but this was not substantiated by another study (3).

In two studies evaluating AgNOR counts, also combining tumors from all gut sites together, the sarcomas as a group had significantly higher counts than did the benign tumors, but even more impressive was the correlation between low counts and prolonged survival and high counts and death from tumor (13,109). It appears that AgNOR counts and PCNA staining may be additional prognostic markers. What makes them so potentially useful is that they are quantitative determinants.

*Grading Sarcomas.* Sarcoma grade has been shown to correlate with prognosis: patients with high-grade tumors have worse outcomes than do patients with low-grade tumors, no matter how the grades are defined. However, no uniform system of grading has been used by all investigators. One three-grade system applied to all gastrointestinal sarcomas, half of which were gastric, separated the grades by a combination of differentiation (although how this was defined was not stated); cellularity (moderate or marked); anaplasia (none, moderate, or marked); and mitoses, with 0 to 4 mitoses/10 high-power fields defining grade I, 5 to 9 for grade II, and 10 or more for grade III (64). In another system, four tumor grades were defined based upon a combination of number of mitoses per 10 high-power fields and separated into 1 to 3, 4 to 6, and over 6; cellularity, defined as either moderate or marked; atypia, which varied from absent to minimal to mild to moderate to marked; and necrosis, which was listed as absent, possible, or present (41). Another study also used a four-grade system, but the mitotic counts per 10 high-power fields were 0 to 4, 5 to 9, and over 10; the other parameters were cellularity (mild, moderate, and marked) and cellular atypia which varied from mild to moderate to marked. In this study, necrosis was not even considered (56). There is no information about how much high-grade sarcoma, in an otherwise low-grade lesion, is needed to impart a high-grade prognosis to the whole tumor. We do not routinely grade sarcomas. Once sarcoma is diagnosed, we use the tumor's size to determine metastatic risk.

*Borderline Malignant Stromal Tumors or Tumors with Indeterminant Malignant Potential.* Since the separation of benign from malignant gastric stromal tumors is dependent upon a number of different morphologic parameters which tend to overlap, it is to be expected that there will be a group of tumors with mixed features of benign and malignant. Such tumors form a heterogeneous group of anecdotal cases, and they may be designated as borderline or of indeterminate malignant potential. No published data have analyzed them. Fortunately, they are rare. The following are examples of such tumors. 1) A small tumor, under 2 cm in diameter, with the dense cellularity of a sarcoma; this is best interpreted as a tiny sarcoma with a minuscule metastatic risk based upon the size. 2) A tumor of any size with the cytologic and histologic features of a benign tumor, but with a high mitotic count. Such tumors occasionally occur, and since there is no published experience with them, and since they are so rare, they probably truly deserve the indeterminate designation. 3) A tumor of any size which is histologically benign except for a small area that looks like a sarcoma. No one knows how much sarcoma is needed to indicate that metastasis is possible.

These examples of borderline tumors are not the same borderline tumors that have been described in a few publications. Those tumors were identified by the combination of a tumor size larger than 5 cm and a mitotic count of less than 5 per 50 high-power fields (57A). It is likely that many of these "borderline" tumors would be diagnosed as benign when the criteria used are those identified earlier in this chapter.

*Summary of Prognosticators.* The best and most useful criteria for distinguishing benign from malignant stromal tumors are mitotic count and cellularity, since these can be evaluated in every tumor. Highly cellular tumors with high mitotic counts are malignant. Gross invasion of an adjacent organ and microscopic invasion of the mucosa are excellent markers of malignancy, but they are present only in a small percentage of cases. Size is an excellent predictor of metastatic risk for sarcomas that are diagnosed by other parameters. Nuclear DNA measurements probably offer little additional information, except that aneuploid sarcomas are more aggressive than diploid ones. Some pathologists grade sarcomas, but the grading schemes differ, and no grading system is offered here.

**Biopsy Diagnosis, including Differential Diagnosis.** Gastric stromal tumors, no matter the type, are predominantly intramural masses. As mentioned earlier in this chapter, the endoscopic appearance is either a smooth bulging mass covered by normal or stretched mucosa or a mass capped by one or more ulcer craters which are commonly deep. If the overlying mucosa is intact, then the only way to sample the tumor is by making a hole in the mucosa with the biopsy forceps and then sampling the tumor through that hole. Taking a biopsy of the covering mucosa is not helpful unless the tumor is situated immediately beneath the mucosa in the most superficial submucosa. A jumbo biopsy forceps is useful in such situations. If the overlying mucosa is ulcerated, then the hole in the mucosa is already present, and the tissue at the ulcer base can be sampled. In addition, sarcomas often invade the mucosa, so multiple samples of the mucosa at the edges of the ulcer may be diagnostic. It is possible that fine-needle aspiration cytology may have a place in diagnosis, once the cytologic features of the tumors have been analyzed.

Certain tumors can be diagnosed from biopsies. Benign spindle cell tumors have the characteristic uniform elongated cells with perinuclear vacuoles; they are unlikely to be confused with anything else. A few cubic millimeters of tumor is enough for a diagnosis (fig. 14-44). Similarly, the same amount from a benign epithelioid cell tumor containing the characteristic round cells with peripheral cytoplasmic clearing is likely to be diagnostic, especially when these cells are arranged in sheets or nests with intervening hyalinized or liquefied stroma. A round or spindle cell tumor that invades the mucosa, separating the glands or pits, is a sarcoma (figs. 14-43, 14-45).

Although the tumor can be identified as stromal in most biopsies, there are a few situations, especially with the epithelioid cell tumors, in which there is a differential diagnosis. Sometimes, the epithelioid cells are arranged in strands that may be accentuated by crush artifact. In this case, the differential diagnosis is a signet-ring cell carcinoma. If the epithelioid cells are arranged in small clusters or nests, a common sarcoma growth pattern, the differential diagnosis includes not only adenocarcinoma but endocrine tumors, including carcinoid tumor (figs. 14-46, 14-47). In both cases, the differential can be resolved by the use of histochemistry or immunohistochemistry. Signet-ring cells contain mucin, so any of the screening mucin stains, such as the combined Alcian blue–periodic acid-Schiff stain will mark these cells, whether they contain acidic or neutral mucins. Any of the all-purpose endocrine markers, either argyrophilic granule staining Grimelius or Churukian-Schenck stains

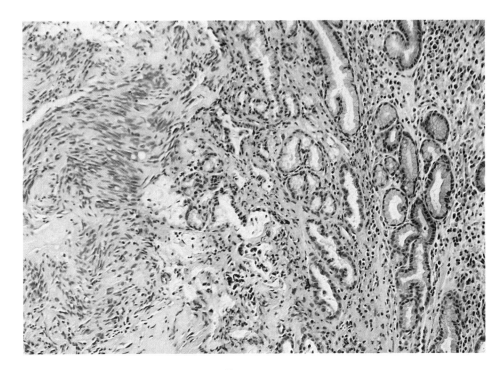

Figure 14-44
LEIOMYOMA/BENIGN SPINDLE CELL STROMAL TUMOR
At the left of this biopsy specimen is a focus of tumor with the characteristic spindled cells that have perinuclear vacuoles. The biopsy came from the edge of an ulcer, so the mucosa adjacent to the tumor is distorted and regenerative.

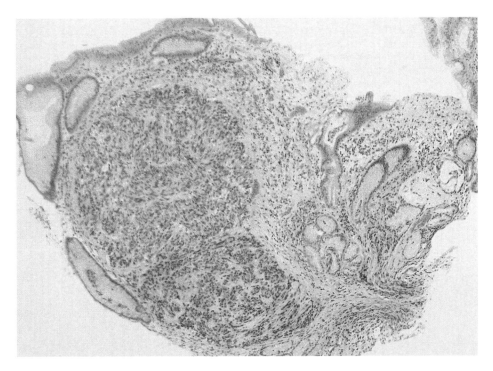

Figure 14-45
LEIOMYOSARCOMA/SARCOMA: BIOPSY
The nodule is a spindled cell sarcoma which has invaded the mucosa.

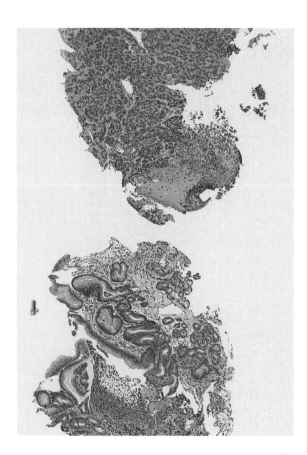
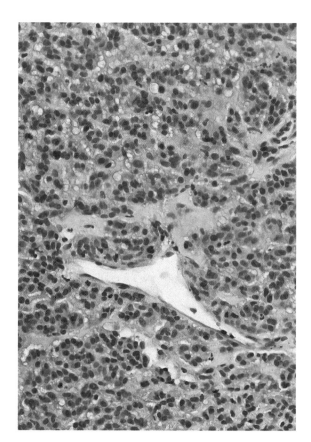

Figure 14-46
EPITHELIOID LEIOMYOSARCOMA/EPITHELIOID CELL SARCOMA: BIOPSY
Left: The biopsy fragment at the top contains the tumor at the base of an ulcer. The ulcer bed is the pale tissue in the center. The fragment on the bottom contains mucosa with distorted pits, which are commonly found at the edges of ulcers and tumors.
Right: In this high-power view the sarcoma cells are arranged in strands and clusters, thus mimicking a carcinoma.

Figure 14-47
EPITHELIOID LEIOMYOSARCOMA/
EPITHELIOID CELL
SARCOMA: BIOPSY

To the left is a gastric gland. The lamina propria is invaded by a tumor with cells that are rounded and arranged in small clusters, much like carcinoma cells.

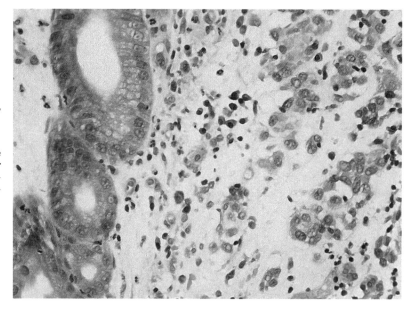

or chromogranin immunostaining, will be positive if the tumor is endocrine, with few exceptions. Immunostaining with antibodies to cytokeratins, particularly those of low molecular weight, detect both carcinoma cells and endocrine cells. However, occasional stromal tumors contain immunoreactive cytokeratin.

Since the treatment of benign and malignant tumors is the same, it is really not necessary to determine if the tumor is a sarcoma from a transmucosal biopsy. Thus a biopsy proving that an intramural mass is any kind of stromal tumor is an indication for surgical removal, if the patient is able to tolerate the procedure.

**Treatment.** The only treatment currently known is gross total surgical removal of the tumor with a narrow rim of nontumorous tissue. Often a stromal tumor looks so discrete that the surgeon may be tempted to shell it out. Since these tumors often appear more circumscribed grossly than microscopically, it seems logical that the shelling out of a tumor might lead to a significant recurrence rate. However, there are no solid data regarding this. In our experience, the tumors rarely recur, no matter what the surgical procedure. Similarly, for sarcomas, there are no data to indicate that any more extensive resection than gross total removal with a rim of uninvolved tissue, possibly about 2 cm on all aspects, is necessary and leads to better survival (10,28,41,56,84). At present, the value of adjuvant chemotherapy or radiation therapy is not established. In order to evaluate these modalities, huge multicenter randomized therapeutic trials have to be undertaken in order to accumulate enough cases. In one recent report, the authors suggest that resection of isolated peritoneal or hepatic metastases improves survival (72).

**Prognosis.** Occasionally, a benign stromal tumor recurs at the resection site, such as in the soft tissues overlying the pancreas. Presumably, this happens because the tumor either was not completely resected, or some of it spilled during handling, thus seeding the operative site. Even less frequently, a tumor that is histologically benign metastasizes, and the metastases become apparent only many years after the primary tumor was resected (8). Most of these metastasizing, histologically benign tumors have some characteristic which suggests that they are

not totally benign, such as an unusually large size or a higher than expected mitotic count (67). This behavior is so uncommon that for all tumors that are histologically benign, it is still justified to diagnose them as benign.

The sarcomas have metastatic capabilities, and as mentioned above, the risk of metastasis is related to the tumor size, although in some studies, metastasis is related to mitotic count (28). Metastases are often present at the time the primary tumor is discovered: one study reported this in 15 percent of tumors, another in 27 percent (10,34). These differences probably reflect the rapidity and accuracy of clinical diagnosis, particularly for those patients with long-duration symptoms. Metastases usually become clinically apparent within the first 18 to 24 months after diagnosis, but there have been cases of late appearance. The most common metastatic sites are the peritoneal surfaces and liver, followed by the retroperitoneal soft tissues (10,28,72,75). Lymph node metastases are unusual, occurring in about 5 percent of patients. These sarcomas tend to stay inside the abdomen. Extra-abdominal metastases, such as to lung or bone, occur in approximately 10 percent of patients. Intra-abdominal recurrences generally become clinically apparent less than 2 years after initial resection.

Survival depends in part upon the type of sarcoma. For instance, the organoid epithelioid cell sarcomas of Carney's triad generally metastasize late, grow slowly, and are infrequently fatal. In contrast, the highly cellular spindled cell sarcomas are aggressive tumors with a 10-year survival rate after diagnosis of about 10 percent (10). Survival also depends upon the study, implying that there are institutional and study design differences. For instance the best survival rates at 5 and 10 years were 56 and 43 percent (84); the next were 45 and 34 percent (34). In contrast, an overall 5-year survival rate of only 19 percent has been reported (56).

## Use of Intraoperative Consultation, including Frozen Section, in the Management of Gastric Stromal Tumors

It has been our experience that when a surgeon finds an intramural gastric mass, of which there has been no previous biopsy diagnosis, then an intraoperative consultation is requested. Since the treatment of both benign and malignant stromal tumors is complete local excision, then the most important information that the pathologist can give the surgeon is that the tumor is stromal.

In most cases, a frozen section is not necessary, since most stromal tumors have gross characteristics, especially circumscription, that easily distinguish them from carcinomas, lymphomas, and endocrine tumors. If a frozen section is performed, it probably will be diagnostic of stromal tumor, but it can be confusing. In most cases, the diagnosis of the particular type of tumor is not as important as the recognition that the tumor is stromal. In addition, in large tumors, there may be both benign and malignant regions, and a single sample taken for frozen section may only capture a benign area in a tumor that has a large sarcomatous component. Therefore, the best frozen section diagnosis is simply "stromal tumor; determination of specific subtype and whether it is malignant must await permanent sections."

When the tumor is an obvious sarcoma, with dense cellularity and many mitoses, simple measurement of the tumor's greatest diameter may offer some instant prognostic information, since the risk of metastasis of a sarcoma is related to its size. A sarcoma less than 5 cm in maximum diameter is unlikely to metastasize, while one with a diameter of 10 cm or more usually will do so, and those with diameters in between have an intermediate risk.

As is true for endoscopic biopsies, occasional cases have a differential diagnosis on frozen section. The cells of some epithelioid cell tumors form strands that tend to be accentuated by the freezing, so they resemble signet-ring cell or diffuse spreading carcinoma (fig. 14-43). This is an important distinction, because the surgical approach for stromal tumors and carcinomas are so different. Carcinomas are usually treated by at least subtotal gastrectomy, while stromal tumors need wide local excision. Usually, the cell strands of an epithelioid leiomyoma or sarcoma are separated by loose liquefied or hyalinized stroma, rather than the dense collagenous desmoplasia that commonly accompanies signet-ring cell carcinomas. When the epithelioid cells are uniform and form nests they then resemble carcinoid tumors.

## Procedure for Pathologic Examination

There are no established rules for handling stromal tumors. The following protocol is based upon what is known about their morphology and behavior.

1. Measure the greatest diameter of the tumor. Remember, size is a predictor of behavior if the tumor is a sarcoma.
2. Photographs may be taken. The best shots include the mucosal aspect and several cross sections.
3. On cross section, note the location within the wall or outside, color, areas of necrosis and hemorrhage, and any variation in consistency from one area to another.
4. Check if the tumor appears to obliterate the mucosal-submucosal interface. If it does, the tumor is probably malignant.
5. If the tumor is received fresh, then samples may be taken for electron microscopic examination. Also samples may be taken for flow cytometry and frozen section immunohistochemistry. These studies are not necessary for diagnosis.
6. Take the following samples for microscopic examination:
   a. The area where the tumor most closely approaches the mucosa, including the edges of any ulcers, to check for mucosal invasion.
   b. Areas of different consistency and color.
   c. Both intramural and extramural components of large tumors.
   d. About one block per centimeter of maximal diameter up to eight blocks. This is a totally arbitrary number, based upon our experience, but there are no data from which to set a standard.
7. Microscopic analysis should include cell type, cellularity, and ease of finding mitoses (compulsive analysts might wish to count mitoses for some number of high-power fields; this is tedious and boring, and not likely to yield information that is any better than an estimate of mitoses, based upon how easy it is to find them).
8. Special microscopic studies may be performed, but they are not necessary.
   a. Immunohistochemistry, using a panel of antibodies, including those against vimentin, desmin, smooth muscle actin, S-100 protein, CD34, cytokeratins of any or all molecular weights, neuron-specific enolase, and chromogranins. Any other immediately available

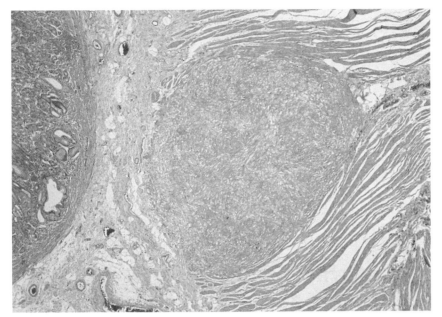

Figure 14-48
TYPICAL LEIOMYOMAS
The muscularis propria contains a discrete tumor, identical to the seedling leiomyoma in the esophagus.

antibodies are also perfectly satisfactory. Any staining reactions, either positive or negative, in any combinations are acceptable, but they will not be of any diagnostic help nor of prognostic importance.

b. Flow cytometry on paraffin-embedded or frozen tissue, image analysis of Feulgen-stained sections, PCNA staining, and silver preparations for counting AgNORs may offer additional limited prognostic information.

9. The final diagnosis requires a name and some indication of potential behavior. Since the "leiomyo" prefix has been used for decades, and is still understood by pathologists and surgeons alike, there is no harm in continuing to designate these generic tumors as smooth muscle tumors. This also allows the behavioral suffix descriptor "-oma" or "-sarcoma" to be included. Additional features may be highlighted, such as epithelioid and spindle cell types. Thus the tumors may be designated as spindle cell or epithelioid cell leiomyomas and leiomyosarcomas. Recently, the designation "stromal tumor" has become popular, so it is acceptable to diagnose these as benign or malignant stromal tumors, adding the cell types, if such designations are understood by the clinician. However, the stromal tumor designation may not be as familiar to surgeons as the smooth muscle name.

## TUMORS COMPOSED OF MATURE SMOOTH MUSCLE CELLS (TYPICAL LEIOMYOMAS)

In spite of the abundant smooth muscle within the stomach in the thin muscularis mucosae, the thick muscularis propria, and the blood vessels in all layers, there are very few gastric leiomyomas composed of mature smooth muscle cells. Almost all are confined to the cardia, and they are probably similar to the more common esophageal leiomyomas which often arise on the proximal side of the cardioesophageal junction (see Leiomyomas of the Esophagus). Most such tumors are too small to produce symptoms, although rare leiomyomas grow large enough to cause obstruction. The tumors are well-circumscribed, nonencapsulated intramural proliferations most commonly situated within the muscularis propria (fig. 14-48). A few cases arise within the muscularis mucosae (fig. 14-49). Often, there are multiple small intramuscularis tumors, comparable to seedling esophageal leiomyomas. Typical leiomyomas are composed of mature, often hypertrophied smooth muscle cells arranged in whorls and fascicles, and they are identical to uterine leiomyomas (fig. 14-50). Ultrastructurally, the cells contain all the characteristic smooth muscle features: prominent cytoplasmic filaments that frequently aggregate to produce

437

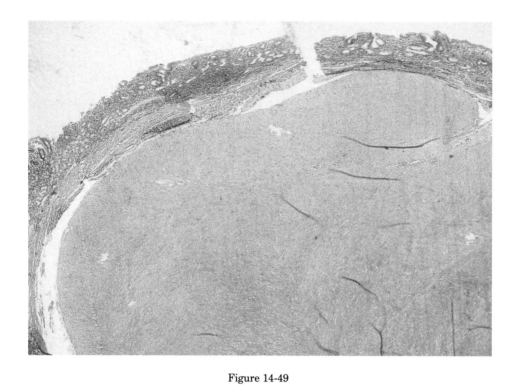

Figure 14-49
LARGE TYPICAL LEIOMYOMA
The bottom of the field contains a large leiomyoma which abuts the mucosa, suggesting that it arose within the muscularis mucosae.

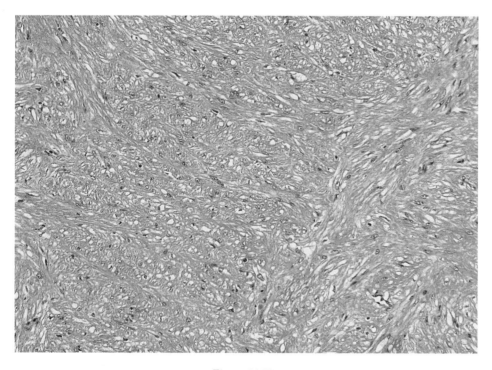

Figure 14-50
TYPICAL LEIOMYOMA
The tumor contains uniform, but hypertrophied smooth muscle cells which are different from the cells in any of the generic tumors. Compare with the tumor cells in figures 14-20, 14-21, 14-28, 14-33, and 14-39.

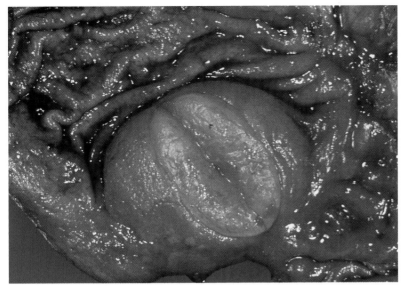

Figure 14-51
BISECTED SUBMUCOSAL LIPOMA
The well-circumscribed pale tumor is situated immediately beneath the flattened mucosa.

dense bodies, subplasmalemmal linear densities, rows of pinocytotic vesicles, and basal lamina. By immunohistochemistry, the cells contain desmin, muscle-specific actin, and smooth muscle myosin, but no vimentin or S-100 protein.

## TUMORS OF ADIPOSE TISSUE

### Lipomas

Rare typical lipomas, identical to those in the soft tissues, occur in the gastric submucosa. The smaller ones are not likely to produce clinical signs and symptoms (82). However, in perhaps half of the lipomas measuring 3 cm or more in diameter, the overlying mucosa ulcerates, resulting in peptic ulcer type symptoms including epigastric pain, bleeding, iron deficiency anemia, and even gastric outlet obstruction. About three quarters are antral. Lipomas appear as endoscopic smooth, round, sharply defined intramural masses that elevate the mucosa. They may be soft and compressible, a hint that they really are lipomas rather than other firmer stromal tumors. This appearance is so characteristic that they are virtually never biopsied. CT may also suggest that the tumor is composed of adipose tissue rather than some denser tissue (60). Similarly, endoscopic ultrasound may define the tumor as having the characteristic hypoechoic character of a soft tissue lipoma (69). Nevertheless, when a lipoma becomes ulcerated, the inflammation and scar from the base of the ulcer may extend

for a considerable distance into the tumor, making it firmer and denser, so that both endoscopic and CT exams may not detect its lipomatous character. Diagnosis is usually made after surgical resection (1,2). However, with the use of jumbo biopsy forceps, a mucosal-submucosal biopsy may be diagnostic when a sheet of adipocytes is found in the superficial submucosa.

Grossly, lipomas are well-circumscribed submucosal nodules with the characteristic yellow cross sectional appearance of lipomas of soft tissue (fig. 14-51). However, if the tumor has ulcerated, then inflammation and scar may extend into the tumor, and if this reaction is very extensive, it may mask the lipomatous characteristics. Almost all lipomas are solitary, but rare cases of multiple lipomas have been reported (82). Microscopically, the submucosa contains a sharply circumscribed mass of mature adipose tissue (fig. 14-52). Inflammation of the ulcer bed with scarring, depending upon the age of the ulcer, may complicate the picture (fig. 14-53). This reaction may be accompanied by fat necrosis with fatty cysts and foamy macrophages. Reactive nuclear hypertrophy and hyperchromatism in the mesenchymal cells may cause the tumor to look like a well-differentiated liposarcoma; however, the diagnostic lipoblasts of the latter are not seen (fig. 14-53). In biopsies, air bubbles in the tissue may resemble adipocytes. Such bubbles are of different sizes, in contrast to the uniform lipid vacuoles in lipomas.

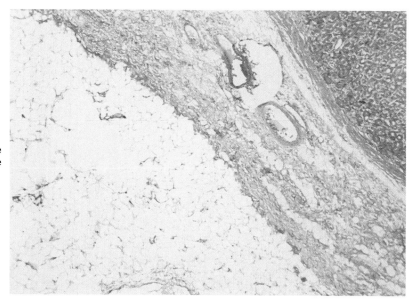

Figure 14-52
SUBMUCOSAL LIPOMA
At the lower left is the edge of the lipoma which is composed of mature adipocytes.

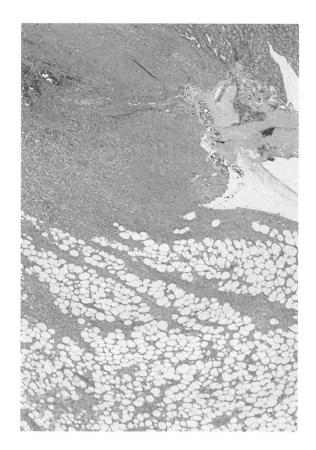 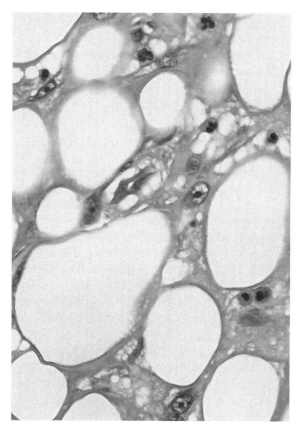

Figure 14-53
ULCERATED LIPOMA

Left: The gastric mucosa is to the upper right. Below that is an ulcer, the inflammatory tissue at the base of which extends into a large collection of adipose tissue which is the submucosal lipoma.

Right: These tumor adipocytes at the base of the ulcer vary in size, and some of their nuclei are unusually large. Such areas as this resemble foci of well-differentiated liposarcoma.

### Liposarcomas

Primary gastric liposarcomas have been reported. From the descriptions, they are probably identical to liposarcomas of the soft tissees (54). There are so few cases that it ic impossible to obtain any meaningful data about clinical and morphologic characteristics.

## NEURAL TUMORS

Although the stomach is richly endowed with nerves in both myenteric and submucosal plexi and in the vagal fibers which spread over the subserosa, proven neural tumors are rare. Some spindle cell stromal tumors have been reported as one type of neural tumor or the other, but usually there is no proof that the component cells are really Schwann cells (23,78,85).

### Common Gastric Stromal Tumors that May Be Neural Neoplasms, including Gastric Autonomic Nerve (GAN) Tumors

In the older literature, a few common gastric stromal tumors were reported as nerve sheath tumors. In these reports, the tumors were given neural names because of the pattern of growth of the spindle cells, particularly the palisades. Recently, based upon both ultrastructural and immunohistochemical findings, a few gastric stromal tumors have been classified as nerve plexus tumors or autonomic nerve (GAN) tumors. One occurred in a patient with Carney's triad; another presented as multiple nodules in a young woman and may also be a Carney's tumor (59,66,92,100). In the largest series of these tumors, 10 were histologically benign and were originally diagnosed as leiomyomas or cellular leiomyomas by light microscopy, while 2 were malignant and originally diagnosed as leiomyosarcomas (106). These tumors have all the light microscopic features of common gastric tumors, but ultrastructurally they have some neural features, such as small dense core granules, long intertwined cytoplasmic processes, and axon-like structures. Immunohistochemically, some tumor cells stain with antibodies to neuron-specific enolase and stain variably with antibodies to S-100 protein, chromogranin, and synaptophysin, depending upon the tumor, the antibodies, the authors, or all three. However, in all cases in which antibodies to vimentin were used, the tumor was diffusely positive, a reaction identical to that in the generic tumors. Perhaps these are nothing more than common tumors that have slight neural differentiation.

In another recent study, five gastric tumors were stained with antibodies to the PGP 9.5 neural marker (91). Three of them were positive, one focally, while none contained immunoreactive desmin. S-100–positive cells were present in four tumors, but the cells were scattered, possibly trapped Schwann cells from one of the nerve plexi. This study offers little help in resolving the complicated issue of differentiation of gastric stromal tumors; instead, it simply adds a new antibody to the many that are sometimes positive in these tumors.

There is a group of tiny spindle cell tumors that arise throughout the gut in the region of the myenteric plexus and outer layer of the muscularis propria, so that their cells seem to blend with cells and fibers both of the plexus and the muscularis propria (fig. 14-54). Initially, these were thought to be small generic tumors, but the association with the nerves of the myenteric plexus was so striking that at one point they were considered to be nerve sheath tumors and were given the name myenteric schwannoma. (5). However, when these tumors were stained with antibody to S-100 protein, the myenteric nerves stained but the tumor cells did not, indicating that these tumors were not schwannomas (74). Probably, they are what they were originally thought to be, namely, small common variety tumors. Typically, these tiny tumors are accidentally picked up during laparotomy. They look to the surgeon like small, hard, round lumps, and in a patient with an intra-abdominal carcinoma, they become grossly suspect as peritoneal metastases. As a result, they are often submitted for frozen section.

### Neuroma/Ganglioneuroma and Neurofibroma with and without Von Recklinghausen's Multiple Neurofibromatosis and Multiple Endocrine Neoplasia Type II

The gastrointestinal tract may contain neural tumors as part of both von Recklinghausen's neurofibromatosis and multiple endocrine neoplasia (MEN) II (73). These include mucosal

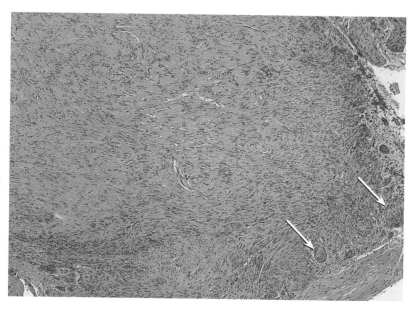

Figure 14-54
SMALL STROMAL TUMOR IN
THE MYENTERIC PLEXUS AREA

This tumor is composed of uniform spindle cells arranged in fascicles with a hint of a storiform pattern. Both the outer muscularis propria (the thick fascicle at the bottom of the field) and a nerve of the myenteric plexus (arrows) are attached to or are even partly within the tumor.

neuromas and ganglioneuromas in both syndromes and plexiform and diffuse neurofibromas in von Recklinghausen's disease. Occasional mucosal neuromas and ganglioneuromas occur in the absence of the syndromes. Gastrointestinal tract tumors occur in about 10 percent of cases of neurofibromatosis (22). The stomach, however, is an unusual site of involvement; the lesions usually occur in the small intestine and colon. Plexiform neurofibromas, the typical neurofibromas of von Recklinghausen's disease, which seem to expand nerves with the proliferation of spindle cells, collagen fibers, and acid mucopolysaccharides, may occur in the stomach, where they expand the fibers of the plexi, mostly the myenteric plexus. However, the most common gastric stromal tumors in this syndrome are not neurofibromas but generic stromal tumors which are often multiple (figs. 14-55, 14-56) (39). Almost all of the syndrome-associated tumors, whatever their type, are benign, but occasional sarcomas have been reported.

## Schwannoma

In a recent report, Daimaru et al. (25) described spindle cell tumors whose cells stained with antibodies to S-100 protein and Leu-7 antigen. Some cells in all of the tumors also stained with antibody to glial fibrillary acidic protein. When antibodies to laminin, a component of basal lamina were used, stained material was found surrounding the tumor cells, suggesting that they were surrounded by basal lamina, much like Schwann cells. These tumors arose within and were mostly confined to the muscularis propria. A peripheral cuff of lymphoid cells was a distinctive feature, and lymphoid septa penetrated and subdivided some of the tumors. The tumor cells had nuclear pleomorphism of the type that is common in schwannomas. Twenty-three of the 24 tumors were in the stomach. The authors of this study dubbed these tumors "benign schwannomas of the gastrointestinal tract." However, these tumors differed from typical schwannomas of peripheral nerves. They lacked the characteristic capsule, the sclerotic vessels, and the usual palisading growth pattern, and they had the peculiar lymphoid cuff, a feature not associated with usual schwannomas. Therefore, although the schwannoma designation may be appropriate, it must be stressed that these gastric tumors are not the same as the usual schwannomas of peripheral nerves. In the study of Mazur and Clark (63), as noted in the discussion of generic stromal tumors, 1 of 28 generic gastric stromal tumors stained intensely with antibody to S-100 protein and had some ultrastructural features of Schwann cells, suggesting that this tumor, at least, was a nerve sheath tumor. Possibly this was an example of the tumor described by Daimaru et al. Such "schwannomas" have not been described in any other reports.

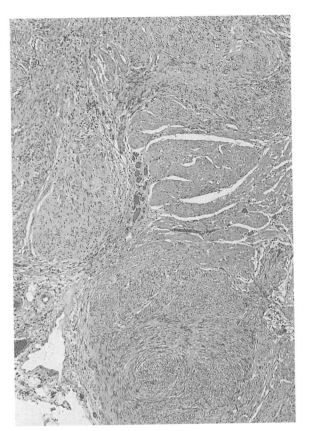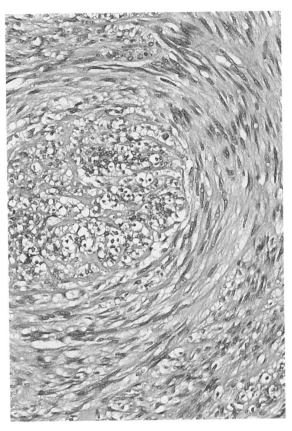

Figure 14-55

LEIOMYOMAS/COMMON TYPE BENIGN SPINDLE CELL STROMAL TUMORS IN NEUROFIBROMATOSIS

Left: At the bottom and center are three spindle cell tumors within the muscularis propria and myenteric plexus area.
Right: High-power view of one of the tumors. The tumor cells are elongate, uniform, and haphazardly arranged.

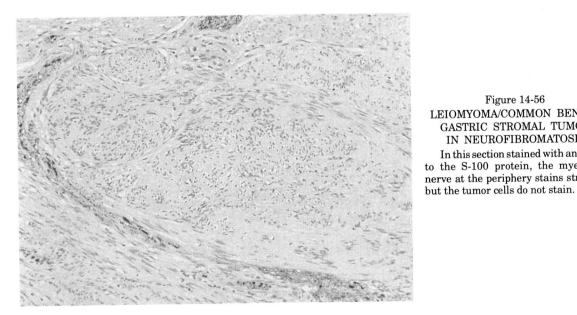

Figure 14-56
LEIOMYOMA/COMMON BENIGN
GASTRIC STROMAL TUMOR
IN NEUROFIBROMATOSIS

In this section stained with antibody to the S-100 protein, the myenteric nerve at the periphery stains strongly, but the tumor cells do not stain.

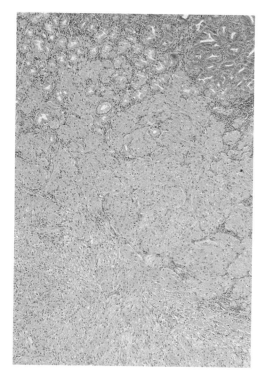
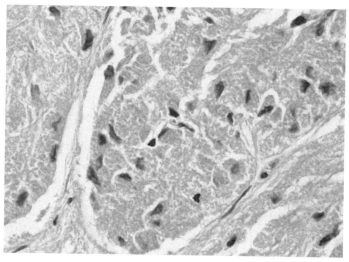

Figure 14-57
GRANULAR CELL TUMOR
Left: This large mass is well circumscribed deeply, but superficially it appears to invade the base of the mucosa. Nests of granular cells extend among the basal gland clusters.
Right: This is a high-power view of the granular cell nests.

## Granular Cell Tumor

Granular cell tumors are proliferations of plump spindled or epithelioid Schwann cells that are full of debris-containing lysosomes; the lysosomes stain with PAS. The cytoplasm and nuclei stain with antibodies to S-100 protein. These tumors infrequently arise throughout the gastrointestinal tract, and most are incidental findings including autopsy findings (48). In the stomach, they are randomly distributed and are situated in the submucosa or muscularis propria. Those in the submucosa may infiltrate or even obliterate the muscularis mucosae and extend into the base of the mucosa between the glands (fig. 14-57). They are histologically identical to their counterparts at other body sites. Most are single tumors, but there are a few reports of multiple lesions confined to the stomach or gastric tumors occurring in patients with tumors elsewhere, such as in the skin (83).

## Gangliocytic Paraganglioma

The peculiar mixed tumor of Schwann cells, ganglion cells, and endocrine cells known as the gangliocytic paraganglioma almost always occurs in the duodenum. One of these occurred in the stomach and was illustrated by Sommers (86) in a textbook covering diseases of the stomach and duodenum. Apparently that is the only gastric gangliocytic paraganglioma recorded.

## TUMORS OF BLOOD AND LYMPHATIC VESSELS

### Glomus Tumors

The most common gastric vascular tumor in immunocompetent patients is the glomus tumor. Although glomus tumors of the skin had been known for many years, it was not until 1951 that they were first documented to occur in the stomach (49). In that paper, Kay et al. reported three cases. That remained the largest published series of gastric glomus tumors until an analysis of 12 cases from the Armed Forces Institute of Pathology was published in 1969 (9). Since then, virtually all published cases have been in the form of single case reports.

The tumors usually occur in the gastric antrum of adults. There is no sex predilection. Symptoms and signs, when attributable to the tumor, are those of peptic disease, including pain, nausea, vomiting, and bleeding. Most are single tumors, although there are a few reports of multiple gastric

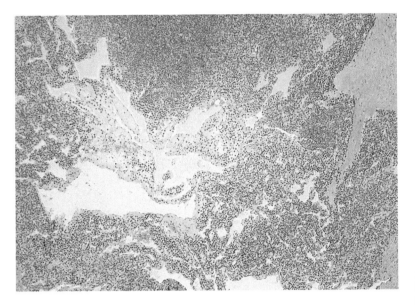

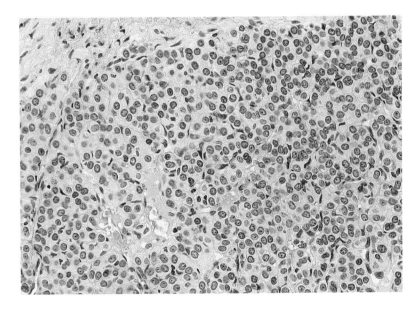

Figure 14-58
GLOMUS TUMOR
Top: Within the muscularis propria (spindle cell fascicle at the right of the field) is a tumor composed of small cells surrounding irregular, often angulated vessels.
Bottom: The glomus cells are round, uniform and have pale cytoplasm, central nuclei, and sharply defined cell borders. (Courtesy of Dr. A. Brian West, New Haven, CT.)

glomus tumors (42). A few cases of malignant glomus tumor have been published, but this diagnosis is impossible to document. Since glomus cells are really modified smooth muscle cells, a malignant variant would be some type of leiomyosarcoma, such as an epithelioid cell type, and it no longer would be a glomus tumor.

Glomus tumors are intramural nodules, mainly situated within the muscularis propria; the latter becomes hypertrophied and collagenized at the margins, forming a pseudo-capsule much like that surrounding many generic stromal tumors. Most are small, with an average size of about 2 to 2.5 cm. There have been a few recent reports of huge or massive tumors, but it is likely that these are really epithelioid leiomyomas rather than glomus tumors (101).

Usually, glomus tumors are highly vascularized with dilated, irregularly shaped, thin-walled vessels; the vessels are probably modified capillaries, lined by endothelium which, in turn,

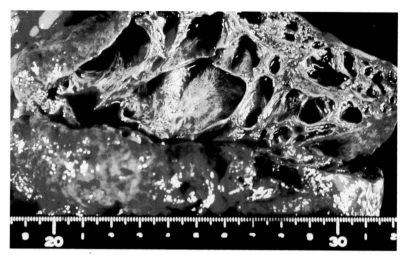

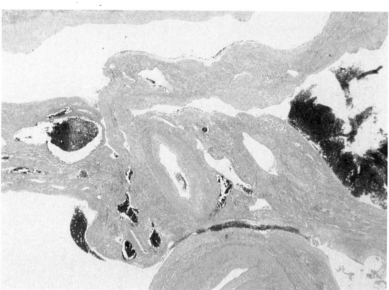

Figure 14-59
CAVERNOUS HEMANGIOMA
OF THE GASTRIC WALL

Top: In this gross photograph, a cut has been made into a submucosal mass composed of huge vascular spaces, essentially a big-holed sponge.

Bottom: Microscopic view of several huge vessels, some of which have smooth muscle in their walls.

is covered by variably thick layers, nests, strands, or sheets of glomus cells (fig. 14-58) (9). Glomus cells are round or epithelioid with pale amphophilic, slightly eosinophilic, or even clear cytoplasm that has typical smooth muscle characteristics by electron microscopi and immunohistochemistry. The nuclei are uniform and round and have coarse chromatin granules. Basement membrane material envelops these cells and can be detected by the PAS stain or by laminin or collagen type IV immunohistochemistry. Reticulin stains also outline individual cells and small clusters with silver-positive fibers. Hyalinization of the stroma is common, and clusters of glomus cells are often trapped in the hyalinized foci.

## Hemangioma, Lymphangioma, and Vascular Malformations

Very few cases of bona fide gastric hemangioma have been described. Most of the published cases have been clusters of dilated or cavernous, thin-walled vessels filling the submucosa and occasionally producing small gross spongy masses, sometimes with phleboliths (fig. 14-59) (108). Some of these, however, are not hemangiomas. Most abnormal gastric vascular proliferations are not neoplasms, but are malformations. For instance, gastrointestinal involvement is common in hereditary hemorrhagic telangiectasia (HHT or Rendu-Osler-Weber syndrome), an inherited systemic vascular abnormality. In fact, gastrointestinal bleeding occurs in about 25 percent of these cases. In an endoscopic study of HHT patients with either overt or occult gastrointestinal bleeding, grossly visible ectasias were found in 80 percent, and of those, almost all (90 percent) had gastric lesions (99). Microscopically, these lesions are dilated, thin-walled vessels, usually veins, in the submucosa. Vascular malformations of the stomach not associated with HHT have also been described. Some of these are referred to as *angiodysplasias* and seem to occur in patients who have aortic valve disease (102).

## Angiosarcoma and Hemangioendothelioma

An angiosarcoma has been reported as a gastric primary. Another vasoformative tumor described as an epithelioid hemangioendothelioma may really be an epithelioid hemangioma (55,90).

## Kaposi's Sarcoma

Kaposi's sarcoma, predominantly a tumor of the skin of the lower extremities in middle-aged men in Western societies, is also known to have visceral expressions, possibly in as many as two thirds of patients. It occasionally is a complication of long-term immunosuppression, such as in patients with organ transplants. Visceral involvement is prominent, especially in parts of Africa where Kaposi's sarcoma affects younger patients, often spares the skin, and is part of a systemic wasting disease. This African manifestation is now recognized as the acquired immunodeficiency syndrome (AIDS), the result of infection with the human immunodeficiency virus (HIV). As this syndrome spread to the West, more and more cases of visceral Kaposi's sarcoma were found. In one series from San Francisco, patients with AIDS and cutaneous or nodal Kaposi's sarcoma had their disease staged by endoscopy (38). Grossly visible esophago-gastric-duodenal lesions consistent with Kaposi's sarcoma were found in 16 of the 50 patients in the study. These endoscopic lesions were either macular with submucosal hemorrhages or nodular and purplish. However, biopsies of the endoscopic lesions were usually not diagnostic, probably because the tumors were predominantly submucosal. There usually are no significant gastroenteric sequela of Kaposi's sarcoma. Although this is a vascular tumor, bleeding is not

a problem in AIDS patients, even after biopsy of the lesions. Possibly this is due to the small size of the lesions and to the fact that they are more solid cellular tumors than vasoformative tumors. Presumably large lesions will result in the same problems that other large tumors cause, such as ulceration with bleeding and obstruction. The presence of gastrointestinal lesions imparts a significantly poorer prognosis for patients with Kaposi's sarcoma than if the lesions are confined to skin or lymph node.

At autopsy of AIDS patients, gastrointestinal lesions are usually 1 to 2 cm in diameter, although occasional large tumors have been documented. In an autopsy study of 45 cases of AIDS, gastrointestinal Kaposi's sarcoma only occurred when there was skin or nodal disease (38). In contrast, in another study, gastric Kaposi's lesions were found in 6 patients infected with HIV who did not have cutaneous disease (12).

Microscopically, the lesions are typical of Kaposi's sarcoma: fascicles and whorls of uniform long spindle cells with scattered mitoses and the characteristic slit-like spaces between the spindle cells which contain erythrocytes. The lesions are mainly submucosal, but some invade the base of the mucosa, insinuating between the basal glands (87). A few hemosiderin granules may be found. In a mucosal biopsy, the lesion is subtle and appears as innocuous-looking spindle cells with small collections of extravasated red blood cells deep in the mucosa between the basal glands (fig. 14-60). The full-blown diagnostic lesion may not be seen. Early or incipient lesions may look like granulation tissue, and they may be confused with the reaction at the edges of healing superficial ulcers. To complicate the biopsy, superimposed prolapse changes with pit hyperplasia, distortion, and excessive smooth muscle fibers high in the lamina propria may occur.

## Hemangiopericytoma

A few gastric stromal tumors designated as hemangiopericytoma have been reported. These are described as containing epithelioid cells arranged around small vessels (24,32). These tumors may not be hemangiopericytomas but simply epithelioid cell variants of generic stromal tumors with a prominent vascular component and perivascular cuffing of the small vessels by the epithelioid tumor cells. However, even if the reported

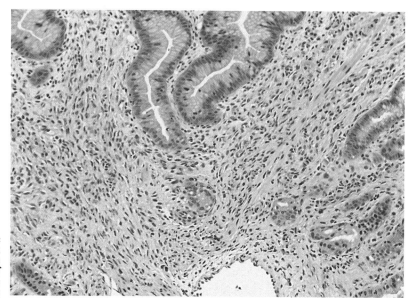

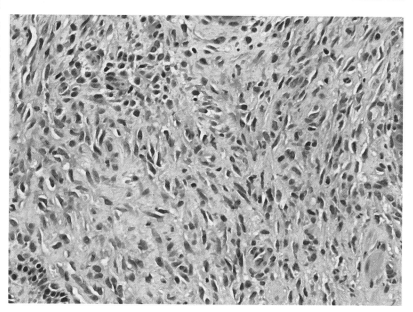

Figure 14-60
KAPOSI'S SARCOMA

Top: This is the base of the gastric mucosa in a biopsy specimen from a patient with AIDS who had endoscopic red nodules. Filling the lower part of the field and extending higher in the lamina propria between the tubules is a proliferation of spindle cells arranged in short fascicles.

Bottom: High-power view shows long spindle cells that are smooth muscle fibers from the muscularis mucosae. The small spindle cells are the tumor cells. The intercellular slits with erythrocytes seen in classic cutaneous Kaposi's sarcoma are often not apparent in gastric lesions.

cases are not hemangiopericytomas, eventually, a real one will be found in the stomach.

## OTHER TUMORS

Probably at least one example of every soft tissue tumor, both benign and malignant, will be described as a gastric primary by the time of publication of this Fascicle. A review of the recent literature uncovered one case report of embryonal rhabdomyosarcoma in a 68-year-old woman with a summary of eight previously re-

ported cases (37); one rhabdomyoma (96); an alveolar soft-part sarcoma (106); and a malignant fibrous histiocytoma which the authors found was only the second such tumor described as primary in the stomach up to the time of publication of the case in March, 1988 (105). An elastofibromatous lesion of the gastric antrum occurred in a woman with bilateral subscapular elastofibroma dorsi in Japan (30). Possibly, there are cases of primary gastric synovial sarcoma, osteosarcoma, chondrosarcomas of various types, and bona fide fibrosarcoma submitted for publication, in press, or already published somewhere. Presumably all of the cases already reported and not yet reported are or will be identical in all morphologic respects to the tumors that commonly occur outside the stomach in the soft tissues.

## TUMOR-LIKE LESIONS

### Inflammatory Fibroid Polyp (Eosinophilic Granuloma, Vanek's Tumor, Granuloblastoma, Fibroma with Eosinophilic Infiltration, Submucosal Granuloma with Eosinophilic Infiltration)

**General Features.** The descriptive name of inflammatory fibroid polyp was given to a proliferation of spindle cells, small blood vessels, and inflammatory cells, often dominated by eosinophils, although it is not clear whether this is an inflammatory phenomenon or a neoplasm. The two most common sites are the distal stomach, particularly the pyloric channel abutting the pyloric sphincter, and the distal ileum (4). In these two sites, the proliferations are somewhat different in terms of the layers of the gastrointestinal tract involved, the size, the pattern of growth, and the cellular constituents. This section deals exclusively with the gastric lesions.

Gastric tumors were first described by Vanek in 1949 (98) as "gastric submucosal granuloma with eosinophilic infiltration." Because of the eosinophils, Vanek suggested that the tumors had an allergic etiology. The currently accepted designation of inflammatory fibroid polyp was coined by Helwig and Ranier in an abstract published in 1952 and in a paper published a year later (44, 45). Similar lesions have been designated as eosinophilic granuloma, granuloblastoma, and as a variety of benign stromal tumor (15). The gastric inflammatory fibroid polyp is situated mainly in the submucosa, although published data suggest that the smallest lesions actually occur at the base of the mucosa (47). Perhaps 80 percent or more are in the pylorus, with occasional lesions occurring in the body and fundus (43). Most are asymptomatic, and as a result of the ever increasing use of upper endoscopy, are likely to be incidental findings during gastroscopy performed for unrelated reasons. They are also incidental findings in distal gastric resections performed for unrelated reasons. Thus some are reported as accompaniments of other lesions, such as carcinomas and adenomas (68). These tumors are found in adults, the age group to have both gastroscopic exams and antrectomies. The reported series indicate a slight male predominance, but that may be artificially skewed because in one large series reported from the Armed Forces Institute of Pathology, 9 of the 10 cases occurred in men (45). They occasionally produce symptoms; as these proliferations enlarge, they become lumps that may compromise the lumen of the pyloric channel, leading to gastric outlet obstruction. A few tumors may become secondarily ulcerated and bleed; however, there is nothing inherent in their growth pattern that indicates that they are destructive lesions, and only infrequently are they large enough to produce these complications. Most are 3 cm or less in maximum dimension when they are discovered. There are no data about their growth characteristics over time: we have no idea if they progressively enlarge or if they reach a certain size and then stop growing. Once they are resected, they do not recur, nor do additional inflammatory fibroid polyps develop in the rest of the stomach.

**Gross Findings.** Gastric inflammatory fibroid polyps are well-circumscribed nodules mainly situated in the submucosa, bulging the mucosa, and obliterating the mucosal-submucosal interface (fig. 14-61). They are firm, as are almost all stromal proliferations, and their color is some variant of homogeneous pale, labeled as gray, tan, yellowish, or pink, depending upon whether they are viewed before fixation or after, and whether the fixation was partial or complete.

**Microscopic Findings.** The well-developed inflammatory fibroid polyp fills the superficial submucosa, although a few tiny ones are in the mucosal base. The tumors have an expansile growth pattern deeply and peripherally, so that the margins within the submucosa are sharp (fig. 14-62). Superficially, the proliferation extends into the base of the mucosa, separating and splitting the smooth muscle bundles of the muscularis mucosae, and spreading apart the basal gland clusters (fig. 14-63). Peculiarly, the tumors do not invade the mucosa above the base, so there is no tendency for them to ulcerate, unless the overlying mucosa has become so stretched by the submucosal mass that it becomes subject to traumatic erosion.

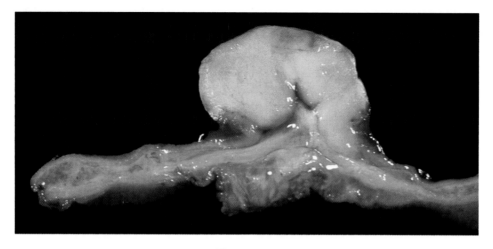

Figure 14-61
INFLAMMATORY FIBROID POLYP
This is an unusually large example of a submucosal tumor. There is a sharp lower border; however, the tumor obliterates the mucosal-submucosal junction superiorly. (Courtesy of Drs. Sharada Hulbanni and Gilbert Herman, Detroit, MI.)

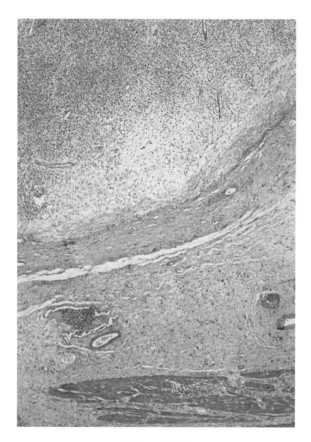

Figure 14-62
INFLAMMATORY FIBROID POLYP
The tumor is the well-circumscribed pale tissue at the top of the field. The lower edge is in the middle of the submucosa. Dark muscle bundles of the muscularis propria are at the bottom.

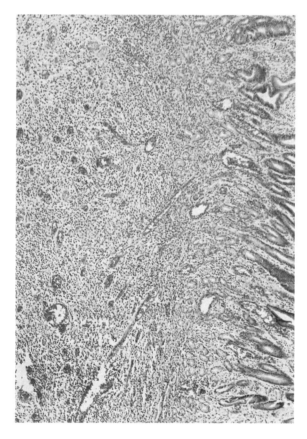

Figure 14-63
INFLAMMATORY FIBROID POLYP
The base of the mucosa is at the right. The abnormal proliferation extends from the submucosa upward between the basal glands.

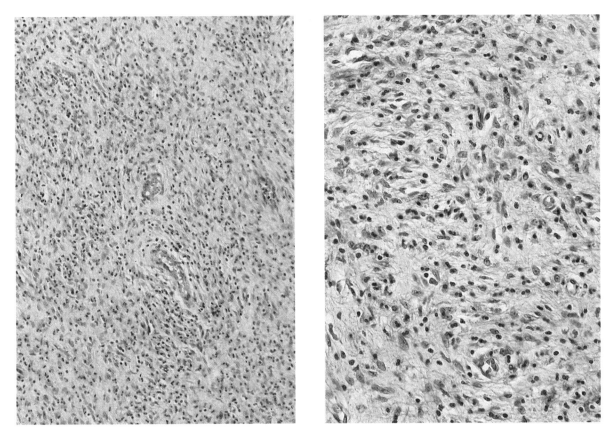

Figure 14-64
INFLAMMATORY FIBROID POLYP
Left: The lesion has a mixture of cells which often wrap concentrically around small vessels.
Right: There is a mixture of large plump spindle and stellate cells, and smaller inflammatory cells.

There are three histologic components (fig. 14-64). The first is a plump spindle cell which, coupled with a loose collagenous background, gives the tumor its fibroid characteristics, the implication being that this cell is a fibroblast. These cells may be round and resemble macrophages, and it is perhaps this quality that led to some of the early descriptions of these lesions as granulomas. Recent electron microscopic and immunohistochemical studies suggest that this cell is a fibroblast, a myofibroblast, or possibly some cell with a mixture of fibroblastic and macrophage features (45,70). Cell marker studies have mostly concentrated on the lack of staining of the spindle cells for S-100 protein and various other neural and endocrine markers including neuron-specific enolase and chromogranin A, factor VIII–related antigen, *Ulex europeus* lectin, desmin, and actin. In fact about the only

antigenic material demonstrated within the cells with any regularity is vimentin, a nonspecific filament common to many stromal and even some epithelial cells. Studies suggest that the spindle cells are not Schwann cells, endocrine cells, muscle cells, or endothelial cells, but are fibroblasts or fibroblast-like cells.

The second component is the inflammatory cell infiltrate. This is usually a mixture of lymphocytes, eosinophils, mast cells, and plasma cells. The eosinophils are likely to dominate the histologic picture, probably because they stand out so well in hematoxylin and eosin–stained sections. No studies have actually quantitated these cells to determine which is the dominant cell numerically. Occasional lymphoid nodules occur in the superficial parts of the tumors. These may not actually be a component of the polyp, but may simply be lymphoid tissue, which is so common in the antrums

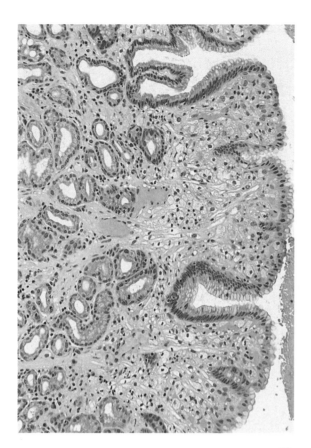 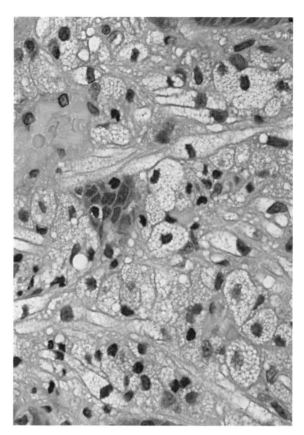

Figure 14-65
XANTHELASMA
Left: The superficial lamina propria is expanded by cells with foamy cytoplasm.
Right: High-power view shows large foam cells filling the lamina propria between the pits.

of adults as part of *Helicobacter pylori* gastritis. The plasma cells and mast cells are less conspicuous and are scattered among the other cells.

The third microscopic component is vascular. These are highly vascularized tumors with a rich network of small vessels, mainly capillaries, around which the spindle and inflammatory cells form concentric lamellae. A recent ultrastructural study revealed that the vessels were composed of a central core of endothelial cells surrounded by a thick basement membrane, around which was a layer of pericytes, an incomplete basal lamina, and a layer of collagen bundles (93). Finally, all these components are embedded in a matrix that is a mixture of acid mucopolysaccharides and fine collagen fibers, presumably types 1 and 3, since there is staining of some of these fibers by reticulin silver stains and staining of others by aniline dyes, such as the aniline blue of the trichrome stain.

## Xanthelasma (Xanthoma, Lipid Island)

Xanthelasmas or lipid islands are collections of large foamy macrophages which fill the lamina propria, usually superficially, and extend deeper into the mucosa or even into the superficial submucosa as they become larger (fig. 14-65). These macrophages are filled with cholesterol, although some may contain neutral lipid. Most islands measure about 1 to 3 mm in diameter and may be grossly, and thus endoscopically, visible as white, yellow, or yellow-white mucosal patches. Smaller ones can be missed endoscopically but may be found in occasional biopsies performed for some other endoscopic abnormality, such as a mucosal polyp. The reasons for their appearance is unknown. although they have been found in several clinical settings. In a study from Japan, xanthelasmas were found in 58 percent of 193 consecutive adult autopsies (51). They were usually multiple, they increased with age, males had them more often than females, they were usually located in the gastric body, and they occurred mostly in stomachs with intestinal metaplasia. In a recent report from China, xanthelasmas were found in 0.8 percent of 3,870 patients who had upper endoscopy (18). In this endoscopic study, in contrast to the autopsy study described above, they were usually single, mostly antral, and were not associated with intestinal metaplasia. In Western societies, xanthelasmas tend to occur in stomachs that have been previously operated upon, such as those in which there has been a partial resection with a gastroenteric anastomosis. In this setting, the islands increase in frequency with postoperative time. In one Swedish study, 60 percent of patients had xanthelasmas at 23 years after antrectomy and gastrojejunostomy (26). Nevertheless, why such localized lipid accumulations occur is a puzzle. In general, they are not associated with hypercholesterolemia, but on rare occasion may be a manifestation of hypercholesterolemia, such as in patients with primary biliary cirrhosis. If there is a microscopic differential diagnosis, it includes signet-ring cell carcinoma, but the foam cells are so characteristic that there should be no confusion. Although xanthelasmas are included with the mesenchymal tumors in this Fascicle, they really are best considered localized, lipid-rich, macrophage-dominant inflammatory reactions.

## REFERENCES

1. Ackerman NB, Chughtai SQ. Symptomatic lipomas of the gastrointestinal tract. Surg Gynecol Obstet 1975;141:565–8.

2. Agha FP, Dent TL, Fiddian-Green RG, Braunstein AH, Nostrant TT. Bleeding lipomas of the upper gastrointestinal tract. A diagnostic challenge. Am Surg 1985;51:279–86.

3. Amin MB, Ma CK, Linden MD, Kubus J, Zarbo RJ. Prognostic value of PCNA index in gastric stromal tumors: correlation with mitotic count and outcome [Abstract]. Mod Pathol 1992;5:40.

4. Appelman HD. Mesenchymal tumors of the gastrointestinal tract. In Ming SC, Goldman H, eds. Pathology of the gastrointestinal tract. Philadelphia: WB Saunders, 1992:310–50.

5. Appelman HD. Stromal tumors of the esophagus, stomach, and duodenum. In: Appelman HD, ed. Pathology of the esophagus, stomach, and duodenum. New York: Churchill Livingstone, 1984:195–242.

6. Appelman HD. Smooth muscle tumors of the gastrointestinal tract. What we know now that Stout didn't know. Am J Surg Pathol 1986;10:83–99.

7. Appelman HD, Helwig EB. Cellular leiomyomas of the stomach in 49 patients. Arch Pathol Lab Med 1977;101:373–7.

8. Appelman HD, Helwig EB. Gastric epithelioid leiomyoma and leiomyosarcoma (leiomyoblastoma). Cancer 1976;38:708–28.

9. Appelman HD, Helwig EB. Glomus tumors of the stomach. Cancer 1969;23:203–13.

10. Appelman HD, Helwig EB. Sarcomas of the stomach. Am J Clin Pathol 1977;67:2–10.

11. Baak JP. Mitosis counting in tumors [Editorial]. Hum Pathol 1990; 21:683–5.

12. Barrison IG, Foster S, Harris JW, Pinching AJ, Walker JG. Upper gastrointestinal Kaposi's sarcoma in patients positive for HIV antibody without cutaneous disease. Br Med J (Clin Res Ed) 1988;296:92–3.

13. Beer TW, Rowlands DC, Crocker J. AgNOR counts and determination of malignancy in stromal tumours of the stomach and small intestine. J Clin Pathol 1992;45:172–4.

14. Blei E, Gonzalez-Crussi F. The intriguing nature of gastric tumors in Carney's triad. Cancer 1992;69:292–300.

15. Bolck F, Katenkamp D. Granuloblastomas of the stomach (so-called eosinophilic granulomas)—a variant of fibrous histiocytomas? Path Res Pract 1981;171:336–44.

16. Byard RW, Barr JR, Naidoo SP, McCaughey WT. Gastric stromal tumors with epithelioid features—clinicopathological features of 22 cases. Surg Pathol 1990;3:281–8.

17. Carney JA. The triad of gastric epithelioid leiomyosarcoma, pulmonary chondroma, and functioning extra-adrenal paraganglioma: a five-year review. Medicine (Baltimore) 1983;62:159–69.

18. Chen YS, Lin JB, Dai KS, et al. Gastric xanthelasma. Chin Med J 1989;102:639–43.

19. Cohen A, Geller SA, Horowitz I, Toth LS, Werther JL. Experimental models for gastric leiomyosarcoma. The effects of N-methyl-N'-nitro-N-nitrosoguanidine in combination with stress, aspirin, or sodium taurocholate. Cancer 1984;53:1088–92.

20. Cooper PN, Quirke P, Hardy GJ, Dixon MF. A flow cytometric, clinical, and histological study of stromal neoplasms of the gastrointestinal tract. Am J Surg Pathol 1992;16:163–70.

21. Cornog JL. Gastric leiomyoblastoma. A clinical and ultrastructural study. Cancer 1974;34:711–9.

22. Cosgrove JM, Fischer MG. Gastrointestinal neurofibroma in a patient with von Recklinghausen's disease. Surgery 1988;103:701–3.

23. Croker JR, Greenstein RJ. Malignant schwannoma of the stomach in a patient with von Recklinghausen's disease. Histopathology 1979;3:79–85.

24. Cueto J, Gilbert EF, Currie RA. Hemangiopericytoma of the stomach. Am J Surg 1966;112:943–6.

25. Daimaru Y, Kido H, Hashimoto H, Enjoji M. Benign schwannoma of the gastrointestinal tract: a clinico-pathologic and immunohistochemical study. Hum Pathol 1988;19:257–64.

26. Domellof L, Eriksson S, Helander HF, Janunger KG. Lipid islands in the gastric mucosa after resection for benign ulcer disease. Gastroenterology 1977;72:14–8.

27. Donner L, de Lanerolle P, Costa J. Immunoreactivity of paraffin-embedded normal tissues and mesenchymal tumors for smooth muscle actin. Am J Clin Pathol 1983;80:677–81.

28. Dougherty MJ, Compton CC, Talbert M, Wood WC. Sarcomas of the gastrointestinal tract. Separation into favorable and unfavorable prognostic groups by mitotic count. Ann Surg 1991;214:569–74.

29. El-Naggar AK, Ro JY, McLemore D, Garnsey L, Ordonez N, MacKay B. Gastrointestinal stromal tumors: DNA flow-cytometric study of 58 patients with at least five years of follow-up. Mod Pathol 1989;2:511–5.

30. Enjoji M, Sumiyoshi K, Sueyoshi K. Elastofibromatous lesion of the stomach in a patient with elastofibroma dorsi. Am J Surg Pathol 1985;9:233–7.

31. Erlandson RA. Cytoskeletal proteins including myofilaments in human tumors. Ultrastruct Pathol 1989;13:155–86.

32. Ernst CB, Abell MR, Kahn DR. Malignant hemangiopericytoma of the stomach. Surgery 1965;58:351–6.

33. Evans HL. Smooth muscle tumors of the gastrointestinal tract. A study of 56 cases followed for a minimum of 10 years. Cancer 1985;56:2242–50.

34. Farrugia G, Kim CH, Grant CS, Zinsmeister AR. Leiomyosarcoma of the stomach: determinants of long-term survival. Mayo Clin Proc 1992;67:533–6.

35. Federspiel BH, Sobin LH, Helwig EB, Mikel UV, Bahr, GF. Morphometry and cytophotometric assessment of DNA in smooth-muscle tumors [leiomyomas and leiomyosarcomas] of the gastrointestinal tract. Anal Quant Cytol and Histol 1987;9:105–14.

36. Flint A, Appelman HD, Beckwith AL. DNA analysis of gastric stromal neoplasms: correlation with pathologic features. Surg Pathol 1989;2:117–24.

37. Fox KR, Moussa SM, Mitre RJ, Zidar BL, Raves JJ. Clinical and pathologic features of primary gastric rhabdomyosarcoma. Cancer 1990;66:772–8.

38. Friedman SL, Wright TL, Altman DF. Gastrointestinal Kaposi's sarcoma in patients with acquired immunodeficiency syndrome. Endoscopic and autopsy findings. Gastroenterology 1985;89:102–8.

39. Fuller CE, Williams GT. Gastrointestinal manifestations of type 1 neurofibromatosis (von Recklinghausen's disease). Histopathology 1991;19:1–11.

40. Goldblum JR, Mandell SH, Appelman HD, Lloyd RV. Proliferating cell nuclear antigen and p53 antigen expression in gastrointestinal stromal tumors [Abstract]. Am J Clin Pathol 1992;98:351–2.

41. Grant CS, Kim CH, Farrugia G, Zinsmeister A, Goellner JR. Gastric leiomyosarcoma. Prognostic factors and surgical management. Arch Surg 1991;126:985–90.

42. Haque S, Modlin IM, West AB. Multiple glomus tumors of the stomach with intravascular spread. Am J Surg Pathol 1992;16:291–9.

43. Harned RK, Buck JL, Shekitka KM. Inflammatory fibroid polyps of the gastrointestinal tract: radiologic evaluation. Radiology 1992;182:863–6.

44. Helwig EB, Ranier A. Inflammatory fibroid polyps of the stomach. Am J Pathol 1952;28:535.

45. Helwig EB, Ranier A. Inflammatory polyps of the stomach. Surg Gynec Obstet 1953;96:355–67.

46. Hjermstad BM, Sobin LH, Helwig EB. Stromal tumors of the gastrointestinal tract: myogenic or neurogenic? Am J Surg Pathol 1987;11:383–6.

47. Ishikura H, Sato F, Naka A, Kodama T, Aizawa M. Inflammatory fibroid polyp of the stomach. Acta Pathol Jpn 1986;36:327–35.

48. Johnston J, Helwig EB. Granular cell tumors of the gastrointestinal tract and perianal region: a study of 74 cases. Dig Dis Sci 1981;26:807–16.

49. Kay S, Callahan WP Jr, Murray MR, Randall HT, Stout AP. Glomus tumors of the stomach. Cancer 1951;4:726–36.

50. Kay S, Still WJ. A comparative electron microscopic study of a leiomyosarcoma and bizarre leiomyoma (leiomyoblastoma) of the stomach. Am J Clin Pathol 1969;52:403–13.

51. Kimura K, Hiramoto T, Buncher CR. Gastric xanthelasma. Arch Pathol 1969; 87:110–7.

52. Kiyabu MT, Bishop PC, Parker JW, Turner RR, Fitzgibbons PL. Smooth muscle tumors of the gastrointestinal tract. Flow cytometric quantitation of DNA and nuclear antigen content and correlation with histologic grade. Am J Surg Pathol 1988;12:954–60.

53. Knapp RH, Wick MR, Goellner JR. Leiomyoblastomas and their relationship to other smooth-muscle tumors of the gastrointestinal tract. An electron-microscopic study. Am J Surg Pathol 1984;8:449–61.

54. Laky D, Stoica T. Gastric liposarcoma. A case report. Path Res Pract 1986;181:112–5.

55. Lee KC, Ng WF, Chan JK. Epithelioid haemangioendothelioma presenting as a gastric polyp. Histopathology 1988;12:335–7.

56. Lindsay PC, Ordonez N, Raaf JH. Gastric leiomyosarcoma: clinical and pathological review of fifty patients. J Surg Oncol 1981;18:399–421.

57. Litzky LA, Brooks JJ. Cytokeratin immunoreactivity in malignant fibrous histiocytoma and spindle cell tumors: comparison between frozen and paraffin-embedded tissues. Mod Pathol 1992;5:30–4.

57a. Ma CK, Amin MB, Kintanar E, Linden MD, Zarbo RJ. Immunohistologic characterization of gastrointestinal stromal tumors: a study of 82 cases compared with 11 cases of leiomyomas. Mod Pathol 1993;6:139–44.

58. Mackay B, Ro J, Floyd C, Ordonez NG. Ultrastructural observations on smooth muscle tumors. Ultrastruct Pathol 1987;11:593–607.

59. MacLeod CB, Tsokos M. Gastrointestinal autonomic nerve tumor. Ultrastruct Pathol 1991;15:49–51.

60. Maderal F, Hunter F, Fuselier G, Gonzales-Rogue P, Torres O. Gastric lipomas—an update of clinical presentation, diagnosis, and treatment. Am J Gastroenterol 1984;79:964–7.

61. Margulies KB, Sheps SG. Carney's triad: guidelines for management. Mayo Clin Proc 1988;63:496–502.

62. Martin JF, Bazin P, Feroldi J, Cabanne F. Tumeurs myoides intra-murales del'estomac. Considerations microscopiques a propos de 6 cas. Ann D'anat Pathol 1960;5:484–97.

63. Mazur MT, Clark HB. Gastric stromal tumors. Reappraisal of histogenesis. Am J Clin Pathol 1983;7:507–19.

64. McGrath PC, Neifeld JP, Lawrence W, Kay S, Horsley JS III, Parker GA. Gastrointestinal sarcomas. Analysis of prognostic factors. Ann Surg 1987;206:706–10.

65. Miettinen M. Gastrointestinal stromal tumors. An immunohistochemical study of cellular differentiation. Am J Clin Pathol 1988;89:601–10.

65a. Monihan JM, Carr NJ, Sobin LH. CD 34 immunoexpression in stromal tumours of the gastrointestinal tract and in mesenteric fibromatoses. Histopathology 1994;25:469–73.

66. Moraleda EP, Gonzalez MA, Carcavilla CB, Castrillon JV. Gastrointestinal autonomic nerve tumours: a case report with ultrastructural and immunohistochemical studies. Histopathology 1992;20:323–9.

67. Morgan BK, Compton C, Talbert M, Gallagher WJ, Wood, WC. Benign smooth muscle tumors of the gastrointestinal tract. A 24-year experience. Ann Surg 1990;211:63–6.

68. Mori M, Tamura S, Enjoji M, Sugimachi K. Concomitant presence of inflammatory fibroid polyp and carcinoma or adenoma in the stomach. Arch Pathol Lab Med. 1988;112:829–32.

69. Nakamura S, Iida M, Suekane H, Matsui T, Yao T, Fujishima M. Endoscopic removal of gastric lipoma: diagnostic value of endoscopic ultrasonography. Am J Gastroenterol 1991;86:619–21.

70. Navas-Palacios JJ, Colina-Ruizdelgado F, Sabches-Parrea MD, Cortes-Cansino J. Inflammatory fibroid polyps of the gastrointestinal tract. An immunohistochemical and electron microscopic study. Cancer 1983;51:1682–90.

71. Newman PL, Wadden C, Fletcher CD. Gastrointestinal stromal tumours: correlation of immunophenotype with clinicopathological features. J Pathol 1991;164:107–17.

72. Ng EH, Pollock RE, Romsdahl MM. Prognostic implications of patterns of failure for gastrointestinal leiomyosarcomas. Cancer 1992;69:1334–41.

73. Petersen JM, Ferguson DR. Gastrointestinal neurofibromatosis. J Clin Gastroenterol 1984;6:529–34.

74. Pike AM, Lloyd RV, Appelman HD. Cell markers in gastrointestinal stromal tumors. Hum Pathol 1988;19:830–4.

75. Ranchod M, Kempson RL. Smooth muscle tumors of the gastrointestinal tract and retroperitoneum. A pathologic analysis of 100 cases. Cancer 1977;39:255–62.

76. Rangdaeng S, Truong LD. Comparative immunohistochemical staining for desmin and muscle-specific actin. A study of 576 cases. Am J Clin Pathol 1991;96:32–45.

77. Roy M, Sommers SC. Metastatic potential of gastric leiomyosarcoma. Path Res Pract 1989;185:874–7.

78. Rutten AP. Neurogenic tumours of the stomach. Brit J Surg 1965;52:920–5.

79. Salazar H, Totten RS. Leiomyoblastoma of the stomach. An ultrastructural study. Cancer 1970;25:176–85.

80. Salmela H. Smooth muscle tumours of the stomach. A clinical study of 112 cases. Acta Chir Scand 1968;134:384–91.

81. Saul SH, Rast ML, Brooks JJ. The immunohistochemistry of gastrointestinal stromal tumors. Am J Surg Pathol 1987;11:464–73.

82. Saunders FC, Gardiner G. Gastric lipoma: a rare cause of GI bleeding. Contemp Gastroenterol 1988;1:15–8.

83. Seo IS, Azzarelli B, Warner TF, Goheen MP, Sentensy GE. Multiple visceral and cutaneous granular cell tumors. Ultrastructural and immunocytochemical evidence of Schwann cell origin. Cancer 1984;53:2104–10.

84. Shiu MH, Farr GH, Papachristou DN, Hajdu SI. Myosarcomas of the stomach: natural history, prognostic factors and management. Cancer 1982;49:177–87.

85. Shivshanker K, Bennetts R. Neurogenic sarcoma of the gastrointestinal tract. Am J Gastroenterology 1981;75:214–7.

86. Sommers SC. Gastric smooth muscle, nerve sheath, and related tumors. In: Rotterdam H, Enterline HT, eds. Pathology of the stomach and duodenum. New York: Springer-Verlag, 1989:271.

87. Stamm B, Grant JW. Biopsy pathology of the gastrointestinal tract in human immunodeficiency virus-associated disease: a 5 year experience in Zurich. Histopathology 1988;13:531–40.

88. Stout AP. Bizarre smooth muscle tumors of the stomach. Cancer 1962;15:400–9.

89. Tauchi K, Tsutsumi Y, Yoshimura S, Watanabe K. Immunohistochemical and immunoblotting detection of cytokeratin in smooth muscle tumors. Acta Pathol Jpn 1990;40:574–80.

90. Taxy JB, Battifora H. Angiosarcoma of the gastrointestinal tract. A report of three cases. Cancer 1988;62:210–6.

91. Thompson EM, Evans DJ. The significance of PGP 9.5 in tumours—an immunohistochemical study of gastrointestinal stromal tumours. Histopathology 1990;17:175–7.

92. Tortella BJ, Matthews JB, Antonioli DA, Dvorak AM, Silen W. Gastric autonomic nerve (GAN) tumor and extra-adrenal paraganglioma in Carney's triad. A common origin. Ann Surg 1987;205:221–5.

93. Trillo AA, Rowden G. The histogenesis of inflammatory fibroid polyps of the gastrointestinal tract. Histopathology 1991;19:431–6.

94. Tsushima K, Rainwater LM, Goellner JR, van Heerden JA, Lieber MM. Leiomyosarcomas and benign smooth muscle tumors of the stomach: nuclear DNA patterns studied by flow cytometry. Mayo Clin Proc 1987;62:275–80.

95. Tsutsumi Y, Kubo H. Immunohistochemistry of desmin and vimentin in smooth muscle tumors of the digestive tract. Acta Pathol Jpn 1988;38:455–69.

96. Tuazon R. Rhabdomyoma of the stomach. Report of a case. Am J Clin Pathol 1969;52:37–41.

97. Ueyama T, Guo KJ, Hashimoto H, Daimaru Y, Enjoji M. A clinicopathologic and immunohistochemical study of gastrointestinal stromal tumors. Cancer 1992;69:947–55.

97a. van de Rijn M, Hendrickson MR, Rouse RV. CD34 expression by gastrointestinal tract stromal tumors. Hum Pathol 1994;25:766–71.

98. Vanek J. Gastric submucosal granuloma with eosinophilic infiltration. Am J Pathol 1949;25:397–411.

99. Vase P, Grove O. Gastrointestinal lesions in hereditary hemorrhagic telangiectasia. Gastroenterology 1986;91:1079–83.

100. Walker P, Dvorak AM. Gastrointestinal autonomic nerve [GAN] tumor. Ultrastructural evidence for a newly recognized entity. Arch Pathol Lab Med 1986;110:309–16.

101. Warner KE, Haidak GL. Massive glomus tumor of the stomach: 20-year follow-up and autopsy findings. Am J Gastroenterol 1984;79:253–5.

102. Weaver GA, Alpern HD, Davis JS, Ramsey WH, Reichelderfer M, Gastrointestinal angiodysplasia associated with aortic valve disease: part of a spectrum of angiodysplasia of the gut. Gastroenterology 1979;77:1–11.

103. Welsh RA, Meyer AT. Ultrastructure of gastric leiomyoma. Arch Pathol 1969;87:71–81.

104. Wick MR, Ruebner BH, Carney JA. Gastric tumors in patients with pulmonary chondroma or extra-adrenal paraganglioma: an ultrastructural study. Arch Pathol Lab Med 1981;105:527–31.
105. Wright JR Jr, Kyriakos M, DeSchryver-Kecskemeti K. Malignant fibrous histiocytoma of the stomach. A report and review of malignant fibrohistiocytic tumors of the alimentary tract. Arch Pathol Lab Med 1988;112:251–8.
106. Yagahashi S, Kimura M, Kurotaki H, et al. Gastric submucosal tumours of neurogenic origin with neuroaxonal and Schwann cell elements. J Pathol 1987;153:41–50.
107. Yagihashi S, Yagihashi N, Hase Y, Nagai N, Alguacil-Garcia A. Primary alveolar soft-part sarcoma of stomach. Am J Surg Pathol 1991;15:399–406.
108. Yamaguchi K, Kato Y, Maeda S, Kitamura K. Cavernous hemangioma of the stomach: a case report and review of the literature. Gastroenterol Jpn 1990;25:489–93.
109. Yu CC, Fletcher CD, Newman PL, Goodland JR, Burton JC, Levison DA. A comparison of proliferating cell nuclear antigen (PCNA) immunostaining, nucleolar organizer region (AgNOR) staining, and histological grading in gastroindestinal stromal tumors. J Pathol 1992;166:!47–52.

✧✧✧

# 15
# MISCELLANEOUS TUMORS

The major classes of gastric tumors, including the adenomas, carcinomas, stromal tumors, lymphomas, and endocrine tumors are described in previous chapters. A small collection of uncommon primary and metastatic neoplasms remain. These are identical to tumors arising in extragastric sites, such as germ cell tumors, metastatic melanomas, metastatic carcinomas of breast and lung, and carcinomas with stromal differentiation. Because they are rare, very little data on either their morphology or clinical characteristics exist.

## GERM CELL TUMORS

Rare teratomas, choriocarcinomas, and yolk sac carcinomas occur as primary tumors in the stomach. The demographics of teratomas differ from those of the two carcinomas, but all these germ cell tumors resemble their counterparts that occur in more traditional sites. To the best of our knowledge, no cases of seminoma, malignant teratoma, or typical gonadal-type embryonal carcinoma have been reported as primary in the stomach.

### Teratoma

Less than 100 primary gastric teratomas have been reported. They tend to occur in newborns, infants, and small children; a few have occurred in young adults. Most patients are male. In a 1981 review of 51 reported cases, only 2 were in females (1). They present as abdominal masses, gastric outlet obstructions, or sources of upper gastrointestinal bleeding. Most are large, but almost any clinically apparent tumor appears large in a newborn or in an infant. Histologically, they contain the usual mix of mature tissue elements derived from the three germ layers: skin, ciliated epithelium, smooth muscle, cartilage, adipose tissue, and neural tissue (6). Resection is curative.

### Choriocarcinoma and Yolk Sac (Embryonal) Carcinoma

Scattered case reports and a few small series of cases of choriocarcinoma, and even fewer cases of yolk sac carcinoma primary in the stomach, have been published. The total number of such cases probably is less than 75. The stomach may be the most common site of origin of nongonadal, nongestational, nonmidline trophoblastic tumors. Most reported cases were tumors composed of both malignant germ cell tumor and adenocarcinoma. In a few tumors, the primary gastric lesion was pure adenocarcinoma; the choriocarcinomatous differentiation only became manifest in the metastases. Approximately one fourth of reported cases are purely choriocarcinoma in the gastric primary; the rest have an adenocarcinomatous component. Teratomatous elements are never present. As a result of these data, most authors have emphasized the theory of "retrodifferentiation" to explain how tumors containing trophoblast can occur in the stomach (2,3,8,10). This theory assumes that since all cells contain the entire genetic material for the whole organism, under certain unexplained circumstances, cancers may differentiate in unusual directions, including the formation of malignant trophoblast and yolk sac epithelium. Metastases from gonadal germ cell tumors occasionally involve the stomach. In a study of 166 primary testicular germ cell tumors, 1 of 43 seminomas and 1 of 123 nonseminomatous tumors metastasized to the stomach (9).

The situation becomes more complex if the presence of human chorionic gonadotrophin (HCG) is considered to be an indication of trophoblastic differentiation. In two Japanese studies, the authors used antibodies against the beta subunit of HCG to detect immunoreactive cells in the neck region of normal antral mucosa (5,10a). One study found a few cells positive for HCG in the body mucosa, while the other did not; in the former, patches of intestinal metaplasia were found in the neck area (5). The cells containing HCG were typical gastric or metaplastic columnar cells or cells at the base of the tubules where endocrine cells are located, but they did not resemble trophoblast. HCG-containing cells have been identified immunohistochemically in about a quarter to half of typical gastric adenocarcinomas (4,5, 10a). In these carcinomas, the tumor cells did not resemble syncytiotrophoblast. Thus there appears to be a group of HCG-producing cells in the stomach: normal antral neck cells, metaplastic cells in atrophic gastritis, adenocarcinoma cells with no trophoblastic features, and carcinoma cells that are identical to trophoblast and are the dominant cell in those tumors designated as primary gastric choriocarcinoma.

Gastric choriocarcinoma occurs in adults of the same age and sex range as typical gastric adenocarcinoma (10). The presenting symptoms and signs are much the same as those of ordinary gastric cancer, including significant bleeding. There are insufficient data to determine if these tumors differ from other gastric carcinomas in clinical course and survival. Grossly, they are more hemorrhagic than gastric carcinomas. Microscopically, they have the typical mix of cytotrophoblastic and syncytial elements, with the syncytial cells containing HCG. Some tumors contain mostly syncytiotrophoblast with very little cytotrophoblast. As is typical for these tumors, they are as hemorrhagic in the stomach as elsewhere. There is a tendency for the choriocarcinomatous component to metastasize via blood vessels to liver and lung, while the adenocarcinomatous component metastasizes via lymphatics to regional nodes.

Yolk sac carcinoma components have been found in rare gastric adenocarcinomas, including one that also had a choriocarcinoma component (2,7). A few seem to be pure yolk sac tumor, without adenocarcinoma (11). The neoplastic cells produce immunoreactive alpha-fetoprotein (AFP). One reported case also had cells with immunoreactive gastrin (11a). In another study, AFP was found in about half of 35 typical gastric carcinomas, but the positive cells did not resemble yolk sac carcinoma cells. Some of the AFP-containing areas were probably the hepatoid variant of gastric carcinoma (4).

## CARCINOSARCOMA (SARCOMATOID CARCINOMA, PSEUDOSARCOMATOUS CARCINOMA)

A few case reports describe gastric tumors with divergent differentiation that includes both carcinomatous and sarcomatous elements (12–15). These tumors occur with the same age and sex distribution as standard gastric carcinoma. They are often polypoid or protruding, and the survival rate is stage related; they are often at a high primary stage at the time of diagnosis. Generally, there is a mix of adenocarcinoma of tubular pattern with a primitive spindle cell stroma that may differentiate into malignant cartilage, smooth muscle, or even skeletal muscle. Dysplasia and intestinal metaplasia in the adjacent mucosa have been reported, further supporting a carcinomatous origin (15). Metastases may be carcinomatous, sarcomatous, or both. Except for the adenocarcinoma component of these gastric tumors, they are identical to comparable esophageal pseudosarcomatous squamous cell carcinoma that is extensively illustrated in chapter 4. These are probably also carcinomas with stromal metaplasia and differentiation. The major difference is that the gastric tumors are usually more advanced when discovered than those in the esophagus.

A single case of a primary gastric adenosarcoma, comparable to those that arise in the uterus, has been reported (16). This was an intramural tumor composed of a cellular, mitotically active, malignant-appearing spindle cell stromal component and a cystic, histologically benign epithelial component. There was no evidence of metastatic or recurrent tumor 15 months after resection.

## METASTATIC NEOPLASMS

Any carcinoma that seeds the peritoneum, such as those arising in the ovary or pancreas, can involve the gastric serosa. On occasion, a large carcinoma of the head of the pancreas invades the gastric wall and extends to the mucosa; it can be seen with endoscopic biopsy. However, there are three neoplasms that periodically produce intramural gastric metastases that may involve the mucosa and produce lesions that mimic primary gastric tumors: these are malignant melanoma, carcinoma of the breast, and carcinoma of the lung (22,26). In a Veterans Hospital study of 1,951 autopsies of patients with nonhematologic malignancies, 57 cases had gastric mucosal metastases (24). Over half of the primary sites were lung, with pancreas and esophagus accounting for about one sixth each. However, this study may not have been representative of the general population with gastric metastases: metastases from melanomas were uncommon, and

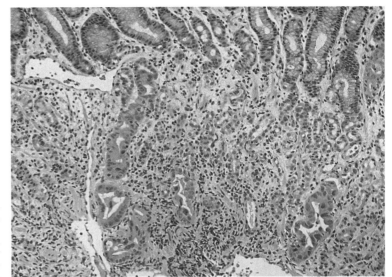

Figure 15-1
METASTATIC ADENOCARCINOMA

A biopsy of metastatic adenocarcinoma to the stomach from a primary in the head of the pancreas.

Top: At the base of the mucosa, mixed with the gastric glands and inflammatory cells, are large calibre carcinomatous tubules, lined by plump columnar cells with large pleomorphic nuclei. These have grown along the contours of the glands. As they reach the surface, they look much like in situ carcinoma or high-grade dysplasia.

Bottom: Higher magnification of the tubules shows the mix of carcinoma, glands, and inflammation.

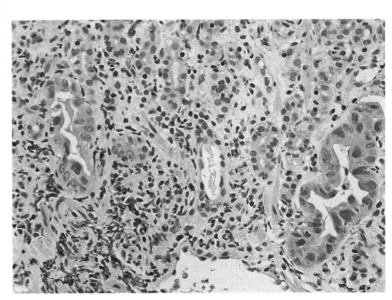

the study population was mostly male, so that breast cancer was not included. The stomach is not nearly as common a site for intramural metastases as is the small intestine.

Metastases often produce expanding mucosal or intramural masses, often with relatively circumscribed margins; many ulcerate. Because of these growth characteristics, metastases commonly appear as ulcer craters surrounded by a round, circumscribed, elevated margin, imparting a "target-like" appearance on mucosal view. A comparable view occurs with barium X ray studies. In about half the cases, the metastases produce multiple lesions. Generally, the primary tumor has already been discovered when the gastric metastases appear, but occasionally, the metastasis may be the presenting problem. In such cases, the metastasis may have the clinical appearance of a primary gastric tumor, especially a stromal tumor. Biopsies should produce samples that allow diagnosis, but some carcinomas and melanomas are composed of anaplastic spindled cells, contributing to confusion with stromal tumors. In mucosal biopsies, metastases may appear as nests or tubules of carcinoma at the base of the mucosa, some of which are in lymphatics (fig. 15-1). In addition, some adeno-carcinomatous metastases to the stomach, especially those from other gastrointestinal or pancreaticobiliary sites, have a peculiar morphology. As they invade the mucosa from the base, they grow toward the lumen, replacing the preexisting glands and pits, and adhering to their contours. In this way they look like an in situ lesion and can mimic primary carcinoma.

## Metastatic Melanoma

It has been estimated that about 60 percent of patients with fatal malignant melanomas have gastrointestinal metastases at the time of death (25). The stomach is involved in about half of these cases, based upon autopsy studies (27). However, very few of these metastases produce symptoms. In cases in which the metastatic tumor produces clinical disease, the most common sites of metastases are the small bowel and colon. Clinically apparent gastric metastases are rare. Nevertheless, on the few occasions when metastatic melanoma to the stomach produces symptoms of pain or bleeding, biopsies of endoscopically visible masses or ulcers usually yield melanoma cells. Melanoma has a variety of histologic expressions which may mimic carcinoma when it is predominantly epithelioid, sarcoma when it is heavily spindled, and lymphoma when it is the small cell variant (18). Unless there is a history of a previous melanoma, the diagnosis of metastatic melanoma is likely to be missed and alternative diagnoses made instead. The tendency of metastatic melanoma to infiltrate the mucosa diffusely and separate the epithelial structures mimics the pattern of mucosal involvement in lymphomas, some signet-ring cell or diffuse spreading carcinomas, and a few sarcomas (fig. 15-2).

## Metastatic Carcinoma of the Breast

The mean time between mastectomy and the development of gastric metastases from mammary carcinoma is between 2 and 4 years. In one report, this lag time was 30 years (20). There have been several reports of lobular carcinoma of the breast metastasizing to the stomach and producing a diffusely infiltrating pattern of involvement, thereby resembling primary signet-ring carcinoma of the stomach (21). There are some morphologic hints which help separate the mucin-containing cells of lobuar carcinoma of the breast from gastric signet-ring carcinoma cells (19): breast signet-ring cells mostly contain intracytoplasmic lumens filled with mucin, whereas gastric signet-ring cells commonly have their mucin within the Golgi apparatus.

## Metastatic Carcinoma of the Lung

One Veterans Hospital studied metastases to the stomach from 35 carcinomas that were primary in lung: half were adenocarcinomas, 30 percent were small cell carcinomas, one sixth were squamous cell carcinomas (24). In an autopsy study of 423 cases of primary lung cancer over a 36-year period, 58 metastasized to the gastrointestinal tract; of the 10 to the stomach, about half metastasized to other gut sites as well (17). Half of the primary carcinomas were either adenocarcinomas or large cell carcinomas, and a third were squamous cell tumors. Primary gastric carcinomas with squamous components are so rare that whenever a squamous carcinomatous epithelium is encountered in a gastric mucosal biopsy of a mass or ulcer, metastases should be considered, especially metastases from primaries in lung or esophagus (23).

## OTHER TUMORS AND TUMOR-LIKE LESIONS

Single case reports of unusual tumors have been published. There is so little information concerning these lesions that it is pointless to try to discuss them. However, they are listed and referenced for the reader. They include squamous cell papilloma, Brunner's gland adenoma, amyloid tumor, benign mesenchymoma, and polypoid histiocytoma (28–31).

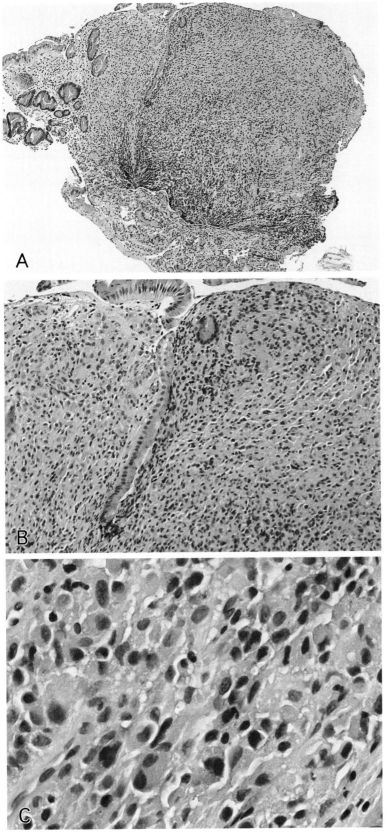

Figure 15-2
METASTATIC MELANOMA

A: This is a mucosal biopsy of the edge of an ulcerated mass. The melanoma cells infiltrate the lamina propria, separating the residual mucosal tubules at the left and totally replacing the mucosa at the right.

B: At this higher magnification, the tumor diffusely infiltrates the tissue without forming any aggregates.

C: The tumor cells are epithelioid, vary slightly in size, and have hyperchromatic nuclei.

## REFERENCES

### Germ Cell Tumors

1. Cairo MS, Grosfeld JL, Weetman RM. Gastric teratoma: unusual cause for bleeding of the upper gastrointestinal tract in the newborn. Pediatrics 1981;67:721–4.
2. Garcia RL, Ghali VS. Gastric choriocarcinoma and yolk sac tumor in a man: observations about its possible origin. Hum Pathol 1985;16:955–8.
3. Jindrak K, Bochetto JF, Alpert LI. Primary gastric choriocarcinoma: case report with review of world literature. Hum Pathol 1976;7:595–604.
4. Kodama T, Kameya T, Hirota T, et al. Production of alpha-fetoprotein, normal serum proteins, and human chorionic gonadotropin in stomach cancer: histologic and immunohistochemical analysis of 35 cases. Cancer 1981;48:1647–55.
5. Manabe T, Adachi M, Hirao K. Human chorionic gonadotropin in normal, inflammatory, and carcinomatous gastric tissue. Gastroenterology 1985;89:1319–25.
6. Ming SC. Adenocarcinoma and other malignant epithelial tumors of the stomach. In: Ming SC, Goldman H, eds. Pathology of the gastrointestinal tract. Philadelphia: WB Saunders 1992:608–10.
7. Motoyama T, Saito K, Iwafuchi M, Watanabe H. Endodermal sinus tumor of the stomach. Acta Pathol Jpn 1985;35:497–505.
8. Saigo PE, Brigati DJ, Sternberg SS, Rosen PP, Turnbull AD. Primary gastric choriocarcinoma. An immunohistological study. Am J Surg Pathol 1981;5:333–42.
9. Sweetenham JW, Whitehouse JM, Williams CJ, Mead GM. Involvement of the gastrointestinal tract by metastases from germ cell tumors of the testis. Cancer 1988;61:2566–70.
10. Wurzel J, Brooks JJ. Primary gastric choriocarcinoma: immunohistochemistry, postmortem documentation, and hormonal effects in a postmenopausal female. Cancer 1981;48:2756–61.
10a. Yakeishi Y, Mori M, Enjoji M. Distribution of beta-human chorionic gonadotropin-positive cells in noncancerous gastric mucosa and in malignant gastric tumors. Cancer 1990;66:695–701.
11. Yano T, Miyamoto U, Mikai T, et al. A case of alpha-fetoprotein producing embryonal carcinoma of the stomach. Gan No Rinsho 1983;29:A–23, 360–3.
11a. Zámecník M, Patriková J, Gomolcák P. Yolk sac carcinoma of the stomach with gastrin positivity. Hum Pathol 1993;24:927–8.

### Carcinosarcomas

12. Aiba M, Hirayama A, Suzuki T, Hamano K, Nomura K. Carcinosarcoma of the stomach: report of a case with review of the literature of gastrectomized patients. Surg Pathol 1991;4:75–83.
13. Bansal M, Kaneko M, Gordon RE. Carcinosarcoma and separate carcinoid tumor of the stomach. A case report with light and electron microscopic studies. Cancer 1982;50:1876–81.
14. Dundas SA, Slater DN, Wagner BE, Mills PA. Gastric adenocarcinoleiomyosarcoma: a light, electron microscopic and immunohistochemical study. Histopathology 1988;13:347–53.
15. Robey-Cafferty SS, Grignon DJ, Ro JY, et al. Sarcomatoid carcinoma of the stomach. A report of three cases with immunohistochemical and ultrastructural observations. Cancer 1990;65:1601–6.
16. Kallakury BV, Bui HX, delRosario A, Wallace J, Solis OG, Ross JS. Primary gastric adenosarcoma. Arch Pathol Lab Med 1992;117:299–301.

### Metastatic Tumors

17. Antler AS, Ough Y, Pitchumoni CS, Davidian M, Thelmo W. Gastrointestinal metastases from malignant tumors of the lung. Cancer 1982;49:170–2.
18. Attanoos R, Griffiths DF. Metastatic small cell melanoma to the stomach mimicking primary gastric lymphoma. Histopathology 1992;21:173–5.
19. Battifora H. Intracytoplasmic lumina in breast carcinoma: a helpful histopathologic feature. Arch Pathol Lab Med 1975;99:614–7.
20. Benfiguig A, Anciaux ML, Eugene CI, Benkemoun G, Etienne JC. Metastase gastrique d'un cancer du sein survenant apres un intervalle libre de 30 ans. Ann Gastroenterol Hepatol 1992;28:175–7.
21. Cormier WJ, Gaffey TA, Welch JM, Welch JS, Edmonson JH. Linitis plastica caused by metastatic lobular carcinoma of the breast. Mayo Clin Proc 1980;55:747–53.
22. Coughlin GP, Bourne AJ, Grant AK. Endoscopic diagnosis of metastatic disease of the stomach and duodenum. Aust N Z J Med 1977;7:52–5.
23. Fletcher MS. Gastric perforation secondary to metastatic carcinoma of the lung: a case report. Cancer 1980;46:1879–82.
24. Green LK. Hematogenous metastases to the stomach. A review of 67 cases. Cancer 1990;65:1596–600.
25. Ihde JK, Coit DG. Melanoma metastatic to stomach, small bowel, or colon. Am J Surg 1991;162:208–11.
26. Menuck LS, Amberg JR. Metastatic disease involving the stomach. Am J Dig Dis 1975;20:903–13.
27. Pector JC, Crokaert F, Lejeune F, Gerard A. Prolonged survival after resection of a malignant melanoma metastatic to the stomach. Cancer 1988;61:2134–5.

### Other Tumors

28. Rubio CA. Rare and secondary (metastatic) tumours. In: Whitehead R, ed. Gastrointestinal and oesophageal pathology. New York: Churchill Livingstone, 1989:726–32.
29. Ikeda K, Murayama H. A case of amyloid tumor of the stomach. Endoscopy 1978;10:54–8.
30. Haqqani MT, Krasner N, Ashworth M. Benign mesenchymoma of the stomach. J Clin Pathol 1983;36:504–7.
31. Costa MJ, Larkin E. Ruebner BH. Polypoid histiocytoma (fibroxanthoma) of the stomach mimicking signet ring adenocarcinoma by endoscopic evaluation. Int J Surg Pathol 1994;2:141–5.

# Index*

---

*Numbers in boldface indicate table and figure pages.